Veterinary Microbiology

*Bacterial and Fungal Agents
of Animal Disease*

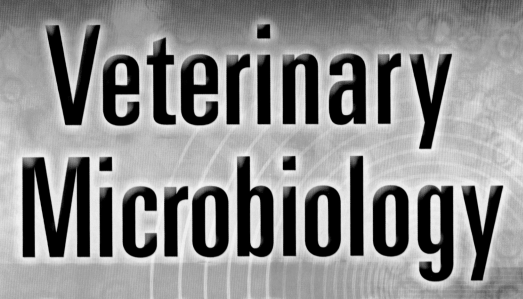

Veterinary Microbiology

Bacterial and Fungal Agents of Animal Disease

J. Glenn Songer, PhD
Professor, Department of Veterinary Science and Microbiology
The University of Arizona
Tucson, Arizona

Karen W. Post, DVM, MS
Diplomate, American College of Veterinary Microbiologists

Veterinary Bacteriologist
North Carolina Department of Agriculture and Consumer Services
Rollins Animal Disease Diagnostic Laboratory
Raleigh, North Carolina

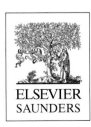

ELSEVIER
SAUNDERS

ELSEVIER
SAUNDERS

11830 Westline Industrial Drive
St. Louis, Missouri 63146

NOTICE

Veterinary medicine is an ever-changing field. Standard safety precautions must be followed, but as new research and clinical experience broaden our knowledge, changes in treatment and drug therapy may become necessary or appropriate. Readers are advised to check the most current product information provided by the manufacturer of each drug to be administered to verify the recommended dose, the method and duration of administration, and contraindications. It is the responsibility of the licensed prescriber, relying on experience and knowledge of the patient, to determine dosages and the best treatment for each individual patient. Neither the publisher nor the author assumes any liability for any injury and/or damage to persons or property arising from this publication.

International Standard Book Number 0-7216-8717-2

Publishing Director: *Linda Duncan*
Acquisitions Editor: *Anthony J. Winkel*
Developmental Editor: *Shelly Dixon*
Publishing Services Manager: *Patricia Tannian*
Senior Project Manager: *Anne Altepeter*
Senior Designer: *Amy Buxton*

Printed in China

Last digit is the print number: 9   8   7   6   5   4   3   2   1

Contributors

Patrick F. McDermott, PhD
Research Microbiologist
Division of Animal and Food Microbiology
U.S. Food and Drug Administration
Center for Veterinary Medicine
Laurel, Maryland

Robert D. Walker, MS, PhD
Director
Division of Animal and Food Microbiology
U.S. Food and Drug Administration
Center for Veterinary Medicine
Laurel, Maryland

David G. White, MS, PhD
Research Microbiologist
Division of Animal and Food Microbiology
U.S. Food and Drug Administration
Center for Veterinary Medicine
Laurel, Maryland

To my parents, Joe and Bettie Songer. With me and their other children, they have been uncompromisingly insistent upon achievement according to ability, and have settled for nothing less in their own lives. I saw early in life the value of this as a personal philosophy, learning only later the cost of living it in daily practice. I admire them for their persistence through thick and thin.

J. Glenn Songer

To Professor Gerald Wilt, Auburn University College of Veterinary Medicine, my major professor, mentor, and friend. His love for veterinary bacteriology was contagious. I also owe a debt of gratitude to my mother, Doris Weden, for her life of love and support.

Karen W. Post

Preface

Seventy years ago, Hans Zinsser said that infectious disease "is merely a disagreeable instance of a widely prevalent tendency of all living creatures to save themselves the bother of building, by their own efforts, the things they require" and that it "remains one of the few sporting propositions left for individuals who feel the need of a certain amount of excitement. It is one of the few genuine adventures left in the world. The dragons are all dead, and the lance grows rusty in the chimney corner."[1] Microbiologists seldom speak of their work in such literary terms, but if pressed (or, in some cases, sufficiently plied with drink), most would accept the truth of the concept.

Infectious diseases in domestic animals have been documented, with greater or lesser clarity, for millennia. One of our professors told us that the first veterinary school was founded centuries ago specifically to deal with what we now know as contagious bovine pleuropneumonia. This may be apocryphal, but I hope it is true, if only because it strengthens my argument: veterinary infectious diseases, old and new, are constants, despite changes in animals and their genetics, changes in production methods, better understanding of the need and methods for sanitation, and development and application of vaccines and antimicrobials.

From Pasteur's crude (by today's standards) but nonetheless elegant work with anthrax and fowl cholera to the molecular pathogenesis and cellular microbiology practiced now in so many veterinary microbiology laboratories, discoveries by veterinary microbiologists have been applied to improving animal production and welfare and to providing a safer and more plentiful source of food for humans. Our motivation for writing this book is the desire to provide a tool, based upon our experiences in diagnostics, research, and clinical medicine, for use by the next generation of veterinarians and microbiologists. We have lived our professional lives in veterinary bacteriology and mycology, and "we love it platonically.....and have sought its acquaintance wherever we could find it"[1] We hope that others will as well.

We have put our best efforts into ensuring the accuracy of the content of this book. Wherever possible, we have updated the taxonomy of the various bacteria and fungi. We have attempted to include the latest information about pathogenesis and diagnosis, with allowances for the primary context of this book, which is in the microbiology curriculum of veterinary colleges. We welcome the critical comments and especially the effusive praise of our readers.

J. GLENN SONGER

KAREN W. POST

---

[1] Zinsser H: *Rats, lice, and history*, Boston, 1934, Little, Brown.

Acknowledgments

This book would not have been possible without the contributions of others. It is based upon the findings of many bacteriologists and mycologists working in research and diagnostics in veterinary and human medical arenas. Photographs provided generously by many of these individuals open a window on the power and stark beauty of microbial interactions with hosts. My daughter, Ashley E. Harmon, patiently tolerated my intrusions into her life as a professional graphic designer, beginning with my incredibly rough drafts and suffering through multiple revisions, to provide the illustrations. Special thanks to Patrick F. McDermott, Robert D. Walker, and David G. White, who made substantial contributions to the chapter on antimicrobials and chemotherapy. Shelly Dixon has proved to be professional in handling the manuscript and illustrations, and almost supernaturally patient with two authors who have been habitually behind schedule. She deserves more credit for the completion of this volume than she is likely to receive. Finally, Durrae Johanek's copy editing ran many inconsistencies to ground, and Anne Altepeter's project management put a final gloss on the entire manuscript. Our sincere thanks to one and all.

Contents

One

Basics of Veterinary Microbiology

Chapter 1

Origin and Evolution of Virulence

Virulence, simply defined, is microbial specialization that facilitates replication in hosts. The resulting damage to the host may be so minimal that it yields no clinical signs, or so great that it results in death. Host and pathogen are often equal players in the initiation, progression, and outcome of the encounter, and are in ceaseless evolutionary conflict.

TRAITS OF PATHOGENS

Frank pathogens cause disease in some proportion of normal hosts and **opportunists** cause disease only in those with compromised defenses; an opportunist in one host may be a frank pathogen in another. A frank pathogen's long-term survival usually depends upon replication in and transmission among members of one or more host species, but opportunists are not bounded by these restrictions.

In either case, the vital events are adherence, entry, avoidance of host defenses, multiplication and spread, and damage to the host. Not all pathogens are equipped for all of these steps. *Clostridium tetani* does not adhere or enter on its own, but often overcomes these deficits by riding into tissue on foreign objects. *Arcanobacterium pyogenes* usually lives a quiet, unobtrusive life on mucous membranes, but given a bit of coaxing (in the form of ruminal acidosis, primary viral or bacterial infection, or injury) it can produce life-threatening infections. Zygomycetes are no threat to the normal rumen, but they invade and do massive damage in cattle with compromised rumen function. Herein lies also the most important

difference between pathogens and commensals: the former can access privileged niches that are normally unavailable to the latter. Pathogens most often gain entry to these sites by relying on their own devices but are sometimes found to be in complicity with the host cell. Opportunistic infections occur when commensals or other nonadapted organisms are provided an advantage in the form of compromised host defenses. It is likely that nearly any microbe, given sufficient help in clearing host-imposed barriers, can cause infection. The common theme is microbial use of available tools and resources to derive a living from the host.

Pathogen entry to an intact host is fraught with challenges (for the pathogen). Crossing of unbroken keratinized epithelium by bacterial pathogens is relatively rare, although "successful" interactions of this type are common among fungi. Encounters with mucosal epithelium are often an extreme change in environment for a pathogen, which needs the specific machinery to deal with unfamiliar pH, osmolarity, redox potential, and other factors. Some pathogens must eventually deal with the intracellular environment, and these organisms cope by way of multiple sets of virulence genes in sometimes-overlapping systems.

Finding and occupying a niche is the next challenge. Multitudes of commensal bacteria, fungi, and protozoa derive their living from residence in or on hosts, and, not surprisingly, make no effort to welcome interlopers. Some opportunistic pathogens cannot succeed in this endeavor without outside assistance, as with *Clostridium difficile* infection

3

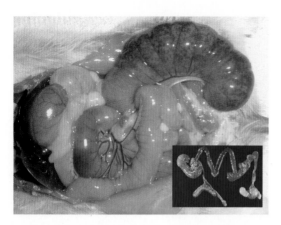

FIGURE 1-1 *Clostridium difficile*, a pathogen of humans and domestic animals, also infects hamsters and other rodents, causing rapidly fatal, antibiotic-associated typhlocolitis. Main photo is of infected hamster at necropsy; inset shows excised hamster gut. (Courtesy J. Glenn Songer.)

in humans subjected to systemic antimicrobial therapy (Figure 1-1).

Having gained a foothold, the pathogen (whether frank or opportunistic) must defend itself, mainly by avoiding, bypassing, or subverting host defenses. The innate and induced components of the immune system, in the form of phagocytes and humoral components, are, by design, hostile to invading microbes. Microbial strategies for dealing with these issues are diverse, inventive, multifaceted, and often elegant.

Having negotiated some sort of understanding with the host immune defenses, the pathogen (if it is to truly earn its stripes) must set about damaging the host. Succeeding chapters relate in some detail myriad methods by which microbial pathogens accomplish this end. Generally speaking, damage is mediated either without production of toxins (as in generation of a self-destructive immune response) or with toxin production, of which there are many examples. An organism that does not consistently cause host damage is unlikely to be a frank pathogen.

ORIGIN AND EVOLUTION OF VIRULENCE

Bacteria are estimated to have emerged as life forms between 3.5 and 3.8 billion years ago and have adapted to numerous microenvironments over the intervening years. Interesting findings of recent studies suggest that evolution may have produced

pathogens long before animals were available as hosts. The principal selective factors affecting microbes seem to have been protozoal predation and environmental stresses in the form of drying and oxidation. Organisms able to cope with both may in fact have been unknowingly assembling the rudiments of a system for survival in animal hosts. They have been left to follow Darwinian principles toward increased overall fitness.

At one time, dogma held that commensal organisms in association with hosts lost the ability to carry out key processes, thus coming to depend on the host to provide essentials for growth and survival. With increased dependence, some organisms "defected," replicating at the host's expense, using host cell machinery and in some cases causing what we recognize as disease. Adaptation of bacteria to the physiologically stable environments of host cells may result in reductive evolution, with loss of genes not essential for this lifestyle. Genomes experiencing reductive evolution often contain large numbers of pseudogenes, as in *Mycobacterium leprae*. Other examples include the absence or inactivation in *Yersinia pestis* of genes of its progenitor *Yersinia pseudotuberculosis*. Large chromosomal regions present in most *Escherichia coli* strains are deleted from enteroinvasive *E. coli* and *Shigella* strains. Loss of *cadA* is virulence associated in *Shigella* and enteroinvasive *E. coli,* in that cadaverine (a product of a CadA-catalyzed reaction) inhibits the enterotoxin activity of these organisms. Despite these supportive data, this "gain of virulence by loss of independence" hypothesis it not completely satisfying in explaining virulence evolution; some commensal organisms (e.g., *Corynebacterium diphtheriae* and perhaps saprophytic neisseriae) *gain* attributes that make them pathogenic.

Another aspect of dogma was that a well-adapted parasite is a benign parasite. Pathogens were believed to evolve uniformly toward a benign coexistence, or mutualism, allowing more effective reproduction in association with a host. Lewis Thomas said, of *C. diphtheriae* relating to human hosts, "It is certainly a strange relationship, without any of the straightforward predator-prey aspects that we used to assume for infectious disease. It is hard to see what the diphtheria bacillus has to gain in life from the capacity to produce such a toxin. Corynebacteria live well enough in the surface of human respiratory membranes, and the production of a necrotic pseudomembrane carries the risk of killing off the host and ending the relationship. It does not, in short, make much sense, and appears more like a biological mix-up than an evolutionary advantage."

The theory behind this statement was widely accepted throughout most of the twentieth century, and has merit in some superficial ways. Ruminants are beautiful examples of beneficial symbiotic relations between host and microbe. Bacteria and protozoa are provided a relatively safe environment with a continuous food supply, whereas the host benefits from microbial transformation of its cellulose-based food intake into ruminant-utilizable nutrients. The skin and gastrointestinal tract also provide residence for microbes that on the whole live harmoniously with their hosts.

However, this theory fails to take into account the basic Darwinian principle of natural selection. Natural selection suggests not peaceful coexistence but competition, in which the genetically superior traits of the stronger, more fit individuals accumulate at the expense of the less fit. Genetically superior pathogens exploit host resources more efficiently and pass on those traits to future generations.

Evolution of microbial virulence is influenced by many factors. One is the selective pressure of the host's defense mechanisms. Rate of pathogen reproduction is equally important. Perhaps most important of all is transmissibility; especially in the case of immobilization and death, the ultimate host disbenefits, and natural selection favors more transmissible genotypes.

Mathematic models describe the dynamics of pathogen transmission in a host population and suggest that the basic reproductive number is pivotal in pathogen transmission. Where host reproduction is continuous and pathogens are transmitted directly from one host to another, the basic reproductive number is:

$$R0 = \frac{bN}{a+m+n}$$

where b is the rate of disease transmission, N is the number of susceptible hosts, a is the rate of pathogen-independent mortality, and n is the rate of recovery of the infected host. This basic reproductive number illustrates the mechanisms by which selection for virulence operates. Selection in the pathogen population favors a high $R0$, achieved by a high rate of transmission, b, or with low rates of pathogen-induced host mortality,

a, or recovery, n. If b, a, and n are independent, selection for high $R0$ will result in the evolution of highly transmissible, benign parasites, an outcome consistent with earlier evolutionary theory. However, if parameters that determine $R0$ are associated with one another, evolutionary endpoints can include evolution toward virulence or toward avirulence. For example, if b increases more than linearly with a, selection favors a pathogen that kills every infected host.

Generation time in the host can dramatically affect the level of virulence; a genotype that reproduces slowly, but immobilizes or kills the host quickly, may not survive. A pathogen that reproduces rapidly and is transmitted may leave many offspring to die with the host but will nonetheless have a fitness advantage. If, however, disease produced by a rapidly reproducing pathogen severely hinders transmission, Darwinian principles might augur toward genotypes with slower reproduction and at least some degree of transmissibility. In general, slowly reproducing pathogens are more likely to cohabit with other slow reproducers because they will fare less well in company with rapidly reproducing pathogens.

Examination of five millennia of human history and patterns of management of domestic animals suggests that what we recognize today as infectious diseases are mainly products of populations large enough to sustain host-to-host pathogen transfer. Pathogens exist in hosts on a fine line between needs for transmission and longevity. Increased transmission contributes to fitness but requires increased growth, which depletes host resources, causes host damage or death, and subsequently pathogen death. Pathogens that optimize this process may be favored by natural selection.

Microbial virulence is on average strongly dependent upon efficient transmission; adding a low infectious dose further increases the efficiency. "Dead-end" hosts are not uncommon, but this is likely not a fully evolved virulence strategy. For example, *Leptospira interrogans* serovar *icterohaemorrhagiae* is commonly found in feral rodents, in which it causes relatively minor pathology (Figure 1-2). However, humans and other species infected by contact with rodent-contaminated environments are likely to develop severe, frequently fatal, disease. Transmission from rodent to rodent and rodent to environment is common, but infected humans (for example) are unlikely to transmit the infection. Another example is provided by

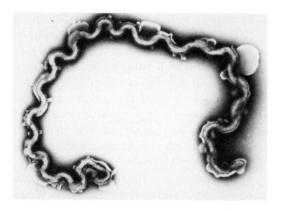

FIGURE 1-2   Pathogenic leptospira may be host adapted or nonadapted and the resulting diseases are less or more severe, respectively. (Courtesy Al Ritchie, deceased.)

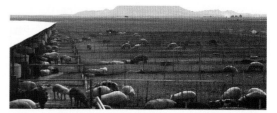

FIGURE 1-3   Desert swine production in the 1970s. Changes in management systems and host genetics influence disease transmission and pathogen evolution. Few changes have been more major or rapidly occurring than those in swine production. (Courtesy J. Glenn Songer.)

the relationship of *Neisseria meningitidis* to human hosts; this organism is a commensal of the human nasopharynx, but can enter the cerebrospinal fluid and produce meningitis. Transmission from the nasopharynx is common, but organisms sequestered in cerebrospinal fluid are not available to other hosts. The host with meningitis is thus a dead-end host.

Mechanisms of transmission are perhaps less understood than any other aspect of microbial virulence. In many cases, transmission is not a passive process, in that many pathogens have developed genetic machinery that specifically addresses aspects of host-to-host transfer.

Routes of excretion, and the extent of excretion by each route, can in theory affect the evolution of host-parasite relationships. Many agents are excreted by more than one route, but one is usually predominant. Control measures may reduce one mode of transmission but fail to deal with others, especially in management of domestic animals. Disease incidence may be reduced overall, but there may be selection for strains that are more capable of transmission by the alternate routes.

Large-scale intensive management systems, such as those used in pig production, are often subject to fewer pathogens than extensive systems, and this number is even smaller with increased biosecurity and age-group segregation (Figure 1-3). These improvements are not without cost; they provide new niches for pathogens and, thus, influence disease evolution. When clinical findings suggest that a microbe is at work in a human or domestic animal population, campaigns for

eradication are often put in place. This may result in unintentional selection for a strain producing fewer cases with less severe symptoms, but that is nonetheless maintained in the population. It is at least theoretically possible to select by this means a highly invasive strain that may achieve its ends of replication and transmission before intervention in the form of treatment or of host defenses. It has been widely stated that microbes abhor a vacuum; the emergence of porcine neonatal enteritis caused by *C. difficile* infection is an illustration of the principle that agents and transmission pathways evolve to take advantage of opportunities, especially in high-health-status herds.

Large group and herd sizes enhance the potential for disease emergence in animal production systems. Pathogens inducing protective immunity in convalescent animals are unlikely to persist in small herds, where the number of susceptible animals may rapidly be reduced below the number required to maintain infection. In such cases, infection is sustained in a herd only by reintroduction. As herd and group sizes increase, it is more likely that the necessary susceptibility threshold will be maintained. Group segregation may influence this positively, but is often accompanied by increased group size, possibly negating beneficial influences of segregation. This system also can encourage emergence of strains that have one or more advantages in a given management scheme. Thus it should be remembered that high-health herds may in fact have their own group of pathogens that have adapted to specific herd characteristics.

Emergence of diseases, especially in high-health-status herds, may actually be a revelation of less obvious problems when more serious ones are dealt with by management. For example, the decline in incidence of swine dysentery has made it more straightforward to recognize other problems, such as infections by *Brachyspira pilosicoli.*

Disease may arise simultaneously in many locations for various reasons, but today the most likely is perhaps the dramatic increase in international trade in animals. Legal and illegal movement of animals can, in a relatively short time, cause widespread dissemination of infectious agents. Recognition of this is important as prevention and control strategies are developed because only by targeting the appropriate source will these efforts be successful.

Establishment and initiation of a disease process may immobilize the host. Organisms infecting such hosts can be transported to new hosts by something mobile or can sit and wait for a susceptible host. The latter must often survive long periods in the environment to develop a high level of virulence in the host. In any case, reduction in mobility has observable, negative effects on the separation of benignity and virulence. This phenomenon is observed to different degrees with different parasites because parasites do not depend equally on host mobility. If a bacterium depends upon host mobility as its primary method of transmission, the overall effect of lost mobility on the bacteria will be great. For example, bacterial infections leading to nasal discharge are typically transmitted via aerosol or direct contact. Thus it would be counterproductive for this type of organism to severely impair its host.

Sexually transmitted bacteria are ill advised to kill or severely disable their hosts because they rely on direct contact for transmission. The pathogen derives no benefit from severe immobilization of the host but *does* profit from remaining longer in situ, to take advantage of what may be limited opportunities for transmission. Cell and tissue tropisms of sexually transmitted parasites may prevent their elimination by the immune response. Two such bacteria are *Neisseria gonorrhoeae* and *Chlamydia trachomatis.*

Bacteria at the other end of this spectrum incur little cost from complete host immobilization. From the parasite's perspective, natural selection should favor increased host exploitation, leading to greater virulence in an immobilized host. Vector-borne diseases are often more likely to immobilize or kill, with minimal negative effects on transmission. Vector-borne pathogens that undergo minimal reproduction and produce

a benign infection in the vector (to avoid decreasing its fitness) have a further advantage. Attendant-borne agents may also increase in virulence, in that there is no requirement for direct host-to-host contact.

Evolutionary studies have demonstrated the correlation between high virulence and water-borne transmission; diarrheal diseases are important causes of morbidity and mortality in humans as well as domestic animals. Not unlike vector-borne agents, water-borne pathogens should benefit from extensive reproduction in their hosts, in that many such infections are accompanied by secretion of water, electrolytes, and pathogens into the environment. Given appropriate conditions (i.e., lack of sanitation), these pathogens find their way into water supplies, from whence they complete the cycle of transmission. Cholera in humans is an example. Pathogens transmitted via water are often also transmitted by flies. Strictly speaking, flies are more often porters (carrying infectious agents that do not replicate in the insect) than vectors. Successful transmission by this route is often associated with a low infectious dose, as is the case with infections by *Shigella* spp.

Environmentally stable pathogens may be associated with higher-than-average virulence. For example, *Bacillus anthracis* in decomposing carcasses forms spores that are remarkably stable in the environment while awaiting another host; this is a classical example of "sit-and-wait" transmission (Figure 1-4). Other pathogens use

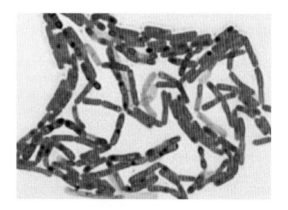

FIGURE 1-4 Persistence of *Bacillus anthracis* as spores in the environment allows it to sit and wait for new hosts. Malachite green spore stain. (Courtesy Public Health Image Library, PHIL #1896, Centers for Disease Control and Prevention, Atlanta, 2002, Larry Stauffer, Oregon State Public Health Laboratory.)

attendant-borne transmission, relying upon healthy mobile hosts to carry agents from one infected, perhaps-immobilized, host to another immobilized host. This is prevalent in hospitals as caregivers unknowingly transport organisms from one patient to another. *C. difficile* nosocomial infection, in humans and domestic animals, is a good example. Attendant-borne pathogens (such as *Staphylococcus aureus*) may have increased virulence in comparison with counterparts outside the hospital environment.

Bacterial genomes are generally considered to contain a universal "core" of genes providing the backbone of genetic information. This includes the "minimal set," which is shared by the majority of bacteria and forms the basic core gene pool. The genome also contains a flexible gene pool consisting of an assortment of strain-specific genetic information that may provide additional power to adapt to special environmental conditions. The immense adaptive capacity of *Pseudomonas aeruginosa* is reflected in its large genome size (6300 kb) and genetic complexity, and much of this results from addition of genomic DNA to the flexible gene pool. Examination of *S. aureus* strains, representing abundant clonal lineages within the species, revealed that more than three quarters of their genes were common to all strains and probably represent a gene complement involved in general cell maintenance and growth. The remaining quarter of the genes is strain specific and may play roles in adaptation to specialized niches. Many of the regions of difference between strains contain genes encoding integrases or transposases (suggesting mobility), and genes that encode virulence determinants or proteins mediating antibiotic resistance.

Regulation of virulence genes and pathways is complex. Pathogens respond in the same general manner as nonpathogens to variations in pH, oxygen tension, nutrients, and availability of iron. Thus virulence-associated regulatory cascades may also control genes not directly associated with virulence. It is important to recognize that regulation of virulence is of paramount importance to the pathogen: untimely expression of virulence genes may have negative consequences for the microbe. During evolution of virulence, defects in regulation are as likely to abort productive (for the pathogen) interactions with the host as shortcomings in availability of effector molecules. For example, invasion of host cells by salmonellae occurs under obligate requirements for appropriate concentrations of oxygen, proper pH and osmolarity, and the proper signal to the PhoP/Q regulon. The host views this interaction as a great inconvenience, with tissue damage to be repaired and foreign objects to be sequestered and removed. The pathogen finds it equally inconvenient because its bottom line is reproduction and, in due time, transmission to other susceptible hosts.

Much of what we know about the evolution of microbial virulence comes from direct comparison of strains. Virulence evolution should, in theory, occur over many generations, but genomics has revealed bacterial acquisition of complex virulence traits in one genetic event. This provides a mechanism for sudden drastic changes in bacterial-host relationships. For example, *E. coli* K12 contains about 500 strain-specific genes, whereas *E. coli* O157:H7 has nearer 1400, many of which encode virulence factors. In contrast, *Mycobacterium tuberculosis* has evolved little over the past few thousand years, as evidenced by negligible variations in *M. tuberculosis* structural genes and even in genes encoding proteins that interact with the host immune system. Lack of evolutionary change suggests that *M. tuberculosis* has reached equilibrium with the host.

Point mutations enable bacterial pathogens to respond, albeit slowly, to pressure applied by the host. Evolution may also be driven by homologous and site-specific recombination events, such as in *N. gonorrhoeae;* expression of an almost-unlimited number of pilus antigens allows it to escape host defense mechanisms. Overall, recombination occurs frequently, and can dominate the long-term evolution of bacterial populations.

Horizontal gene transfer is also extremely important in evolution of virulence. It has been said that we incriminate the bacterium for the sins of the virus, in specific reference to the virulence of *C. diphtheriae.* Lewis Thomas said, "The diphtheria bacillus would not be in any sense a pathogen were it not for its toxin.… Moreover, the toxin is not…the bacillus' own idea; it is made by the bacterium under instructions from a virus, the bacteriophage.…" In fact, plasmids, phages, and other mobile genetic elements *do* play important roles in transfer of virulence attributes among bacteria. Horizontal transfer often results in formation of *genomic islands,* which are seen as gene clusters in the chromosome. These clusters are often called *pathogenicity islands,* and can transform an avirulent strain to virulence in a single step. Most pathogenicity islands are 10 to 200 kb pairs in size, have a G+C content that differs from the average for the genome, are usually associated with a tRNA locus, contain direct repeats at each end, and may have genes encoding genetic mobility.

Pathogenicity islands have been described in *E. coli, Salmonella* spp., *Yersinia* spp., *Shigella* spp., *Vibrio cholerae,* and many other pathogens. They contain genes that encode adherence molecules, machinery for host cell entry and nutrient competition, toxins, secretion systems, and other factors. For example, in some species of *Salmonella*, genes in island SPI-1 govern epithelial cell invasion, whereas those in island SPI-2 mediate intramacrophage survival. The locus of enterocyte effacement (LEE) in enteropathogenic and enterohemorrhagic *E. coli* encodes the adherence factor intimin, and an island in *V. cholerae* encodes a type 4 pilus. Type III secretion systems in many species act like a needle and syringe, injecting effector molecules into host cells; the genetic machinery for this and other types of secretion systems is often found on pathogenicity islands. Smaller regions of DNA with the characteristics of pathogenicity islands are known as pathogenicity islets, and a system of islands may be referred to as a pathogenicity archipelago.

Plasmids carrying virulence genes are found in many pathogenic bacteria, including *Y. pestis, Yersinia enterocolitica, Y. pseudotuberculosis, Shigella* spp., and diarrheagenic *E. coli.* A plasmid of enteropathogenic *E. coli* (EPEC) carries genes encoding bundle-forming pili (BFP) that facilitate formation of densely packed, three-dimensional clusters on host enterocytes. In many other instances virulence-associated genes are plasmid-borne.

Bacteriophages can also carry virulence genes among pathogenic bacteria. Phage-associated genes encode proteins important in colonization, inactivation of host defense mechanisms, damage to tissues, and other factors. Strains of *E. coli* produce Shiga toxin as a result of lysogeny by *stx*-bearing phages. The gene for toxic shock syndrome toxin of *S. aureus* is not an integral part of a bacteriophage genome, but is transported strain to strain by transduction. Toxins produced by *V. cholerae* and *C. diphtheriae* are also encoded by bacteriophage-borne genes.

In sum, microbial virulence is dependent on numerous overlapping characteristics, of which a key factor appears to be mode of transmission. Highly virulent pathogens are often water- or vector-borne, using animal hosts as a part of their life cycles. Overall virulence is probably inversely proportional to the need for host mobility in transmission, and genetic transfer often explains rapid evolution of microbial virulence. Like other microbes, pathogens have the ingenuity to fill open niches, sometimes after contributing to making them available.

SUGGESTED READINGS
Achtman M, Zurth K, Morelli G et al: *Yersinia pestis,* the cause of plague, is a recently emerged clone of *Yersinia pseudotuberculosis, Proc Natl Acad Sci U S A* 96:14043-14048, 1999.

Anderson RM, May RM: Coevolution of hosts and parasites, *Parasitology* 85:411-426, 1982.

Boots M, Sasaki A: "Small worlds" and the evolution of virulence: infection occurs locally and at a distance, *Proc R Soc London* 266:1933-1938, 1999.

Bull JJ, Molineux IJ, Rice WR: Selection of benevolence in a host-parasite system, *Evolution* 45:875-882, 1991.

Ewald PW: Host-parasite relations, vectors, and the evolution of disease severity, *Ann Rev Ecol System* 14:465-485, 1983.

Ewald PW: Waterborne transmission and the evolution of virulence among gastrointestinal bacteria, *Epidemiol Infect* 106:83-119, 1991.

Ewald PW: *Evolution of infectious disease,* New York, 1994, Oxford University Press.

Ewald PW: The evolution of virulence: A unifying link between parasitology and biology, *J Parasitol* 81:659-669, 1995.

Ewald PW: Guarding against the most dangerous emerging pathogens: insights from evolutionary biology, *Emerg Infect Dis* 2:245-257, 1996.

Levin BR, Bull JJ: Short-sighted evolution and the virulence of pathogenic microorganisms, *Trends Microbiol* 2:76-80, 1994.

Maurelli A, Fernandez RE, Bloch CA et al: "Black holes" and bacterial pathogenicity: a large genomic deletion that enhance the virulence of *Shigella* spp. and enteroinvasive *Escherichia coli, Proc Natl Acad Sci U S A* 95:3943-3948, 1998.

Ochman H, Moran NA: Genes lost and genes found: evolution of bacterial pathogenesis and symbiosis, *Science* 292:1096-1098, 2001.

Pfenning KS: Evolution of pathogen virulence: the role of variation in host phenotype, *Proc R Soc London* 268:755-760, 2001.

Thomas L: On disease. In *The medusa and the snail,* New York, 1979, Viking Press.

Chapter 2

General Principles of Bacterial Disease Diagnosis

SPECIMEN SELECTION, COLLECTION, AND TRANSPORT

Results obtained from veterinary diagnosticians are in large part a direct reflection of the quality of specimen that was submitted. It is not always easy to obtain optimal specimens from animals, but application of a few basic principles should yield acceptable specimens that in turn yield high-quality microbiology results.

The first principle seems self-evident, but transgressions against it are common: specimens must be obtained aseptically from a site that is representative of the disease process. In some instances, the appropriate course is obvious; for example, urine culture is unlikely to yield clinically relevant information in a dog manifesting clinical signs of otitis externa. However, in some instances the choice of correct specimen may not be quite so straightforward; a swab of nasal drainage might seem suitable for diagnosis of pneumonia, but in most cases a transtracheal wash is more appropriate (Table 2-1).

Swabs are the most commonly collected specimens, but they are generally not specimens of choice. They may become contaminated with commensal bacteria, and they provide a small sample volume when compared with aspirates, tissues, or body fluids. Bacteria may adsorb to fibers in swabs, further decreasing effective sample volume. Swabs can be useful for obtaining specimens from skin pustules, ears, conjunctivae, deep draining tracts or wounds, soft tissue infections, and the reproductive tract. It is advisable to avoid the wooden-shafted cotton-tipped variety because residual fatty acids and other potentially toxic substances in the fibers may inhibit recovery of bacteria, including chlamydiae. Plastic-shafted calcium alginate, rayon, or Dacron swabs are preferred.

Thorough microbiologic testing should include a direct microscopic examination as well as culture of the specimen, so it is important to collect a sufficient quantity of material to permit adequate examination. This requires, depending on the type of lesion, approximately 0.5 ml of aspirate or fluid, at least two swabs, 5 to 10 ml of blood, or about 1 cm³ of tissue.

Specimens must be collected at the proper time in the disease process, generally during the acute stage of infection and before initiation of antimicrobial therapy. Bacteria are often present throughout the course of the disease, such as in infections of the genitourinary tract. Other infections may be cyclical in nature and require planning to maximize recovery of the etiologic agent; for example, in animals suspected of having septicemia, blood cultures should be collected during a febrile spike.

Specimens should be placed in appropriate transport devices to maintain a buffered and nonnutritive environment to prevent metabolic damage to organisms of interest and overgrowth of contaminants (Table 2-2). It is imperative to keep swabs moist to prevent bacterial desiccation and loss of viability. If samples are to be cultured aerobically, swabs should be placed in Stuart's, Cary-Blair, or Amies medium for transport.

TABLE **2-1** Specimen Selection by Infection Site and Transport Devices

Site	Acceptable Specimen	Transport Device	Comments
Central nervous system	Spinal fluid	Blood culture medium	Hold, ship at RT
Blood	Whole, unclotted blood Minimum of 3 ml	Blood culture medium	Hold, ship at RT Submit ≤3 samples per 24 hr collected during febrile spike
Eye	Conjunctival swab Corneal scrapings Ocular fluid	Amies or semisolid reducing medium Syringe	Hold, ship at RT Inoculate plated media directly with corneal scrapings if fungal keratitis suspected
Bone and joints	Joint aspirate Bone marrow aspirate, bone	Blood culture medium Sterile tube	Hold, ship at RT
Urinary tract	Urine by cystocentesis Catheterized urine Midstream urine	Sterile tube	Hold, ship under refrigeration
Upper respiratory tract	Nasopharyngeal swab Sinus washings Biopsy specimen	Semisolid reducing medium Sterile tube	Ship refrigerated except washings, biopsies (RT)
Lower respiratory tract	Transtracheal wash Lung aspirate or biopsy	Sterile tube Semisolid reducing medium	Hold, ship at RT
Gastrointestinal tract	Feces Rectal swab	Sterile cup or bag Cary-Blair or semisolid reducing medium	Feces: hold, ship at RT; refrigerate *Campylobacter, Brachyspira* suspects
Skin	Aspirate or swab, if superficial Deep swab of draining tract Tissue biopsy Scabs, hairs, scrapings	Sterile syringe Semisolid reducing medium Sterile tube with saline Paper envelope	Anaerobe suspects not refrigerated
Milk	Remove milk from teat cistern; collect 5-10 ml aseptically	Sterile tube	Freeze
Necropsy tissues	Lesions, including adjacent, normal tissue Minimum of 1 cm³ to maximum of 35 cm³ Include one serosal or capsular surface intact	Whirl-Pak bags Screw-cap jars	Individual containers to prevent cross-contamination; ship refrigerated
Reproductive tract	Prostatic fluid, raw semen Uterus Vagina Abortion	Sterile tube Biopsy or swab Swab Fetal lung, liver, kidney, stomach contents, placenta in separate Whirl-Pak bags or screw-capped containers	Guarded swabbing for uterine cultures; hold, ship at RT Ship refrigerated

RT, Room temperature.

They should not be placed in sterile containers with bacteriostatic saline solutions or ethylenediaminetetraacetic acid (EDTA), which is bactericidal. Aspirated specimens may be left in the syringe (with the needle removed), or may be placed into sterile tubes. Tissue specimens may be transported in sterile tubes or in Whirl-Pak bags. Fecal specimens should be collected in sterile cups or bags, but if *Campylobacter* spp. is suspected, feces should be placed in Cary-Blair transport medium.

Use of a transport system is critical to avoid exposure to oxygen of specimens intended for anaerobic culture. Semisolid reducing medium is available in a variety of forms for the transport of fluids, swabs, and tissues, and is useful for recovery of aerobic, anaerobic, and microaerobic bacteria.

TABLE **2-2** Specimen Transport Systems

Transport System and Manufacturer	Comments
Swab Transport System (Stuart's medium) Culturette (Becton Dickinson, Franklin Lakes, NJ) Bacti-Swab (Remel, Lenexa, Kan)	Rayon or Dacron-tipped swabs in plastic sleeves with crushable ampule of Stuart's transport medium; recommended for most aerobic and aerotolerant organisms
Swab Transport System (Cary-Blair medium) Anaerobic culturette (Becton Dickinson, Franklin Lakes, NJ) Cary-Blair Agar Gel Swab (Copan, Corona, Calif)	Specimens suspected to contain anaerobes: mycobacteria and *Campylobacter* spp.
Swab Transport System (Amies medium with charcoal) Amies Agar Gel Swab with charcoal (Copan, Corona, Calif)	Charcoal neutralizes toxins, growth inhibitors; recommended medium for *Taylorella equigenitalis* and *Brachyspira* spp.
Semisolid reducing medium A.C.T. system (Remel, Lenexa, Kan) Port-a-Cul tubes, vials, or jars (Becton Dickinson, Franklin Lakes, NJ)	Semisolid medium for transport of swabs, fluids, small pieces of tissue; useful for aerobic, anaerobic, microaerobic bacteria; reazurin eH indicator
Nasopharyngeal/urethrogenital swabs Fisherbrand calcium alginate swabs Calgiswab (Spectrum; Remel, Lenexa, Kan)	Small, Dacron or calcium alginate tips on flexible wire shafts; useful for obtaining specimens from small orifices; no transport medium
Sterile tubes Vacutainer tubes without additives	Sterile fluids, transtracheal washes, biopsy specimens
Paper envelope, sterile Petri dish	Hairs, scabs, skin scrapings for *Dermatophilus* spp.
Guarded culture systems Tiegland tubes (Jorgensen, Loveland, Colo) Accu-CulShure (MLA Systems, Pleasantville, NY)	Swab in flexible plastic tube; specimen (nasal, uterine) pulled into self-contained transport medium, avoiding contamination from external surfaces
Sterile, plastic screw-cap cups	Feces, urine, biopsies; add 1 ml sterile, nonbacteriostatic saline to small biopsies
Blood culture medium BBL Septi-chek (Becton Dickinson, Franklin Lakes, NJ)	Culture bottles, tubes with liquid medium under vacuum; most contain sodium polyanetholesulfonate (anticoagulant, antiphagocytic, anticomplement); useful for collection of cerebrospinal and joint fluids
Syringe or needle aspirates	Express air from syringe; remove needle, cap with original seal; anaerobes survive $\leq$24 hr at RT if specimen volume >2 ml
Bio-Bag Environmental System (Becton Dickinson, Franklin Lakes, NJ)	Ampules of indicator, hydrogen-CO_2 generator, catalyst crushed in bag, creates anaerobic environment; useful for swabs, tubes, plates

RT, Room temperature.

Refrigeration usually preserves viability and reduces overgrowth by extraneous organisms, but fastidious organisms (such as anaerobes) will sometimes die rapidly when exposed to low temperatures. Specimens likely to contain these organisms, or samples of body fluids other than urine, should be held at room temperature.

Legible labeling of specimens, with an indelible marker, is critical. Note the source and/or specific body site, and provide relevant clinical information on the submittal form to facilitate appropriate specimen handling and interpretation of results. Information regarding the animal species and anatomic site of origin, the suspected causative agent, previous antimicrobial therapy, and clinical signs will help the laboratory make the best choices regarding media and incubation conditions. Delivery to the laboratory should be within 48 hours of collection. Regulations governing the shipment of clinical specimens are changing rapidly, and compliance with prevailing laws may be facilitated by consulting the U.S. Department of Transportation (www.dot.gov).

LABORATORY DIAGNOSIS

The specific procedures for diagnosis of bacterial or fungal diseases vary widely, but usually include direct examination of clinical materials by microscopy, isolation of agents from diagnostic specimens, and detection of agents by immunologic or molecular methods.

Direct Examination

The initial step in a microbiologic workup is often direct microscopic examination; brightfield, darkfield, and fluorescence microscopy is routine in most diagnostic laboratories. In brightfield microscopy, a specimen is illuminated by visible light. A condenser focuses the light on the specimen and objective, and ocular lenses magnify the image. Three different objective lenses are used: low power (10×), high dry (40×), and oil immersion (100×). Low power (10×) is used to scan specimens; filamentous fungi (with india ink and/or potassium hydroxide [KOH] as a mounting medium) are best visualized with the high dry objective (40×), and the oil immersion objective (100×) is needed to observe stained bacteria and yeasts. Examination of Gram-stained smears is important, especially in specimens procured from normally sterile sites because it provides an inventory of morphologic types of bacteria that can be followed up during bacteriologic culture.

The darkfield microscope uses a specific type of condenser that applies light to the specimen in an oblique manner. It is particularly useful with specimens that are difficult to visualize by conventional lighting methods, including bacteria whose length-to-width ratio is large; examples are *Brachyspira hyodysenteriae,* leptospires, and *Borrelia burgdorferi,* which are illuminated against a black background (Figure 2-1).

Microbes can also be stained with fluorescent dyes and examined under ultraviolet illumination. Typically, organisms are brightly illuminated against a black background (Figure 2-2). In veterinary microbiology, this method is used extensively for detection of histotoxic clostridia and leptospires in tissue preparations.

As noted, direct examination of specimens can use wet mounts or stained smears. Samples for wet mounts can be suspended in sterile saline for examination by brightfield or darkfield microscopy. If fungi are suspected, specimens are suspended in 10% KOH or, in the case of cryptococci, in india ink. Differential stains are indispensable tools.

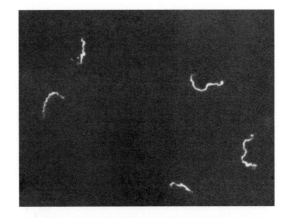

FIGURE 2-1   Darkfield photomicrograph of *Treponema pallidum,* the causative agent of human syphilis. (Courtesy Public Health Image Library, PHIL #2335, W. Hubbard, Atlanta, 1971, Centers for Disease Control and Prevention.)

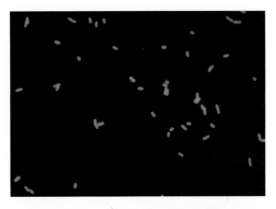

FIGURE 2-2   *Legionella pneumophila* stained using a direct immunofluorescence method. (Courtesy Public Health Image Library, PHIL #2015, William Cherry, Atlanta, 1978, Centers for Disease Control and Prevention.)

Gram stains are the basis for phenotypic characterization of bacteria (Figure 2-3), and acid-fast stains such as Kinyoun's or Ziehl-Neelsen's, are used primarily to detect *Nocardia* and *Mycobacterium* spp. (Figure 2-4). Many fluorescent dyes have been used to stain specimens, including calcofluor white, which stains chitin in the fungal cell wall. Examination with hematologic stains (Diff Quik or Wright-Giemsa) is performed when specimens may contain *Pneumocystis, Ehrlichia, Borrelia,* or *Rickettsia* spp. (Figure 2-5).

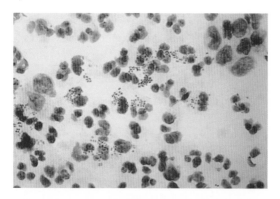

FIGURE 2-3   Gram-stained smear of urethral exudate, revealing *Neisseria gonorrhoeae* as gram-negative cocci. (Courtesy Public Health Image Library, PHIL #2309, Norman Jacobs, Atlanta, 1974, Centers for Disease Control and Prevention.)

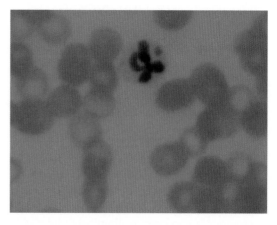

FIGURE 2-5   Hematologic stain, showing *Ehrlichia* in association with a neutrophil. (Courtesy Karen W. Post.)

Bacteriologic and Fungal Culture

Clinical microbiology generally requires that both liquid (broth) and solid (agar) media be inoculated for isolation of microorganisms. Solid media facilitate isolation of individual microbial colonies, quantitation of bacteria, and selection or differentiation of normal flora from potential pathogens. Broth media allow recovery of small numbers of organisms or those that are more fastidious,

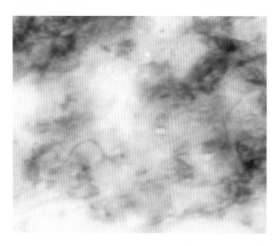

FIGURE 2-4   Stained smear of pus, with acid-fast *Nocardia* spp. (Courtesy Public Health Image Library, PHIL #2797, Leanor Haley, Atlanta, 1969, Centers for Disease Control and Prevention.)

whereas some may enrich for a particular pathogen (e.g., tetrathionate broth for salmonellae).

A few drops of liquid specimen are placed via syringe or pipette onto a quadrant of plated medium and into broth. Urine and bulk tank milk are plated for quantitation, often by use of a calibrated loop. Swabs are generally plated directly and then placed into enriched broth. Fecal specimens are sampled by swabbing, followed by inoculation of solid and liquid media. The surface of tissue specimens is decontaminated by searing with a hot spatula, and a portion is then removed and touched to the agar surface. Eventual identification of bacteria depends upon obtaining isolated colonies by some type of specimen dilution. The most common technique is streaking of plates, with wire or plastic loops. Specific methods are numerous, but the end goal is to obtain individual colonies of the subject organism.

Inoculated media are placed in incubators with the appropriate environmental conditions. Plates are inverted for incubation to prevent dripping of condensate onto the agar surface and the resulting confluent bacterial growth. Optimal growth temperature for most organisms is 35° C to 37° C. Exceptions are *Campylobacter jejuni*, which grows optimally at 42° C, and most fungi, which grow best at 25° C to 30° C. Relative humidity of 70% to 80% is desirable, and although many bacteria grow well in ambient air, growth of some is enhanced by or impossible without CO_2 concentrations greater than those in air. These include many of the fastidious organisms in the genera *Brucella*, *Taylorella*, and *Haemophilus*.

The first step in culture evaluation is the visual examination of plated media. Most bacteria produce visible colonies in 24 to 48 hours, although some require longer incubation periods. Inspection includes examination of colonial morphology, noting both the types and numbers of each morphologic set, as well as hemolytic reactions on blood-based agar. Experienced microbiologists learn to visually classify colonial types into various groups and to distinguish normal flora from potential pathogens. Further classification is based on the presence or absence of growth on differential or selective media.

Gram stains of each colony morphotype may allow presumptive identification. Colonies of potentially significant organisms should be subcultured to a nonselective plated medium to produce a pure culture for biochemical characterization and antimicrobial susceptibility testing. Figures 2-6 through 2-9 summarize laboratory procedures for specimen processing and presumptive identification of bacteria.

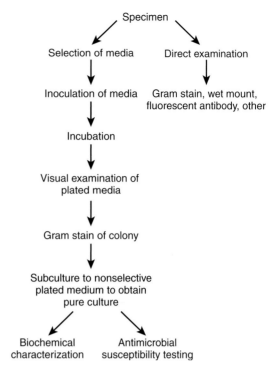

FIGURE 2-6   Microbiologic examination of clinical specimens. (Courtesy Ashley E. Harmon.)

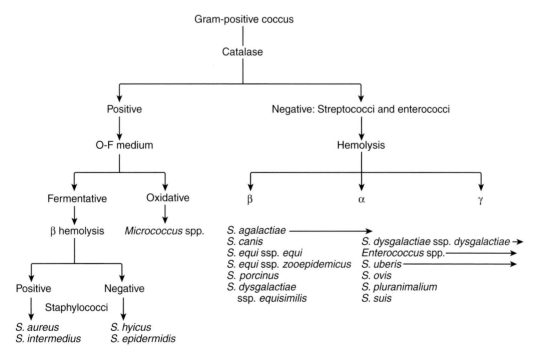

FIGURE 2-7   Presumptive identification of aerobic gram-positive cocci. *O-F,* Oxidative-fermentative. (Courtesy Ashley E. Harmon.)

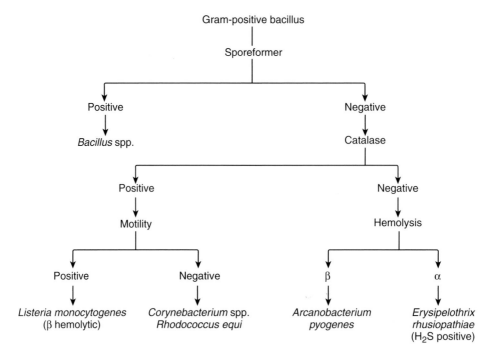

FIGURE 2-8 Presumptive identification of aerobic gram-positive bacilli. (Courtesy Ashley E. Harmon.)

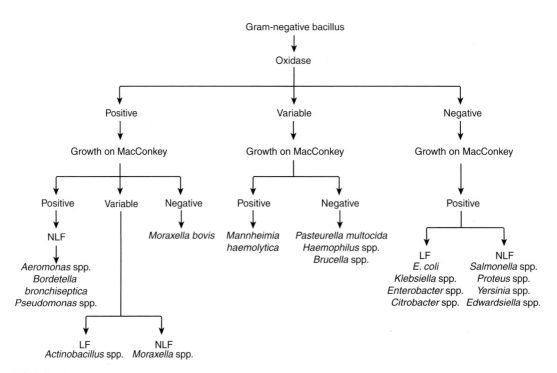

FIGURE 2-9 Presumptive identification of aerobic gram-negative bacilli. *LF,* Lactose fermenter; *NLF,* non–lactose fermenter. (Courtesy Ashley E. Harmon.)

Immunologic Methods of Diagnosis

Tests that detect antigens or antibodies are collectively referred to as immunoassays. Commonly used techniques are precipitation, agglutination, complement fixation, immunofluorescence, and enzyme-linked immunosorbent assay (ELISA). These methods are valuable tools in disease diagnosis, in that they can be specific and sensitive.

Precipitation reactions occur when soluble antigens are mixed with specific antibodies, generally of the immunoglobulin G (IgG) class. When appropriate concentrations of antigen and antibody are present, these mixtures become cloudy and flocculent, and a fine precipitate is formed. Antibodies involved in these reactions are sometimes referred to as precipitins. Precipitation tests can be performed in tubes or on slides, but diffusion in agar or agarose is often more convenient. Wells punched in the agar surface are filled with a known antigen and a test serum suspected to contain antibody (or antigen of unknown composition and serum against a specific antigen). Antigen and antibody molecules diffuse toward one another until equal amounts of each mix, at which point a visible line forms in the agarose. In veterinary diagnostic medicine, this test is used routinely for detection of antibodies against viruses such as equine infectious anemia, bovine leukemia, and bluetongue. Immunodiffusion tests have also been used for the diagnosis of systemic fungal infections in animals, as well as for definitive identification of those agents in culture (exoantigen tests) (Figure 2-10).

Agglutination occurs when antibodies are mixed with and bind to particulate antigens, resulting in visible clumping of particles. Agglutination is more sensitive than precipitation, and although both immunoglobulin M (IgM) and IgG can cause agglutination, the former, with its pentameric structure, is more efficient. Agglutination may be detected macroscopically or microscopically; macroscopic slide and tube agglutination tests are used extensively in monitoring for brucellosis, and the microscopic agglutination test is widely used for diagnosis of leptospirosis (Figure 2-11). Rapid latex agglutination tests are used for direct detection of bacterial or fungal antigens in cerebrospinal fluid, serum, and urine. For example, latex particles coated with anticryptococcal antibodies interact with antigens liberated by the organism into blood or body fluids, causing agglutination and facilitating diagnosis of cryptococcosis in cats.

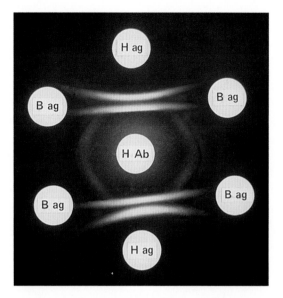

FIGURE 2-10 Double immunodiffusion as applied to exoantigen testing for systemic fungi. *B ag, Blastomyces dermatitidis* extract; *H Ab,* antibodies to *Histoplasma capsulatum; H ag,* histoplasmin or fungal extract. (Courtesy Public Health Image Library, PHIL #459, Errol Reiss, Atlanta, date unknown, Centers for Disease Control and Prevention.)

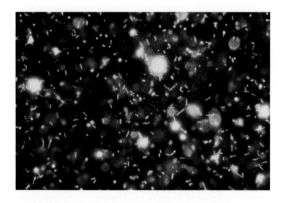

FIGURE 2-11 Photomicrograph of leptospiral agglutination. (Courtesy Public Health Image Library, PHIL #2888, M. Gatton, Atlanta, 1961, Centers for Disease Control and Prevention.)

The complement fixation test is based on the principle that complement components become depleted in the presence of antigen-antibody complexes. Antigen is added to test serum and complement, usually from guinea pigs. Complement is bound (or "fixed") by interaction with immune complexes that form when antigens and antibodies match. Sheep red blood cells (SRBCs) sensitized

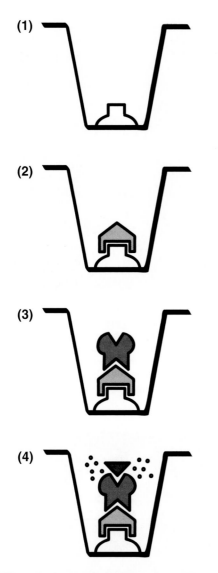

FIGURE 2-12 Schematic of direct enzyme-linked immunosorbent assay (ELISA). **(1)** Wells of the assay plate are coated with capture antibody, which has specificity for antigen (polyclonal antibody) or antigenic epitope (monoclonal antibody) of interest. If the assay is intended to *detect* antibodies, coating is with antigen specific for those antibodies. **(2)** Antigen (or antibody) in test solution combines with capture molecule. **(3)** A second antibody, recognizing one or more other epitopes of the captured antigen or antibody, and labeled to allow detection, is added and allowed to bind. **(4)** Substrate interacts with detection molecule, producing an observable reaction. (Courtesy Ashley E. Harmon.)

with rabbit anti-SRBCs lyse in samples in which complement has not been fixed, indicating lack of specific antigen-antibody reaction. Complement fixation tests are quite difficult to standardize, and in many laboratories have been replaced by ELISA methods. However, the test is still useful for diagnosis of brucellosis, anaplasmosis, and systemic mycoses.

Immunofluorescence assays employ fluorescent dyes, the most common of which is fluorescein isothiocyanate (FITC); when irradiated by ultraviolet light, FITC emits an apple-green fluorescence. Direct fluorescent antibody tests detect antigen by application of labeled antibody against a microorganism or subunits of it. Tissue or impression smears are fixed to a glass slide and after incubation with the labeled antibody and washing, examination by fluorescence microscopy reveals positive reactions as bound particles of fluorescing antigen. Indirect fluorescent antibody tests may be used to demonstrate antigens in tissues or antibodies in serum. For antibody detection, antigen fixed to a slide is incubated with test serum and then to FITC-labeled antiglobulin. When examined under ultraviolet illumination, fluorescence indicates that antibody is present in the test serum.

Enzyme immunoassays may be used to detect and quantitate antibody or antigen. These tests use antibodies conjugated with an enzyme (such as horseradish peroxidase or alkaline phosphatase). Like indirect fluorescent antibody assays, indirect ELISAs are often directed toward detection of antibodies, and antigen-capture or direct ELISAs are commonly used for detection of viruses (Figure 2-12).

Molecular Methods

The advent of molecular diagnostic testing for infectious diseases has changed the basic methods of operation in microbiology laboratories around the world. Molecular methods are based upon detection of DNA or RNA of microorganisms present in clinical specimens, and in general, molecular assays offer better performance and shorter testing times than traditional methods. They are especially useful for rapid detection of microorganisms that are uncultivable or slowly growing, such as mycoplasmas, mycobacteria, spirochetes, and ehrlichiae. Molecular methods may have drawbacks, including lack of necessary sensitivity and specificity and failure to differentiate live and dead organisms, but they also have many advantages over traditional methods.

Nucleic acid probes are usually relatively small segments of DNA or RNA that, in sequence, are complementary to some part of the genome of an organism of interest. Probes may be synthetic, or derived from cloned nucleic acid, often produced in a plasmid and suitable host. Labeling with radioactive or chemically modified nucleotides permits detection and quantitation. Separation of DNA strands by heating or chemical treatment and provision of appropriate conditions of pH, temperature, and osmolarity allows the probes to hybridize, and any labeled DNA in the specimen is detected (Figure 2-13). The sensitivity of the assay varies directly with the size and composition of the probe as well as the nature of the clinical

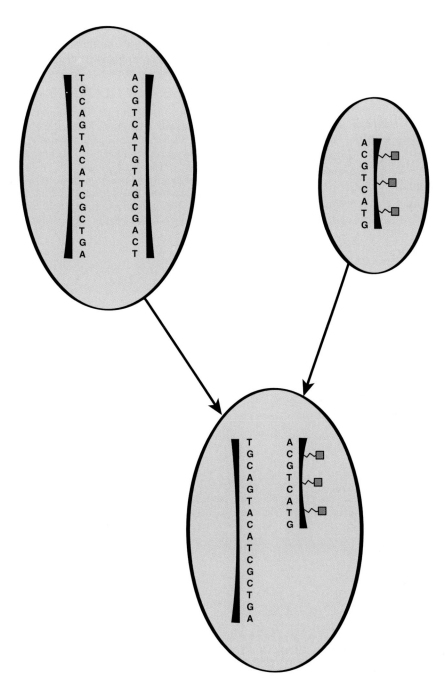

FIGURE 2-13 Schematic of gene detection by nucleic acid probe. A probe is synthesized to correspond in nucleotide sequence to the target for detection. It is labeled, often with fluorescent or radioactive substances, to allow detection of binding. If the target nucleic acid is double-stranded, it is denatured by heating and placed on a support matrix (usually a nylon or nitrocellulose membrane). The probe is applied and, under proper conditions of temperature and osmolarity, binds to its target. Detection of the label confirms binding to the appropriate target. (Courtesy Ashley E. Harmon.)

specimen, but in general, probing of clinical specimens has a low sensitivity.

The polymerase chain reaction (PCR) and PCR-derived techniques are the best developed and the most widely used methods of nucleic acid detection. They allow for amplification of a specific sequence many millions of times in a few hours, and can theoretically detect single copies of a sequence. An important part of the enabling technology is the automated thermal cycler, which heats and cools the reaction mixture (DNA polymerase, oligonucleotide primers, deoxynucleotides, $MgCl_2$) through multiple cycles of denaturation (typically at 94° C), annealing (at various temperatures, in keeping with the composition of the target sequence and the primers), and extension (usually at 72° C, to accommodate the polymerase). Amplification is exponential. PCR assays are used extensively in veterinary microbiology for detection of bacteria and fungi in clinical materials and for characterization of microorganisms (e.g., toxinotyping of *Clostridium perfringens Pasteurella multocida,* and *Escherichia coli*).

Molecular applications can also be utilized for definitive identification of microorganisms. Sequence analysis of the highly conserved stable bacterial 16S ribosomal ribonucleic acid (rRNA) gene has evolved as the gold standard for identification. The major limitation of this approach in the veterinary arena is expense.

SUGGESTED READINGS

Mahony JB, Chernesky MA: Immunoassays for the diagnosis of infectious diseases. In Murray PR, Baron EJ, Pfaller MA, et al, eds: *Manual of clinical microbiology,* ed 7, Washington, DC, 1999, ASM Press.
Persing DH, Smith TF, Tenover FC, White TJ, eds: 1993. *Diagnostic molecular microbiology: principles and applications,* Washington, DC, 1993, ASM Press.
Tenover FC: Diagnostic deoxyribonucleic acid probes for infectious diseases, *Clin Microbiol Rev* 1:82-101, 1988.

Chapter 3

Antimicrobial Agents, Mechanisms of Resistance, and Susceptibility Testing

The veterinarian attending to a domestic animal with a bacterial infection must identify and eliminate predisposing factors (e.g., foreign bodies or stress), reduce the numbers of the etiological agent and its toxic products from the site of infection when possible (usually by drainage or some other form of surgical intervention), and reduce proliferation of the agent to allow host defenses to gain control at the infected site (most often by use of antimicrobial chemotherapeutic agents). Administration must be in a manner that exploits a drug's pharmacodynamic parameters relative to the target pathogen; successful outcomes are most common when an effective drug concentration is maintained for an appropriate time at the site of infection, allowing specific and nonspecific defenses to eliminate the offending pathogen. Knowledge of natural resistance traits of common pathogens is a key component of antimicrobial susceptibility testing and the practice of veterinary therapeutics.

Many factors contribute to a successful outcome of antimicrobial therapy. Intrinsic resistance is not uncommon (e.g., resistance of *Salmonella typhimurium* to vancomycin), and antimicrobial therapy will not be effective in such instances. Other organisms can become resistant through acquisition of resistance elements or through mutation. Antimicrobials in the same chemical class may have similar in vitro activities against bacterial pathogens (e.g., ampicillin and amoxicillin), and a representative antimicrobial can often be used as a predictor of susceptibility to other members of the same class. However, this is not always the case, as in the differing efficacies of ciprofloxacin and enrofloxacin against infections by *Pseudomonas aeruginosa*. Natural resistance traits of common pathogens and members of each antimicrobial drug class are key components in antimicrobial susceptibility testing and the practice of infectious disease medicine.

ANTIMICROBIAL AGENTS

Antimicrobial agents may be based on fungal or higher bacterial metabolites or may be wholly synthetic. They may have a broad or narrow spectrum of activity, as in the case of cephalexin (a first-generation cephalosporin, which has a narrow spectrum of activity, directed primarily against gram-positive bacteria) and tetracyclines (which are active against a broad range of bacteria, including some mycoplasmas, rickettsiae, and chlamydiae) (Tables 3-1 and 3-2). Antimicrobials may also be classified by their ability to kill the target organism or simply inhibit growth. Bactericidal agents kill at or near the same concentration that inhibits bacterial growth (the minimal inhibitory concentration, MIC). Bacteriostatic drugs inhibit multiplication at the MIC, but a higher concentration, the minimal bactericidal concentration (MBC), is necessary to kill bacteria.

Classes of Antimicrobials

Aminoglycosides include amikacin, gentamicin, kanamycin, neomycin, streptomycin, tobramycin, and apramycin and are derived from either

TABLE **3-1** Sensitivity of Various Bacteria to Major Classes of Antimicrobial Agents

Antimicrobial Agent	Gram-Positive Aerobes	Gram-Negative Aerobes	Gram-Positive Anaerobes	Gram-Negative Anaerobes	Mycoplasmas	Chlamydiae	Rickettsiae
Aminoglycosides/ Aminocyclitols	Most neg	Pos	Neg	Neg	Pos	Neg	Neg
β-lactams	Pos	Most neg	Pos	Most pos	Neg	Neg	Neg
Chloramphenicol/ Florfenicol	Pos	Pos	Pos	Pos	Pos	Pos	Pos
Fluoroquinolones	Most pos	Pos	Neg	Neg	Pos	Pos	Pos
Lincosamides	Pos	Neg	Pos	Pos	Pos	Neg	Neg
Macrolides	Pos	Most neg	Pos	Pos	Pos	Pos	Neg
Pleuromutilins	Pos	Most neg	Pos	Pos	Pos	Pos	Neg
Potentiated sulfas	Pos	Pos	Most neg	Pos	Neg	Pos	Neg
Sulfonamides	Pos	Most pos	Most neg	Most neg	Neg	Pos	Neg
Tetracyclines	Pos	Most pos	Pos	Most pos	Most pos	Pos	Pos

Neg, Negative; *Pos,* positive.

TABLE **3-2** Mechanism of Action of Various Antimicrobial Agents

Agent	Mechanism of Action
Aminoglycosides/aminocyclitols	Inhibit protein synthesis via irreversible binding to 30S ribosomal subunit
β-lactams	Inhibit enzymes essential for peptidoglycan synthesis
Chloramphenicol/florfenicol	Inhibits protein synthesis via irreversible binding to 50S ribosomal subunit
Fluoroquinolones	Inhibit DNA gyrase (involved in synthesis and maintenance of DNA)
Lincosamides	Inhibit protein synthesis via binding to 50S ribosomal subunit
Macrolides	Inhibit protein synthesis via reversible binding to 23S rRNA of 50S ribosomal subunit
Pleuromutilins	Inhibit protein synthesis by effects on peptidyl transferase center of 50S ribosomal subunit
Potentiated sulfonamides	Inhibit folic acid metabolism, interfering with DNA synthesis
Sulfonamides	Inhibit folic acid synthesis via competition with para-aminobenzoic acid for dihydropteroate synthetase
Tetracyclines	Inhibit protein synthesis via reversible binding to 30S ribosomal subunit

DNA, Deoxyribonucleic acid; *rRNA,* ribosomal ribonucleic acid.

Streptomyces spp. or *Micromonospora* spp. These agents inhibit protein synthesis by binding to the 30S subunit of the ribosome, rendering it unavailable for translocation of mRNA during protein synthesis, and can cause mistranslation of genes and production of defective proteins. Their activity is directed mainly against aerobic, gram-negative bacilli, *Staphylococcus aureus,* and mycoplasmas. Aminoglycosides may be both nephrotoxic and ototoxic, but these toxic effects are mitigated with appropriate dosing regimens.

Aminocyclitols differ from aminoglycosides in that they lack an amino sugar and a glycosidic bond. Spectinomycin, derived from *Streptomyces spectabilis,* is the only aminocyclitol used in veterinary medicine. It is commonly considered to be bacteriostatic, but higher concentrations may be bactericidal for specific pathogens. The mechanism of action of spectinomycin is similar to that of aminoglycosides except that it does not cause mistranslation. It is active against a broad range of pathogens, and is used for treatment of bovine respiratory disease, porcine neonatal colibacillosis, and for control of avian salmonellosis, mycoplasmosis, colisepticemia, and fowl cholera. Unlike the aminoglycosides, spectinomycin is relatively nontoxic.

β-Lactam antimicrobials include penicillins, cephalosporins, carbapenems, and monobactams and are named for their β-lactam ring structure. Carbapenems and monobactams have limited use in veterinary medicine. The β-lactam's bactericidal effect is exerted through interference with cell wall synthesis, specifically by preventing transpeptidation, thus depriving the peptidoglycan layer of its rigidity. The specific targets of the β-lactams are the penicillin-binding proteins located on the outside of the cytoplasmic membrane.

Penicillins may be divided into several classes. These include the benzylpenicillins, aminobenzyl penicillins, isoxazolyl penicillins, carboxypenicillins, and ureidopenicillins. The benzylpenicillins, such as penicillin G, are active mainly against gram-positive bacteria and are widely used in veterinary medicine, especially in large animals. In ruminants they are used to treat clostridial and corynebacterial infections, pneumonic pasteurellosis, and listeriosis. Penicillin is the drug of choice for treatment and control of swine erysipelas and *Streptococcus suis* infections. Equine infections by β-hemolytic streptococci and *Clostridium*

tetani may be effectively treated with penicillin, as are necrotic enteritis, erysipelas, and ulcerative enteritis in poultry. The aminobenzyl penicillins (e.g., ampicillin and amoxicillin) exhibit increased activity against gram-negative bacteria while retaining their activity against the gram-positive bacteria. Newer β-lactam agents, such as carboxypenicillins (e.g., ticarcillin) and ureidopenicillins (e.g., piperacillin), have increased activity against gram-negative pathogens, at the expense of activity against gram-positive bacteria. The isoxazolyl penicillins are β-lactamase resistant and are active only against staphylococci, including those that are β-lactamase producers.

Cephalosporins are less susceptible to hydrolysis by β-lactamases, especially those that degrade penicillins, but are susceptible to hydrolysis by cephalosporinases. They are classified into groups, or "generations," based on their structure and antibacterial activity. First-generation cephalosporins include drugs such as cefazolin and cefadroxil, which exhibit activity against gram-positive bacteria, including penicillin-resistant staphylococci and many gram-negative bacteria. They are also active against many anaerobic bacteria, but enterococci are intrinsically resistant to all cephalosporins. Second-generation drugs, such as cefaclor, have additional activity against gram-negative bacteria. The cephamycins (e.g., cefoxitin and cefotetan) are closely related to the second-generation cephalosporins, and of these, cefoxitin is most commonly used in companion animal medicine. Third-generation cephalosporins have a broad activity spectrum, exhibiting good to excellent efficacy against a variety of pathogens. Ceftiofur is the only one marketed specifically for use in veterinary medicine. It is approved for treatment of bovine respiratory disease associated with *Mannheimia haemolytica, Pasteurella multocida,* and *Histophilus somni,* swine respiratory disease caused by *Actinobacillus pleuropneumoniae* and *P. multocida,* and infections by *Salmonella choleraesuis* and *S. suis.* In addition, the drug may be used for control of poultry enteric disease, is indicated for treatment of equine respiratory infections with *Streptococcus equi* ssp. *zooepidemicus* and canine urinary tract infections, and is being evaluated for intramammary therapy of bovine mastitis. The fourth-generation cephalosporins are primarily marketed for use in human medicine, although cefquinome is being investigated for use in veterinary medicine.

Chloramphenicol, a bacteriostatic agent originally isolated from *Streptomyces venezuela*, is now produced as a derivative of dichloroacetic acid. The drug binds irreversibly to the 50S ribosomal subunit and prevents peptide chain elongation. It has a broad spectrum of activity against gram-positive and gram-negative aerobes, anaerobes, chlamydiae, rickettsiae, and many mycoplasmas. Use of this drug in food animals is prohibited in the United States. Eukaryotic mitochondrial ribosomes are also subject to the effects of chloramphenicol, and bone marrow suppression with irreversible aplastic anemia and neutropenia may be a consequence of chloramphenicol therapy.

Florfenicol is a synthetic thiamphenicol analog with broad-spectrum activity and a mechanism of action equivalent to that of chloramphenicol. It lacks the chloramphenicol nitrobenzene moiety, which has been associated with aplastic anemia. Florfenicol is used exclusively in veterinary medicine, and is approved for treatment of bovine infections by *M. haemolytica*, *P. multocida*, and *H. somni* and porcine disease associated with infection by *A. pleuropneumoniae*, *P. multocida*, *S. choleraesuis*, and *S. suis* type 2.

Fluoroquinolones are bactericidal and have activity against gram-negative bacteria, chlamydiae, rickettsiae, and mycoplasmas; they are moderately active against staphylococci and have fair to poor activity against streptococci and anaerobes. As with cephalosporins, fluoroquinolones are divided into classes based on chemical structure and spectrum of activity. The first quinolone, nalidixic acid, has a limited spectrum of activity, perhaps due to restricted absorption following oral administration and finite tissue distribution, and second-generation quinolones (e.g., flumequine) have similar limitations. However, third-generation fluoroquinolones (e.g., ciprofloxacin and enrofloxacin) are markedly improved in spectrum of antibacterial activity and in absorption and distribution, but toxic effects on articular cartilage make fluoroquinolones contraindicated in growing animals. Additionally, fluoroquinolone therapy in livestock has been controversial because of common use of these antimicrobials for treatment of human infections (especially in the gastrointestinal tract) and concerns that resistant bacteria may be transmitted to humans via the food chain. Danofloxacin, difloxacin, enrofloxacin, marbofloxacin, and orbifloxacin are approved for use in veterinary medicine. Danofloxacin is a synthetic fluoroquinolone available for treatment of bovine respiratory disease associated with *M. haemolytica* and *P. multocida* infection. Difloxacin is approved only for managing bacterial infections of the canine urinary tract, respiratory tract, and skin. It is especially useful for treating canine otitis caused by members of the Enterobacteriaceae, *S. aureus*, or *Staphylococcus intermedius*. Enrofloxacin, the first fluoroquinolone marketed exclusively for use in veterinary medicine, is approved for treating gastrointestinal, soft tissue, and respiratory infections, including bovine respiratory disease associated with *M. haemolytica*, *P. multocida*, and *H. somni*. It has been approved for control of *Escherichia coli* infections in chickens and *E. coli* and *P. multocida* infection in turkeys. However, this has recently undergone an administrative review because of human food safety concerns associated with the selection of ciprofloxacin-resistant *Campylobacter*. Marbofloxacin was also specifically developed for veterinary medical applications, and is used for treatment of soft tissue infections and cystitis in dogs and cats. Orbifloxacin is indicated for managing canine skin, soft tissue, and urinary tract infections.

Lincosamides (clindamycin, lincomycin, and pirlimycin) are bacteriostatic, interfering with protein synthesis by binding to the 50S subunit of the 70S ribosome. Specifically, this binding occurs at the L15 protein in the peptidyltransferase region. During translocation the growing peptide chain with its tRNA moves from an "acceptor site" to a "donor site." The exact mechanism is unknown, but lincosamides probably bind to the donor site on the ribosome, interrupting completion of the peptide chain.

Lincosamides have a moderate spectrum of activity. Clindamycin, a semisynthetic derivative of lincomycin, is used primarily in small animal medicine for treatment of anaerobic or staphlylococcal soft tissue infections. Lincomycin is used to control dysentery, erysipelas, and mycoplasmosis in swine. Pirlimycin is veterinary specific and has activity against gram-positive organisms, especially staphylococci and streptococci. It is used as an intramammary infusion for treatment of mastitis due to infection with *S. aureus*, *Streptococcus agalactiae*, *Streptococcus uberis*, and *Streptococcus dysgalactiae* ssp. *dysgalactiae* infection in lactating dairy cattle. Lincosamides are toxic for sheep, horses, rabbits, and laboratory rodents, and may induce pseudomembranous colitis as a result of overgrowth of *Clostridium difficile* in laboratory animals.

Erythromycin, tylosin, and tilmicosin are the most common macrolide antibiotics and are derived from various *Streptomyces* spp. These agents are bacteriostatic and act similarly to lincosamides. Their spectrum of activity is relatively broad, including gram-positive aerobes, anaerobes, mycoplasmas, and chlamydiae. Use of erythromycin in large animals is limited by the fact that it is irritating if injected intramuscularly and is toxic for ruminants if given orally. It is commonly associated with gastric upset in small animals but is the drug of choice for treatment of diarrhea caused by *Campylobacter jejuni*. It is used for treatment of *Rhodococcus equi* pneumonia in foals and is administered to poultry for prevention or treatment of infections caused by *S. aureus, Clostridium* spp., *Haemophilus paragallinarum,* or mycoplasmas.

Tylosin and tilmicosin are used exclusively in veterinary medicine. The former is for treatment of pneumonia, pinkeye, mastitis, and footrot in ruminants and mycoplasmal pneumonia, erysipelas, atrophic rhinitis, and proliferative/hemorrhagic enteropathy caused by *Lawsonia intracellularis* in swine. Tylosin is also used in poultry for treating and controlling mycoplasmosis and spirochetosis. Tilmicosin is a semisynthetic macrolide with efficacy against swine respiratory infection caused by *A. pleuropneumoniae* and *P. multocida,* and bovine respiratory infection caused by *M. haemolytica.* The drug can be lethal in swine, horses, or humans injected intramuscularly. Azithromycin and clarithromycin are macrolide-like compounds used in human medicine; they are seeing some application in veterinary medicine such as the use of azithromycin for the treatment of *R. equi* infections in horses.

Pleuromutilin is a product of the basidiomycete, *Clitopilus scyphoides* (formerly *Pleurotus mutilus*). The semisynthetic pleuromutilin derivatives tiamulin and valnemulin are not used in human medicine. They have a unique diterpine chemical structure and are bacteriostatic by binding to the 50S ribosomal subunit and inhibition of protein synthesis. They inhibit peptidyl transferase and interact with the rRNA in the peptidyl transferase slot on the ribosomes, in which they prevent correct positioning of the CCA ends of tRNAs for peptide transfer. In the United States, tiamulin is approved for treatment of *A. pleuropneumoniae* and *Brachyspira hyodysenteriae* infections in swine. Valnemulin is used in Europe for treating various swine diseases.

Potentiated sulfa drugs are combinations of sulfonamides and diaminopyrimidines, trimethoprim, or ormetoprim, which have broad-spectrum, synergistic bactericidal activity against many aerobic gram-positive and gram-negative bacteria, anaerobes, and chlamydiae. Potentiated sulfas prevent folic acid synthesis and diaminopyrimidines inhibit the enzyme that converts dihydrofolate into tetrahydrofolic acid. Sulfonamides compete with para-aminobenzoic acid (PABA) for incorporation into dihydrofolate. Veterinary preparations include ormetoprim-sulfadimethoxine, trimethoprim-sulfaquinoxaline, trimethoprim-sulfamethoxazole, and trimethoprim-sulfadiazine. They are effective in treatment of genitourinary tract infections, otitis externa, and enteritis in small animals, and for prophylaxis and treatment of respiratory infections caused by *E. coli, P. multocida,* and *H. paragallinarum* in poultry. Potentiated sulfas are used extensively in equine medicine to treat respiratory, genitourinary, skin, and gastrointestinal infections, as well as applications for treatment of pneumonia and enteritis in cattle and swine.

Sulfonamides are broad-spectrum bacteriostatic antimicrobials derived from sulfanilamide. Examples are sulfamethoxazole, sulfisoxazole, sulfachlorpyridazine, sulfamethazine, sulfadiazine, and sulfaquinoxaline. As noted, they interfere with folic acid synthesis. Widespread resistance has limited recent use of these drugs, and clinical applications include treatment of nocardiosis, urinary tract infections, and infectious coryza.

The tetracycline group comprises the bacteriostatic antibiotics oxytetracycline, chlortetracycline, tetracycline, minocycline, and doxycycline, produced by various *Streptomyces* spp. These drugs inhibit bacterial protein synthesis by preventing peptide bond formation. The binding site is on the 30S ribosomal subunit, where the drugs interfere with binding of tRNA to the ribosome. Tetracyclines have broad-spectrum activity against gram-positive and gram-negative aerobes, anaerobes, mycoplasmas, chlamydiae, and rickettsiae. They are used widely in food animal and small animal medicine. They are also primarily indicated for treatment of tick-borne infections, chlamydiosis, mycoplasmosis, and bordetellosis.

Mechanisms of Resistance

Antimicrobial resistance limits use of many of these agents. *Constitutive* resistance is nonacquired and inherent, and exemplified by streptomycetes that have genes responsible for resistance to their own antibiotics. Examples of intrinsic resistance include gram-negative bacteria whose outer membranes are permeability barriers, bacteria that lack antimicrobial transport systems, and bacteria that lack the antimicrobial's target site.

Acquired resistance can arise from chromosomal mutations or through acquisition of genetic elements. A single random mutation can impart resistance, and rapid multiplication leads to predominance of organisms that survive in the presence of antibiotic. Combination therapy decreases the chance that such organisms will become dominant in the population.

Bacteria can acquire exogenous resistance genes via transformation, transduction, conjugation, and transposition. *Transformation* occurs when DNA released from one bacterial cell is acquired directly from the environment by another organism, with insertion into the new genome by recombination. An example is resistance of some strains of *Streptococcus pneumoniae* to penicillin because of production of altered penicillin-binding proteins.

In *transduction,* a bacteriophage transfers resistance genes among bacteria. Transfer of penicillinase genes to *S. aureus* best exemplifies this mechanism.

Conjugation involves DNA transfer following cell-to-cell contact via sex pili. This process may result in the exchange of chromosomal or plasmid-borne resistance genes. The latter commonly contain genes for resistance to multiple unrelated antimicrobials.

Transposons also play a role in transfer of resistance genes. These DNA elements insert themselves into bacterial DNA independently of recombination because they do not require homologous DNA in the recipient strand. Transposons can also move from plasmid to plasmid, which may explain in part the progressive development of multiple antimicrobial resistance phenotypes.

Genes (usually plasmid-borne) encode enzymes that inactivate aminoglycosides. Natural resistance to the aminocyclitol spectinomycin is common especially among Enterobacteriaceae, and chromosomal mutations typically arise within a few days of initiation of antimicrobial therapy. Resistance to β-lactam antibiotics is mainly through the production of specific β-lactamases, enzymes that destroy the β-lactam ring. Genes for enzymes are often acquired by transfer of plasmids, and resistance is widespread among gram-negative bacteria. Bacterial penicillin-binding proteins may also be altered as a result of chromosomal mutations.

Phenicol resistance is most commonly plasmid mediated and results from drug inactivation by chloramphenicol aceytltransferase. Florfenicol is not subject to this resistance mechanism, and resistance to other phenicols may be by selective drug efflux pumps and ribosomal mutations.

A single-step chromosomal mutation is the most common mechanism of resistance to fluoroquinolones. This mutation leads to a change in the affinity with which the drug binds to the target enzyme, DNA gyrase. High-level resistance may occur uncommonly through a multiple-step mutation process, resulting in both a change in binding affinity and a decrease in drug penetration into the bacterial cell.

Resistance among the lincosamides occurs primarily in gram-positive bacteria and is usually associated with cross-resistance to macrolides and streptogramin type B antimicrobials (macrolide-lincomycin-streptogramin [MLS$_B$] phenotype). Both chromosomal and plasmid-mediated resistance is seen. The former develops in a stepwise manner, whereas in the latter, methylation of the adenine residue in the 23S rRNA of the 50S ribosome inhibits drug binding to the target site.

Chromosomal mutation to high-level macrolide resistance develops readily, although it is fairly unstable. Resistance may even develop during therapy. Plasmid-mediated resistance is also common and is a result of methylation of the drug's target site. Frequently cross-resistance among macrolides and lincosamides occurs.

Natural resistance to tiamulin appears to be the result of a penetration barrier rather than development of tiamulin-resistant ribosomes. Acquired resistance does not occur rapidly or in a single-step process and no cross-resistance to other antimicrobials has been shown.

Resistance to both diaminopyrimidine and sulfonamide drugs is mediated by plasmid-borne resistance and to a lesser degree by chromosomal mutations. Plasmids encode proteins that interfere with drug penetration, enzyme affinity, or high production of PABA. Resistance to either diaminopyrimidine or to one sulfonamide will impart resistance to all potentiated sulfa drugs.

Bacterial resistance to the tetracyclines can follow introduction of a variety of plasmid-borne genes. Most of these are inducible, suggesting that exposure to tetracyclines actually encourages development of resistant strains. The plasmid-borne genes encode a number of proteins that prevent the antibiotics from accumulating within the bacterium. Cross-resistance among tetracyclines is common.

ANTIMICROBIAL SUSCEPTIBILITY TESTING: PAST TO PRESENT

Historically, many infectious disease processes could be treated based on clinician experience. This empirical therapy is based on the expectation that the bacterium causing the disease is susceptible to the chosen antimicrobial agent and that it is not likely to acquire resistance during the course of therapy. Although some bacterial pathogens remain predictably susceptible to certain antimicrobial agents (e.g., susceptibility of *Arcanobacterium pyogenes* to penicillin), this is becoming more the exception than the rule. Resistance to essentially all antimicrobial agents approved for human and veterinary clinical use has been documented, and the proportion of strains resistant to multiple antimicrobial agents has increased significantly for many pathogens. This in combination with the escalating variety of available antimicrobials makes the selection of an appropriate agent an increasingly challenging task. This has made clinicians more dependent on data from in vitro antimicrobial susceptibility testing, and highlights the importance of the diagnostic laboratory in clinical practice.

However, with this said, it is not necessary to subject all bacteria recovered from a clinical specimen to antimicrobial susceptibility testing. Samples frequently are contaminated with normal flora, and the testing of these contaminants and bacteria with known susceptibility to certain agents (e.g., uniform susceptibility of β-hemolytic streptococci to penicillin) is unwarranted.

In vitro antimicrobial susceptibility testing, when performed properly, may be a reliable predictor of the efficacy of a specific antimicrobial agent against a specific pathogen in vivo. To optimize the benefits of in vitro antimicrobial susceptibility testing, care must be taken to perform the tests exactly as described in the standards reference manual. The results are then interpreted

qualitatively or quantitatively, and the drug is administered at the correct dose, at a dosing interval that maximizes its effectiveness and for the appropriate length of time. Even if these conditions are met, therapeutic failures may still occur as a result of incorrect or delayed diagnosis or lack of appropriate nonantimicrobial interventions (e.g., removal of foreign material) to prevent reinfection.

The use of data from in vitro antimicrobial susceptibility testing is only appropriate when performed according to standardized and validated methods. Constraints imposed to ensure reliability differ, but each method requires the use of quality control (QC) organisms and specific QC ranges for each drug, a standardized test medium, appropriate organism concentration, and suitable growth conditions (atmosphere, incubation temperature, and time). Most bacteria are tested under the same in vitro conditions, but some require longer incubation times, different incubation temperatures or atmospheric conditions, or a different growth medium. When conditions differ it may be necessary to validate specific QC organisms for those test conditions. For example, *C. jejuni* requires a different growth medium and different atmospheric conditions than those applied to *Escherichia coli*. Testing of *H. somni (Haemophilus somnus)* requires specific incubation conditions and QC organism.

It is not uncommon for veterinary laboratories to generate their own variation of the relatively simple in vitro antimicrobial susceptibility test. However, data generated under nonstandardized testing conditions should not be interpreted using criteria from standardized testing methods because the result will most likely be misleading. In the United States, the National Committee for Clinical Laboratory Standards (NCCLS) provides standardized reference methodology for testing of animal and human pathogens, specifying appropriate QC organisms and QC ranges for approved antimicrobials. Adherence to antimicrobial susceptibility testing standards and application of prudent use guidelines (e.g., those published by the American Veterinary Medical Association [AVMA]) and pharmacokinetic/pharmacodynamic principles increases the therapeutic success rate. Data generated by standardized susceptibility testing methods also serve surveillance purposes and can be applied to development of appropriate antimicrobial use policies.

Methods

NCCLS-approved methods for in vitro anti-microbial susceptibility testing include disk diffusion, agar dilution, broth macrodilution, and broth microdilution. Other methods producing comparable results include automated systems (Vitek and Microscan), dehydrated microtiter formats (Sensititre), and variations of the disk diffusion test (Etest and BioMic). Selection of testing method is based on the specific requirements of the test organism, cost and ease of use, and flexibility in light of the needs of the laboratory's clientele. If NCCLS recommended testing methods, including QC organisms and appropriate QC ranges, are used NCCLS interpretive criteria can be applied.

The Subcommittee on Veterinary Antimicrobial Susceptibility Testing (VAST) was established as a part of NCCLS to address testing issues unique to animal pathogens. Its main objective is to enable laboratories to assist clinicians in selecting antimicrobial therapy, through promotion of appropriate antimicrobial susceptibility testing methodologies, endorsing quality control data, establishing interpretive criteria, and educating users in routine laboratory testing and reporting. The VAST subcommittee developed consensus documents that serve as guidelines for drug sponsors in development of quality control information and interpretive criteria for veterinary-specific drugs and compendia of standardized testing procedures, quality control information, and interpretive criteria for bacterium-antimicrobial agent combinations specific for animal pathogens and veterinary-specific antimicrobial agents. Included are specific methods for susceptibility testing of *A. pleuropneumoniae*, *H. somni*, *Campylobacter* spp., *Staphylococcus hyicus*, *Enterococcus* spp., *S. pneumoniae*, and *Listeria* spp.

Diffusion Susceptibility Testing

The disk diffusion (Kirby-Bauer) test (Figure 3-1) is the most common testing method in the clinical veterinary setting because of its flexibility, simplicity, and relatively low cost. A plate of standardized growth medium (commonly Mueller-Hinton agar) is inoculated as a lawn with a pure culture of the test bacterium (derived from liquid or solid medium), using a standardized inoculum of approximately 1×10^8 colony-forming units (CFU)/ml. Within 15 minutes of inoculating the agar surface with the bacterial suspension, a paper disk impregnated with antimicrobial agent is applied to the surface of the agar. The antimicrobial agents immediately begin to diffuse out of the paper disk and into the surrounding medium, producing a concentration gradient around the disk. When the concentration of antimicrobial agent for the disk becomes too dilute to inhibit the bacterial growth, a zone of inhibition forms around the disk. The size of the zone is inversely proportional to the MIC of the test organism; the larger the zone of inhibition, the lower the concentration of drug required to inhibit the bacterial growth. Susceptibility or resistance is determined by comparing the diameter of the zone of inhibition with established ranges for each antimicrobial agent for the pathogen in question.

There are several factors that affect the outcome of this testing method. Medium composition, bacterial growth rate, and the chemical nature of the antimicrobial can affect results. For example, too dense an inoculum may produce artificially small zones of inhibition, resulting in a false perception of resistance. An inoculum that is too dilute or a slow bacterial growth rate may result in larger zones of inhibition and false conclusions of susceptibility. Differences in molecular size and charge (and resulting differences in rates of diffusion) may result in smaller zones of inhibition for some agents relative to others, but does not necessarily indicate lower activity in vivo.

Interpretive criteria for disk diffusion tests are based on data generated under standardized testing conditions and are best applied to testing done according to the same standards. Bacterial suspensions should be used within 15 minutes to prevent an increase in the number of organisms from cell division. Variation in agar thickness influences

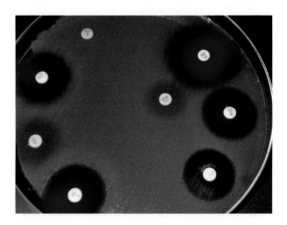

FIGURE 3-1 Kirby-Bauer plate, illustrating the disk diffusion antimicrobial susceptibility test method. (Courtesy Robert D. Walker.)

lateral diffusion of the drug and, as a consequence, zone size. Increased lateral diffusion occurs in agar that is thinner than the recommended 4 mm, with a corresponding increase in the size of the zone of inhibition. Downward diffusion in thicker agar matrices limits lateral diffusion and may result in a smaller zone of inhibition. Use of nonstandardized agar media may also affect the diffusion rate and or the activity of the drug.

Anaerobes and some other bacteria (e.g., *Campylobacter* spp. and *Helicobacter pylori*) cannot be tested by disk diffusion, and other methods (e.g., agar dilution and broth microdilution) have been adopted by NCCLS for testing these organisms. Another potential disadvantage is qualitative reporting of results, which limits rational use of lower therapeutic doses for infection caused by organisms that are acutely susceptible, or to increase the dose for treatment of infections by organisms that are less susceptible but in which clinical cure can still be achieved by higher therapeutic doses.

The epsilometer test (Etest, AB BIODISK) is a variation of disk diffusion that allows determination of an MIC. The antimicrobial diffuses from a concentration gradient on one side of a plastic strip (Figure 3-2) and the MIC is the value where the zone of inhibition intersects the interpretive scale printed on the strip. Etests are simple to perform and have been adapted for use with a variety of organisms, including slow growers, anaerobes, fastidious pathogens, and fungi. The use of a continuous antimicrobial drug gradient correlated with an MIC scale provides intermediate MIC increments between twofold serial dilution values. A potential disadvantage is reagent cost per isolate, especially when testing multiple antimicrobial agents. Some may consider it a drawback that, as a proprietary technology provided by a single company, it has not received formal NCCLS endorsement.

A computerized caliper-based system (BioMic) allows generation of quantitative results from zone sizes in standard disk diffusion assays. Zone size determined precisely by use of digital technology standardizes endpoints, speeds quantitative measurements, and eliminates the tedious task of individual antibiotic disk zone measurement. This method has not been validated for many of the bacterial pathogens encountered in a veterinary practice or diagnostic laboratory.

Dilution Susceptibility Testing Methods

Dilution susceptibility tests generate quantitative data based on twofold dilutions of antimicrobials (centering on 1 µg/ml [i.e., 0.25, 0.5, 1, 2, 4 µg/ml]) incorporated into agar (agar dilution) or broth (broth dilution). The MIC is expressed as the lowest concentration of antimicrobial agent that completely inhibits growth of the organism.

Broth dilution can be performed in tubes (usually 1 to 2 ml volume), in which case it is called broth macrodilution, but is usually performed in 96-well plates containing twofold dilutions of freshly made, frozen, or dehydrated antimicrobials (microdilution). *Broth microdilution* is the most widely used method, and it can be semiautomated for higher sample throughput. Microtiter plates usually contain several antimicrobial agents that are tested against a single isolate. Wells are inoculated with 5×10^4 CFU of the test organism, and plates are incubated under standard conditions for a standard time. The MIC is the lowest concentration of antimicrobial that completely inhibits bacterial growth, as detected by the unaided eye, and application of interpretive criteria enables the clinician to select the most suitable antimicrobial for treatment.

Microdilution provides more information than disk diffusion tests, but is more expensive to conduct. It also lacks the day-to-day flexibility of disk diffusion, agar dilution, and Etests, in terms of the need to change antimicrobial agents tested.

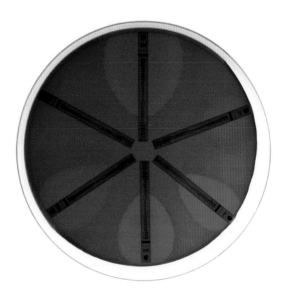

FIGURE 3-2 Use of the Etest method for antimicrobial susceptibility testing. (Courtesy Robert D. Walker.)

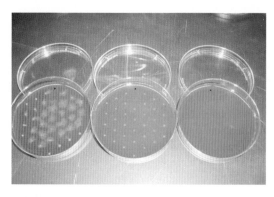

FIGURE 3-3 Antimicrobial susceptibility determined by agar dilution. (Courtesy Robert D. Walker.)

Agar dilution is considered the gold standard, and is currently the only standardized method for some fastidious organisms such as certain species of anaerobes or *Helicobacter* and *Campylobacter* (Figure 3-3). Agar plates containing 8 to 10 serial dilutions of an antimicrobial agent, as well as control plates without antimicrobial, are inoculated with the test organism by use of a commercial inoculum-replicating apparatus. Inoculated plates are allowed to dry and are then inverted and incubated. The MIC is the first dilution that inhibits growth, although as with other methods, some experience is needed to interpret occasional ambiguities in the endpoint. The main drawback to agar dilution is its labor intensity, and it is best suited to batch-processing large numbers of samples.

Quality Control of Dilution Testing

Inclusion of QC organisms ensures precision and accuracy in susceptibility test development and use. They provide sentinel data on performance of reagents, potency of antimicrobials being tested, possible deviations from the standard protocol, viability of organisms being tested, and interpretation of results. Choice of QC organisms is based on stable, defined, antimicrobial susceptibility phenotypes and MICs that fall near the midrange of values for susceptible clinical isolates. They must be suited to the incubation conditions used for testing clinical isolates, and should be recertified frequently. It may be necessary to use several different QC organisms when performing dilution susceptibility tests on multiple antimicrobial agents in the same plate to ensure that each drug is appropriately monitored for QC.

In all dilution-based methods, dilution ranges should encompass concentrations similar to those obtained in serum and tissue at recommended doses. It is also important that the dilution range for each agent span the susceptibility range of QC organisms, including one dilution below the lowest MIC of the QC organism and one greater than or equal to the highest MIC. This can be a challenge when designing microdilution plate formats; if the upper end of the QC range is much lower than the resistance breakpoint, the broad dilution range for a single drug may limit the number of drugs that can be incorporated into a single panel. Higher-density plate arrays may overcome this problem in the future.

Breakpoint formats have been used to reduce the cost associated with dilution testing. These usually consist of testing over a two- or three-dilution range, usually including one dilution below the susceptible breakpoint, the susceptible breakpoint itself, and sometimes one dilution above the susceptible breakpoint. This allows more compounds to be included in a microdilution tray. The usefulness may be limited by its reliance on NCCLS interpretive criteria and not allow for the needed quality control dilution ranges. In addition, results generated by breakpoint testing are essentially qualitative and thus similar (although more expensive) to those generated by disk diffusion.

Data Interpretation

Results generated in susceptibility testing are either in zones of inhibition (in mm), which are *qualitative* (allowing the test organism to be designated susceptible [S], resistant [R], or intermediate [I]), or MICs (in µg/ml, the lowest concentration of antimicrobial required to inhibit growth, as determined by the unaided eye), which are *quantitative*. MIC values by themselves may be of little value to the clinician, who needs to know if an isolate is susceptible or resistant in vivo to the antimicrobial agents tested. The susceptible or resistant breakpoints are the zone size or MIC value at which an organism is categorized as susceptible or resistant to a particular antimicrobial. Designation of susceptibility or resistance is based on (1) the population distributions of clinical isolates targeted by the specific antimicrobial agent, (2) achievable serum concentrations of the drug administered at approved doses in the target animal species and its pharmacodynamic properties, and (3) results of clinical efficacy trials. *Susceptible* implies that administration of the tested drug at the recommended dose will yield a sufficiently high serum or tissue concentration to inhibit the bacterium's growth at the site of infection. *Resistant* strains are those not inhibited by systemic concentrations of the agent usually achieved with normal dosage schedules. Strains with *intermediate* MIC values or zone sizes fall between the susceptible and resistant breakpoints and have traditionally represented a "buffer zone" to avoid misclassification of organisms because of the possibility of technical problems in the laboratory. However, this category may also include potentially susceptible organisms, in which antimicrobial agents can be administered at higher than normal doses or are concentrated at the site of infection (e.g., amoxicillin for treating cystitis).

Interpretive criteria have not been established for all antimicrobials and pathogens (e.g., *Haemophilus parasuis*). Increasing antimicrobial resistance often drives veterinary practitioners toward application of therapeutic agents for which the NCCLS testing standardization process has not been completed. When no guidance is available from the NCCLS, selection of antimicrobial therapy is based on clinical judgment and inference from activity of related drugs and similar pathogens. Tentative susceptibility and resistance breakpoints, based on those established for other organisms, should be used with caution.

SUGGESTED READINGS

National Committee for Clinical Laboratory Standards. Performance standards for antimicrobial disk and dilution susceptibility tests for bacteria isolated from animals; Approved standard, ed 2, NCCLS Document M31-A2, Wayne, Pa, 2002, National Committee for Clinical Laboratory Standards.

Prescott JF, Baggot JD, Walker RD, eds: *Antimicrobial therapy in veterinary medicine,* ed 3, Ames, Iowa, 2000, Iowa State University Press.

Two

Veterinary Bacteriology

Chapter 4

The Genus *Staphylococcus*

THE GENUS *STAPHYLOCOCCUS*

The gram-positive aerobic cocci are conveniently divided into two groups based on catalase production. The family Micrococcaceae (genera *Micrococcus*, *Staphylococcus*, and *Rothia* [*Stomatococcus*]) are catalase positive, whereas the genera *Streptococcus*, *Enterococcus*, *Eremococcus*, *Gemella*, *Globicatella*, *Helcococcus*, and *Vagococcus* are catalase negative.

Staphylococci are the most commonly isolated Micrococcaceae from veterinary clinical specimens. They occur in pairs, in grapelike clusters, or singly, and colonies are generally white to off-white, with smooth surfaces and butyrous consistency; many strains of *Staphylococcus aureus* have a golden pigment from which the organism derives its name. Members of the genus *Staphylococcus* can usually be differentiated from micrococci based on cell morphology (the latter form tetrads and cells tend to be larger than those of the staphylococci) and pigment production on solid media. *Rothia (Stomatococcus)* species are found infrequently in veterinary specimens, and a weak catalase reaction, ovoid cell shape, and sticky colonies are useful phenotypic features (Table 4-1). *Rothia* species are further distinguished from other members of the Micrococcaceae by the low G+C content of its DNA (30%-38%), the presence of teichoic acid in their cell walls, and the ability to tolerate high levels of NaCl (15% to saturated).

There are 32 recognized species of staphylococci (Table 4-2), 13 of which are indigenous to humans, with the remainder associated with various nonprimate animals. They are aerobic or facultatively anaerobic, and are capable of generating energy by respiratory and fermentative pathways. Staphylococci are nutritionally fastidious, with complex nitrogen requirements; most species require several amino acids, vitamins (thiamine and niacin), and uracil (to grow anaerobically). In complex, nutritionally complete media, the organism has a generation time of approximately 20 minutes.

The staphylococcal cell wall is composed primarily of peptidoglycan complexed with teichoic acid, and is resistant to lysozyme digestion by virtue of O-acetylation of muramic acid residues. In *S. aureus* the teichoic acid backbone is ribitol based, whereas in *Staphylococcus epidermidis* it is glycerol based. In other species, glycerol teichoic acids are more common than their ribitol counterparts.

Eleven capsular polysaccharide serotypes have been described for *S. aureus*, and the most common in clinical isolates are types 5 and 8. The main capsular components are *N*-acetylaminouronic acids and *N*-acetylfucosamine. The genes for capsule production are in a single chromosomal operon.

The genome of *S. aureus* is circular and consists of approximately 2.8 Mb. In addition to the normal complement of housekeeping genes, the chromosome contains many accessory genetic elements that are not necessary for growth under laboratory conditions. The genes and genomic organization are so strikingly similar to those of *Bacillus subtilis* that some have referred to *S. aureus* as a morphologically degenerate *Bacillus* sp.

Staphylococci are also equipped with copious plasmids, ranging in size up to approximately 50 kb pairs. Most of the smaller plasmids encode resistance to one or more antibiotics, and the majority of large plasmids encode resistance to penicillin or heavy metals; a few have conjugative functions by which they can mobilize themselves and other plasmids. Dogma holds that plasmids are exchanged among staphylococci, streptococci, and bacilli, accounting for the presence of the same or similar plasmids in each genus.

TABLE **4-1** Differentiation of the Micrococcaceae

	Micrococcus	*Staphylococcus*	*Rothia (Stomatococcus)*
Catalase	Positive	Positive	Weak positive
Oxidase	Positive	Negative	Negative
Sticky colonies	Negative	Negative	Positive

TABLE **4-2** Species of *Staphylococcus* Important in Veterinary Medicine

Staphylococcus Species	Veterinary Importance
S. aureus	Wound infections in all animals; mastitis, skin infections; joint infections, especially in chickens; diarrhea in pet birds; vaginal infections in dogs and horses
S. aureus ssp. *anaerobius*	Isolated occasionally from ovine caseous lymphadenitis
S. epidermidis	Opportunistic pathogen; bovine mastitis, skin abscesses in other animals
S. warneri	Septicemia in lovebirds
S. saprophyticus	Possible opportunist in urinary tract infections
S. kloosii	Normal skin and mucous membrane flora in squirrels and opossums
S. intermedius	Skin and ear infections in dogs, occasional bovine mastitis; isolated occasionally from birds and horses
S. hyicus	Skin infections, arthritis in pigs; skin, milk of cattle; avian arthritis
S. chromogenes	Bovine milk, skin of pigs and cattle; normal skin and mucous membrane flora in cattle
S. sciuri	Normal skin and mucous membrane flora in squirrels
S. lentus	Normal skin and mucous membrane flora in sheep and goats
S. gallinarum	Normal skin and mucous membrane flora in turkeys
S. caprae	Normal skin and mucous membrane flora in goats
S. equorum, arlettae	Normal skin and mucous membrane flora in horses
S. felis	Otitis externa, cystitis, abscesses and wounds in cats only
S. auricularis, S. capitis, S. carnosus, S. caseolyticus, S. cohnii, S. haemolyticus, S. hominis, S. lugdenensis, S. muscae, S. pasteuri, S. piscifermentans, S. saccharolyticus, S. schlieferi, S. simulans, S. vitulus, S. xylosus	None known

Staphylococcal bacteriophages were among the first demonstrated, and this has led to the establishment of a bacteriophage typing method for epidemiologic studies. Most pathogenic strains belong to phage groups II and III, but all are capable of causing disease.

Phage typing can be complicated by the fact that virtually all strains of *S. aureus* are lysogenized by one or more temperate bacteriophages. Phage insertion can alter the phenotype of a strain by introduction of genes and by integration at specific attachment sites within chromosomal genes; thus both negative conversion (inactivation of genes, such as those for lipase and β-toxin) and positive conversion (introduction of genes such as those for enterotoxin A and staphylokinase) are common. Transduction to penicillin resistance was reported more than 40 years ago. Most staphylococcal bacteriophages are now known to be capable of transferring approximately 40 kb of DNA.

Diseases and Pathogenesis

Staphylococci may be transient contaminants, short-term replicating residents, or long-term colonizers of the skin of mammals. Most that cause infection do so when the skin or mucous membranes are compromised in some way. Infections by S. *aureus* often begin at some breach in the epithelial barrier, whether keratinized, mucosal, or conjunctival, and establishment of infection is facilitated by foreign bodies, such as catheters, sutures, or even debris.

Virulence of staphylococci for domestic animals is almost always multifactorial, but interaction with animal hosts usually includes a few common steps. They produce *microbial surface components recognizing adhesive matrix molecules* (MSCRAMMs), which comprise the main adhesins of the organism and include collagen-binding protein, fibronectin-binding proteins, fibrinogen-binding protein, elastin-binding protein, clumping factor, and the matrix adhesin factor. As many as 12 other surface proteins may contain membrane anchor domains and potentially qualify as MSCRAMMs. Roles in virulence have been postulated but not confirmed for infections of domestic animals.

Staphylococci are killed by neutrophils, so many of their virulence attributes are focused upon avoiding phagocytosis or intracellular killing. This is mediated in large part by production of capsules and protein A. Capsules, produced in

12 immunotypes, are antiphagocytic and those of type 1 are associated with enhanced virulence. Those strains not producing a type 1 *macro*capsule may produce a polysaccharide *micro*capsule (for example, strains from mastitis); nonencapsulated strains are substantially more susceptible to phagocytosis and, in bovine mastitis and other in vivo models, less virulent. Protein A, which is found on the surface of the vast majority of strains of *S. aureus,* binds immunoglobulins by their Fc portion, limiting the degree of opsonization for phagocytosis. Mutants have reduced virulence in some in vivo systems. In a similar vein, teichoic acids and peptidoglycan fragments may serve as decomplementation antigens, exhausting in free solution the supply of complement components that would ordinarily be available for bacterial surface deposition (and thus opsonization). There are clearly two sides to this bacterial approach in host interaction: peptidoglycan interaction with host factors leads to complement activation (by classical or alternate pathways) and neutrophil chemotaxis.

Coagulase activates thrombin, with subsequent conversion of fibrinogen to fibrin. Some staphylococci produce coagulase (S. *aureus, Staphylococcus intermedius, Staphylococcus schlieferi* ssp. *coagulans,* and *Staphylococcus delphini*), while most do not; coagulase production by *Staphylococcus hyicus* is variable. The dogma that coagulase production distinguished pathogenic from nonpathogenic species held until coagulase-negative staphylococci (CoNS) were recognized as a major cause of wound infections and infections associated with foreign bodies including catheters, prosthetic heart valves, joint prostheses, and pacemaker electrodes; thus coagulase is no longer an exclusive indicator of pathogenicity. Coagulase mutants and parent strains are of equivalent virulence in various animal models of infection; nonetheless, some speculate that the enzyme participates in the infectious process by walling off the site of infection (limiting leukocyte infiltration and protecting the organisms against phagocytosis) or cloaking staphylococci in host proteins and preventing recognition as nonself.

Intracellular survival and spread are mediated in large part by production of toxins. Membrane-active toxins, some of which are enzymes, protect the organism against the host response and provide access to host-derived nutrients. Many of

TABLE **4-3**   Virulence Factors of *Staphylococcus aureus*

Virulence Factor	Effects
Capsule	Inhibits phagocytosis; promotes adherence
Peptidoglycan	Leukocyte chemoattractant; decomplementation
Teichoic acid	Fibronectin binding
Protein A	Immunoglobulin binding
Toxins (α, β, others)	Antiphagocytic; cytotoxic
Exfoliative toxins	Serine proteases; split cellular bridges in stratum granulosum
Enterotoxins	Superantigens; nauseogenic, diarrheagenic
Toxic shock syndrome toxin	Superantigen; endothelial damage
Coagulase	Converts fibrinogen to fibrin
Hyaluronidase	Hydrolyzes hyaluronic acid in connective tissue
Lipase	Hydrolyzes lipids
Nuclease	Hydrolyzes deoxyribonucleic acid (DNA)

the approximately 30 extracellular proteins pro-duced by *S. aureus* are plasmid encoded, provid-ing an armada of potential virulence factors that varies from strain to strain (Table 4-3). A single bacterial product is rarely of overriding impor-tance in development of disease. Alpha toxin sub-units bind to cell membranes, oligomerize, and form pores, leading to necrosis. Prostaglandins and other inflammatory mediators are released from some target cells, and macrophage function is compromised. Systemic effects of alpha toxin are most pronounced on cardiac and central nervous system tissue. Most bovine isolates of *S. aureus* produce β-toxin, a sphingomyelinase that lyses susceptible cells by enzymatic degradation of phospholipids in the outer leaflet of the membrane. Its role in pathogenesis is less clearly understood, but it augments staphylococcal growth in vivo. Hyaluronidase is a putative virulence attribute that may contribute to spread of the organism in the host.

Staphylococcus aureus causes suppurative infec-tions and septicemia (Figure 4-1) in all species, and a few examples are illustrative. Arthropod bite wounds in lambs and other animals may become infected, and these animals may also develop lameness and bacteremia. Abscesses form in kidney, liver, joints, and brain, and death is rapid. The organism may also be associated with ovine periorbital eczema.

Botryomycosis is an uncommon problem, char-acterized by chronic granulomagenesis involving the udder of various animals or the stump of the spermatic cord of geldings. The tissue becomes thickened and hardened, with multiple small abscesses containing actinomycosis-like granules.

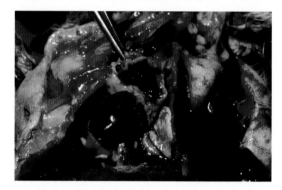

FIGURE 4-1   Staphylococcal septicemia in a chinchilla. (Courtesy Raymond E. Reed.)

Poultry are also affected, with arthritis and sep-ticemia, as well as bumblefoot (Figure 4-2). Birds develop lameness, foot swellings, and occasionally spondylitis. Staphylococcal urinary tract infections are not uncommon in humans and animals.

Staphylococcal mastitis occurs in goats, sows, and ewes; in cattle it is most often chronic and subclinical, but can be acute or even gangrenous, especially in postparturient cows (Figure 4-3). *Staphylococcus aureus* is the most common mam-mary pathogen in many dairying regions, and transmission by insufficiently sanitized milking machines is common. Mastitis is initiated when organisms colonize areas of the teat tip that have been damaged in some way. Binding to ductular and alveolar epithelial cells is an important step in pathogenesis, and the infection eventually progresses through the teat duct, teat and udder cisterns, and into the milk ducts. The outcome from this stage depends upon mainly unknown

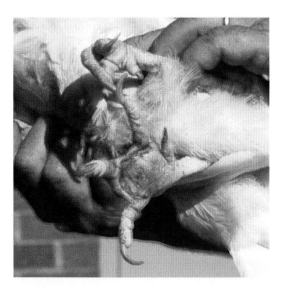

FIGURE 4-2 *Staphylococcus aureus* infection in a chicken (bumblefoot). (Courtesy Raymond E. Reed.)

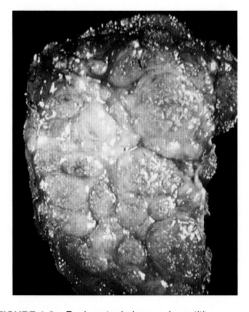

FIGURE 4-3 Bovine staphylococcal mastitis. (Courtesy J. Glenn Songer.)

factors that affected bacterial multiplication, the immune status with regard to alpha toxin, the vigor of the neutrophil response, the frequency of milking, and perhaps the ability of the organism to produce β-toxin and coagulase. Bovine peripheral blood neutrophils effectively kill *S. aureus* in vitro, whereas neutrophils from the mammary gland are less effective, perhaps because of the presence of fat globules in the milk. Casein may also

limit bactericidal activity of neutrophils by effects on the lactoperoxidase system. On the other hand, cows subclinically infected with *S. epidermidis* are less susceptible to infection by *Escherichia coli* or *Streptococcus agalactiae,* suggesting nonspecific stimulation of the mammary immune response.

In any case, the resulting disease varies from subclinical to gangrenous. Most cases are the former, and in toto the negative economic impacts are in lost milk production. Chronic infection results in induration of the udder, with passage of occasional clots and elevated cell counts in milk. When it occurs, peracute gangrenous mastitis is most common in first-calf heifers infected with *S. aureus,* and usually results in loss of one or more quarters. Alpha toxin plays an important role in development of gangrene (much the same as in "blue breast" of domestic rabbits); circulation is damaged by toxin effects on blood vessels, and ischemic coagulative necrosis develops in affected adjacent tissue. The case fatality rate is high, with death from toxemia in 24 to 48 hours. Experimental α- and β-toxoids are partially efficacious against *S. aureus* mastitis in goats, sheep, and rabbits.

Pyoderma affects dogs and horses, and may progress to subcutaneous abscesses and cellulitis. It is a common, generalized skin infection of dogs, characterized by erythema, vesicle formation, pustules, yellowish exudates, yellow-brown crusts, and disappearance of the keratinized layer of the epidermis. These clinical features resemble those of staphylococcal scalded-skin syndrome (SSSS) in humans and exudative epidermitis (EE) in pigs. *Staphylococcus intermedius* is the predominant type of coagulase-positive staphylococci on normal canine skin, and is a causative agent of pyoderma and otitis externa in dogs. *Staphylococcus schlieferi* ssp. *coagulans,* a coagulase-positive staphylococcus that is newly recognized in veterinary medicine, is another cause of canine pyoderma. This organism is not isolated from dogs with first-time pyoderma, but is frequently found in dogs with recurrent disease. It has also been isolated from dogs with otitis externa and from human wound infections. Hypersensitivity to staphylococcal peptidoglycan is mediated by IgE sensitization of skin mast cells. Degranulation in the presence of staphylococcal antigens yields a local inflammatory response, with erythema and pruritus. Clinical features resemble those of SSSS in humans and EE in pigs. Exfoliative toxins (exfoliative toxin A [ETA], from a chromosomal locus, and exfoliative toxin B [ETB], from a plasmid locus) are approximately 30 kD proteins that target epidermal cells in the granular layer and the upper spinous layer of the epidermis. They disrupt cellular attachment at the level of the stratum granulosum, with so-called Nikolsky's sign (lateral extension of a bulla with flanking pressure, suggesting detachment of the epidermis from the skin); in humans, this is SSSS. Exfoliative epidermitis has also been associated with infection by exfoliative toxin (Exhs)–producing strains of *S. hyicus*. Three toxin serotypes (ExhA, ExhB, and ExhC) are heat labile and are produced from plasmid-based or chromosomal genes. Like the ETs, the Exhs are metalloproteins which target epidermal cells in the skin's granular layer. Nikolsky's sign is observed in inoculated piglets and young chickens. It has been speculated that *S. intermedius* also produces an exfoliative toxin that functions as a virulence factor in the pathogenesis of canine pyoderma.

Exudative epidermitis (greasy pig disease) is characterized by excess sebaceous secretion and exfoliation in young pigs. Loss of the various functions of the skin predisposes to other infections; the mortality rate may be as high as 90% in some herds, but affected animals survive in most herds. Epidermitis can be produced by subcutaneous inoculation with the organism or its exfoliative toxin.

Staphylococcal toxic shock syndrome occurs in humans, but is of unknown importance in domestic animals. Horses may develop pulmonary infections with strains similar to those from humans, manifesting shock, vasculitis, and fever that is not responsive to nonsteroidal antiinflammatory drugs. Isolates may be susceptible in vitro to β-lactam antimicrobials, but aggressive, long-term treatment with trimethoprim-sulfamethoxazole and gentamicin may be indicated.

Toxic shock syndrome toxin (TSST-1) is a 22 kD protein that is absorbed into circulation from a focus of production. Augmented by endotoxin, TSST-1 produces multisystemic effects, including disseminated intravascular coagulation, not infrequently resulting in death. TSST-1 is a member of the superfamily of toxins, including also staphylococcal enterotoxin, that bind to major histocompatibility complex class II antigens on host cells and induce immoderate production of lymphokines and tumor necrosis factor, with extensive tissue damage and shock.

Enterotoxins have immunomodulatory effects similar to those of TSST-1. Six heat-stable, structurally similar but antigenically different types of enterotoxins (A, B, C_1, C_2, D, and E) may be produced by *S. aureus*. They are formed during staphylococcal multiplication in foods, and cause nausea, projectile vomiting, and explosive diarrhea in humans. Studies of enterotoxin action have been limited by the extraordinary resistance of most animal species to their gastrointestinal effects. Enterotoxins are perhaps more accurately referred to as neurotoxins because toxic effects on nerve centers in the stomach and intestine, relayed to the vomit center in the brain, are the basis for the vomitory effect. They may also downregulate humoral and cell-mediated immune responses in staphylococcal infections, perhaps explaining the lack of immune response in severe infections. We understand little of the role, if any, of these toxins in animal infections.

The expression of extracellular proteins is largely under the influence of a master genetic circuit called *agr* (accessory gene regulator). This signaling arm of the operon (AgrBDCA) is activated by a quorum sensing mechanism that depends on the accumulation of an activating octomeric peptide (processed from the AgrD precursor by AgrB).

Epidemiology

The broad distribution of staphylococci as normal flora of domestic animals is perhaps the most important epidemiologic factor in staphylococcal disease. Ready availability of virulent organisms, combined with factors related to host resistance and health management, encourage the development of most infections. Opportunities for occurrence of staphylococcal mastitis are provided by the widespread use of the milking machine, although hand-milked, suckled, and dry cows are also affected. Dogs are predisposed to pyoderma by underlying conditions such as immunodeficiency, preexisting dermatosis, and allergy.

The epidemiology of porcine exudative epidermitis may involve vaginal colonization of sows and gilts as the source for infection of neonates. Introduction of infected piglets, including by cross-fostering, may spread the disease between and within herds. Chickens and turkeys are predisposed to staphylococcal infections by concurrent viral infections, husbandry deficits, and other factors that may compromise resistance.

TABLE **4-4** Differentiation of Animal Pathogenic Staphylococci

Characteristic	S. aureus	S. intermedius	S. hyicus*	S. saprophyticus	S. felis
Coagulase	Pos (4 hr)	Pos (24 hr)	Var	Neg	Neg
β-hemolysis	Pos	Pos	Neg	Neg	Pos
Maltose	A	(A)	Neg	A	Neg
Mannose					A
Mannitol	A	Var	Neg	Var	(A)
TNase	Pos	Neg	Pos	Neg	
Voges-Proskauer	Pos	Neg	Neg		Neg
Hyaluronidase	Pos	Neg	Pos		

* *Staphylococcus hyicus* suspects should be examined on thermonuclease (TNase) agar.
A, Acid produced; *(A)*, delayed acid production; *Neg*, negative; *Pos*, positive; *Var*, variable.

Diagnosis

Primary culture for staphylococci is best accomplished on bovine blood agar, although selective media (e.g., mannitol salt agar, Staph 110 agar) are available. An enzyme immunoassay for detection of *S. aureus* has been developed, but comparative study has revealed that microbiologic culture of a single milk sample remains the most effective means for diagnosis of staphylococcal mastitis. Colonies are generally white to off-white with shiny to smooth surfaces and butyrous (butter-like) consistency. *Staphylococcus aureus* may have a golden pigment. Microscopic examination of isolated colonies will reveal gram-positive cocci in singles, pairs, or grapelike clusters. Coagulase testing and determination of hemolytic pattern are important initial tests, and isolates can usually be identified based on tests in Table 4-4. Rapid commercial methods are available for identification of most of the staphylococci.

Control and Prevention

Repeated exposure to *S. aureus* and *S. epidermidis* leads to a high prevalence of antibodies to various somatic and soluble staphylococcal components, although prior infection fails to elicit immunity to reinfection. However, only in the cases of α-toxin in mastitis and toxic shock syndrome toxin in human disease have antibodies proven to be an important factor in immunity. The capsule is a prime vaccine target, as anticapsular antibodies are prophagocytic, and MSCRAMM antigens are also under evaluation.

More than 95% of human patients with *S. aureus* infections worldwide do not respond to first-line antibiotics such as penicillin and ampicillin, and the picture is much the same for infections of domestic animals. About 30% are methicillin resistant, and vancomycin is the most effective treatment for multiply resistant strains. The emergence of vancomycin resistance has excited interest in antibiotic discovery and vaccine development.

Control of staphylococcal mastitis is based mainly on prevention. A typical program would include pre- and postmilking teat dipping, immediate treatment of clinical cases, culling of chronically infected cows, and dry cow therapy. Other aspects of milking hygiene, including routine disinfection of milking machines, are equally important.

SUGGESTED READINGS

Berg JN, Wendell DE, Vogelweid C, Fales, WH: 1984. Identification of the major coagulase-positive *Staphylococcus* sp. of dogs as *Staphylococcus intermedius, Am J Vet Res* 45:1307-1309, 1984.

Cole JR: *Micrococcus* and *Staphylococcus.* In Carter GR, Cole JR, eds: *Diagnostic procedures in veterinary bacteriology and mycology,* ed 5, San Diego, 1990, Academic Press.

Hesselbarth J, Flachsbarth MF, Amtberg G: Studies on the production of an exfoliative toxin by *Staphylococcus intermedius, J Vet Med B* 41:411-416, 1994.

Higgins R: Isolation of *Staphylococcus felis* from cases of external otitis in cats, *Can Vet J* 32:312-313, 1991.

Iandolo JJ: Genetic analysis of extracellular toxins of *Staphylococcus aureus, Ann Rev Microbiol* 43:375-402, 1989.

Iandolo JJ, Bannantine JP, Stewart GC: Genetic and physical map of the chromosome of *Staphylococcus aureus.* In Crosley KB, Archer GL, eds: *The staphylococci in human disease,* New York, 1997, Churchill Livingstone.

Kloos WE: The genus *Staphylococcus, Annu Rev Microbiol* 34:559-592, 1980.

Leung DYM, Huber BT, Schlievert PM: Historical perspectives of superantigens and their biological activities. In Leung DYM, Huber BT, Schlievert PM, eds: *Superantigens: molecular biology, immunology, and relevance to human disease,* New York, 1997, Marcel Dekker.

Novick RP: Genetic systems in staphylococci, *Meth Enzymol (Bacterial Genetics)* 204:587-636, 1991.

Watts JL, Yancey RJ: Identification of veterinary pathogens by use of commercial identification systems and new trends in antimicrobial susceptibility testing of veterinary pathogen, *Clin Microbiol Rev* 7:346-356, 1994.

Chapter 5

The Genera *Streptococcus* and *Enterococcus*

THE GENUS STREPTOCOCCUS

Streptococci are gram-positive, facultatively anaerobic, catalase negative, non–spore-forming, nonmotile spherical bacteria. Cell division in a single plane leads to formation of chains. Their nutritional requirements are complex and variable, reflecting adaptation as commensals or parasites of a wide variety of vertebrates. For the first third of the twentieth century, streptococci were differentiated only based on hemolysis, fermentation of carbohydrates, and tolerance of various chemicals. In the early 1930s, Rebecca Lancefield developed a grouping scheme based upon species-specific carbohydrate cell wall antigens, with groups designated A through H and K through V. Animal pathogenic streptococci are in groups A, B, C, D, E, G, L, and V, although some (*Streptococcus uberis*, *Streptococcus parauberis*, and *Streptococcus pneumoniae*) are not groupable. During the past decade, streptococci have been reclassified by 16S rDNA sequencing, but can be identified in the clinical laboratory by examination of hemolytic properties, biochemical activities, and characterization of carbohydrate and protein antigens. Accurate identification of β-hemolytic streptococci cannot be achieved by Lancefield grouping alone; except for the *Streptococcus bovis* group and *Streptococcus suis*, Lancefield grouping is of little value in identification of the non–β-hemolytic streptococci.

Diseases and Pathogenesis

Streptococcus pyogenes (group A) is a paradigmatic extracellular gram-positive pathogen causing pharyngitis, impetigo, rheumatic fever, and acute glomerulonephritis in humans; it is a rare cause of bovine mastitis, often contracted from carriers among the milkers. Invasive streptococcal diseases (the so-called flesh-eating bacteria) and rheumatic fever in humans have become prominent over the decade of the 1990s.

Humans are the major reservoir hosts for group A streptococci. It is worth noting that although pediatricians frequently implicate companion animals as a source of infection for children, the evidence supports the opposite conclusion: pets are more likely to become culture positive by contact with infected children.

Streptococcal virulence is based in large part on antiphagocytic surface components, including the M protein. Its hypervariable N-terminal portion gives rise to different types, which may be determined by serologic methods or, more accurately, by *emm* typing, based upon the sequence of the hypervariable region of *emm*. The *emm* superfamily includes antiphagocytic molecules and immunoglobulin-binding proteins. Pyrogenic exotoxin A is one of nine superantigens that contribute to the pathogenesis of streptococcal toxic shock syndrome by stimulating cytokine production by T cells, with subsequent endothelial cell damage, hypotensive shock, and ischemia-based necrosis.

Enzymes that dissolve fibrin clots and other somatic and soluble toxic molecules also participate. Binding of plasma components may enable the organisms to evade host immune detection or to avoid the opsonophagocytic effects of complement. Factor H and fibrinogen binding by M protein are important virulence attributes, as is degradation of complement component C5a by the C5a peptidase. Mimicry of host molecules not only allows the organism to escape detection as foreign but may prompt the autoimmune responses associated with rheumatic fever; proteins in some strains are involved in immune-mediated acute glomerulonephritis, which sometimes follows streptococcal infection in humans. Production of capsular hyaluronic acid may be coregulated, with M protein and C5a peptidase, by *virR*. Loss of capsule is associated with reduction in virulence in the range of 100-fold.

Streptolysin O (SLO), produced by streptococci of groups A, C, and G, is a cholesterol-binding toxin with potent membrane-damaging effects. Individual SLO molecules associate with cholesterol in cell membranes and then oligomerize, inserting into the membrane and forming a hydrophilic channel. Toxicity is expressed against neutrophils, platelets, myocardial cells, and membrane-enclosed subcellular components.

Streptococcus agalactiae, the only member of group B, is best known as a cause of chronic bovine mastitis. In cattle, its nearly exclusive localization to the mammary gland facilitates eradication of the organism from affected herds. The organism also causes mastitis in sheep, goats, and camels, and has been associated with folliculitis in elephants, neonatal death, endocarditis, and vaginal and skin infections in dogs, and kidney and uterine infections in cats. *Streptococcus agalactiae* also causes rare infections in horses (genital tract) and monkeys.

In humans it is found in the vagina and in the oropharynx, and epidemiologic evidence suggests that this may be perpetuated by mixing and matching of mucous membranes. Early or late-onset meningeal sepsis in human neonates follows infection of the fetus in the birth canal, and *S. agalactiae* is in fact the most common cause of this type of human infection. Animal-to-human transmission probably does not occur, and substantial differences in phenotype suggest that bacteria from each host are distinct. Most isolates of *S. agalactiae* can be typed based on polysaccharide capsular antigens (types Ia, Ib Ic, II, and III).

Most study of virulence of S. *agalactiae* has focused upon human isolates and infections, and knowledge of the role of specific virulence factors in bovine mastitis is largely derivative. Human strains produce sufficient capsular polysaccharide to inhibit complement activation and C3 deposition, but bovine strains usually do not. Capsular polysaccharide is antiphagocytic, and type-specific antibody is protective in both the mouse model and in human infants. Anti–group B antibodies are opsonic in concert with complement.

Colonization of the mammary gland by *S. agalactiae* is facilitated by adhesion to gland sinus epithelium. Progressive inflammation and fibrosis result from multiplication on the teat epithelium and in duct sinuses. Isolation of the organism from supramammary lymph nodes early in the infection is evidence of transient invasiveness, but a strong neutrophil response clears these organisms rapidly. Contents of dead neutrophils accentuate the inflammatory process and formation of fibrin plugs in milk ducts may lead to loss of milk-producing capacity. The host response alone is not sufficient to clear the infection, so without treatment it often becomes chronic.

Strains of *S. agalactiae* augment the hemolytic activity of staphylococcal β-toxin via the action of the CAMP factor (Figure 5-1), a ceramide-binding protein. CAMP factor is lethal for laboratory rodents, and mutants lacking it have a 50-fold increased LD_{50}. The question of CAMP factor toxicity for the mammary gland remains open. Neuraminidase and hemolysin may also play a role in development of mastitis.

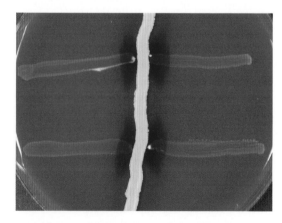

FIGURE 5-1 Augmentation of staphylococcal β-hemolysis by *Streptococcus agalactiae* CAMP protein (CAMP reaction). (Courtesy Karen W. Post.)

Streptococcus canis (group G) comprises large-colony β-hemolytic organisms that produce β-galactosidase but not hyaluronidase (by which they are distinguished from *Streptococcus dysgalactiae*) and cause genital, skin, and wound infections in dogs. Dogs and cats can be genital or oral carriers of *S. canis,* but the main source of the organism, especially in dogs, is the anal mucosa. Infections are opportunistic and consist of abscesses, mastitis, prostatitis, lymphadenitis, pyometra, pyoderma, and "puppy strangles." *Streptococcus canis* is commonly isolated from feline abscesses, metritis, mastitis, and kitten septicemia. Although *Streptococcus zooepidemicus* ssp. *equi* infection is more common, *S. canis* lymphadenitis has been reported in rats. Group G streptococci from humans and domestic animals are genetically distinct, but *S. canis* has nonetheless been associated with caretaker-associated bovine mastitis.

Streptococcal toxic shock, with or without necrotizing fasciitis, is apparently emerging as a disease problem in dogs. Organisms isolated from these cases are group G, and although most are *S. canis,* strains characteristic of those from human disease have also been found. The most common primary source of infection in toxic shock cases is the lung, with dogs experiencing acute or peracute suppurative bronchopneumonia. The case history sometimes includes failed attempts to treat with enrofloxacin; corticosteroids or nonsteroidal anti-inflammatory drugs also have been associated with infection. Septicemia and toxic shock are uniformly fatal, whereas most dogs with necrotizing fasciitis alone survive with radical treatment. Most isolates have the genetic machinery for production of SLO and M protein, but lack genes with homology to other virulence genes found in *S. pyogenes.*

Neonatal kittens are infected via the umbilicus, with the organisms originating from vaginal or oral colonization of the queen. *Streptococcus canis* is distributed hematogenously, and disseminated microabscesses result, with death following in the first week of life. This form of the disease occurs only in litters from young queens. Young cats can also be infected when maternal antibody titers decrease below effective levels, at 2 to 4 months of age. Organisms invading from the oral cavity cause purulent lymphadenitis involving the mandibular lymph nodes.

Little is known of the virulence factors of *S. canis.* Hyaluronidase and streptokinase are not involved, but large amounts of SLO and M protein

are produced by low-passage clinical isolates. Antiserum against M protein is opsonic.

The taxonomy of *S. dysgalactiae* has changed substantially in recent years. The genetic similarity of the former *Streptococcus equisimilis* to *S. dysgalactiae,* as well as strains in groups G and L, led to their placement in *S. dysgalactiae,* with subspecies *dysgalactiae* and *equisimilis.* Strains identified as *Streptococcus dysgalactiae* ssp. *equisimilis* are mainly of group C, with some of group G (Figure 5-2); a not-insignificant number have group A and L antigens. *Streptococcus dysgalactiae* ssp. *dysgalactiae* has not been isolated from humans, despite the fact that it produces M-like proteins and other virulence attributes similar to those of *S. pyogenes.* Subspecies *equisimilis* also has such virulence factors, including *emm* homologs. When *S. dysgalactiae* ssp. *equisimilis* had species status, it was often referred to as "the human C."

Subspecies *dysgalactiae* (Figure 5-3) infects the bovine mammary gland, originating in the mouth and vagina, and in skin lesions on the udder,

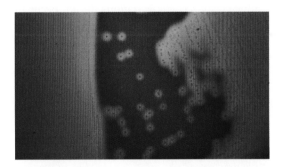

FIGURE 5-2 Growth of *Streptococcus dysgalactiae* ssp. *equisimilis* on blood agar. (Courtesy J. Glenn Songer.)

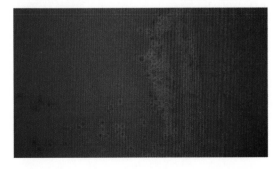

FIGURE 5-3 Growth of *Streptococcus dysgalactiae* ssp. *dysgalactiae* on blood agar. (Courtesy J. Glenn Songer.)

producing sporadic cases of acute bovine mastitis; initiation of infection requires only a very low infectious dose, and it often occurs in synergy with *Arcanobacterium pyogenes*. These organisms also are a cause of arthritis, septicemia, and meningitis in goats and lambs. Human group G strains resembling *S. dysgalactiae* can also cause mastitis in cattle. Little is known about the virulence of *S. dysgalactiae* ssp. *dysgalactiae,* although most strains produce fibronectin-binding protein, streptokinase, and hyaluronidase. The role of M proteins in virulence of *S. dysgalactiae* ssp. *equisimilis* is not known, although at least four M types are produced.

Other strains in *S. dysgalactiae* ssp. *dysgalactiae* cause abortion, dermatitis, and septicemia in cattle and dogs, and abortion and a strangleslike syndrome in horses. It is perhaps most common in piglets; organisms carried by the sow infect by way of wounds, the umbilicus, or tonsil and produce suppurative arthritis.

Streptococcus equi ssp. *equi* (group C) causes strangles, as well as genital and mastitic infections, in horses. It has also been associated with suppurative omphalophlebitis in foals (Figure 5-4). Antigenic and genetic variations do not occur in *S. equi* ssp. *equi,* whereas the more cosmopolitan *S. equi* ssp. *zooepidemicus* is genetically heterogeneous. Survival of *S. equi* ssp. *equi* outside the host is limited (perhaps as much as 2 months under optimum conditions), so its distribution follows that of equids.

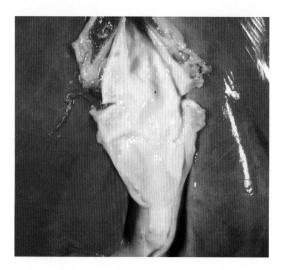

FIGURE 5-4 *Streptococcus equi* ssp. *equi*–associated suppurative omphalophlebitis in a foal. (Courtesy Lisa LaFranco-Scheuch.)

Partially immune animals (for example, those with residual maternal immunity or with a previous infection) may develop a catarrhal infection, with cough, fever, and mild nasal discharge. Lymph node abscessation is uncommon.

Strangles is a highly communicable infection of the upper respiratory tract and associated lymph nodes. The asymptomatic carrier state in horses is apparently quite rare, and the most important source of infection is a clinically affected horse shedding the organism in nasal discharges or from a draining abscess. Encapsulated abscesses, which later rupture to initiate shedding, may be a means of introducing the disease into a herd. The incubation period can be as short as 3 days or as long as 2 weeks. *Streptococcus equi* ssp. *equi* attaches to tonsillar crypt cells and adjacent lymphoid nodules. Within a few hours the organism translocates into the local lymphatics and cannot be detected on the mucosal surface. The influx of neutrophils is, in sum, inefficacious in phagocytosing and killing the organisms, so smears of lesion material reveal large numbers of streptococci in chains among degenerating neutrophils. Affected horses manifest fever, malaise, nasal discharge, cough, and swelling associated with the mandibular lymph node. Progressive lymph node abscessation causes pressure on the airway and respiratory difficulty, giving rise to the common name of the disease. Metastatic abscessation, with spread via circulation or the lymphatic route to lungs, abdomen, or brain, is not uncommon. The clinical course is usually short and uneventful, but myocarditis and purpura hemorrhagica can follow; immune complex formation can lead to acute leukocytoclastic vasculitis and glomerulonephritis.

Virulence factors of *S. equi* ssp. *equi* include a nonantigenic hyaluronic acid capsule, hyaluronidase, SLO, streptokinase, IgG Fc-receptor proteins, peptidoglycan, and the antiphagocytic M protein. Isolate-to-isolate variation in virulence is related, for the most part, to the amount of antiphagocytic M protein produced. M proteins project as fibrils from the cell wall surface, and are composed of a coiled central region flanked by a short, coiled sequence at the N-terminus and a highly conserved region of hydrophobic and charged amino acids at the C-terminus. Its antiphagocytic activity lies in its ability to bind fibrinogen and complement control factor H, masking bacterial C3b-binding sites and inhibiting C3 and C5 convertases. Antibodies against

N-terminal epitopes are opsonizing. *Streptococcus equi* ssp. *equi* M protein is uniform in size and antigenic properties, unlike those of *S. pyogenes* or *S. equi* ssp. *zooepidemicus*. In vitro passage results in diminished M protein production.

Isolates from cases of strangles produce mucoid colonies, indicative of encapsulation; virulence is reduced, but not abrogated, by loss of capsule. Peptidoglycan of *S. equi* ssp. *equi* activates complement by the alternate pathway, generating neutrophil chemotactic factors, and induces release of pyrogenic cytokines (such as interleukin [IL]-6). This accumulation of neutrophils at the site of infection and the febrile response contributes to the characteristic clinical signs of strangles.

Streptococcus equi ssp. *equi* also has Fc receptors on its surface, similar to protein A of *Staphylococcus aureus*, hypothetically allowing the organism to avoid opsonization by binding of the Fc portion of the antibody.

Streptokinase acts on the serine protease domain of equine plasminogen, forming plasmin, which in turn hydrolyses fibrin. Thus streptokinase may aid in dissemination of *S. equi* ssp. *equi* in tissue. SLO is produced, but its role in virulence of *S. equi* ssp. *equi* for horses has not been investigated.

Streptococcus equi ssp. *zooepidemicus* (group C) has a high degree of DNA sequence homology with *S. equi* ssp. *equi*. *Streptococcus equi.* ssp. *zooepidemicus* is a mucosal commensal, especially in the horse, but it is promiscuous in its selection of hosts, causing opportunistic respiratory, wound, and genital infections in most species. It is a frequent cause of mastitis in cattle and goats. Lambs infected with *S. equi* ssp. *zooepidemicus* can develop wound infections, pneumonia, and septicemia; puppies may be similarly affected. Chicken infections manifest as septicemia, and guinea pigs in rodent colonies develop epidemic lymphadenitis. Equine wound infections are quite common, as are joint ill, lymphatic abscesses approximating those caused by *S. equi* ssp. *equi*, and pneumonia in foals (Figure 5-5). *Streptococcus equi* ssp. *zooepidemicus* is the most common pathogen from the mare reproductive tract. Unlike *S. equi* ssp. *equi*, *S. equi* ssp. *zooepidemicus* is recovered from human infections, most of which follow consumption of contaminated dairy products.

Streptococcus equi ssp. *zooepidemicus* has the same virulence factors as *S. equi* ssp. *equi*, but

hyaluronic acid production is variable and most nondisease isolates are nonencapsulated. Hyaluronidase production by some strains has an uncertain role in virulence because it might be predicted to reduce virulence by removing the capsule. M proteins of *S. equi* ssp. *zooepidemicus* from horses are variable in molecular weight and antigenic composition.

Streptococcus pneumoniae (not groupable) is the cause of primary lobar pneumonia in primates, and remains the most important cause of community-acquired pneumonia in humans. Multidrug resistance is increasingly prevalent, and major effort has been focused on development of vaccines for humans. *Streptococcus pneumoniae* also causes pneumonia in rats, mice, guinea pigs, and calves, and is isolated rarely from cases of bovine mastitis. It has been associated with lower respiratory tract disease in young horses, which experience fever, bronchitis, and tracheitis.

A polysaccharide capsule provides resistance to phagocytosis, specifically through interference with complement binding and by mediating complement inactivation. Phagocytosis does occur, and this may explain the self-limiting nature of the naturally occurring disease in horses. Alveolar necrosis may be explained by production of pneumolysin, and neuraminidase may decrease the viscosity of mucus and expose receptors for bacterial attachment. Large numbers of *S. equi* ssp. *zooepidemicus*

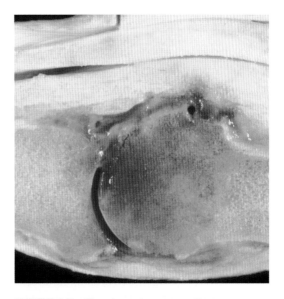

FIGURE 5-5 Chronic equine suppurative osteomyelitis and arthritis caused by *Streptococcus zooepidemicus*. (Courtesy Rob Fairley.)

sometimes accompany *S. pneumoniae* in tracheal aspirates, perhaps because IgA protease produced by the latter destroys anti–M protein antibodies against the former.

Streptococcus porcinus (groups E, P, U, and V) isolated from the genitourinary tract of human females typically agglutinate with commercially prepared group B antisera, making misidentification as *S. agalactiae* an issue in the human clinical laboratory. *Streptococcus porcinus* is also isolated from opportunistic infections of horses and cats, but is primarily associated with abscesses and lymph node infections in young pigs. Tonsillar carriage leads to transmission by nose-to-nose contact, as well as by contamination of drinking water and feces. The frequency of cervical lymphadenitis in swine in the United States has decreased in the face of routine antimicrobial use and modern methods of management. Experimental infection is accomplished by feeding, rather than injection, of infectious materials. Enlarged mandibular, parotid, and retropharyngeal lymph nodes rupture and drain, often into feed, leading to spread of infection. *Streptococcus porcinus* is encapsulated and produces a porcine plasminogen-specific streptokinase. An M-like protein may be required for virulence.

Streptococci from groups D, R, S, and T are of a single genetic type and have been assigned to the taxon *S. suis*. This species is an occasional cause of septicemia in birds, and has been isolated infrequently from ruminants and horses. However, it is most widely known as a cause of encephalitis, meningitis, arthritis, septicemia, abortion, and endocarditis in swine (Figures 5-6 and 5-7). The palatine tonsil carrier rate can approach 100%, and infection of piglets may occur at birth. Most carriers do not develop clinical disease, but they transmit *S. suis* by respiratory and oral routes to susceptible contacts. Typing has identified 35 antigenic carbohydrate types; group R, the most common strain, is type 2, and group S is type 1. Types 1 and 2 are associated with septicemia, meningitis, arthritis, bronchopneumonia, and other lesions typical of generalized septicemia. Human infection has been limited to type 2 strains, which cause mainly meningitis, occasionally septicemia without meningitis, and rarely endocarditis; most cases carry the suggestion of zoonotic disease. Agglutination with group D antisera likely represents cross-reactivity with type R antigens. Some strains are β-hemolytic on horse blood agar, but

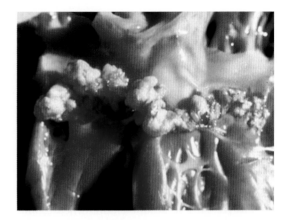

FIGURE 5-6 Porcine valvular endocarditis associated with *Streptococcus suis* infection. (Courtesy J. Glenn Songer.)

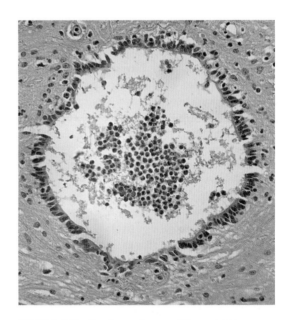

FIGURE 5-7 Porcine syringomyelitis caused by *Streptococcus suis* infection. (Courtesy M. Kevin Keel.)

all are α-hemolytic on sheep blood agar. As such, *S. suis* may be misidentified in human clinical laboratories, perhaps explaining the lack of cases in the United States.

Capsular polysaccharide is antiphagocytic, possibly through prevention of complement deposition. Nonencapsulated isolates are readily phagocytosed without opsonization. A 100-kD soluble protein is apparently necessary for full virulence. The events that culminate in *S. suis* bacteremia are often stress associated and originate in the tonsil. Subsequent invasion of regional lymphatics (e.g., the mandibular lymph node) may be followed by escape to the bloodstream. Sustained, high-grade bacteremia is the predecessor of meningoencephalitis. Organisms survive in mononuclear cells and are carried to the joints and meninges.

Streptococcus uberis and *S. parauberis* are phenotypically similar but genetically distinct mucosal and epithelial commensals of cattle; they become pathogens under poor hygienic conditions, causing as many as 20% of the cases of clinical bovine mastitis in North America. Environmental contamination and soiling of the udder are important predisposing factors. Neither organism has been isolated from human infections; isolates of *S. uberis* from humans are now identified as *Globicatella sanguinis*. This organism is isolated from human bacteremia, sepsis, endocarditis, and urinary tract infections, and little is known of its importance in domestic animals. Many strains of *S. uberis* produce a hyaluronic acid capsule but a role for capsule in virulence is equivocal. Virulence factors may also include hyaluronidase and a *uberis* factor analogous to the CAMP factor.

Streptococcus equinus (group D, a member of the *S. bovis* group) causes bovine mastitis, as well as septicemia and arthritis in pigeons. *Streptococcus phocae* appears to be related to group C streptococci and is a cause of secondary septicemia in seals; *Streptococcus didelphis* has been isolated from opossums. *Streptococcus iniae* (not groupable) has been isolated from skin abscesses of dolphins and is a common pathogen of fish; isolation from cases of bacteremia in fish handlers suggests zoonotic potential. *Streptococcus pluranimalium* has been isolated from bovine mastitis, and from the normal bovine vagina, cervix, and tonsils. It has also been found in canary lung lesions, but has not been isolated from humans.

The so-called nutritionally variant streptococci (NVS), recovered from corneal ulcers in horses, are recognized by their growth as satellites around colonies of staphylococci. These have been moved recently to the genus *Abiotrophia*.

Diagnosis

Diagnosis of streptococcal and enterococcal disease should include isolation and identification of the causative organisms (Table 5-1). Significant progress toward identification can be made by examination of colonial morphology and hemolytic pattern of isolates (Table 5-2). Cellular morphology, determined by microscopic examination of Gram-stained smears, and ability to produce catalase, are also essential parts of identification. The genera *Streptococcus* and *Enterococcus* are accompanied among the gram-positive, aerobic, catalase-negative cocci by newly recognized veterinary pathogens in the genera *Eremococcus, Gemella, Globicatella, Helcococcus,* and *Vagococcus* (Table 5-3), from which they must be differentiated. Other gram-positive cocci, such as *Lactococcus, Aerococcus, Rothia,* and *Leuconostoc,* may be encountered among the resident flora on the mucous membranes of animals and must be separated from the potential pathogens.

Immunity

Streptococcus agalactiae. Infections are not cleared by most cattle, despite the presence of agglutinating antibodies in milk. However, if antibodies preexist infection, especially antibodies specific for the group B polysaccharides, they may moderate the disease process. Success in dealing with the disease by improved hygiene, antimicrobial therapy, and culling of affected cows has augured against the initiation of definitive work on aspects of the host-parasite interaction.

Streptococcus equi ssp. *equi.* The antiphagocytic M protein is the major protective antigen of *S. equi* ssp. *equi.* Most horses recovering from strangles are immune to subsequent infection, and the remainder become immune if they experience a second infection. Protection is mediated by nasopharyngeal IgG and IgA, directed in large part against M protein and forming early in convalescence. Milk from recovered mares contains antibodies against M protein, and foals of immune mares are resistant to infection until weaning. Parenteral vaccines containing M protein give rise to serum opsonic antibodies but do not protect fully against natural exposure. Attenuated live vaccines that stimulate mucosal responses have been developed; an avirulent nonencapsulated strain has been used widely in North America as an intranasal vaccine. Antibodies to the M protein of *S. equi* ssp. *zooepidemicus* are not as effective as *S. equi* ssp. *equi* antibodies in clearing the infection from the nasopharynx.

TABLE **5-1** Identification of Streptococci

Streptococcus Species	Group	Hemolysis	6.5% NaCl	Fermentation of: Sorbitol	Trehalose	Other Tests
S. agalactiae	B	α, β, γ	–	–	+	Inulin neg, CAMP pos, esculin neg, hippurate hydrolyzed
S. canis	G	β	–	–	+	
S. didelphis		β	Neg	Pos	Pos	Catalase pos
S. dysgalactiae ssp. dysgalactiae	C	α	–	–	+	Inulin neg, CAMP neg, esculin neg, hippurate hydrolyzed
S. dysgalactiae ssp. equisimilis		β				
S. equi ssp. equi	C	β	–	–	–	Salicin pos
S. equi ssp. zooepidemicus	C	β	–	+	–	
S. equines	D	α	–	–	Var	
S. gallinaceus		α	ND	Neg	Pos	Mannitol pos, melibiose pos
S. iniae	None	β	Var	–	+	Esculin pos, mannitol pos, CAMP pos, starch hydrolyzed, Voges-Proskauer neg
S. ovis		α	Neg	Pos	Pos	Esculin pos, Voges-Proskauer neg, hippurate not hydrolyzed
S. phocae	C?	β	–	–	–	Salicin neg
S. pluranimalium		α	Var	(Neg)	Pos	Esculin pos, Voges-Proskauer neg, hippurate hydrolyzed
S. porcinus	E, P, U, V	β	+	+	+	Mannitol pos, Voges-Proskauer pos, pyrrolidony-larylamidase pos, CAMP pos, bile esculin neg
S. pneumoniae	None	α	–	–	+	Optochin sensitive
S. pyogenes*	A	β	–	–	+	Hippurate not hydrolyzed
S. suis	D, R, S, T	α	–	–	+	Voges-Proskauer neg, starch hydrolyzed; capsular serotyping
S. uberis	None	α, γ	–	+	+	Inulin pos, CAMP v, esculin pos, hippurate hydrolyzed

*Best identified by demonstration of the group A antigen on the cell.
ND, Not determined; *Neg*, negative; *(Neg)*, most negative; *Pos*, positive; *Var*, variable.

TABLE **5-2** Colonial Morphology of Streptococci of Veterinary Importance

β-Hemolytic Streptococci	
S. pyogenes	Three colony types: mucoid, matte, glossy
S. agalactiae	1-2 mm, entire, translucent, convex, moist
S. dysgalactiae ssp. dysgalactiae	1-2 mm, entire, translucent, convex, moist; may be α- to nonhemolytic
S. dysgalactiae ssp. equisimilis	Small, entire, translucent waxy to mucoid
S. equi ssp. equi	Small, watery; dry rapidly, leaving flat, glistening colony
S. equi ssp. zooepidemicus	Small, entire, translucent waxy to mucoid
S. canis	Small, matte
S. porcinus	Small, waxy, circular, entire
S. iniae	≤1 mm with opaque centers, translucent borders
S. phocae	Pinpoint to 1 mm
S. didelphis	Small, translucent, β-hemolytic
Non–β-Hemolytic Streptococci	
S. pneumoniae	Small, mucoid; some rough; may be domed
S. equinus	Small, entire, circular, smooth
S. suis	Small, entire, circular; may be very wet in appearance
S. uberis	1-3 mm, entire, translucent, convex, moist; dense centers

TABLE **5-3** Morphology of Cells and Colonies of *Eremococcus, Gemella, Globicatella, Helcococcus,* and *Vagococcus*

Organism	Cellular and Colonial Morphology
Eremococcus coleocola	Gram-positive cocci, some elongated; single, pairs, short chains; α-hemolytic on sheep blood agar, pinpoint, shiny, entire, circular, convex colonies after 24 hr
Gemella cuniculi	Gram-positive cocci; β-hemolytic, nonpigmented
Gemella palaticanis	Gram positive, ovoid; small pinpoint colonies on blood agar after 72 hr
Globicatella sanguinis	Gram positive, tend to form chains; α-hemolytic, may be satellitic; colonies resemble viridans streptococci
Globicatella sulfidifaciens	Gram-positive cocci; single, pairs, short chains; colonies dry, corroding, α-hemolytic with 2 days' incubation
Helcococcus ovis	Gram positive, resemble staphylococci; ovoid, single; usually nonhemolytic, grow slowly, resemble viridans streptococci
Vagococcus spp.	Gram positive, ovoid; single, pairs, chains; small (0.1-0.2 mm), smooth, α-hemolytic

Streptococcus canis. M protein–neutralizing antibodies develop following natural exposure to *S. canis,* resulting in decreased reproductive tract colonization rates in older cats.

Streptococcus suis. Inactivated vaccines have been largely disappointing in the field, although repeated, experimental vaccination with either live or formalin-killed *S. suis* gives rise to a strong protective response.

Streptococcus porcinus. Opsonic antibodies neutralizing the M protein–like antiphagocytic factor arise as a result of infection, and oral avirulent vaccines probably stimulate mucosal immunity.

Streptococcus pneumoniae. Anticapsular antibody is protective, but there is limited cross-protection among antibodies against the various capsular types.

Streptococcus uberis. Specific immunity is involved in clearance of *S. uberis* from the udder, although the antigens involved have not been characterized. After mammary infection, milk is opsonic for *S. uberis.*

THE GENUS ENTEROCOCCUS

Enterococci have emerged as pathogens of several domestic species, causing enteritis, septicemia, mastitis, respiratory disease, and urinary tract infections (Table 5-4). These organisms are of

TABLE **5-4** Enterococci as Pathogens of Domestic Animals

Enterococcus Species	Disease
E. avium	Septicemia in birds
E. durans	Septicemia in birds; neonatal diarrhea in calves, puppies, foals, pigs; diarrhea in an adult cat
E. faecalis	Septicemia, diarrhea in birds; chronic tracheitis in canaries; urinary tract infections in dogs; mastitis in cattle
E. faecium	Septicemia in birds
E. gallinarum	Septicemia in birds
E. hirae	Septicemia in psittacine birds; growth depression, septicemia, brain infection in chicks; hepatic, pancreatic infection in kittens
E. porcinus	Neonatal diarrhea in pigs
E. ratti	Diarrhea in neonatal rats
E. villorum	Enteritis in neonatal pigs
Enterococcus spp.	Temporomandibular joint arthritis in pet birds

particular concern because of the role of various *Enterococcus* spp. in human disease; antimicrobial resistance is another aspect of the human–enterococcus interaction.

In domestic animals, enterococcal disease is most commonly seen as urinary tract infection or, in chickens, endocarditis. *Enterococcus durans, Enterococcus porcinus,* and *Enterococcus villorum* may be emerging causes of sporadic enteritis in pigs. It is common to see large numbers of gram-positive cocci aligning on villus tips from mid-jejunum through the ileum. Diagnoses are based on culture and histologic demonstration of associated organisms.

The pathogenesis of enterococcal infections is based in part on intrinsic, but largely unknown, properties of the organism. However, enterococci often establish in patients receiving antibiotic therapy for other illnesses; effects on endogenous bacterial flora promote colonization, and the ensuing infections can become serious as a result of enterococcal accumulation of resistance elements.

Levels of resistance in isolates from animals in a given geographic locale in some cases appear to correspond to the amounts of antimicrobial agents used in animal production. Pathogenesis of enterococcal infections in domestic animals has not been studied. Characterization of the various infections that have been reported suggests that hosts are immunologically intact but that the infecting organisms may nonetheless be opportunistic.

Diagnosis

The best source of new information on the role of enterococci in disease of domestic animals is probably careful characterization of potential cases as part of the diagnostic process. Colonies of *Enterococcus* spp. are small (1-3 mm), gray, smooth, round, and usually α- to γ-hemolytic. About 80% are group D, and all species grow in the presence of 6.5% NaCl and ferment sorbitol and trehalose. Leucine aminopeptidase, pyrrolidonylarylamidase, and bile esculin tests are positive. Identification of the animal pathogenic species is by standard biochemical tests (Table 5-5).

OTHER CATALASE-NEGATIVE AEROBIC COCCI

As mentioned, other catalase negative aerobic cocci may also be isolated from specimens of veterinary origin. *Eremococcus coleocola* is found in vaginal discharges of mares. *Gemella cuniculi* has been recovered from rabbit abscesses and *Gemella palaticanis* from an inflammatory gum lesion in a dog. *Globicatella* spp. have caused an outbreak of meningoencephalitis in lambs *(Globicatella sanguinis)* and been associated with purulent lung and joint infections in calves, a lung lesion in a sheep, and joint infections in pigs *(Globicatella sulfidifaciens).* *Helcococcus ovis* has been isolated from cases of ovine mastitis and from bovine endocarditis. *Vagococcus* spp. are mainly from water-dwelling animals, including *Vagococcus salmoninarum* from rainbow and brown trout and Atlantic salmon with peritonitis and *Vagococcus lutrae*

TABLE **5-5** Identification of Animal-Pathogenic Species of Enterococci

Enterococcus Species	Characteristic						
	Fermentation					Hippurate Hydrolysis	H$_2$S*
	Arabinose	Glycerol	Inulin	Melibiose	Sucrose		
E. avium	Pos	Pos	Neg	Neg	Pos	Var	Pos
E. durans	Neg	Neg	Neg	Neg	Neg	Pos	Neg
E. faecalis	Neg	Pos	Neg	Neg	Pos	Most Pos	Neg
E. faecium	Pos	Pos	Neg	Var	Var	Pos	Neg
E. gallinarum†	Pos	Pos	Pos	Pos	Pos	Pos	Neg
E. hirae	Neg	Var	Neg	Pos	Pos	Neg	Neg
E. villorum	Neg	Pos (w)	Neg	Pos	Neg	Neg	Neg
E. porcinus	Neg	Neg	Neg	Pos	Neg	Neg	Neg
E. ratti‡	Neg	Neg	Neg	Neg	Neg	Var	Neg

*Production of H$_2$S over a cysteine-containing medium.
†*E. gallinarum* is motile and nonpigmented.
‡Differentiate *E. ratti* (unreactive) from *E. durans* (acid, clot) by inoculation of litmus milk.
Neg, Negative; *Pos,* positive; *Var,* variable; *w,* weak reaction.

and *Vagococcus fessus,* isolated from otters and porpoises but of unknown significance in disease. Nothing is known of the pathogenesis of these infections in domestic animals.

SUGGESTED READINGS

Beall B, Facklam R, Thompson T: Sequencing emm-specific PCR products for routine and accurate typing of group A streptococci, *J Clin Microbiol* 34:953-958, 1996.

Bisno AL, Collins CM, Turner JC: M proteins of group C streptococci isolated from patients with acute pharyngitis, *J Clin Microbiol* 34:2511-2515, 1996.

Bruckner DA, Colonna P: Nomenclature for aerobic and facultative bacteria, *Clin Infect Dis* 25:1-10, 1997.

Cole JR: *Streptococcus* and related cocci. In Carter GR, Cole JR, eds: *Diagnostic procedures in veterinary bacteriology and mycology,* ed 5, San Diego, 1990, Academic Press.

Cunningham MW: Pathogenesis of group A streptococcal infections, *Clin Microbiol Rev* 13:470-511, 2000.

Devriese LA, Ceyssens K, Hommez J, et al: Characteristics of different *Streptococcus suis* ecovars and description of a simplified identification method, *Vet Microbiol* 26:141-150, 1991.

Facklam RR, Elliott JA: Identification, classification, and clinical relevance of catalase-negative, gram-positive cocci, excluding the streptococci and enterococci, *Clin Microbiol Rev* 8:479-495, 1995.

Hardie JM: The genus *Streptococcus.* In Sneath PHA, ed: *Bergey's manual of systematic bacteriology,* vol 2, Baltimore, 1986, Williams & Wilkins.

Schuchat A: Epidemiology of group B streptococcal disease in the United States: shifting paradigms, *Clin Microbiol Rev* 11:497-513, 1998.

Whitney CN, Farley MM, Hadler J et al: Increasing prevalence of multidrug-resistant *Streptococccus pneumoniae* in the United States, *N Engl J Med* 343:1917-1924, 2000.

Chapter 6

The Genera *Actinomyces* and *Arcanobacterium*

THE GENUS ACTINOMYCES

Members of the genus *Actinomyces* are gram-positive, non–acid-fast, non–spore-forming rods. They are facultatively anaerobic, and most species prefer a reduced oxygen environment; CO_2 enhances the growth of aerotolerant species. *Actinomyces* spp. grow poorly, if at all, on Sabouraud's dextrose agar, a characteristic that differentiates them from *Nocardia* and *Streptomyces* spp. Most species in the genus produce a true mycelium, and angular branching is common. They are nonmotile and the mycelium breaks into irregularly sized elements.

The species most often associated with disease in domestic animals are *Actinomyces bovis*, *Actinomyces viscosus*, and *Actinomyces suis*. Other species are presented in Table 6-1.

Diseases and Pathogenesis

Actinomyces bovis causes actinomycosis, or lumpy jaw, in cattle (Figure 6-1), as well as occasional similar human infections. Bovine actinomycosis usually affects bony structures, and is most commonly seen in the mandible, or lower jaw. Pulmonary infections may occur in cattle and swine. The organism has also been associated with equine fistulous withers and similar conditions, sometimes in company with *Brucella abortus* or *Brucella suis*. Disease in other ruminants has also been reported, and dogs often develop actinomycotic spondylitis as a consequence of migration of foxtails from the upper respiratory tract. *Actinomyces hordeovulneris* is a newly described species that is more common than *A. bovis* in these canine infections. Actinomycosis can also occur concurrently with lung adenocarcinomas in dogs.

Actinomyces bovis is a normal resident of bovine oropharyngeal and digestive tract tissues. Organisms gain access to deeper tissues of the jaw by way of the dental alveoli or paralveoli, or through mucosae damaged by rough feed or foreign bodies. Mandibular granulation and chronic rarefying osteomyelitis follow. Suppurative necrosis can occur in the esophagus and reticulum, and thick green to yellow pus moves to the surface by way of fistulous tracts. Palpable masses can be found in normally soft tissues. Macrocolonies of *A. bovis* up to 5 mm in diameter, often called sulfur granules, are found in pus.

Pathogenesis of *A. bovis* infection is poorly understood. The pyogranulomatous response is a hallmark of infection, but it occurs by unknown mechanism. Areas of suppuration are surrounded by granulation, fibrosis, and infiltration of mononuclear cells.

TABLE **6-1** Animal-Pathogenic *Actinomyces* Species Other Than *Actinomyces bovis*, *Actinomyces viscosus*, and *Actinomyces suis*

Actinomyces Species	Conditions
A. hordeovulneris	Canine pleuritis, peritonitis, arthritis, abscesses; associated with grass awns
A. howelli	Dental plaque of cattle; questionable pathogen
A. hyovaginalis	Porcine purulent vaginitis and other lesions; isolated from aborted swine fetuses
A. israelii	Actinomycosis in cattle and swine; important human pathogen
A. naeslundii	Isolated from porcine abortions
A. bowdenii	Recent isolate from dogs and cats; resembles *A. viscosus*

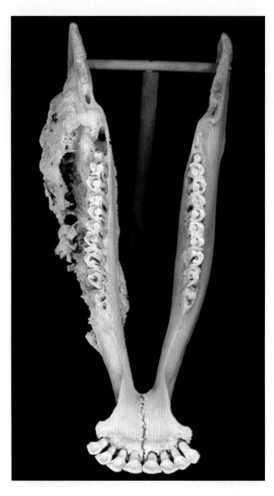

FIGURE 6-1 Bone damage in *Actinomyces bovis* infection (lumpy jaw). (Courtesy J. Glenn Songer.)

Bone honeycombed with pus-filled sinus tracts replaces normal bone (see Figure 6-1), and affected animals may lose teeth, become unable to chew, and develop mandibular fractures. Jaw lesions are often impressive in extent, but if vascular dissemination occurs, infection does not establish in other tissues. Circulating antibody developed as a result of infection has no impact on recovery, and it is likely that resistance is cell mediated.

Actinomyces viscosus infection in dogs manifests as cutaneous, noduloulcerative lymphangitis. The organism also causes periodontal disease in hamsters and other rodents. The normal habitat of *A. viscosus* is likely the same as that of *A. bovis,* but it invades wounds in dogs and produces abscesses and pedunculated cysts. *Actinomyces viscosus* is commonly associated with thoracic infections in dogs, but abdominal infections and osteomyelitis also occur.

Actinomyces suis is frequently recovered from opportunistic mammary infections in sows, probably from a source among the normal inhabitants of the porcine oropharynx. Infection may begin in superficial teat wounds caused by piglets during suckling. Formation of a mammary actinomycotic granuloma results in enlargement and induration of the gland, and the suppurative exudate contains typical sulfur granules.

Actinomyces spp. are prominent in the human oral cavity and are important factors in plaque development. Extensive study has revealed unique attributes that favor colonization and persistence in this environment. Fimbrial adhesins are perhaps the most important of these in that they enable adherence to receptors on tooth and mucosal surfaces and interaction with other plaque bacteria. Sialidase may amplify the adhesion process by exposing host cell receptors. Diverse enzymatic activities of *Actinomyces* spp. enhance its own lifestyle and that of other oral bacteria, possibly exerting a positive selective effect on the actinomycetes. Such information is not available for the *Actinomyces* spp. associated primarily with animal diseases, but the same selective pressures may apply. Application of similar genetic systems and methods of approach to animal pathogenic *Actinomyces* spp. provides many opportunities, perhaps leading to better methods for prevention.

Epidemiology

As noted, *Actinomyces* spp. are found on oral mucous membranes and in the gastrointestinal tract. Thus most actinomycoses have an endogenous origin and are noncommunicable, except via bites.

Diagnosis

Actinomycetes can usually be demonstrated in the "sulfur granules" associated with draining lesions. Colonies surrounded by a border of clublike structures (composed of mineral and the detritus of inflammatory and immune responses) are called rosettes. The radiating, somewhat distended clublike filaments may be found more commonly in tissue sections than in pus. Some staphylococcal lesions, especially in horses, contain sulfur granulelike structures; these are usually much smaller than true actinomycotic granules, and definitive differentiation can usually be accomplished by examination of the gram reaction and morphology of bacteria comprising the granules. Granules (not pus) should be washed and crushed under coverslips on a clean slide.

In such preparations, *A. bovis* appears as a tangled mass of filaments, with acidophilic capsular material at the periphery. The filaments are gram positive and basophilic. It is important to note, however, that diverse forms can be observed in crushed granules; *A. bovis* can appear as cocci, pleomorphic and branched rods, filaments, diphtheroidal forms, and even spirals. In vitro, *A. bovis* usually takes the diphtheroidal forms, although extended incubation, especially in a CO_2 atmosphere, drive the morphology toward branching filaments and clubs.

Actinomyces bovis is facultatively anaerobic and when cultivated aerobically, subsurface colonies predominate; the organism prefers an atmosphere containing 10% to 15% CO_2. Like all animal *Actinomyces* spp., *A. bovis* requires rich media, preferably containing serum or blood. Growth on blood-containing media is evident after 48 to 72 hours of incubation, although maximum colonial size is usually reached only after 5 to 6 days' incubation. The organism is nonhemolytic.

Lesion-associated granules in *A. viscosus* infection contain the typical filamentous masses

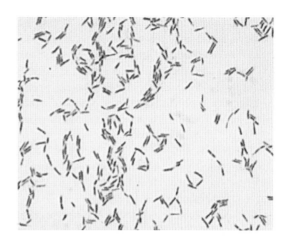

FIGURE 6-2　Gram stain of *Actinomyces viscosus.* (Courtesy Public Health Image Library, PHIL #1256, William A. Clark, Atlanta, 1977, Centers for Disease Control and Prevention.)

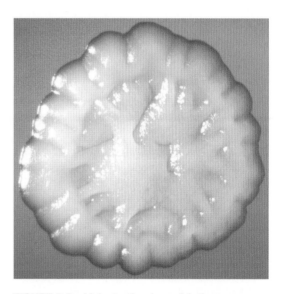

FIGURE 6-3　Molar tooth colony of *Actinomyces* sp. (Courtesy Public Health Image Library, PHIL #2846, Dr. Georg, Atlanta, 1963, Centers for Disease Control and Prevention.)

and diphtheroidal forms, but the clubs that are characteristic of *A. bovis* are absent (Figure 6-2). It produces flat, smooth-to-granular "molar tooth" colonies (Figure 6-3), which, at approximately 2 mm in diameter, are perhaps twice as large as those of *A. bovis*. Microcolonies, after 24-hour incubation in an atmosphere enriched for CO_2, have a dense center and filamentous fringe, and after 72 to 96 hours are circular, convex, smooth and white to cream. *Actinomyces viscosus* is catalase positive, unlike other members of the genus. The organism is relatively uncommon in purulent exudates, and cultural false negatives may result. Granules may be cultured in thioglycollate broth.

Colonies of porcine isolates of *A. suis* are granular with filamentous extensions, and when grown on blood-containing media are brown or reddish brown. Cells of medium length and uniform thickness predominate in smooth colonies, whereas those from rough colonies are long, curved, and frequently branched.

Differential characteristics of *Actinomyces* spp. are presented in Table 6-2 and colony morphologies in Table 6-3.

Control and Prevention

The cellular response to infection suggests that cell-mediated immunity is the critical component of the host response, but this has not been characterized and vaccine development has not been attempted.

Actinomyces bovis is sensitive to penicillin, streptomycin, tetracyclines, cephalosporins, lincomycin, and sulfonamides. Local lesions have often been treated with Lugol's iodine and sodium iodide has been administered intravenously (IV) (~75 mg/kg weekly) in cases of lumpy jaw, but must be stopped with the appearance of signs of toxicity. Concurrent therapy with penicillin and streptomycin has also been recommended.

Actinomyces viscosus is sensitive to penicillin, chloramphenicol, erythromycin, and tetracyclines. Effective therapy often requires high doses of antimicrobials, such as penicillin or sulfonamides, administered long term; thoracic involvement is a risk factor for relapse, usually after several months. Extensive fistulated lesions may require some form of surgical intervention, especially in companion animals, with drainage and removal of foreign bodies.

Actinomyces suis is sensitive to penicillin, erythromycin, and chloramphenicol, but less so to chlortetracycline and streptomycin. Large lesions

TABLE **6-2** Differential Characteristics of Important *Actinomyces* Species

| Characteristic | Actinomyces Species | | | | | |
	A. bovis	*A. hordeovulneris*	*A. hyovaginalis*	*A. israelii*	*A. suis*	*A. viscosus*
Catalase	Neg	Most pos	Neg	Neg	Neg	Pos
Nitrate reduction	Neg	Neg	Pos	Neg	Most pos	Most pos
Urease	Neg	Neg	Neg	Most neg	Pos	Most pos
Esculin hydrolysis	Most neg	Pos	Pos	Most neg	Most pos	Pos
Gelatinase	Neg	Weak pos	Neg	Neg	Neg	Neg
β-hemolysis	Most neg	Pos 7 days	Neg	Neg	Variable	Neg
Arabinose fermentation	Neg	Neg	Unknown	Neg	Most neg	Neg
Mannitol fermentation	Neg	Neg	Pos	Most neg	Most neg	Neg
Raffinose fermentation	Neg	Weak pos	Neg	Neg	Pos	Pos
Xylose fermentation	Neg	Pos	Neg	Pos	Neg	Neg

Neg, Negative; *Pos,* positive.

TABLE **6-3** Colonial Morphology of *Actinomyces* Species

Actinomyces Species	Colonial Characteristics
A. bovis	White, darker center; 0.5-1 mm; circular; smooth and nonfilamentous or filamentous with irregular edges
A. hordeovulneris	White agar-adherent molar-toothed colonies; may become conical or domed; 0.5-1 mm; may be filamentous
A. howelli	White, smooth, shiny, translucent, entire, convex; ≤2 mm diameter
A. hyovaginalis	Flat with outrunning edges
A. israelii	Gray or white; 0.5-2 mm; filamentous or spiderlike
A. suis	Small, smooth, opaque; short, radiating filaments
A. viscosus	White to gray; rough, dry, and crumbly or soft to mucoid; 0.5-5 mm

require surgical excision followed by antimicrobial therapy, but relapses are common.

THE GENUS *ARCANOBACTERIUM*

The genus *Arcanobacterium* began with a single member, *Arcanobacterium (Corynebacterium haemolyticum)*, but now includes the animal pathogens *Arcanobacterium hippocoleae*, *Arcanobacterium phocae*, *Arcanobacterium pluranimalium*, and *Arcanobacterium pyogenes*. *Arcanobacterium* spp. are gram-positive nonmotile coccoid rods (Table 6-4).

Diseases and Pathogenesis

Arcanobacterium (Actinomyces, Corynebacterium) pyogenes is the predominant animal pathogen in the genus. It commonly inhabits mucous membranes of the upper respiratory, gastrointestinal, and genital tracts of domestic animals, but is perhaps the most common opportunistic pathogen of domestic ruminants and other animals (Figure 6-4).

Virulence factors of *A. pyogenes* enable adherence, colonization, and in vivo multiplication, with accompanying damage to the host (Table 6-5). The organism is β-hemolytic as a result of production of pyolysin (PLO), which is dermonecrotic and lethal. PLO has 35% to 41% amino acid identity with cholesterol binding cytolysins (CBCs) that are produced by many species of gram-positive bacteria. Toxin monomers apparently interact with cholesterol and assemble in the outer leaflet of the eukaryotic cell membrane. The resulting multimers undergo a conformational change and insert through the hydrophobic core of the membrane, forming pores; *plo* mutants have reduced virulence, but the specific function of PLO is not known. Effects on immune cells may be important, but may also involve modulation of the immune response through the alteration of cytokine expression.

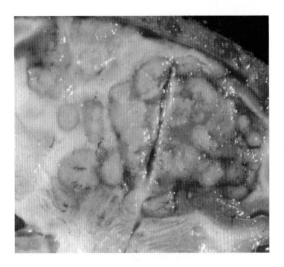

FIGURE 6-4 Kidney infection by *Arcanobacterium pyogenes*. (Courtesy Raymond E. Reed.)

TABLE **6-4** Disease Production by *Arcanobacterium* Species

Arcanobacterium Species	Condition
A. bernardiae	Human abscesses, septicemia
A. haemolyticum	Human pharyngitis, wound infections
A. hippocoleae	Equine vaginitis
A. phocae	Seal septicemia
A. pluranimalium	Deer lung abscess; porpoise splenic abscess
A. pyogenes	Bovine liver abscesses, mastitis, endometritis, abortion, endocarditis; caprine mastitis; porcine pneumonia, septic arthritis, endocarditis; poultry osteomyelitis, nephritis; ovine pneumonia, abortion, endometritis

TABLE **6-5** Virulence Factors of *Arcanobacterium pyogenes*

Attribute	Activity
PLO	Cell damage by pore formation
Collagen-binding protein	Adhesion to collagen-rich tissues
Fibrinogen-binding	Phagocytosis by neutrophils protein
Fibronectin-binding protein	Adhesion
DNase	Degrades host nucleic acids
Neuraminidases	Exposure of receptors; reduced mucus viscosity; decreases half-life of sIgA
Proteases	Nutrient acquisition; possible degradation of sIgA

DNase, Deoxyribonuclease; *PLO,* pyolysin; *sIgA,* secretory immunoglobulin A.

Arcanobacterium pyogenes binds collagen and fibronectin, and mutation of genes for collagen-binding proteins reduces the organism's ability to bind to cells in vitro. DNase may depolymerize DNA released from neutrophils, allowing bacterial access to nucleotides and perhaps facilitating invasion. Neuraminidase activity, encoded by two different genes, also facilitates binding to cells, perhaps by removal of sialic acid and exposure of receptors. Proteases with caseinase or gelatinase activity may also be involved in pathogenesis, although there is as yet no compelling experimental evidence.

Physical or microbial damage allows establishment of the normally commensal organism in various systems, including mammary gland, reproductive tract, joints, skin, and viscera. Liver abscesses can affect 60% to 80% of feedlot cattle fed high-energy rations, resulting in reduced feed conversion and condemnation of livers at slaughter. *Fusobacterium necrophorum* is perhaps somewhat more commonly isolated from these abscesses, but *A. pyogenes* is found in approximately 90%, including a proportion without *F. necrophorum*. Nutrient-rich feeds induce ruminal acidosis, and bacteria grow in the damaged papillar tissue. Microcolonies escape into portal circulation and shower down the liver with septic thrombi, with subsequent abscess formation.

Arcanobacterium pyogenes–associated suppurative mastitis frequently affects dry cows, but also other animals, especially if teats are injured. Spread is facilitated by contaminated milking machines and biting flies. Bovine uterine infections are also common, resulting in endometritis and infertility, especially in postpartum cows.

Diagnosis

Diagnosis of *A. pyogenes* infections is by isolation and identification of the organism from lesion material. It produces 0.5 mm colonies, surrounded by a zone of β-hemolysis.

Control and Prevention

Prognosis is poor in cases of mastitis, because of frequent ineffectiveness of antimicrobial therapy, and loss of function in affected quarters is not unusual. Thus economic impact of *A. pyogenes* can be great, even with relatively low incidence. Therapy of liver abscesses is not practical, and tylosin is widely used as an effort at prevention.

Vaccination with inactivated cells or culture filtrates has been largely unsuccessful in protecting domestic animals against *Arcanobacterium pyogenes* infection. PLO has potential as a subunit vaccine, in that it produces high titers in immunized animals and protects mice against challenge. No commercial products are currently available in the United States.

SUGGESTED READINGS

Billington SJ, Jost BH, Cuevas WA, et al: The *Arcanobacterium (Actinomyces) pyogenes* hemolysin, pyolysin, is a novel member of the thiol-activated cytolysin family, *J Bacteriol* 179:6100-6106, 1997.

Billington SJ, Jost BH, Songer JG: Thiol-activated cytolysins: structure, function and role in pathogenesis, *FEMS Microbiol Lett* 182:197-205, 2000.

Jost BH, Songer JG, Billington SJ: An *Arcanobacterium (Actinomyces) pyogenes* mutant deficient in production of the pore-forming cytolysin pyolysin has reduced virulence, *Infect Immun* 67:1723-1728, 1999.

Chapter 7

The Genus *Bacillus*

Bacilli are strictly aerobic or facultatively anaerobic, spore-forming rods (Figure 7-1). Most are catalase positive and motile, many are gram variable, and all are medium to large. Spores may be readily visualized or may require induction by incubation at 42° C or for an extended period at 37° C.

The *Bacillus anthracis* genome comprises an approximately 5.3 Mb chromosome and two plasmids, pX01 and pX02. The genome of at least two strains has been sequenced, and genetic analysis has focused mainly on the structural genes for toxin proteins (*pagA, lef,* and *cya,* located on pX01, see later) and the capsular biosynthetic genes (*capB, capC,* and *capA,* in a putative operon on pX02). The plasmids carry regulatory genes *atxA* (on pX01) and *acpA* (on pX02), which control toxin and capsule synthesis, respectively. A chromosomal gene, *abrB,* controls phase-specific transcription of the toxin genes.

Genetic exchange can occur among *B. anthracis* strains, as well as between *B. anthracis* and closely related species; pX01 and pX02 are not self-transmissible, but can be transferred by conjugative plasmids of *Bacillus thuringiensis. Bacillus anthracis* is genetically indistinguishable from *Bacillus cereus* and *B. thuringiensis;* evolution of *B. anthracis* and *B. thuringiensis* from *B. cereus,* with subsequent gain of plasmid-based genes and loss of chromosomal genes or gene function may explain the emergence of the anthrax bacillus.

Diseases and Epidemiolgoy

There are more than 40 species in the genus *Bacillus,* but only a few are animal pathogens. *Bacillus cereus* may cause gangrenous mastitis in cattle and, rarely, abortion in cattle, sheep, and horses. It has been associated with infertility in mares. *Bacillus licheniformis* is a rare cause of bovine abortion. *Paenibacillus (Bacillus) larvae* var. *larvae* is the agent most often associated with American foulbrood, a disease of larval honeybees.

In terms of disease, the genus is dominated by *B. anthracis.* This organism causes anthrax, which occurs primarily as septicemia in domestic and wild ruminants and horses. Dogs, cats, and other carnivores may also be infected, but they usually experience pharyngitis rather than septicemia. Humans are also susceptible, and the type of human disease depends on the route of exposure.

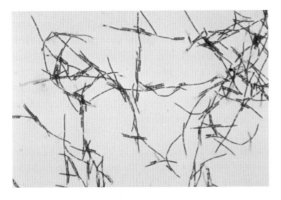

FIGURE 7-1 *Bacillus anthracis* gram-stained smear from pure culture. (Courtesy Public Health Image Library, PHIL #1064, William A. Clark, Atlanta, date unknown, Centers for Disease Control and Prevention.)

61

Egyptian and Mesopotamian writings from approximately 5000 BC describe a cattle disease that very much resembles anthrax, and may have been the cause of two of the plagues on the Egyptians and their cattle, described in Exodus 9 (the "murrain of beasts…" and the "plague of boils and blains…"). In his treatise on agriculture, Virgil describes a disease of domestic animals and man that is almost certainly anthrax.

Anthrax in Domestic Animals

Anthrax continues to be reported among domestic and wild animals in the United States. The incidence of anthrax in U.S. animals is unknown; however, reports of animal infection have occurred among the Great Plains states from Texas to North Dakota and from eastern New York to California.

Signs of anthrax appear following a highly variable incubation period, which is usually 3 to 7 days, but may be as short as 24 hours or greater than 2 weeks. The course of peracute anthrax in cattle and sheep may be as little as 1 to 2 hours, with sudden death a result of rapidly developing cerebral anoxia and pulmonary edema; fever (≤107° F), respiratory distress, and convulsions may be observed, but death is often reported as due to lightning strike. Epistaxis is common, and rigor mortis is often absent. One or two animals may die, followed by many others after several days. Acute anthrax in ruminants, with a clinical course of 24 to 48 hours, is characterized by an abrupt rise in temperature, anorexia, excitement followed by depression, and convulsions; in some cases there is evidence of pharyngeal involvement (lingual edema, with fluid accumulation in the throat and sternum) and respiratory distress. Animals may hemorrhage from the mouth, nose, and anus before death.

The course of equine anthrax is usually acute to subacute, with affected animals often surviving for 96 hours. Ingestion of spores results in septicemia, with enteritis and colic; disease following transmission by insect bite is initiated after the manner of human cutaneous anthrax, but the local subcutaneous edema spreads, often affecting the throat, ventral thorax, and abdomen. It is important to distinguish this syndrome from *Corynebacterium pseudotuberculosis* infection in the horse, which can also be associated with insect bites.

In the 1990s, *B. anthracis* was found during repair work in King's Cross and Liverpool Street Stations in London. This should not have been surprising; the organism was associated with horse hair used in wall plaster in stations that were built in the nineteenth century. Decontamination is routine in these situations, and there is little or no risk to the public. Similar situations were encountered in the past; use of saddle blankets woven from contaminated materials has led to equine anthrax, and manufacture of shaving brushes with *B. anthracis*–contaminated bristles resulted in cases of human cutaneous anthrax.

Omnivores and carnivores may have natural resistance to anthrax, and are more likely than other species to recover from the disease. Anthrax is typically subacute to chronic, and usually occurs after ingestion of contaminated meat or, in the case of swine, meat-and-bone meal. Lingual and pharyngeal edema, a common manifestation of infection in regional lymph nodes, may cause dyspnea and dysphagia, with discharge of serosanguineous fluid from the mouth and death due to asphyxia. Necrosis in the upper gastrointestinal tract, as well as mesenteric lymphadenopathy, occurs in carnivores. Cats may develop jowl and lingual carbuncles, cranial swelling, and severe gastroenteritis. An intestinal form of chronic anthrax has also been reported in swine.

Anthrax is not uncommon among wild carnivores. This is almost always associated with consumption of meat from animals dead of anthrax, sometimes when moribund, and presumably anthrax-affected, animals are shot as food for carnivores in game farms. In these cases, antimicrobial therapy, as well as antimicrobial prophylaxis and immunoprophylaxis, carry the obvious risks associated with patient ingratitude.

Human Anthrax

Spores remain viable for decades, and, as such, soil is the usual source of infection for ruminants. Human infection following contact with contaminated soil usually takes the *cutaneous* form. *Gastrointestinal* and *inhalation* anthrax result from contact with products from affected animals, and, of course, may arise from laboratory exposure. Human anthrax is noncommunicable, regardless of the form of the disease.

Cutaneous anthrax (Figure 7-2) follows entry of the organism into a cut or abrasion. The incubation period is usually 24 to 72 hours, but can range up to 2 weeks. Signs begin with a painless papule, which becomes vesicular in 1 to 2 days, and can be surrounded by an extensive area of edema. The vesicle ulcerates by day 5 or 6 and the lesion dries, leaving a blackened necrotic area, the so-called black eschar. Affected individuals may also experience fever, malaise, headache, and swelling of draining lymph nodes. About 20% of untreated cases will progress to fatal septicemia. The case fatality rate with timely antimicrobial therapy is less than 1%, although treatment does not stop the progression of lesions.

Gastrointestinal anthrax follows consumption of contaminated meat. A recent outbreak in Russia was associated with meat given to farm workers in lieu of wages; exposure of more than 1500 people led to 23 hospitalizations and 1 death. The incubation period of gastrointestinal anthrax is approximately 1 to 7 days. Pharyngeal lesions appear on the base of the tongue and tonsils and are accompanied by sore throat, dysphagia, and regional lymphadenopathy. Inappetence, nausea and vomiting, and fever, followed by abdominal pain, vomiting of blood, and bloody diarrhea are signs of acute colonic inflammation. Dissemination of *B. anthracis* from the initial site of infection leads to massive septicemia and toxemia. The case fatality rate is 25% to 60%, and even prompt antimicrobial therapy is not always sufficient to prevent mortality.

Cutaneous and gastrointestinal anthrax in humans may follow naturally occurring animal anthrax, but aerosol exposure is most likely to take place in laboratories, textile mills, or following a biological weapons attack. *Pulmonary,* or *inhalation, anthrax* results from respiratory exposure to spores. The infectious dose has been estimated variously as 8000 to 50,000 spores, and the incubation period is uncertain; recent experience suggests that it can be quite short (as little as 1-2 days), but some cases associated with the Sverdlovsk outbreak

of 1979 (see Suggested Readings) were apparently as along as 43 days. The length of the incubation period may be inversely related to the dose. Spores do not all germinate immediately, but may in fact remain dormant until engulfed by pulmonary alveolar macrophages. This phenomenon is of particular importance in regard to duration of administration of therapy or prophylaxis; spores are not susceptible to antimicrobials, so these drugs must be present throughout the period in which germination may occur. Delayed onset does not appear to be an issue with cutaneous or gastrointestinal infections.

As spores germinate in macrophages and are carried to mediastinal lymph nodes, the patient may experience sore throat, mild fever, and muscle aches, which progress rapidly to severe respiratory difficulty. Organisms originating in the lungs and, later, those in the bloodstream, are temporarily removed by the reticuloendothelial system; however, *B. anthracis* ultimately escapes the lymphatics to produce overwhelming septicemia, usually with meningitis (Figures 7-3 through 7-5). Sudden onset of acute symptoms, including hypotension, edema, and fatal shock follow in 2 to 5 days. Estimates of the case-fatality rate are based upon limited data, but are probably at least 90% and, without therapy, are more nearly 100%. Therapeutic intervention is of little use unless initiated quite early in the clinical course.

In the United States, as many as 130 cases of human anthrax occurred each year at the beginning of the twentieth century, but this declined to zero annual incidence through most of the 1990s. Most infections have been cutaneous, although 18 were

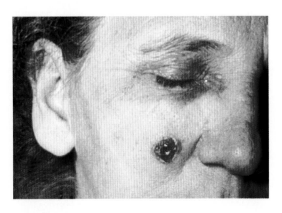

FIGURE 7-2   Facial lesion of cutaneous anthrax (day 11) on employee of the spinning department of a goat-hair processing mill. (Courtesy Public Health Image Library, #1804, Atlanta, date unknown, Centers for Disease Control and Prevention.)

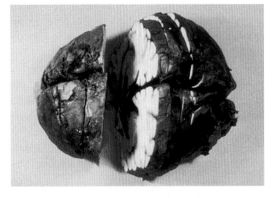

FIGURE 7-3   Meningitis in human systemic *Bacillus anthracis* infection. (Courtesy Public Health Image Library, PHIL #1121, Atlanta, 1966, Centers for Disease Control and Prevention.)

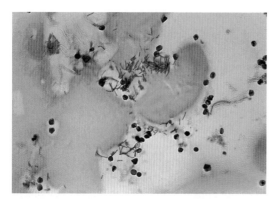

FIGURE 7-4 *Bacillus anthracis* in cerebrospinal fluid of patient with meningitis. (Courtesy Public Health Image Library, PHIL #1782, Marshal Fox, Atlanta, 1976, Centers for Disease Control and Prevention.)

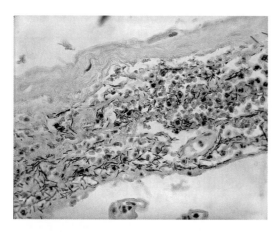

FIGURE 7-5 Meningeal tissue, showing large numbers of *Bacillus anthracis*. (Courtesy Public Health Image Library, PHIL #1791, Dr. LaForce, Atlanta, 1967, Centers for Disease Control and Prevention.)

pulmonary, the last in 1976 in a weaver. Worldwide, human anthrax is particularly common in agricultural regions with inadequate programs for control of livestock anthrax; in South and Central America, southern and eastern Europe, Asia, Africa, the Caribbean, and the Middle East, where animal anthrax occurs frequently, human cases are common and more than 95% are cutaneous. A recent epidemic in Zimbabwe comprised nearly 10,000 cases, with a case fatality rate of less than 2%.

Bacillus anthracis and Biological Warfare and Bioterrorism

Manufacture of biological weapons involving *B. anthracis* has been mentioned. It has, in fact, been a focus of biological warfare (BW) programs for decades, in the West before the establishment of biological weapons treaties in the late 1960s and, by all indications, into the 1990s in the former Soviet Union.

Evidence of this is provided by the unusual anthrax epidemic that occurred in Sverdlovsk (Ekaterinburg), Russia, in April and May 1979. It was officially attributed to consumption of contaminated meat, but there was considerable international sentiment that it resulted from an accidental release of spores from a military microbiology facility in the city. Examination of prevailing winds during the period preceding the outbreak revealed that the pattern of deaths, humans and domestic animals alike, was correlated with what would have been the plume from the facility. Necropsies revealed lesions typical of inhalation anthrax, including hemorrhagic necrosis of thoracic lymph nodes and hemorrhagic mediastinitis; gastrointestinal submucosal hemorrhagic lesions were nearly universal and mesenteric lymphadenitis occurred in a few cases. In most, edema was demonstrable adjacent to sites of infection and hemorrhagic meningitis indicated hematogenous dissemination. Subsequent investigation, which included testimony by defectors formerly involved in the illicit Soviet biological weapons program, established the reality of this epidemic, the occurrence of which is still officially denied by the Russian government.

B. anthracis is a likely BW and biological terrorism (BT) agent because of the stability of its spores, transmission by the respiratory route, and the high mortality of the resulting disease. Release of 50 kg of spores upwind of a city of a half million people would cause an estimated 220,000 cases of anthrax, with 95,000 deaths.

Putative release of anthrax spores has, on several occasions before September 11, 2001, and on many occasions since, proven to be a hoax; law enforcement agencies dealt with an average of 1 or 2 cases per week through the summer of 2002. Targets have included abortion clinics, public officials, and others. Cornstarch and baby powder seem to be the most commonly chosen stand-ins for anthrax spores.

Anthrax and Agricultural Bioterrorism

Little has been said about the possible role of *B. anthracis* in agricultural bioterrorism, but such efforts date back at least to the early part of the twentieth century. Widespread germ warfare in World War I has been widely attributed to Germany, with particular attention to Allied horses, which were crucial factors in many aspects of the war. Their BW campaign, using glanders and anthrax in Argentina, the United States, Romania, and France, is well documented, but nonetheless vehemently denied. In one specific instance, a German message to an agent in Buenos Aires, deciphered by the British Admiralty, described a shipment from Madrid of cultures in sugar cubes. Of unknown meaning at the time, it has since come to light that this was part of an attempt by the Germans, working through a Swedish aristocrat, to produce anthrax in horses and reindeer used to carry British arms across northern Norway and into Russia. Baron Otto Robert Karl von Rosen was arrested near the Finnish frontier in January 1917. Police found among the baron's possessions tins labeled "Swedish meat" that contained, in reality, dynamite; they also found curare, microbial cultures, and 19 sugar cubes, some containing small glass vials. Political pressure led to the baron's expulsion from Norway, and the cubes eventually were placed in a police museum in Trondheim. The curator of the museum recently rediscovered two of the cubes, together with a label claiming that they contained anthrax. They were passed for testing to the Norwegian Defence Microbiological Institute in Oslo and then to the Chemical and Biological Defence Establishment at Porton Down in the United Kingdom, and did, indeed, contain *B. anthracis*.

The British used the same idea during World War II; they drilled holes into pelleted dairy cattle feed and inserted capillary tubes filled with anthrax spores, with the intention of dropping them from bombers. They were, fortunately, never used.

PATHOGENESIS

Basic principles of pathogenesis of anthrax apply across species, but there are also specific aspects to occurrence of disease in each species. Pigs may experience a form of cutaneous anthrax, known as bullnose, when lesions acquired through rooting behavior become contaminated with spores. Carnivores are especially likely to experience pharyngeal anthrax, through exposure to spores in infected meat. Ruminants have almost exclusively a septicemic form of anthrax, but initiated by gastrointestinal exposure to spores (Figure 7-6). Circumvention of host defenses is facilitated by breaks in the keratinized epithelial barrier;

and much attention has been given to the physical aspects of spore retention in the lung and the spore-macrophage interaction. Relatively little is known of the specific steps by which spores cross the pharyngeal or intestinal mucosal epithelium.

Following inhalation, spores can remain dormant for months, based upon findings of studies in nonhuman primates, and, as mentioned, this delayed germination can result in prolonged incubation periods; this phenomenon has not been reported with infection by routes other than respiratory. In monkeys exposed to four spore $LD_{50}s$, 15% to 20% survived in lung tissue after 42 days, 2% remained after 50 days, and less than 1% (still a substantial number) were recovered after 75 days. No such studies have been performed in humans, for reasons that may be obvious, but the apparently prolonged incubation period in the Sverdlovsk outbreak suggests that lethal numbers of spores persisted for more than 6 weeks after exposure.

Regardless of route of exposure, spores of *B. anthracis* are engulfed by and germinate in macrophages; the resulting vegetative cells escape from the phagocytic vesicles and replicate within the cytoplasm. To escape the vesicle, strains must carry the genetic information found on the toxin plasmid (pX01). Interestingly, the toxin genes themselves are not required for phagosomal escape, but another genetic element on pX01, *atxA*, is required. The product of *atxA* activates transcription of *pag*, *cya*, and *lef*, the genes for protective antigen, edema factor, and lethal factor, respectively; it may regulate one or more of the genes, whether chromosomal or pX01 associated, that are necessary for release of *B. anthracis* from macrophages. *atxA* mutants are avirulent for mice, and these mice have a diminished immunologic response to the toxin proteins. As might be expected, neither capsule nor products of any other genes on capsule plasmid pX02 play a role in release.

Even with repeated phagocytosis, phagosomal escape, and release from the macrophage, the infection may remain localized, as in cutaneous anthrax; however, by virtue of the local antiphagocytic effects of toxins and capsule, it may spread to local and regional lymph nodes, as with gastrointestinal anthrax. Bacterial multiplication in the lymph nodes leads to toxemia and bacteremia, especially in pulmonary anthrax. Temperature and bicarbonate serve as host signals to the organism, upregulating transcription of toxin and capsule genes.

Lethal toxin and edema factor cause local necrosis and extensive edema, respectively, both of which are major pathologic processes associated with anthrax. Increased toxin production is the basis for increasingly widespread necrosis and, as a consequence, organ failure.

As noted, capsule production by *B. anthracis* is a key aspect of virulence. Vegetative cells released by dead or dying macrophages are protected from further phagocytosis by capsule, which is composed of a polymer of D-glutamic acid. Capsule production in vitro is enhanced by inclusion of bicarbonate and serum in growth media and incubation in at least 5% CO_2. Membrane-associated capsule biosynthetic enzymes are encoded by *capA, capB,* and *capC,* found on pX02. AcpA (encoded by *acpA,* found on pX02) and AtxA (encoded by *atxA,* found on pX01) regulate capsule production by effects on *capB*. Nonencapsulated isolates are essentially avirulent

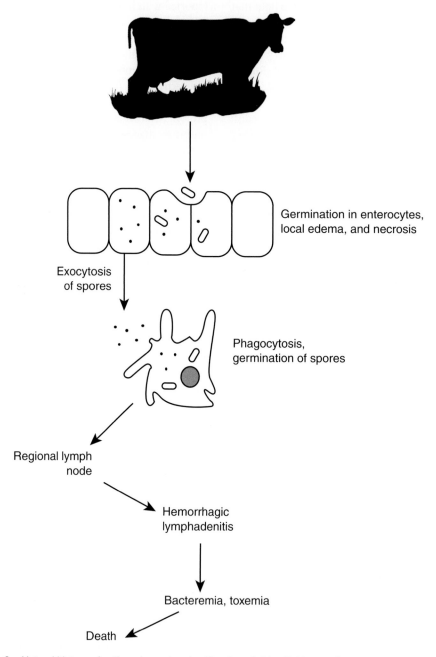

FIGURE 7-6 Natural history of anthrax in ruminants. (Courtesy Ashley E. Harmon.)

and are, in fact, the basis for active immunization of animals against anthrax (see Control and Prevention later in this chapter).

Evidence for toxin production by *B. anthracis* was based initially upon the finding that antibiotic-mediated termination of late-stage bacteremia in guinea pigs did not prevent death. The toxin, isolated from the plasma of *B. anthracis*–infected guinea pigs and from in vitro cultures of the organism, was lethal on intravenous injection of mice and guinea pigs and edemagenic when injected intradermally; its activities were neutralized by antisera. Three proteins, now known as edema factor (EF, or factor I), protective antigen (PA, or factor II), and lethal factor (LF, or factor III),

were purified, and when administered to experimental animals in specific combinations, they mimicked the features of infection with *B. anthracis*. Intradermal injection of EF and PA produced edema, and together are called edema toxin. Intravenous injection of LF and PA yielded symptoms seen in infection, including lethality; this combination is called lethal toxin.

Different regions of PA (MW 82,684 Da) mediate binding to the cell receptor, binding LF and EF, membrane insertion, and translocation to the cytosol (Figure 7-7). As such, PA is the major immunogen in anthrax vaccines.

The characteristic edema observed in anthrax results from the adenylate cyclase activity of EF

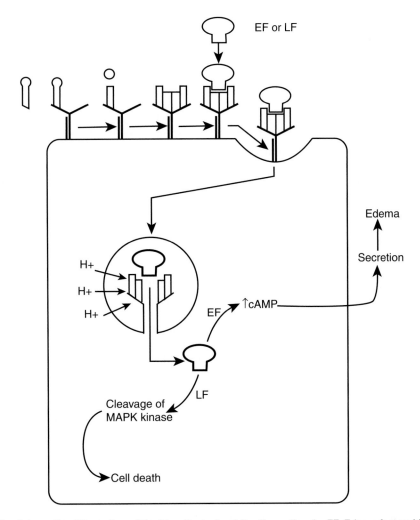

FIGURE 7-7   Schematic of the action of the tripartite toxin of *Bacillus anthracis*. *EF*, Edema factor; *LF*, lethal factor; *H+*, hydrogen; *cAMP*, cyclic adenosine monophosphate; *MAPK*, mitogen-activated protein kinase. (Courtesy Ashley E. Harmon.)

(MW 88,808 Da). The carboxyl-terminal region of EF catalyzes production of intracellular cyclic adenosine monophosphate (cAMP), in the presence of calcium and the eukaryotic calcium-binding protein calmodulin. EF may indirectly increase host susceptibility to infection by disrupting the cytokine response of monocytes and by suppressing neutrophil function: accumulation of cAMP induces interleukin (IL)-6 production and inhibits TNF-α production by monocytes, and neutrophil function is also compromised, through inhibition of both phagocytosis and the respiratory burst.

Amino-terminal amino acid sequence homology between EF and LF (MW 90,237 Da) is probably related to the ability of these molecules to competitively bind to PA. LF also has carboxyl-terminal catalytic activity and functions as a metalloprotease, cleaving mitogen-activated protein kinase (MAPK) kinases; this compromises the activation of downstream substrates, perhaps inhibiting one or more signaling pathways, altering the ability of the cell to respond to extracellular stresses, and driving it toward lysis. Hypotension, shock, and death seen in systemic *B. anthracis* infection can be duplicated by injection of LF and PA. Its level of toxicity, compared with other bacterial toxins, is low; the rat minimum lethal dose (MLD) is 600 mg LF and 3 g PA.

EF, LF, and PA act in binary combinations. Most cells possess 8000 to 50,000 PA receptors, and after binding, a 20 kD fragment of PA is removed by proteolysis. This allows oligomerization of the remaining approximately 63 kD portion of PA, into heptamers (called the "prepore"), and exposes the EF/LF binding site. The PA/EF and PA/LF toxin complexes enter cells by receptor-mediated endocytosis. Acidification of the endosome triggers insertion of the prepore into the endosomal membrane, forming ion-conductive channels and allowing translocation of LF or EF into the cytosol.

The adenylate cyclase activity of EF affects all cell types, but toxicity of LT is apparently limited to macrophages; resistant cells have PA receptors and bind and internalize LF, but are not lysed. Cultured macrophages are uniquely sensitive to LF and appear to mediate anthrax toxicity. Macrophage depletion makes mice resistant to LF toxicity and reconstitution with LF-sensitive macrophage cell lines restores their sensitivity to LF. Thus LF effects on macrophages may be ultimately responsible for the death of the host. Sublytic levels of LF induce hyperproduction of IL-1 and TNF-α production by macrophages, and mice can be passively protected against LF challenge by administration of IL-1 antiserum. Furthermore, lysis of macrophages exposed to lytic levels of LF correlated with production of elevated levels of superoxide anion, the reactive oxygen intermediate produced in greatest quantity by macrophages; LF is not lethal for some macrophage cell lines, even if injected into the cytosol, perhaps because no reactive oxygen intermediates were produced. Thus it may be that low concentrations of LF upregulate superoxide anion production, which in turn induces cytokine production; IL-1 would be expected to accumulate in macrophages and TNF-α would be released. Increased concentrations of LF and, concomitantly, superoxide anion, lead to macrophage lysis and sudden release of IL-1, causing shock and death. In sum, the pathogenesis of anthrax is probably related to the unique sensitivity of macrophages to the activity of LF, the adenylate cyclase activity of EF, and the antiphagocytic effect of the capsule.

CONTROL AND PREVENTION

Nearly 125 years ago, Louis Pasteur developed a heat-attenuated anthrax vaccine that we now know to have resulted from selective curing of the toxin plasmid, pX01. Although concurrent work was conducted in the United Kingdom, the public field trials of his vaccine at Pouilly-le-Fort, France, in 1881, led to apportionment of primary credit to Pasteur. The Pasteur vaccine was used widely in Europe and South America, and even earned passing mention in the Mel Brooks western spoof, *Blazing Saddles*. However, in 1939, Sterne isolated a strain that carried pX01 but not pX02; it carries the full complement of genetic machinery for production of toxins, but is nonencapsulated and thus avirulent. Vaccines based upon the Sterne strain were so immunogenic that they remain the standard veterinary product today. Colorado Serum Company is the sole North American producer of animal anthrax vaccines. In contrast to the strictly regulated possession and shipping of virulent strains of *B. anthracis*, the vaccine is available to anyone with money. In some countries (for example, China and some states of the former Soviet Union), similar strains have been used to immunize humans.

Reduction of incidence and prevalence of animal anthrax is a key part of controlling human infection. In endemic areas, veterinary supervision of slaughter is necessary to minimize contact between affected animals and abattoir workers and to prevent entry of infected meat into the food supply. It hardly seems necessary to comment that in these areas it is wise to avoid consumption of meat of uncertain origin, and especially meat from animals that have experienced sudden death. It is also important to be circumspect about importation of hides and wool from endemic countries.

Vaccination of humans has become a high-profile topic mainly because of the controversy over immunization of military personnel. The first suggested use of acellular vaccines, nearly 100 years ago, forms the basis for today's licensed vaccines. Research in this area has been aimed primarily at PA, and PA-based vaccines are now produced in the United States and England. An alum-precipitated cell-free culture filtrate vaccine was developed in 1954, and has been improved through use of a strain producing more PA, cultivated in protein-free medium, adjuvanted with aluminum hydroxide rather than alum. The current product, called AVA (anthrax vaccine adsorbed) is a cell-free filtrate of cultures of *B. anthracis* strain V770-NP1-R, which is toxigenic and nonencapsulated, and the product contains all three toxin components. Primary vaccination is relatively intensive, consisting of subcutaneous injections at zero, 2, and 4 weeks, and 6, 12, and 18 months, with annual boosters thereafter. The correlation between level of anti-PA antibodies and degree of protection is poor. However, epidemiologic study of cutaneous anthrax among workers processing imported goat hair revealed that PA-based vaccination is more than 90% effective. There is good evidence that the humoral response to PA is the key element in protection. Results of recent studies suggest that inclusion of inactivated spores in PA vaccination regimens greatly increases the efficacy of the response.

Local reactions (tenderness, erythema, induration, and nodule formation), which have been much publicized in the processing of military vaccination, are less common following intramuscular vaccination, and there may be future changes in routes and numbers of immunizations. About 95% of those vaccinated seroconvert, but it is not known if this has any bearing on protection in humans. However, rhesus monkeys (*Macaca mulatta*) immunized with the AVA vaccine are protected against inhalation anthrax following pulmonary spore challenge.

Penicillin and doxycycline are the drugs of choice for treatment of naturally occurring anthrax, and ciprofloxacin has been approved to prevent development or progression of inhalation anthrax in humans. Short courses of postexposure antibiotic therapy do not prevent disease when large numbers of spores are inhaled; rhesus monkeys treated with penicillin or doxycycline for 30 days following aerosol exposure to spores may die up to 4 weeks after antibiotics are discontinued. Thus postexposure antimicrobial prophylaxis might provide an opportunity for effective vaccination.

DIAGNOSIS

In numerous examples, hindsight has suggested mishandling of cases that were later found to be anthrax. In one case, a cow was buried in a city landfill before the establishment of a diagnosis; in another, a veterinarian performed a necropsy on an anthrax suspect cow, packaged tissues and other specimens in a 5-gallon plastic bucket, and shipped them to a diagnostic laboratory by way of a public bus. Application of sound principles of case management provides the necessary degree of safety, for other animals and for personnel, and minimizes the number of opportunities for public hysteria.

Recognition of clinical signs of anthrax (see earlier) and knowledge of diagnostic protocols are vital. Carcasses should not be opened and exposed to air. If opened, lesions observed will be typical of septicemia, including hemorrhages on serosal surfaces and red-tinged effusions. Disposal of affected carcasses should *always* be by incineration, preferably on site. Burial, with or without quicklime, may serve only to increase the pH and the amount of calcium in the soil, both of which have been associated with extended spore persistence. Furthermore, spores probably have a slight positive buoyancy and therefore may float upward when soil is wet. Pasteur himself demonstrated that after burial of cows dead of anthrax, earthworms brought spores of *B. anthracis* to the surface.

The general change from on-farm to laboratory diagnosis introduces a delay between sample collection and obtaining results. Risk of environmental contamination increases significantly if incineration and site control are not initiated quickly, especially if a necropsy has been performed. In the wake of the malicious dissemination of *B. anthracis* spores in the United States in the autumn of 2001, a surfeit of attention has been given to the need for and development of rapid diagnostic methods. The exponential increase in the extent of technology applied to detection of spores or vegetative cells of *B. anthracis* may be a necessary part of the frenzied response to increased potential for use of the organism as a tool of bioterrorism. However, diagnosis of livestock infections can usually be accomplished by refreshingly low-tech methods. A presumptive diagnosis can be based on carcass-side demonstration of morphologically compatible rod-shaped bacteria in a peripheral blood smear. This is, unfortunately, rarely done today, if only because veterinarians seldom carry a microscope and stains. Smears (preferably of peripheral blood but also from lymph nodes or splenic tissue) are air dried, stained with polychrome methylene blue for 30 to 60 seconds, and examined microscopically for bacilli in chains, with pink-staining capsules. Capsules are not present on organisms grown aerobically on routine solid media. It is important to recognize that wash fluids should be collected in a disinfectant solution (such as 10% bleach), and that slides and blotting paper should be likewise disinfected or autoclaved.

Bacteriologic culture should, of course, still be performed for confirmation of the diagnosis. Colonies of *B. anthracis* are white to gray and non-hemolytic (or weakly α-hemolytic with extended incubation) when cultivated on blood agar. Older colonies or those of nonencapsulated strains have the characteristic ground glass aspect; wisps of growth at the edges, trailing back in unison toward the parent colony, give rise to the "Medusa head" appearance (Figure 7-8). In contrast, *B. cereus* has large, rough, dry colonies, often with "hairy" edges, but always β-hemolytic (as are environmental *Bacillus* spp., such as *B. subtilis*). *Bacillus licheniformis* produces opaque colonies with dull to rough surfaces; they are usually tightly attached

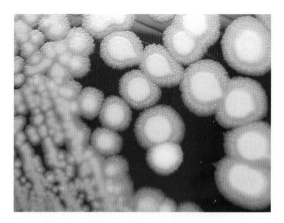

FIGURE 7-8 Medusa-head colonies of *Bacillus anthracis* (avirulent Pasteur strain). (Courtesy Public Health Image Library, PHIL #1897, Atlanta, 2002, Larry Stauffer, Oregon State Public Health Laboratory.)

to the agar and may accumulate large amounts of slime, reminiscent of isolates of *Pseudomonas aeruginosa* producing alginate. *Paenibacillus larvae* requires thiamine for growth, and its colonies are flat, white, rough, granular, and nonhemolytic.

The identity of an isolate of *B. anthracis* can be confirmed by a variety of additional tests (Table 7-1). Capsule production can be induced by cultivation in defibrinated equine blood or on bicarbonate-containing media. The "string of pearls" takes advantage of the fact that *B. anthracis*, in the presence of penicillin, is more coccoid than rod shaped. The organism is also lethal for mice injected intraperitoneally; impression smears should be made of liver tissue from mice that die within 24 hours. Polymerase chain reaction (PCR) assays, based on amplification of fragments of capsule or toxin genes, may be useful not only in confirming an identification but also in detecting the organism in the environment or in cases of anthrax.

TABLE **7-1** Differential Characteristics of *Bacillus* and *Paenibacillus*

Species	β-Hemolysis	Motility	Penicillin	7% NaCl	Voges-Proskauer	Nitrate Reduction
B. anthracis	Neg	Neg	Sensitive	Pos	Pos	Pos
B. cereus	Pos	Pos	Resistant	Neg	Pos	Pos
B. cereus ssp. *mycoides*	Var	Var	Resistant	Var	Pos	Pos
B. licheniformis	Neg	Pos	Resistant	Neg	Pos	Pos
B. thuringiensis	Pos	Pos	ND	Pos	Pos	Pos
*P. larvae**	Neg	Pos	ND	Neg	Neg	Var

*Cultivate on tryptose phosphate glucose agar to satisfy requirement for thiamine; also hydrolyzes casein and gelatin.
ND, Not determined; *Neg,* negative; *Pos,* positive; *Var,* variable.

SUGGESTED READINGS

Abramova FA, Grinberg LM, Yampolskaya OV, Walker DH: Pathology of inhalational anthrax in 42 cases from the Sverdlovsk outbreak of 1979, *Proc National Acad Sci U S A* 90:2291-2294, 1993.

Brachman PS, Friedlander AM: Anthrax. In Plotkin SA, Mortimer EA, eds: *Vaccines,* Philadelphia, 1994, WB Saunders.

Dixon TC, Fadl AA, Koehler TM, et al: Early *Bacillus anthracis*–macrophage interactions: intracellular survival and escape, *Cell Microbiol* 2:453-463, 2000.

Friedlander AM: The anthrax toxins. In Saelinger CB, ed: *Trafficking of bacterial toxins,* Boca Raton, Fla, 1990, CRC Press.

Hambleton P, Turnbull PCB: Anthrax vaccine development: a continuing story, *Adv Biotechnol Proc* 13:105-122, 1990.

Hanna P: Anthrax pathogenesis and host response, *Curr Top Microbiol Immunol* 225:13-35, 1998.

Hedlund KW: Anthrax toxin: history and recent advances and perspectives, *J Toxicol* 11:41-88, 1992.

Huxsoll DL: Narrowing the zone of uncertainty between research and development in biological warfare defense, *Ann N Y Acad Sci* 666:177-901, 1992.

Koehler TM: *Bacillus anthracis* genetics and virulence gene regulation, *Curr Top Microbiol Immunol* 271:143-164, 2002.

Leppla SH: The anthrax toxin complex. In Alouf JE, Freer JH, eds: *Sourcebook of bacterial protein toxins,* New York, 1991, Academic Press.

Leppla SH: Anthrax toxins. In Moss J, Iglewski B, Vaughan M, Tu AT, eds: *Bacterial toxins and virulence factors in disease,* New York, 1996, Marcel Dekker.

Little SF, Ivins BE: Molecular pathogenesis of *Bacillus anthracis* infection, *Microbes Infect* 1:131-139, 1999.

Meselson M, Guillemin J, Hugh-Jones M, et al: *The Sverdlovsk anthrax outbreak of 1979,* Science 266:1202-1208, 1994.

Petosa C, Liddington RC: The anthrax toxin. In Parker MW, ed: *Protein toxin structure,* Austin, Texas, 1996, RG Landes.

Pratt-Rippin K, Pezzlo M: Identification of commonly isolated aerobic gram-positive bacteria. In Isenberg HD, ed: *Clinical microbiology procedures handbook,* vol 1, Washington, DC, 1992, ASM Press.

Quinn CP, Turnbull PCB: Anthrax. In Collier L, Balows A, Sussman M, eds: *Topley and Wilson's microbiology and microbial infections,* London, 1998, Arnold.

Thorne CB: *Bacillus anthracis.* In Hoch JA, Losick R, eds: *Biochemistry, physiology, and molecular genetics,* Washington, DC, 1993, ASM Press.

Turnbull PCB: Anthrax vaccines: past, present and future, *Vaccine* 9:533-539, 1991.

Chapter 8

The Genus *Corynebacterium*

Members of the genus *Corynebacterium* are actinomycetes that are related to the genera *Mycobacterium, Nocardia,* and *Rhodococcus.* The genus comprises aerobic gram-positive pleomorphic rods (Figure 8-1), often with a coccoid or club-shaped appearance, called diptheroidal after *Corynebacterium diphtheriae,* the agent of human diphtheria. *Corynebacterium aquaticum* is motile, but the remaining species in the genus are nonmotile. They are aerobic or facultatively anaerobic, catalase positive, non–spore forming and non–acid fast, with little tendency to branch. The cells walls of corynebacteria are singular in structure and composition; they are, in large part, the basis for the organism's ability to survive under adverse environmental conditions, including the skin. They contain corynemycolic acids, which are granulomagenic and may mediate intracellular survival.

Corynebacterium diphtheriae and *Corynebacterium ulcerans* are prominent human pathogens. *Arcanobacterium (Actinomyces, Corynebacterium) pyogenes, Actinobaculum (Actinomyces, Eubacterium, Corynebacterium) suis,* and *Arcanobacterium (Corynebacterium) haemolyticum* are former members of the genus. The notable animal pathogens (Table 8-1) are *Corynebacterium pseudotuberculosis,* a cause of lymphadenitis and lymphangitis in small ruminants and horses, respectively, and *Corynebacterium renale (cystitidis, pilosum),* opportunist agents of urinary tract infections in cattle and occasionally other species. *Corynebacterium pseudotuberculosis* and *C. ulcerans* can produce diphtheria toxin when lysogenized by corynephage β-bearing *tox.*

DISEASES, EPIDEMIOLOGY, AND PATHOGENESIS

For many members of the genus there is little more information than that presented in Table 8-1, especially regarding pathogenesis.

Corynebacterium renale Group (*C. renale, Corynebacterium pilosum, Corynebacterium cystitidis*)

Corynebacterium renale is considered to be normal flora of the lower urogenital tract, and, based upon incidence of disease, is the most important member of the group. *Corynebacterium pilosum* is also normal flora, and is a less common cause of cystitis and, quite infrequently, pyelonephritis (Figure 8-2).

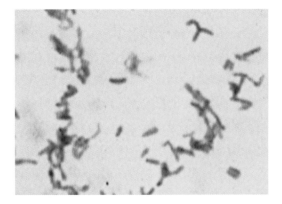

FIGURE 8-1   Gram-stained cells of *Corynebacterium diphtheriae*. (Courtesy J. Glenn Songer.)

TABLE **8-1**   Corynebacteria Encountered in Veterinary Medicine

Corynebacterium Species	Disease
C. diphtheriae	Human diphtheria; bovine mastitis and dermatitis (infrequent); isolated from an equine wound infection
C. renale	Bladder, kidney infections in cattle and swine; penis infections (pizzle rot) in castrated sheep; rare bladder infections in the dog; osteomyelitis in goats
C. cystitidis	Bovine bladder and kidney infections
C. pilosum	Bovine bladder and kidney infections
C. kutscheri	Lung, lymph node, liver, kidney abscesses in rats, mice
C. pseudotuberculosis	Ovine and caprine abscesses, lymphadenitis, abortion, arthritis; equine ulcerative lymphangitis, abscesses; bovine abscesses, mastitis (uncommon)
C. ulcerans	Bovine mastitis, abscesses: gangrenous dermatitis in rodents
C. bovis	Bovine mastitis (rare)
C. minutissimum	"Skin scalding" syndrome (tail, brisket, interdigital space in lambs); rare cause of bovine mastitis
C. camporealensis	Subclinical ovine mastitis
C. mastitidis	Subclinical ovine mastitis
C. capitovis	Isolated from skin scrapings of the infected head of a sheep
Group D2	Canine urinary tract infections
C. auriscanis	Canine otitis, dermatitis, and vaginitis
C. amycolatum	Bovine mastitis (rare)
C. testudinoris	Necrotic mouth lesions in tortoises

Corynebacterium cystitidis is usually associated with chronic pyelonephritis, but can cause more severe cystitis than the other members of the group; isolation from normal animals is rare.

Thus members of the *C. renale* group are opportunistic pathogens of the urinary tract of cattle and other domestic animals. These organisms cause cystitis and ascending pyelonephritis, a sporadic but nonetheless widespread problem in cattle. Herd incidence greater than 5% is apparently uncommon, and is typically nearer 1%.

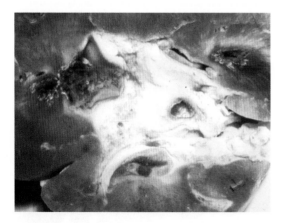

FIGURE 8-2   Bovine nephritis associated with *Corynebacterium renale* infection. (Courtesy Raymond E. Reed.)

Major risk factors are the shortness of the female urethra, effects of pregnancy and parturition, anatomic anomalies, physical damage, and obstruction of the urinary tract. Disease occurs most frequently in mature cows, and one quarter to one third of cases are fatal. Frequent relapses require additional treatment. Transmission may be venereal, but *C. renale* survives well in soil, possibly facilitating indirect transmission.

Colonization is pilus mediated, and the rapidly urease-positive nature of the organism leads to production of ammonia, with resulting mucosal inflammation. Cows with basic urine pH are at greater risk of developing pyelonephritis.

The clinical presentation of acute pyelonephritis includes fever, anorexia, polyuria, hematuria, pyuria, and abnormal posture (arched back). Infections that go untreated can become chronic, with weight loss, anorexia, and decreased milk production.

Posthitis (pizzle rot, sheath rot) is a form of preputial ulcerative dermatitis that occurs primarily in entire and castrated sheep and goats. The attack rate is rarely greater than 20%, and cases are often sporadic. The etiologic agents are *C. pilosum* and *C. cystitidis,* which are normal preputial inhabitants of these animals. Diets high in protein favor production of alkaline urine, with excretion of urea and production of ammonia by urease.

This leads to ulceration of the preputial epithelium, with predisposition to secondary bacterial infections. Wethers grazing rich pastures are at risk, as are breeding rams and bucks on high-protein forages. Ewes may develop ulcerative vulvovaginitis after exposure to diseased rams at breeding.

Mild ulcers develop at the preputial orifice, often within 1 to 2 weeks of a dietary change. If left unattended, the lesions may spread into the preputial mucosa, with subsequent crusting, swelling, and pain. Painful urination may mimic urolithiasis. Pooled urine and purulent exudate inside the prepuce may lead to necrosis, development of sinus tracts draining through the prepuce to the skin, and, ultimately, to chronic scarring of the preputial orifice. Sequelae include fly-strike, occasional obstructive uremia, and, rarely, death.

The first step in pathogenesis of pyelonephritis is corynebacterial attachment to the urethral epithelium. Bacteria grow readily in urine, producing cystitis and ascending (through vesiculo-urethral reflux) to the kidney, where in most cases infection spreads chronically and relentlessly. Virulence factors of *C. renale* and their roles in pathogenesis have, except possibly of pili, not been explored in depth. Renalin, a *C. renale* extracellular protein with a strong nonenzymatic affinity for ceramide (one product of the action of phospholipase C on sphingomyelin), may play a role in lysis of cell membranes. This protein is apparently not produced by *C. pilosum* or *C. cystitidis*.

Pili are produced by all three of these species. Rare and apparently minor antigenic cross-reactions have been demonstrated between pili of *C. renale* and *C. pilosum*. Piliated organisms are more resistant to phagocytosis by mouse neutrophils in vitro than nonpiliated organisms (in the absence of opsonizing antibodies), but are phagocytosed at a rate equal to that of nonpiliated bacteria in the presence of antipilus serum and complement. Phagocytosis of piliated bacteria by mouse peritoneal macrophages is likewise enhanced by complement and by antipilus polyclonal serum. Curiously, polyclonal antibodies prepared against nonpiliated bacteria also enhance phagocytosis of piliated bacteria, suggesting that nonpilus factors may play an antiphagocytic role.

Loss of pili upon repeated in vitro passage in the presence of antipilus antibodies has been reported. In vivo growth of *C. renale* in mice is apparently also selective for nonpiliated organisms that are present as approximately 0.1% of piliated cultures. This selection is evidently not significantly influenced by growth in mice with naturally or passively acquired antipilus antibodies. Furthermore, in mice infected with *C. renale,* no significant differences in mortality, number of culture-positive mice, or numbers of bacteria recovered from the urinary tract have been found in mice infected with piliated and nonpiliated bacteria, suggesting that pili are not an obligate factor in virulence of *C. renale* or perhaps that the mouse is not an appropriate model of bovine infection.

The role of humoral and cellular immunity in these conditions has not been investigated thoroughly. Circulating antibodies are present in cows that develop pyelonephritis rather than cystitis, but humoral antibodies in mice immunized with killed organisms are apparently not protective because these mice develop pyelonephritis upon challenge. Data suggesting a selection for nonpiliated clones in mice may explain this lack of protection. In a rat model, IgG is apparently the major component of the immune response to *C. renale* infection.

Corynebacterium (ovis) pseudotuberculosis

Corynebacterium pseudotuberculosis (Figure 8-3) is a facultative intracellular parasite that is most widely recognized as the cause of caseous lymphadenitis (CLA) in sheep and goats (Figure 8-4), ulcerative lymphangitis and ventral abscess in horses, and abscesses and mastitis in cattle. Disease in horses is sporadic in nature, except in geographically limited areas.

CLA, which is economically significant worldwide, is characterized by chronic abscessation of peripheral lymph nodes. Abscesses are lamellar

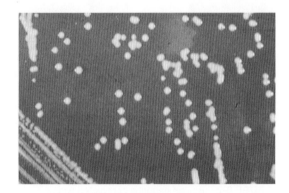

FIGURE 8-3 *Corynebacterium pseudotuberculosis* cultivated on blood agar. (Courtesy J. Glenn Songer.)

and filled with thick caseous exudate that may be slightly greenish. Extension to internal lymph nodes, particularly those associated with lungs, occurs at a variable rate and may be involved in transmission.

Prevalence rates of 30% to 50% in affected herds and flocks are not unusual, and the rate typically increases with advancing age. Lambs and kids are rarely affected beyond certain specific epidemiologic conditions (e.g., shearing and dipping of lambs with groups of infected ewes). Economic losses due to CLA arise from deaths (often following development of the "thin ewe syndrome"), carcass condemnations at slaughter, decreased wool and milk production during at least the first year of disease, decreased value of hides, and decreased reproductive performance.

Transmission occurs primarily through direct contact with contaminated shears, sheep dip, feeders, and feed. Recent findings suggest that congregation of sheep during shearing and dipping provides opportunities for aerosol transmission of *C. pseudotuberculosis* from lung abscesses to shearing wounds and abrasions. Organisms entering superficial tissues in this manner are phagocytosed and transported to regional lymph nodes, where uncontrolled intracellular multiplication leads to abscess formation. Phospholipase D (PLD) aids in the dissemination from primary to secondary sites, and anti-PLD antibodies are protective.

About 20 human cases of *C. pseudotuberculosis* infection have been documented, but anecdotal reports of axillary lymphadenitis in sheep handlers and veterinarians suggest that human cases may be more common than is realized.

Pathogenesis of CLA begins when bacteria, entering the host via skin wounds, multiply and are phagocytosed. Phagosome-lysosome fusion takes place, but *C. pseudotuberculosis* multiplies in the phagolysosome. If multiplication is sufficient, or if large numbers of organisms are engulfed, phagocytic cells die. Permeability of local blood vessels increases, encouraging spread of the infection from the initial site to other locations, often the regional lymph nodes. Abscesses may develop at either primary or secondary sites. Eventually these rupture and discharge a thick caseous pus containing large numbers of viable bacteria; direct transmission via these discharges (through animal-to-animal contact or via shears) and indirect transmission through survival of the organism in the environment probably represent the primary means of spread of the infection. Humoral and cell-mediated immune responses develop, and immune macrophages that infiltrate and engulf small numbers of *C. pseudotuberculosis* are able to kill them. Collectively the cells control and sometimes eliminate the infection, at least at the primary focus, although abscesses may recur at the same site. In some instances, lesions become metastatic (Figure 8-5)

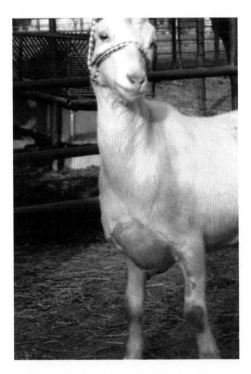

FIGURE 8-4   Caseous lymphadenitis manifesting as a chest abscess in a goat. (Courtesy J. Glenn Songer.)

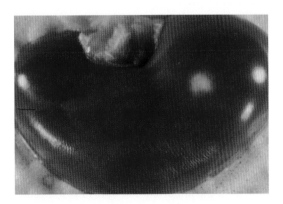

FIGURE 8-5   Kidney pyogranuloma in systemic caseous lymphadenitis ("thin ewe syndrome"). (Courtesy J. Glenn Songer.)

and, as they increase in number, the thin ewe syndrome develops, resulting in progressive debilitation and death. Generally the clinical and pathologic picture in CLA illustrates the dual role of granulomatous lesions in chronic bacterial infections: dissemination, but not persistence, is limited, and localized tissue damage occurs.

Intracellular survival by *C. pseudotuberculosis* is pivotal to eventual formation of abscesses and may be mediated by one or both of the organism's two major putative virulence attributes. Concurrent changes in bacterial viability and in the morphology of bacterial lipid external to the cell wall suggest that this lipid may facilitate survival in activated macrophages. However, the lipid is not systemically toxic for guinea pigs, which are highly susceptible to *C. pseudotuberculosis* or its exotoxin, suggesting that the lipid may be similar to mycobacterial cord factor in its toxicity for cells, but different in not being systemically lethal. Its exact role in pathogenesis remains unclear.

The second putative virulence attribute is a toxic PLD that is apparently produced by all isolates of *C. pseudotuberculosis* and *C. ulcerans*. Production of PLD in the early phase of infection apparently has profound effects on survival and multiplication of *C. pseudotuberculosis* in the host. This may be because of effects on phagocytic cells (inhibition of chemotaxis, degranulation, and lethality in PLD-treated neutrophils have been demonstrated) or complement depletion (PLD inactivates complement, reducing amounts available for opsonization of *C. pseudotuberculosis*). PLD-induced increases in vascular permeability may also play a role because increased permeability increases the extravascular circulation of fluid and facilitates spread of infection both locally and via the lymphatics. In fact, active or passive immunization of sheep against PLD limits movement of *C. pseudotuberculosis* from inoculation sites to regional lymph nodes in natural and experimental infections. If increased lymph node infection increases the incidence of lymph node caseation, then anti-PLD antibodies, by neutralizing the permeability-promoting effect of PLD, should have protective value against the disease in field situations. In fact, a number of workers have addressed the importance of anti-PLD immunity in protection of sheep or goats against *C. pseudotuberculosis* infection, and the results generally support the contention that neutralization of the effects of PLD has value in prevention of lesion development in sheep and goats. Cloning and characterization of the PLD gene and development of methods for genetic manipulation of *C. pseudotuberculosis* have facilitated the construction of isogenic Pld− mutants, which do not produce lesions of CLA in sheep or goats. Thus a direct and vital role for PLD in pathogenesis of *C. pseudotuberculosis* infections has been established; the exact nature of this role, particularly as it pertains to intracellular survival and multiplication, remains to be defined.

Corynebacterium ulcerans is best known as a cause of pharyngitis in humans, but is isolated with surprising frequency from cases of bovine mastitis. This organism is approximately 50% DNA–DNA homologous with *C. pseudotuberculosis*, and all strains examined by sensitive methods produce a PLD that is antigenically similar to that produced by *C. pseudotuberculosis;* the genes are approximately 80% DNA homologous. A matter of concern to public health officials is the capacity of *C. ulcerans* to produce diphtheria toxin when lysogenized by a phage carrying *tox*. Naturally occurring *tox*-positive isolates of *C. ulcerans* have been obtained from a variety of sources, including mastitic bovine milk. Infected cows may shed *C. ulcerans* for months or years in milk from a diseased quarter, and sporadic human cases of *C. ulcerans* infection associated with raw milk have also been reported. In a recent study, nearly 50% of isolates from milk samples produced diphtheria toxin. Clinical signs in affected cows were minor, but cell counts were high ($\geq 5 \times 10^6$/ml). In most of these cases, a sequel to the inflammation was permanent loss of the affected quarter.

Corynebacterium bovis

Corynebacterium bovis is a commensal of the bovine udder, where it adheres to the squamous epithelium of the teat duct. Up to 20% of the quarters of cattle in most dairy herds carry *C. bovis*. Growth of *C. bovis* is apparently enhanced in milk during lactation, but inhibited by mammary secretions during the nonlactating period. Inflammatory changes occur in the teat cisterns, Furstenberg's rosettes, and mammary parenchyma, but not consistently in teat canals. The basis of the negligible virulence of *C. bovis* has not been explored, but there is some interest in its ability to persist as a low-grade irritant in the udder, which, by provoking a mild neutrophil response, may protect the udder against infection by more virulent bacteria.

DIAGNOSIS

Bacteriologic culture and identification of isolates is appropriate in all forms of corynebacterial disease in domestic animals (Tables 8-2 and 8-3).

Pyelonephritis

Rectal palpation (to detect left-kidney infections) and vaginal examination (as a more sensitive measure of ureteral enlargement) can contribute to diagnosis. Demonstration of proteinuria and hematuria is useful; corynebacteria are sometimes isolated from urine, but *Escherichia coli* and other gram-negative bacteria are more likely to be found in chronic cases. Gross pathology includes multifocal kidney abscessation, dilated and thickened ureters containing purulent exudate, and cystitis.

Posthitis

Diagnosis is based on history, assessment of feeding practices, and examination of lesions. The differential diagnosis would include urolithiasis,

contagious ecthyma, and ulcerative dermatosis (lip and leg disease). The painful stance adopted by blocked males with urolithiasis is similar to that seen in moderate posthitis, but in the former, other signs indicative of urethral blockage will be seen, and ulcers will be absent. Lesions of contagious ecthyma typically involve the face and mouth, and ulcerative dermatosis is venereally transmitted and usually manifests as an epidemic, with animals developing ulcers on the face, prepuce, penis, vulva, and feet. Flock morbidity with ulcerative dermatosis can be high, and is not necessarily associated with high-protein feeding.

Caseous Lymphadenitis

Typical clinical signs and bacteriologic culture of abscesses allow unequivocal establishment of a diagnosis. *Arcanobacterium (Actinomyces) pyogenes* and *Staphylococcus aureus* may be isolated with *C. pseudotuberculosis,* or in pure culture from similar-appearing abscesses. The thin-ewe syndrome, and its equivalent in goats, may result from infection with other agents (e.g., internal parasitism, ovine progressive pneumonia, caprine arthritis-encephalitis, and paratuberculosis). The excellent sensitivity and specificity of an enzyme-linked immunosorbent assay may allow better

TABLE **8-2**   Colonial Morphologies of Corynebacteria of Veterinary Importance
(after 48 Hours' Incubation on Blood Agar)

Corynebacterium Species	Colonial Morphology
C. diphtheriae	Variable size, appearance; usually 1-3 mm diameter, gray, convex, translucent; narrow hemolytic zone possible
C. renale	Small, yellowish, circular, entire opaque
C. cystitidis	White, entire, circular, semitranslucent, usually very small
C. pilosum	Cream to pale yellow, entire, circular, opaque, ≈1 mm diameter
C. kutscheri	Small, yellowish or grayish white
C. pseudotuberculosis	β-hemolytic; white to gray; waxy, crackle in flame
C. ulcerans	Slightly hemolytic, tiny, staphylococcal in appearance
C. bovis	White to cream, circular, entire, slightly powdery or granular; 1-2 mm diameter
C. minutissimum	Circular, slightly convex, shiny, moist; ≤2 mm diameter
C. camporealensis	Nonhemolytic; 1-2 mm diameter; slightly convex, smooth, creamy consistency
C. capitovis	Circular, entire, convex, nonhemolytic; lemon pigmented, ≈0.5 mm diameter
Group D2	Nonhemolytic; pinpoint colonies after 48 hr incubation
C. mastitidis	Nonhemolytic, <1 mm diameter; rough, whitish, low, convex after 72 hr incubation
C. auriscanis	Not reported
C. amycolatum	Dry, waxy; crenate edges, whitish elevated centers
C. testudinoris	Entire, yellow

TABLE 8-3 Identification of Corynebacteria of Veterinary Importance

Corynebacterium Species	β-Hemolysis	Hydrolysis of: Esculin	Hydrolysis of: Gelatin (25° C)	Nitrate Reduction	Urease	Acid from: Glucose	Acid from: Maltose	Acid from: Sucrose	Acid from: Xylose
C. renale	Neg	Neg	Neg	Neg	Pos	Pos	Neg	Neg	Neg
C. pseudotuberculosis*	Pos	Neg	Neg	Var†	Neg (rare Pos)	Pos	Pos	Neg	Neg
C. bovis	Neg	Neg	Neg	Neg	Neg	Pos	Neg	Neg	Neg
C. kutscheri	Var	Pos	Neg	Pos	Pos	Pos	Pos	Pos	Neg
C. minutissimum	Neg	Neg	Neg	Neg	Neg	Pos	Pos	Var	Neg
C. cystitidis	Neg	Neg	Neg	Neg	Pos	Pos	Pos	Neg	Pos
C. pilosum	Neg	Pos	Neg	Pos	Pos	Pos	Pos	Neg	Neg
C. ulcerans*	Pos	Neg	Pos	Pos	Pos	Neg	Pos	Neg	Neg
C. capitovis	Neg	Neg	Neg	Neg	Neg	Neg	Neg	Neg	Neg
C. camporealis	Neg	Neg	Neg	Neg	Neg	Var	Neg	Neg	Neg
C. mastitidis	Neg	Neg	Neg	Neg	Var	Neg	Var	Var	Neg
Group D2	Var	Neg	Var	Var	Pos	Neg	Neg	Neg	Neg
C. diphtheriae	Var	Neg	Neg	Neg	Neg	Pos	Pos	Neg	Neg
C. auriscanis	ND	Var	Neg	Neg	Neg	Pos	Neg	Neg	Neg
C. amycolatum	Neg	Neg	Neg	Neg	(Neg)	Pos	(Pos)	(Neg)	Neg
C. testudinoris	Neg	Pos	Neg	Neg	Neg	Pos	Pos	Pos	Neg

*Further differentiate this species from other corynebacteria by streaking perpendicular to a β-hemolysin–producing strain of *Staphylococcus aureus*; *C. pseudotuberculosis* and *C. ulcerans* inhibit staphylococcal β-hemolysin (a reverse CAMP test).

†Equine and bovine strains are usually nitrate positive, whereas ovine and caprine strains are negative.

ND, Not determined; *Neg*, negative; *(Neg)*, most negative; *Pos*, positive; *(Pos)*, most positive; *Var*, variable.

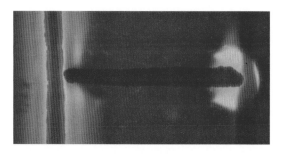

FIGURE 8-6 Inhibition of staphylococcal β-hemolysin (left) and synergistic hemolysis with *Rhodococcus equi* (right). (Courtesy J. Glenn Songer.)

management of the disease, detecting animals with internal abscesses or inapparent disease and in the screening of new introductions. *Corynebacterium pseudotuberculosis* produces synergistic hemolysis with products of *Rhodococcus equi* and inhibits β-hemolysis of *Staphylococcus aureus* (Figure 8-6).

Corynebacterium bovis Infection

Mastitis is a low-grade inflammatory process, and diagnosis by assessment of clinical signs or by somatic cell counts is not possible. The organism is isolated from affected quarters and identified by standard means. Standards for diagnosis are vague at best, in that the organism is so commonly found in the normal mammary gland.

CONTROL AND PREVENTION

Pyelonephritis

Penicillin or trimethoprim-sulfamethoxazole should be administered intramuscularly twice daily for at least 3 weeks. Urine should be examined by bacteriologic culture about 1 week after termination of antibiotic therapy.

Posthitis

Treatment should begin with reduction of total protein in ration to less than or equal to 12%, typically by switching from legume hay to grassy or mixed hay. Given this as a first step, mild lesions resolve spontaneously within a few weeks. In those requiring individual treatment, the wool should be clipped from the preputial opening and an antibacterial ointment or spray applied (5% copper sulfate solution flushed into the prepuce twice per week; penicillin-based ointments; 90% ethanol). Those severely affected should be given systemic penicillin. For scarring and phimosis,

a V section of the scarred portion of prepuce should be surgically removed. The prepuce of wethers, and of individual rams and bucks with recurrent problems, may be infused several times annually with an antiseptic solution to reduce the number of resident coryneforms.

Caseous Lymphadenitis

Infected animals should be isolated and the abscesses lanced, collecting the contents to prevent environmental contamination. The abscess should be flushed with 2% iodine or 30% hydrogen peroxide, and if it is large, it may be packed with rolled gauze soaked in 2% iodine. A portion of gauze is removed daily to facilitate drainage and proper healing. If not packed, the abscess should be cleaned with chlorhexidine or iodine soap and then flushed with iodine or peroxide. Antibiotic therapy is not generally recommended because of poor penetration of antibiotics into the abscess. If needed for a specific clinical presentation, penicillin is the antibiotic of choice.

The often difficult clinical diagnosis of CLA, as well as the poor prognosis for recovery, suggests the need for implementation of control measures. Regular disinfection of shearing blades in a cold sterilization solution is recommended. Fomites with the potential to cause wounds should be removed from the environment, and chronically infected animals should be culled. Two commercially available vaccines are Caseous DT (Colorado Serum Company, Denver) and Glanvac (CSL, Parkville, Victoria, Australia), both of which are sold as combination products with clostridial toxoids. Efficacy can be greater than 90% with natural challenge. Vaccination will often not eliminate the disease from a herd, but may decrease both incidence and prevalence.

SUGGESTED READINGS

Eggleton DG, Haynes JA, Middleton HD, Cox JC: Immunisation against ovine caseous lymphadenitis: correlation between *Corynebacterium pseudotuberculosis* toxoid content and protective efficacy in combined clostridial-corynebacterial vaccines, *Aust Vet J* 68:322-325, 1991.

Eggleton DG, Doidge CV, Middleton HD, Minty DW: Immunisation against ovine caseous lymphadenitis: efficacy of monocomponent *Corynebacterium pseudotuberculosis* toxoid vaccine and combined clostridial-corynebacterial vaccines, *Aust Vet J* 68:320-321, 1991.

Hayashi A, Yanagawa R, Kida H: Adhesion of *Corynebacterium renale* and *Corynebacterium pilosum* to the epithelial cells of various parts of the bovine urinary tract from the renal pelvis to vulva, *Vet Microbiol* 10:287-292, 1985.

Hodgson ALM, Krywult J, Corner LA, et al: Rational attenuation of *Corynebacterium pseudotuberculosis:* potential cheesy gland vaccine and live delivery vehicle, *Infect Immun* 60:2900-2905, 1992.

McNamara PJ, Bradley GA, Songer JG: Targeted mutagenesis of the phospholipase D gene results in decreased virulence of *Corynebacterium pseudotuberculosis, Mol Microbiol* 12:921-930, 1994.

Pepin M, Fontaine JJ, Pardon P, et al: Histopathology of the early phase during experimental *Corynebacterium*

pseudotuberculosis infection in lambs, *Vet Microbiol* 29:123-34, 1991.

Pepin M, Pardon P, Lantier F, et al: Experimental *Corynebacterium pseudotuberculosis* infection in lambs: kinetics of bacterial dissemination and inflammation, *Vet Microbiol* 26:381-392, 1991.

Sheldon IM: Suspected venereal spread of *Corynebacterium renale, Vet Rec* 137:100, 1995.

Songer J Glenn, Libby SJ, Iandolo JJ, Cuevas WA: Cloning and expression of the phospholipase D gene of *Corynebacterium pseudotuberculosis* in *Escherichia coli, Infect Immun* 58:131-136, 1990.

Chapter 9

The Genera *Dermatophilus* and *Nocardia*

THE GENUS DERMATOPHILUS

Members of the genus *Dermatophilus* are aerobic, gram-positive, branching, filamentous rods. They produce motile zoospores, and aerial mycelia are ordinarily absent (Figure 9-1). The substrate mycelium consists of long filaments that branch laterally at right angles. Septa are formed in transverse and horizontal planes and give rise to parallel rows of coccoid cells, often referred to as "railroad tracks." These organisms are catalase positive and non–acid fast.

Diseases, Epidemiology, and Pathogenesis

Dermatophilus congolensis is an obligate parasite of animals and affects many species, causing generalized exudative dermatitis in livestock. Dermatophilosis occurs in cattle in tropical and subtropical regions (Figure 9-2); disease in sheep is especially common in areas of high rainfall. Temperate breeds of cattle are more severely affected than tropical breeds. Economic losses derive from effects on production of beef, mutton, milk, hides, skins, and wool, and are especially notable in relation to cattle production in West and Central Africa and in the Caribbean, and sheep production in Australia.

The life cycle of the organism involves germination of cocci and production of hyphae that elongate through the epidermis and then undergo transverse and longitudinal division to produce filaments that release cocci. Motile zoospores develop from cocci and are released from wet

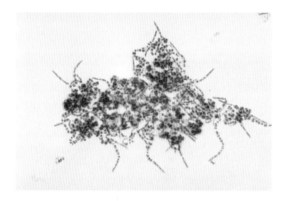

FIGURE 9-1 Clustering of *Dermatophilus congolensis* (Giemsa stain). (Courtesy Public Health Image Library, PHIL #2986, Atlanta, date unknown, Centers for Disease Control and Prevention.)

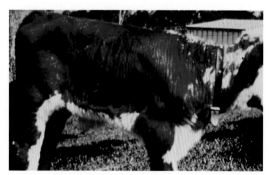

FIGURE 9-2 Bovine dermatophilosis. (Courtesy Raymond E. Reed.)

crusts to establish new sites of infection on the same animal or new hosts.

The infection is spread by contact (direct or via fomites) or by biting insects. Establishment of infection is affected by host genetic factors, and there is good evidence for effects of immunosuppression by *Amblyomma variegatum* ticks. Skin infections in sheep occur worldwide, and are basically mycotic dermatitis. Clinical disease is characterized by matting of hair or wool, and scab and crust formation, which can be substantial in chronic cases and lead to loss of hair or even skin. Crust forms by about 4 days after experimental inoculation and lesions resolve without treatment in about 4 weeks. Dermatitis of wool-covered areas is commonly called "lumpy wool." Infection can also involve the face and scrotum, and the sometimes severe ulcerative dermatitis of lower legs and feet is called "strawberry footrot." In its more severe forms, infection may result in deaths. Moist conditions promote disease development in sheep, and the same can be said of the disease in cattle, goats, and horses. "Rain rot" involves the superficial layers of skin and is characterized by the formation of crusts and scabs, varying in size from quite small to about 2.5 cm in diameter. In advanced cases, smaller lesions may coalesce, leaving large areas of skin affected. When examined microscopically, crusts have a palisaded appearance, with layers of keratinocytes, serous exudate, and neutrophil infiltrates, suggesting cycles of epidermal proliferation, invasion by *D. congolensis*, exudation, and influx of neutrophils. Intensity of cellular infiltration correlates with lesion severity.

Various factors, including pre-rainy season malnutrition, predispose to *D. congolensis* infection. Infection begins at sites where skin defenses are compromised by intense rainfall or by mechanical trauma, and wet weather facilitates dispersal of the organism from affected to healthy skin. Biting flies cause skin damage and initiate inflammatory exudation, which encourages bacterial growth and attracts flies that mechanically vector *D. congolensis* to new hosts.

Dermatophilus congolensis is hemolytic, and produces phospholipases and proteolytic enzymes. Infectivity has been correlated with production of extracellular proteases; most isolates produce these enzymes, with isolate-to-isolate variation in the number of enzymes and the quantity of each produced. Studies with inhibitors suggest that these are serine proteases; their alkaline pH optima may enable them to function in lesion development. Bovine skin is normally pH 5.6, but it becomes alkaline in the face of humoral components of the inflammatory response. Lipases and proteases may play a role in penetration of the epithelial barrier, including perhaps nutrient acquisition, inactivation of host inflammatory protease cascades, or hydrolysis of cytokines and other immune effector molecules.

A progressive, chronic form of bovine dermatophilosis occurs in animals infested with the ixodid tick *Amblyomma variegatum*; ticks and disease have similar seasonal and geographic distribution; tick control reduces the prevalence of disease. This association probably involves more than simple transmission of *D. congolensis* by *A. variegatum,* especially in that molting of larvae and nymphs between hosts augurs against mechanical transfer of *D. congolensis*. It seems likely that development of progressive disease is related to immunosuppression by factors in tick saliva.

Dogs, rabbits, deer and other ungulates, foxes, seals, and pigs are affected by scabs and hair loss. Cats are often infected by way of puncture wounds, and the resulting abscesses involve the subcutis, muscles, and lymph nodes, with chronic draining fistulas. The organism is also associated with ulcerative lymphangitis in cattle and ulcerative and hyperkeratotic skin diseases in lizards and alligators (Figure 9-3), and has been isolated sporadically from various skin diseases in monkeys, ground squirrels, and polar bears. Several cases acquired from animals have occurred in humans. *Dermatophilus chelonae* is a newly characterized organism isolated from skin lesions in chelonids (turtles and tortoises).

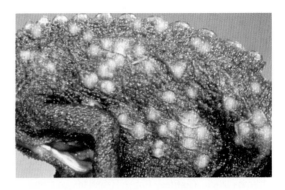

FIGURE 9-3 *Dermatophilus congolensis* infection in a lizard. (Courtesy Raymond E. Reed.)

Diagnosis

Diagnosis is based on the finding of morphologically compatible organisms in stained smears from clinical materials; conventional or fluorescent antibody stains may be useful. Gram-positive, branching segmented hyphae are seen, with hyphal elements larger and less regularly shaped than those of members of the genera *Streptomyces* and *Nocardia*. After 24 hours of incubation on solid media, *D. congolensis* produces tiny, grayish white round colonies that pit and adhere to the agar. Colonies may become orange after 2 to 5 days, and they are frequently β-hemolytic. Stains reveal segmenting, longitudinal and transverse filaments and coccoid spores that are often deep purple and in packets. Septation of hyphal elements results in formation of zoospores that are motile by way of polar flagella. Differentiation is by standard phenotypic assays (Table 9-1).

Immunodiagnosis of *D. congolensis* infections has been based upon crude and partially purified antigens derived from various morphologic phases of in vitro cultivated organisms. Results of such assays are often poorly reproducible, perhaps because of variation in preparation methods or among strains used as the antigen source.

Dermatophilus chelonae produces small, dry, adherent, umbonate colonies with two zones of hemolysis (an inner β and an outer α) after 72 hours of incubation on solid media. This species has a characteristic putrid odor.

Control and Prevention

Scabs should be removed with mild soap and water, followed by topical application of iodine or copper sulfate. Mild cases may resolve with grooming alone. The clinical course of dermatophilosis can be quite long, but when cleared of infection, reinfection does not occur. Vaccination has not been effective, but antimicrobial therapy is useful; penicillin and streptomycin, used together, are effectual, as are tetracyclines and chloramphenicol. Severely infected cattle may not respond to antimicrobial therapy, and the secondary bacterial infections or starvation that follows culminates in death.

Immunodominant proteins have been described, including one of 28 kD that may play a role in humoral immunity. Differences in resistance by different breeds of cattle may be the result of immunity to ticks or their effects, and efforts to develop a vaccine have been hampered by the strain-specific nature of acquired immunity to *D. congolensis*. Nonetheless, immunity, measured as an increased infectious dose and a shortened clinical course, has been demonstrated after infection or vaccination.

THE GENUS *NOCARDIA*

The suprageneric group of nocardioform actinomycetes are prominent causes of disease in humans and domestic animals. Nocardiae were first described by Edmond Nocard, a French veterinarian who isolated the organism in 1888 from cattle with farcy. Nearly a century later, reexamination of the original culture revealed both a nocardia and a mycobacterium. Subsequently, the etiology of farcy was attributed to the latter, which may have been *Mycobacterium farcinogenes*.

Members of the genus *Nocardia* were originally classified as fungi, based on presence of cell wall muramic acid, lack of a membrane-bound nucleus and mitochondria, and sensitivity to antibacterials. Nocardiae are strictly aerobic, nonmotile, pleomorphic gram-positive organisms. They do not form spores, and may take the form of rods, cocci, or diphtheroids, although they sometimes produce branching filaments and aerial hyphae. Nitrate reduction and catalase production are characteristic, and sugars are oxidized. Some are partially acid fast.

Like other aerobic actinomycetes, nocardiae are found commonly in soil, decaying vegetation, compost, fresh and salt water, and in animal feces. Approximately 12 species comprise the genus, including *Nocardia amarae*, *Nocardia brevicatena*, *Nocardia carnea*, *Nocardia pinensis*, *Nocardia*

TABLE **9-1** Differentiation of *Dermatophilus* species

| | *Dermatophilus* Species | |
	D. congolensis	*D. chelonae*
Acid from glucose	Pos	Pos
Growth at 25° C	Less	More
Nitrate reduction	Neg	Wk pos
Double-zone hemolysis	Neg	Pos
Putrid odor	Neg	Pos
Capsule	Neg	Pos

Neg, Negative; *Pos*, positive; *Wk pos*, weak positive.

seriolae, Nocardia transvalensis, Nocardia vaccinni, Nocardia brasiliensis, and *Nocardia otitidis-caviarum (Nocardia caviae); Nocardia asteroides,* the type species, together with *Nocardia farcinica,* and *Nocardia nova,* constitute the *N. asteroides* complex. *Nocardia asteroides* is found frequently in temperate regions, whereas *N. brasiliensis* is more common in tropical and subtropical areas.

Disease, Epidemiology, and Pathogenesis

Nocardia asteroides is the most frequently reported pathogen of humans and other animals, followed by *N. brasiliensis* and *N. otitidis-caviarum. Nocardia farcinica* has gained greater medical importance in recent years. *Nocardia brasiliensis* has been isolated from horses with pneumonia and pleuritis. *Nocardia salmonicida* is found in salmonid fish with granulomas in muscles and internal organs, and *N. seriolae* causes granulomatous disease in other fresh- and saltwater fish. *Nocardia otitidis-caviarum* is recovered most often from bovine mastitis and from ear infections in guinea pigs, but has also been associated with pneumonia and disseminated infections in other animals. Nocardioform actinomycetes isolated from cases of placentitis and abortion in horses in some areas of the United States have been placed in the genus *Crossiella,* as *Crossiella equi.*

Clinical signs of *N. asteroides* infection begin with the appearance of an indurated nodule or pustule, which ruptures and suppurates. Discrete lesions are often joined by sinuses, and chronic progressive disease follows in untreated cases. The organism is isolated from cases of acute or chronic mastitis in cows, with granulomatous lesions and draining fistulous tracts. Dogs and cats often develop localized infections, with subcutaneous lesions, mycetomas, and lymphadenitis (Figure 9-4). Nocardial stomatitis usually manifests as gingivitis and ulceration of the oral cavity, with the added gratification of severe halitosis. Thoracic nocardiosis in dogs often involves suppurative pleuritis or peritonitis, and abscessation of heart, liver, and kidneys; dissemination to the central nervous system (CNS), with multiple brain abscesses, is common. In horses, skin infection and lymph node abscessation are common presentations, with occasional respiratory or disseminated disease in immunosuppressed animals (Figure 9-5). Nocardial abortion occurs in horses and pigs, and infections in birds, foxes, koalas, fish, and monkeys have been reported sporadically. In humans,

nocardiosis takes subcutaneous and pulmonary forms; some human strains are neurotropic, and systemic disease often involves the CNS, frequently with fatal outcome. The incidence of pulmonary nocardiosis may be increasing because of decreased average immunocompetence in the population in general, and to a higher degree of clinical recognition. Nocardiosis is often associated with chronic obstructive pulmonary disease

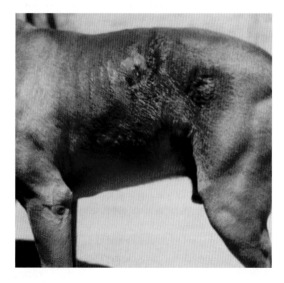

FIGURE 9-4 Canine nocardiosis. (Courtesy Raymond E. Reed.)

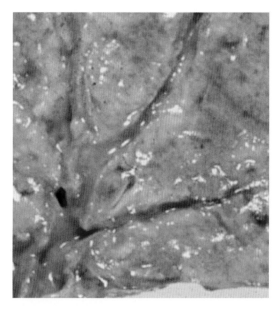

FIGURE 9-5 Nocardial infection in monkey lung. (Courtesy Raymond E. Reed.)

and acquired immunodeficiency syndrome (AIDS). Corneal infection sometimes follows trauma, and may be associated with contact lens wear and laser-assisted in situ keratomileusis (LASIK). Nocardiosis is not communicable.

Populations of cell wall mycolic acids, including trehalose 6,6'-dimycolate, contribute to virulence, perhaps by inhibition of phagosome-lysosome fusion in macrophages. Filamentous forms prominent in log phase are more virulent than the coccoid forms of stationary phase, perhaps relating to invasiveness. Membrane-bound catalase and superoxide dismutase are probably involved in resistance of nocardiae to killing by neutrophils. A secreted product of *N. otitidis-caviarum* is toxic for mice and may be involved in pathogenesis. Resistance to nocardial infection is poorly understood, but is likely primarily cell mediated.

Diagnosis

Presumptive diagnosis can be based on pathology and the presence of compatible organisms in clinical materials. The presence of gram-positive, acid-fast, branching beaded filaments in smears is suggestive of nocardial infection. Specimens for diagnosis of nocardiosis should be cultivated on blood or Sabouraud agar and incubated at 25° C and at 37° C for 4 to 5 days. The resulting cultures have an odor that can be described no better than "wet dirt," although this is unfortunately insufficient to differentiate nocardiae from many other organisms.

Microscopic morphology of nocardial cultures is best observed by in situ observation of undisturbed colonies in slide cultures on tapwater agar or corn meal agar without dextrose, incubated at 25° C for 2 to 3 weeks. Subsurface hyphae are fine filaments that are dichotomously branched at right angles. The presence of aerial hyphae differentiates the genus *Nocardia* from related genera; subsurface hyphae branching at acute angles are characteristic of some rapidly growing mycobacteria that do not produce aerial hyphae.

Colonies of nocardiae on blood or chocolate agar are small and indistinct after 48 hours of incubation. With extended incubation, colonies adhere to the surface of the medium, with the leading edge embedded in the agar. Isolates may be hemolytic on sheep or bovine blood agar, but most strains of *N. asteroides* are nonhemolytic. Colonies of *N. asteroides* may be salmon colored or orange-tan, with fringes of white to pinkish sparse aerial mycelium. *Nocardia brasiliensis* is much the same, but with a moderate amount of nonfragmenting aerial hyphae and soluble dark pigments.

Aerial hyphae of *N. otitidis-caviarum* are sparse and off-white; colonies are usually pale tan but may vary from cream colored to gray, peach, tan, or even purplish. *Nocardia salmonicida* produces an extensively branched substrate mycelium that fragments into rod- or coccoid-shaped elements, and diffusible pigments are absent.

Speciation is based upon phenotypic properties (Table 9-2). Tentative identification can be based

TABLE **9-2** Differentiation of *Nocardia* Species

	N. asteroides	N. brasiliensis	N. farcinica	N. otitidiscaviarum	N. salmonicida	N. seriolae
Esculin hydrolysis	Pos	Pos	Pos	Pos	Pos	Pos
Nitrate reduction	Pos	Pos	Pos	Pos	Pos	Neg
Urease	Pos	Pos	Pos	Pos	Pos	Neg
Casein hydrolysis	Neg	Pos	Neg	Neg	Neg	Neg
Decomposition of:						
Xanthine	Neg	Neg	Neg	Pos	Neg	Neg
Tyrosine	Neg	Pos	Neg	Neg	Pos	Neg
Growth at 45° C	Neg	Pos	Pos	Pos	Neg	Neg
Middlebrook's agar opacity	Neg	Neg	Pos	Neg	Neg	Neg
Growth in lysozyme broth	Pos	Pos	Pos	Pos	Pos	Pos

Neg, Negative; *Pos,* positive.

on their abilities to decompose casein, xanthine, hypoxanthine, and tyrosine. Mycolic acid–based speciation has been reported.

Diagnostic serology lacks specificity and sensitivity, in part due to antigenic heterogeneity among nocardial pathogens. Detection of antibodies in patients with systemic disease can be accomplished by indirect immunofluorescence microscopy and, more recently, by enzyme-linked immunosorbent assay (ELISA) or Western blot analysis against specific antigens.

Control and Prevention

Management of cases of nocardiosis often requires surgical débridement and draining of suppurative lesions. Antimicrobial susceptibility must be determined by a broth microdilution method, rather than by use of antimicrobial-impregnated disks in a conventional Kirby-Bauer test. Penicillin is not an effective therapeutic for any nocardial infection, and there is no effective antimicrobial therapy for nocardial mastitis. For other conditions, it is often possible to treat with trimethoprim-sulfamethoxazole, sulfonamides, novobiocin, ampicillin, or tetracyclines. It is often necessary to continue therapy for 12 weeks or longer.

SUGGESTED READINGS

Flores M, Desmond E: Opacification of Middlebrook agar as an aid in identification of *Nocardia farcinica, J Clin Microbiol* 31:3040-3041, 1993.

Isik K, Chun J, Hah YC, Goodfellow M: *Nocardia salmonicida* nom. rev., a fish pathogen, *Int J System Evol Microbiol* 49:833-837, 1999.

Masters AM, Ellis TM, Carson JM: *Dermatophilus chelonae* sp. nov., isolated from chelonids in Australia, *Int J Syst Bacteriol* 45:50-56, 1995.

McNeil MM, Brown JM: The medically important aerobic actinomycetes: epidemiology and microbiology, *Clin Microbiol Rev* 7:357-417, 1994.

Chapter 10

The Genera *Listeria* and *Erysipelothrix*

Members of the genera *Listeria* and *Erysipelothrix* are gram-positive, non–spore-forming, facultatively anaerobic rods. *Listeria monocytogenes* are small coccoid rods that occur frequently in chains. *Erysipelothrix rhusiopathiae* and *Erysipelothrix tonsillarum* are short rods with rounded ends, but also grow as long, nonbranching filaments. *Listeria monocytogenes* is catalase positive and motile, whereas *E. rhusiopathiae* is catalase negative and nonmotile (Table 10-1).

DISEASES, EPIDEMIOLOGY, AND PATHOGENESIS

Listeria monocytogenes

The natural habitat of members of the genus *Listeria* is probably decomposing plant matter, where they live as saprophytes. However, they are isolated from many environmental sources, and ruminants probably maintain environmental populations by continuous fecal-oral enrichment.

Until the mid-1980s, *L. monocytogenes* was, to human medical microbiologists, nothing more than a part of the arcane province of veterinary microbiologists and a model organism for study of the cell-mediated immune response. However, in 1985, listeriae in general moved to national prominence because of their role in extensive outbreaks of food-borne disease in humans. *Listeria monocytogenes* remains one of the most important causes of human food-borne illness; overall, it is the fifth most common cause of bacterial meningitis in the United States, but is second most important in neonates and in individuals older than age 60.

In the veterinary arena, *L. monocytogenes* is still a common pathogen; listeriosis has been described in more than 40 species of animals, but it is particularly in domestic ruminants. It causes central nervous system (CNS) infections in cattle, sheep, goats, horses, fowl, and dogs, as well as abortions and mastitis in cattle, sheep, and goats. Systemic listeriosis occurs in laboratory rodents, poultry, swine, cattle, and sheep. It is not uncommon as a cause of abortions and septicemia in horses.

Our understanding of the pathophysiology of listeriosis is mainly a synthesis of epidemiologic,

TABLE **10-1** Differentiation of *Listeria* and *Erysipelothrix* from Closely Related Gram-Positive Bacilli

Genus	Catalase	Motility	Esculin Hydrolysis	H$_2$S
Listeria	Pos	Pos	Pos	Neg
Corynebacterium	Pos	(Neg)	Var	Neg
Erysipelothrix	Neg	Neg	Neg	Pos
Lactobacillus	Neg	Neg	Var	Neg

Neg, Negative; *(Neg)*, most negative; *Pos*, positive; *Var*, variable.

clinical, and pathologic findings in natural cases and study of experimental infections in laboratory rodents; statements about events occurring in humans and domestic animals before association of *L. monocytogenes* with epithelial cells are mainly based on interpolation and extrapolation.

Disease in monogastrics is often mild or even asymptomatic. It commonly manifests as febrile gastroenteritis, a mild, influenza-like disease. More serious effects of infection occur in the form of invasive disease, especially in patients who are immunocompromised (in particular, those suffering from acquired immunodeficiency syndrome [AIDS], diabetes, or alcoholism). Renal transplantation and lymphoreticular malignancies are also associated with increased risk of infection. Such individuals develop meningoencephalitis, often accompanied by an ultimately fatal bacteremia.

Listeria monocytogenes–associated puerperal sepsis in humans is a flulike illness that occurs during pregnancy. Many cases in the 1985 food-borne disease outbreak in the southwestern and western United States were in pregnant women, most with disastrous consequences for the fetus. The organism is usually ingested and after crossing the intestinal mucosal barrier, causes bacteremia. It crosses the placenta (Figure 10-1), causing in utero fetal infection, resulting in stillbirths, preterm labor, and the birth of infants with systemic infection. Neonatal meningeal sepsis caused by *L. monocytogenes* occurs in two forms. Early onset disease is predominantly septicemic, with affected infants having low birthweight. These cases are often associated with obstetric complications and colonization of the maternal genital

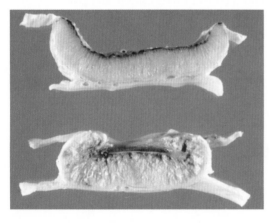

FIGURE 10-1 Placentitis caused by *Listeria monocytogenes* in the mouse model. (Courtesy Raymond E. Reed.)

tract by *L. monocytogenes*. Late-onset disease manifests mainly as meningitis and occurs in children of normal birthweight, usually without obstetric complications or genital tract colonization. Outside the neonatal period, the incidence of neural listeriosis increases with advancing age.

Disease in domestic ruminants mainly takes the form of meningoencephalitis, called circling disease in its most common form (Figure 10-2). The organism is found commonly in poor-quality silage (pH ≥5). Affected animals circle, in one direction only, and display unilateral facial paralysis, difficulty in swallowing, fever, blindness, and head pressing; paralysis and death follow in 2 to 3 days. If treated, less than 40% of animals will recover, most with permanent brain damage (Figure 10-3).

In pregnant animals, *L. monocytogenes* may localize in the placentomes and cross over to amniotic fluid. It multiplies there and is ingested by the fetus, eventually causing fetal death and abortion. Listerial abortion usually occurs in late gestation.

Although ingestion seems to be the most common route of infection, *L. monocytogenes* can also enter via the nasal mucosa and conjunctivae. It may find direct access to the nervous system by way of the dental plates of the trigeminal ganglia.

In milking cows, the mammary gland can become involved, resulting in subclinical mastitis and contamination of milk. The organism may then be spread to humans in unpasteurized dairy products; *L. monocytogenes* may also survive low-temperature pasteurization from its place of residence inside macrophages, and its lengthy survival in nature makes postpasteurization contamination a continual threat. The ability of *L. monocytogenes* to grow at 4° C is useful in diagnosis (see p. 92), but is an additional food-borne disease risk, in that the organism can multiply during production, storage, shipping, and marketing of dairy products.

Comparison of endemic and epidemic rates for human listeriosis suggests that in the gastroenteric form of infection, *L. monocytogenes* has lower virulence than other food-borne pathogens. This is consistent with the relatively high oral LD_{50} rates in mice and the large numbers often detected in outbreak-associated foods. However, the lengthy incubation period preceding invasive disease (suggesting amplification of a small inoculum), as well as the expectation of strain-to-strain variability in virulence and differences in host susceptibility, suggest that the infectious dose need not always be large.

Listeriosis can be usefully modeled in rodents and in cell cultures. As noted, murine listeriosis

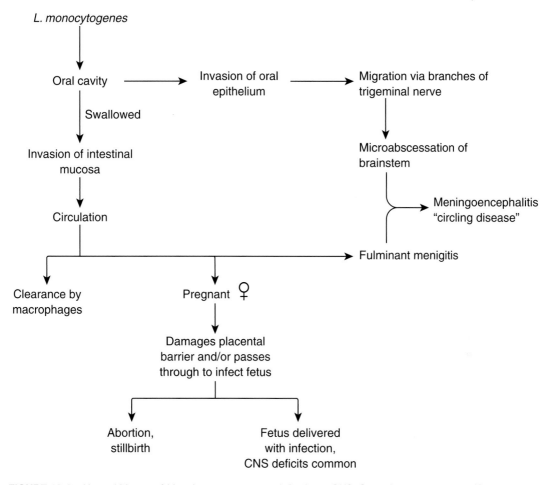

FIGURE 10-2　Natural history of *Listeria monocytogenes* infections. *CNS,* Central nervous system. (Courtesy Ashley E. Harmon.)

has been an important model of the cell-mediated immune response to bacteria; discovery of the activated macrophage response, as well as natural killer cells and cytotoxic T-cell activity against

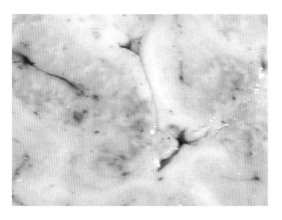

FIGURE 10-3　Ovine brain with focal lesions of listeriosis. (Courtesy Raymond E. Reed.)

intracellular organisms came from the study of *L. monocytogenes* infection in mice. The mouse model has also been used extensively in the study of pathogenesis. Infection by oral or intraperitoneal routes, in pregnant or nonpregnant conventional or gnotobiotic mice, has provided an exceptional platform for investigation of invasion, intracellular survival, and general pathogenesis of listeriosis. Listeriae invade intestinal and macrophage cell lines and produce plaques in fibroblast monolayers; much of our knowledge of cell invasion, intracellular survival, and cell-to-cell spread comes from studies in cultured cells.

As noted, exposure to listeriae is primarily by ingestion. In its gastroenteric form, invasion beyond the mucosa is limited, but when *L. monocytogenes* crosses this barrier, the liver is probably the first target organ. Multiplication there is eventually controlled by a cell-mediated immune response, which is probably maintained in most individuals by continual exposure to listerial antigens. Low-level bacteremia may result from uncontrolled multiplication in the liver of debilitated and immunocompromised patients, allowing invasion of brain and gravid uterus.

Virulence of *L. monocytogenes* is mediated by many factors. Flagella-mediated motility is unlikely to be important virulence factor, although actin-based motility is very important (see later). Little is known about adherence of the organism to target cells, although bacterial α-D-galactose residues may bind to receptors on intestinal cells.

Listeria monocytogenes and *Listeria ivanovii* are facultative intracellular parasites, surviving in macrophages and invading nonprofessional phagocytes, including epithelial cells, hepatocytes, and endothelial cells. M cells may be a target in vivo, although the organism may enter intestinal crypt cells, the only undifferentiated mucosal cells. Cellular uptake of listeriae is by induced phagocytosis, mediated by listerial membrane proteins called internalins. Specific mutation in the structural gene, *inlA*, eliminates invasion, and this deficit can be complemented by supplying *inlA* in trans. InlA has sequence similarity with the M protein of *Streptococcus pyogenes*, although functionally it *stimulates*, rather than inhibits phagocytosis, and may interact in similar ways with host proteins that have shared domains but dissimilar functions. Cell-to-cell spread, in cell monolayers or in the endothelium in vivo, apparently does not involve internalins.

Pathogenic listeriae have an intracellular life cycle involving escape from the phagosome, intracytosolic multiplication, actin-based motility, and lateral spread to adjacent cells. After entering epithelial cells, *L. monocytogenes* escapes the phagosome and multiplies in the cytoplasm. Exocytosis from the epithelial cell is followed by phagocytosis, by macrophages and neutrophils; multiplication in these cells is eventually lethal, and is followed by secondary phagocytosis and, in some proportion of infections, systemic spread. Beyond the epithelium, relatively little is known about pathogenesis of listeriosis.

The major virulence factor mediating intracellular survival is a cholesterol-binding cytolysin called listeriolysin (LLO). It shares 40% to 50% amino acid sequence similarity to other members of a family, sometimes referred to as thiol-activated toxins, and including streptolysin O, pneumolysin, perfringolysin, alveolysin, pyolysin, and others.

Common characteristics of this group are binding to cholesterol in cell membranes and oligomerization and insertion to form a transmembrane pore. An undecapeptide near the C-terminus is involved in these activities, as well as reversible inactivation by oxygen in most members of the group.

LLO is produced in varying quantities by all virulent strains of *L. monocytogenes*. Its importance in the process of invasion and spread of the organism is in its facilitation of escape from the phagocytic vesicle. The LD_{50} of LLO mutants is 5 logs higher than that of the wildtype, and the mutants do not survive in macrophages. *Bacillus subtilis* (which, in the wildtype, does not survive intracellularly) engineered to express LLO escapes the phagocytic vesicle and enters the cytoplasm of macrophages.

Regulation of production of LLO production and activity are important in that *L. monocytogenes* prefers to maintain intracellular residence; producing LLO at the same rate and with the same activity *after* phagosomal escape would be roughly the equivalent of an arsonist taking his work home. In fact, the rate of synthesis and secretion of LLO by extracellular bacteria (which includes the interior of the phagosome) is approximately 50 times higher than cytosolic bacteria, which secrete approximately 1 molecule per bacterium per minute. LLO is a major protective antigen, giving rise to major histocompatibility complex (MHC) class I–restricted cytotoxic T-lymphocytes (CTLs) in mice; it is immunodominant because it is rapidly degraded and efficiently processed into an MHC class I–associated epitope.

Listerial phospholipases also participate in the interaction of *L. monocytogenes* with cells. A phosphatidylinositol-specific (called PI-PLC, and encoded encoded by *plcA*) and a so-called broad-activity phospholipase C (PC-PLC, encoded by *plcB*) can hydrolyze most phospholipids in host cells. PI-PLC mutants are less efficient than wild-type organisms in phagosomal escape, which may account for the limited replication of *plcA* mutants in mouse peritoneal macrophages. PC-PLC is apparently involved in cell-to-cell spread of *L. monocytogenes*, enabling the organism to escape from the double-membraned vesicle in which it is enclosed after moving from one cell to another. Thus the functions of the two phospholipase Cs overlap during intracellular infection.

Many virulence genes of *L. monocytogenes* are regulated by a protein, PrfA, that may be a temperature sensor; genes controlled by *prfA* are expressed to a greater extent at 37° C than at lower temperatures, suggesting upregulation when the organism comes into contact with a mammalian host.

Bacteria, freed of the phagosome and living in the cytosol, polymerize actin, forming a tail and facilitating motility. A hollow mesh, formed on the bacterial surface, is left behind as the organism moves forward; actin is depolymerized and thus turned over. With this propulsion system, *L. monocytogenes* can move through the cytoplasm at the blistering pace of 1.5 μm/second. Actin polymerization is mediated by a bacterial protein, ActA, that localizes to the end of the organism on which the tail forms.

Bacteria encountering a plasma membrane continue to move forward, producing protrusions that extend into the adjacent cell. This eventually progresses to release of the organism in a double-membraned vesicle (one for each cell membrane); escape from this vesicle involves the action of PC-PLC, as mentioned. This lateral spread of the organism is seen in the plaques produced in monolayers of cultured cells. In vivo it probably serves to increase the population of listeriae, which escape to the gut lumen, returning to a saprophytic lifestyle, or are exocytosed on the basolateral surface of the epithelium, to participate in possible systemic disease.

Listeria ivanovii behaves in much the same manner as *L. monocytogenes*, except that it lacks the extraordinary degree of promiscuity in host selection; it is exclusively (or nearly so) a pathogen of ruminants. Human cases are rare. Other species, such as *Listeria seeligeri*, *Listeria grayi*, *Listeria innocua*, and *Listeria welshimeri*, may occasionally be isolated from clinical specimens (including at least one case of human listeriosis due to *L. seeligeri*), but they are considered to be soil contaminants.

Erysipelothrix rhusiopathiae

Erysipelothrix rhusiopathiae is found worldwide in tonsils and intestines of many species, including pigs, turkeys, sheep, and cattle. At one time the organism was thought to multiply in alkaline soil, but that now seems unlikely. Transmission is by way of direct contact with infected animals and fomites, and the mode of infection may be ingestion. The occurrence of *E. rhusiopathiae* in the surface slime of fish may imply its presence in fish

meal and suggests an additional means by which infection could be acquired by domestic animals.

Erysipelas affects mainly swine and poultry but is also found, in a variety of forms, in other species. The type of disease that follows entry of *E. rhusiopathiae* to the bloodstream of pigs probably depends to a considerable extent on immune status of individual. Swine 3 to 18 months of age are subject to outbreaks of bacteremia, with high case fatality rates if untreated. Diamond skin disease (also called the urticarial form of erysipelas) is characterized by the appearance of red to purple rhomboidal patches on the skin, and may be concurrent with, or may follow, the septicemic phase (Figure 10-4). Older pigs may experience arthritis, characterized by chronic, proliferative, nonsuppurative polysynovitis and polyarthritis (Figure 10-5). Cardiac involvement, usually in the

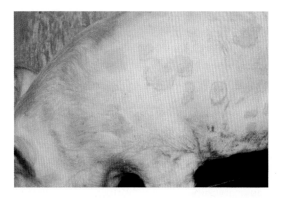

FIGURE 10-4 Typical rhomboid urticarial skin lesions ("diamond skin disease") in a pig inoculated intramuscularly with *Erysipelothrix rhusiopathiae*. (Courtesy U.S. Department of Agriculture, Ames, Iowa, National Animal Disease Center.)

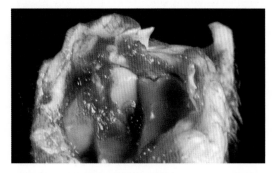

FIGURE 10-5 Synovitis and arthritis of hock joints of swine, with pannus extending across the articular surface. (Courtesy U.S. Department of Agriculture, Ames, Iowa, National Animal Disease Center.)

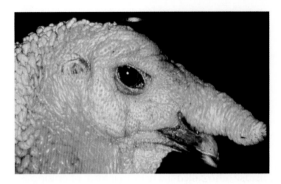

FIGURE 10-6 Swollen snood in acute turkey erysipelas. (Courtesy U.S. Department of Agriculture, Ames, Iowa, National Animal Disease Center.)

form of endocarditis, adds to the panoply of clinical presentations of erysipelas in swine. Urogenital erysipelas may occur in sows in herds where vaccination is allowed to lapse; in addition to pre- and postparturient vulval discharge in sows, evidence of disease includes longer farrowing interval and a reduction in the number of pigs born live.

Erysipelothrix rhusiopathiae is also an important cause of disease in fowl; turkeys, chickens, ducks, geese, and wild birds are susceptible. The infection in growing turkeys is acute, characterized by septicemia (Figure 10-6).

Sheep develop septicemia, as well as postdipping lameness as a result of extension of focal cutaneous infections to the laminae. The organism also causes nonsuppurative polyarthritis in lambs and calves; cattle can develop polyserositis, septicemia, and arthritis. Infected dogs experience arthritis and endocarditis, but infection is rare. Cetaceans and pinnipeds develop fatal septicemias.

In humans, *E. rhusiopathiae* infection is called erysipeloid, and usually occurs following occupational exposure of veterinarians, abattoir workers, butchers, and fish handlers. Infection leads to erythematous swelling at the site of entry, often followed by ulceration. Although infection usually remains localized, it can become systemic, taking the form of septicemia, endocarditis, or septic arthritis. Predisposing factors include malignancy, alcoholism, or concurrent use of steroids.

Pathogenesis of diamond skin disease may be the result of deposition of antigen-antibody complexes in the subcutaneous vasculature, with subsequent thrombus formation; the periarticular fibrosis that follows arthritis supports this contention. Activation of macrophages by cell wall

peptidoglycan may promote release inflammatory cytokines (such as tumor necrosis factor [TNF]-α), possibly potentiating generalized coagulopathy.

Toxins have not been demonstrated, but hyaluronidase and neuraminidase are produced by some strains. The latter may be involved in the etiology of the widespread hyaline thromboses that follow septicemia, by cleaving sialic acid on endothelial cell surfaces and promoting vascular damage.

Erysipelothrix tonsillarum has been isolated from the tonsils of healthy swine and must be differentiated from *E. rhusiopathiae*.

DIAGNOSIS

Infections by *Listeria* Species

Tissue from aborted fetuses, placenta, brain, mastitic milk, visceral organs (with lesions), and animal feed, as well as human food, is macerated and mixed 1:10 with a liquid nutrient medium (such as *Listeria* enrichment broth). This is incubated at 4° C, and subcultures are made (after 1, 3, 6, and 12 weeks) onto blood agar with phenylethanol (to inhibit swarming by *Proteus* spp.) or colistin and nalidixic acid as selective agents (Columbia CNA agar). Differentiation among species is made on the basis of standard phenotypic characteristics (Table 10-2).

Listeria monocytogenes produces a narrow zone of β-hemolysis around colonies that are translucent, 0.5 to 1 mm in diameter, and have a dewdrop appearance. Colonies of *L. ivanovii* are similar but with a more pronounced zone of β-hemolysis.

Infections by *Erysipelothrix rhusiopathiae*

A diagnosis of erysipelas can be confirmed by observation of compatible clinical signs, demonstration of small gram-positive rods in stained smears, and isolation of *E. rhusiopathiae* from appropriate specimens. Colonies of *E. rhusiopathiae* may be rough (usually from chronic infections) or smooth (from acute infections). They are small, mildly convex, circular, and transparent, with α-hemolysis (Figure 10-7). Identification is on the basis of phenotypic characteristics (Table 10-2).

The organism can be placed into three groups (A, B, and N), based upon agglutination reactions to detect somatic antigens. Group A organisms are usually found in acute disease in pigs, whereas groups B and N are found in cases of chronic disease. A typing scheme based upon cell wall

TABLE **10-2** Differentiation of *Listeria* and *Erysipelothrix* Species

Listeria and Erysipelothrix Species	Catalase	Motility (25° C)	β-Hemolysis	Camp Test: Staphylococcus aureus	Camp Test: Rhodococcus equi	Acid from: Rhamnose	Acid from: Xylose	Acid from: Sucrose	H$_2$S
L. monocytogenes	Pos	Pos*	Pos	Pos	Neg	Pos	Neg		Neg
L. seeligeri	Pos	Pos	Pos	Pos	Neg	Neg	Pos		Neg
L. innocua	Pos	Pos	Neg	Neg	Neg	Var	Neg		Neg
L. welshimeri	Pos	Pos	Neg	Neg	Neg	Var	Pos		Neg
L. ivanovii	Pos	Pos	Pos	Neg	Pos	Neg	Pos		Neg
L. grayi	Pos	Pos	Neg	Neg	Neg	Var	Neg		Neg
E. rhusiopathiae	Neg	Neg	Neg	Neg	Neg	Neg	Neg	Neg	Pos
E. tonsillarum								Pos	

Listeria spp. have a characteristic umbrella-shaped pattern of motility in sulfide-indole-motility (SIM) tubes incubated at room temperature; tumbling motility is apparent upon microscopic examination of wet mounts of cultures incubated for less than 20 hours; growth of *Erysipelothrix* spp. in gelatin stabs incubated at room temperature exhibit a "pipe cleaner" appearance

Neg, negative; *Pos,* positive; *Var,* variable.

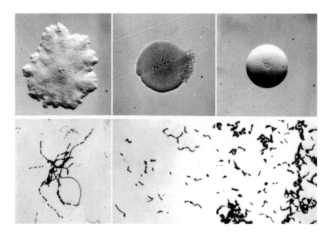

FIGURE 10-7 Colonial and microscopic appearance of rough *(left),* intermediate *(center),* and smooth *(right)* cultures of *Erysipelothrix rhusiopathiae.* (Courtesy U.S. Department of Agriculture, Ames, Iowa, National Animal Disease Center.)

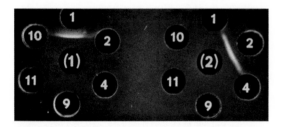

FIGURE 10-8 Serotyping of *Erysipelothrix rhusiopathiae* by immunodiffusion. Cell extracts are placed in the center well and specific antisera in the surrounding wells. Photo shows cultures of serotypes 1 and 2. (Courtesy U.S. Department of Agriculture, Ames, Iowa, National Animal Disease Center.)

antigens divides the species into 22 serotypes (group A is serotype 1 and group B is serotype 2), and is the preferred method for intraspecies differentiation (Figure 10-8).

CONTROL AND PREVENTION

Prevention of listeriosis is achieved primarily by management of silage quality. Some cases of listeriosis will respond to antimicrobial therapy; sulfonamides and penicillin may be of use for therapy or prophylaxis, but tetracyclines at maximum dosages are best. Therapy is often of little use, especially in animals that have begun to show neurologic signs.

Immunity to swine erysipelas is thought to be primarily humoral, and control of the disease is by vaccination with an attenuated live or killed vaccine. Turkeys may also be vaccinated. Hyperimmune equine serum can be used for therapy in outbreaks. *Erysipelothrix rhusiopathiae* is relatively resistant to environmental insults, especially for a non–spore former, and disinfection limits its accumulation in the environment.

Penicillin is the antimicrobial of choice for treatment of swine or turkeys. Erythromycin, cephalosporins, or clindamycin may be used to treat erysipeloid in humans allergic to penicillin.

SUGGESTED READINGS

Vazquez-Boland JA, Kuhn M, Berche P, et al: *Listeria* pathogenesis and molecular virulence determinants, *Clin Microbiol Rev* 14:584-640, 2001.

Wilkins PA, Marsh PS, Acland H, Del Piero F: *Listeria monocytogenes* septicemia in a Thoroughbred foal, *J Vet Diagn Invest* 12:173-176, 2000.

Chapter 11

The Genus *Mycobacterium*

Mycobacteria cover the range from saprophytes to opportunists to obligate pathogens, and have close relatives in other genera of pathogenic bacteria (Table 11-1). All members of the genus are aerobic, acid-fast, non–spore-forming, nonmotile gram-positive rods. They often stain irregularly and appear somewhat beaded. They are catalase positive. Many produce pigments, which are a means of classification and differentiation; scotochromogenic organisms produce pigments whether incubated in light or dark, whereas in photochromogenic organisms, light is required for pigment production (Figure 11-1). Most mycobacteria have relatively simple growth requirements. *Mycobacterium tuberculosis,* for example, can be cultivated in a synthetic liquid medium with only trace metals, asparagine, and glycerol. Rapidly growing mycobacteria produce colonies on solid media in less than 7 days, and slow growers require 7 to 14 days (or longer, if growth must be initiated from low-titer inocula), and, in some cases, as long as several months, to exhibit recognizable colonial growth. To put this in perspective, the generation time of *Escherichia coli* is usually accepted to be about 15 to 20 minutes, whereas that of *Corynebacterium diphtheriae* is closer to 60 minutes. *Mycobacterium tuberculosis,* on the other hand, completes a single round of cell division in about 300 minutes; *Mycobacterium avium* ssp. *paratuberculosis* is perhaps the most slow-growing of all the mycobacteria, in that cultures for diagnosis of Johne's disease are not discarded as negative until they have incubated for greater than or equal to 5 months.

Acid fastness refers to the ability of mycobacterial cells to bind phenol-based dyes (for example,

TABLE **11-1** Differentiation of *Mycobacteria* from Closely Related Genera

	Mycobacterium	Nocardia	Rhodococcus	Corynebacterium
Acid fastness	Pos	Weak	Neg	Neg
Aerial vegetative filaments	Neg	Pos	Neg	Neg
Growth rate	2-40 days	1-5 days	1-3 days	1-2 days
Mycolic acids	Pos	Pos	Pos	Pos
Arylsulfatase	Pos	Neg	Neg	Neg
Growth in lysozyme	Neg	Pos	Var	Neg
Sugars found in whole cells	Arabinose, xylose	Arabinose, galactose	Arabinose, galactose	Arabinose, galactose

Neg, Negative; *Pos,* positive; *Var,* variable.

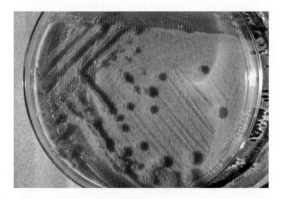

FIGURE 11-1 *Mycobacterium marinum,* cultivated on Middlebrook's 7H10 agar. (Courtesy J. Glenn Songer.)

carbol fuchsin in 5% phenol), typically when heated while staining; the dye is retained when the smear is subsequently treated with acidified alcohol. Whereas characteristic of mycobacteria, acid-fastness occurs in other genera of bacteria and even in certain life stages of some eukaryotes.

Complex lipids in mycobacterial cell walls include the mycolic acids, which are also found in related genera (Figure 11-2; see Table 11-1); acid fastness relates to the presence of peptidoglycan and glycolipids. This cell wall composition is also responsible for resistance of mycobacteria to drying, extremes of pH, and other environmental stresses. The complex, lipid-rich cell wall also protects the organism in the phagolysosome, and probably plays a major part in mycobacterial survival in macrophages. Furthermore, components of the cell wall are immunostimulatory, and are the basis for adjuvants, including Freund's complete and N-acetyl-muramyl-L-alanyl-D isoglutamine, or muramyl dipeptide (MDP).

Some mycobacteria are major pathogens of domestic animals, whereas others are encountered only occasionally (Table 11-2).

MYCOBACTERIUM TUBERCULOSIS COMPLEX

Members of the *M. tuberculosis* complex differ widely in host preference, phenotype, and virulence, despite 99.9% nucleotide sequence similarity and identical 16S ribosomal ribonucleic acid (rRNA) sequences. They are assumed to be derived from a common ancestor, yet some (*Mycobacterium tuberculosis, Mycobacterium africanum,* and *Mycobacterium canettii*) are almost exclusively human pathogens, whereas others *(Mycobacterium bovis)* are more cosmopolitan in host preference.

Mycobacterial evolutionary dogma has held that *M. bovis* infecting humans became host adapted, giving rise to what we now know as *M. tuberculosis,* and that conservation of housekeeping genes within the *M. tuberculosis* complex suggests that these organisms have been caught in an evolutionary bottleneck since the time of differentiation into species, possibly about 15,000 to 20,000 years ago. However, the availability of whole genome sequences for many of these organisms, and the advent of comparative genomics, promises to bring major changes in our view of evolutionary relationships among pathogenic mycobacteria.

Infection by *M. tuberculosis* is primarily a problem in humans and subhuman primates, but dogs, canaries, psittacine birds, swine, and many other species are susceptible to human tuberculosis. Feline cutaneous tuberculosis is associated with infection by *M. tuberculosis* or *M. bovis* and presents as multiple exudative ulcers and abscesses, in the form of pyogranulomatous dermatitis with

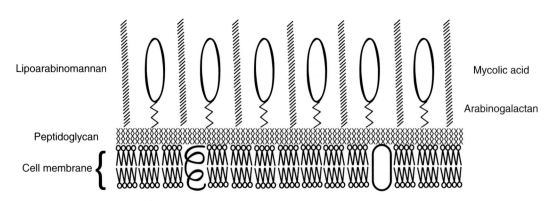

FIGURE 11-2 Schematic representation of mycobacterial cell wall composition. (Courtesy Ashley E. Harmon.)

TABLE 11-2 Mycobacteria of Veterinary Significance

Mycobacterium Species	Disease	Cultural Features
M. tuberculosis	Human tuberculosis	Rough, raised, thick; nodular or wrinkled surfaces; white to buff, very light yellow
M. africanum	Human tuberculosis (Africa); tuberculosis in primates, hoofed animals, dogs, swine, other species	
M. bovis	Tuberculosis in cattle, other ruminants; humans, dogs, cats, swine, rabbits, subhuman primates	Small, rounded, white, irregular edges, granular surface
M. bovis ssp. caprae	Caprine tuberculosis	
M. microti	Vole tuberculosis	
M. avium ssp. avium	Avian tuberculosis, swine mycobacteriosis (lymphadenitis); granulomatous disease (usually lymphadenitis) in cats, dogs, ruminants; disease in cold-blooded species; lymphadenitis, progressive disease in humans; rare intestinal lesions in horses, pigs, others	Transparent to opaque, smooth, "asteroid" margins; may become yellow with age
M. intracellulare	Swine mycobacteriosis, avian tuberculosis; isolated from mesenteric lymph nodes of cattle; granulomatous enteritis in subhuman primates (resembles paratuberculosis)	
M. avium ssp. paratuberculosis	Ruminant paratuberculosis (Johne's disease); associated with human Crohn's disease	Colorless to white, translucent
M. genavense	Tuberculosis in psittacine birds	Smooth, thin to transparent, nonchromogenic
M. scrofulaceum	Porcine lymphadenitis	Raised, rounded, pale orange
M. porcinum	Porcine lymphadenitis	Rough, buff-to-whitish colonies
M. simiae	Tuberculosis-like disease in monkeys, humans	Smooth, usually photochromogenic
M. ulcerans	Feline ulcerative/nodular skin lesions	
M. xenopi	Feline ulcerative/nodular skin lesions; porcine cervical, mesenteric lymphadenitis	
M. kansasii	Human lymphadenitis, lung disease; lymphadenitis in cattle, swine	Smooth to rough, colorless to buff; photochromogenic (bright yellow pigment)
M. marinum	Granulomatous disease in fish, other species (marine and freshwater); human granulomatous disease	Smooth to rough colonies; appear in approximately 7 days incubation at 30° C, more quickly at 25° C; brilliant yellow
M. fortuitum	Bovine granulomatous mastitis; piscine granulomatous disease; feline ulcerative pyogranulomatous skin disease; canine granulomatous lung and skin disease; porcine granulomatous joint and lung disease	Small, rough, buff colored, waxy, convex; entire edges; peculiar odors
M. peregrinum		
M. chelonae	Piscine granulomatous disease; tuberculosis-like lung lesions in turtles; bovine granulomatous lymphadenitis; feline, porcine abscesses, ulcerative lesions; lymph node abscesses, disseminated disease in monkeys	Small, rough, buff colored, waxy, convex; entire edges; peculiar odors
M. abscessus		
M. farcinogenes	Bovine farcy (Africa)	
M. senegalense	Bovine farcy (Africa)	
M. vaccae	Bovine skin disease	
M. smegmatis	Bovine granulomatous mastitis; feline ulcerative skin disease	Rough, wrinkled or coarsely folded, butyrous, glistening; nonpigmented or creamy white
M. phlei	Feline ulcerative skin disease (rare)	
M. leprae	Human leprosy; granulomatous disease in armadillos, other species	
M. lepraemurium	Possible cause of feline, murine leprosy	

caseous necrosis. *Mycobacterium tuberculosis* should be part of the differential diagnosis in any granulomatous disease of warm-blooded animals.

In the early 1800s, tuberculosis was an epidemic disease in the United States and Europe, with an annual death rate approaching 1% of the population in some cities. The incidence and prevalence of disease declined with improved living conditions, screening, and aggressive case studies to identify and deal with contacts; the availability of antimicrobials in the early 1950s provided another tool for dealing with the disease.

However, even at the times when the incidence and prevalence were lowest, tuberculosis made a major impact on human health worldwide: about 2 billion people were infected, with 8 million new cases per year. Tuberculosis caused more than 5% of the infant deaths, nearly 20% of adult deaths, and, perhaps worst of all, more than 25% of avoidable deaths.

Regardless, success in decreasing incidence of tuberculosis pushed it into the shadows of the public health enterprise in the United States; research, screening, and drug discovery were essentially halted in favor of topics considered more important. Dismantling of antituberculosis programs left physicians and public health officials unprepared to deal with the disease, in large part because of an erosion of diagnostic capabilities. In this environment of neglect, the incidence of tuberculosis has made well-publicized increases, and is once again a major focus of public health concern and infectious disease research. Part of this is a result of failures in management of screening programs for tuberculosis in immigrants from endemic countries; at one time, fully one quarter of new tuberculosis cases in United States were in immigrants. The increase in prevalence was encouraged by crowded conditions in homeless shelters and prisons, and by the increased susceptibility of substance abusers and patients with acquired immunodeficiency syndrome (AIDS). In developing countries, the incidence of tuberculosis is higher in AIDS patients than in the noninfected population, and the time from exposure to shedding is greatly shortened, facilitating rapid spread of infection. Drug resistance had been a problem since the early days of streptomycin use, but this became worse with the emergence of multidrug resistance. The case fatality rate of untreated tuberculosis can be as high as 50%, and the arising of untreatable strains through mutation to drug resistance presents a serious public health concern. Other infectious diseases have received significantly greater press coverage and political attention, but few have had the sustained negative impact on human health of *M. tuberculosis* infection.

Pathogenesis

Mycobacterium tuberculosis can infect any area of body, including bones, joints, liver, spleen, gastrointestinal tract, and brain. In these sites its preferred residence is within cells of the reticuloendothelial system. Tuberculosis is not normally a rapidly developing disease, but is rather, if untreated, associated with years of declining health, culminating in death. The pace of the clinical course is more rapid in the immunocompromised, often lasting only a few months, and with a case fatality rate of nearly 80%. The disease is also not highly contagious, but transmission occurs with prolonged contact between susceptible individuals and an active case. Transmission is usually by the airborne route, and bacteria-bearing droplets must be of a size and mass to allow them to penetrate deep into the respiratory tree and impinge into mucus overlying the epithelium. Infection can occur by other routes, as well; ingestion of the organism can lead to infection through cervical or mesenteric lymph nodes. Individuals developing tuberculosis experience fever, cough (often with bloody sputum), malaise, and anorexia, with progressive, irreversible lung destruction.

Regardless of the route of infection, the organism is phagocytosed by macrophages, probably following complement-mediated opsonization. Defense of the lungs centers, of course, on the work of pulmonary alveolar macrophages; survival and multiplication of *M. tuberculosis* in phagocytes is the key factor in development of disease. Phagosome-lysosome fusion occurs, but the organisms either escape to the cytoplasm or simply multiply within the phagolysosome, eventually causing it to burst. Part of the success of *M. tuberculosis* in this endeavor lies in its ability to prevent acidification of the phagosome, which decreases the killing capacity of phagocytes. Mycobacteria in general are relatively resistant to the bactericidal mechanisms of professional phagocytes, with resistance to reactive oxygen intermediates associated with catalase, peroxidase, and alkyl hydroperoxidase reductase production; the last also mediates resistance to reactive nitrogen intermediates. Mycobacterial sulfolipids may inhibit phagosome:lysosome fusion and potentiate the cord factor–induced inhibition of oxidative phosphorylation in mitochondria. Phenolic glycolipids in the cell wall scavenge and detoxify oxygen radicals. Furthermore, *M. tuberculosis* produces compounds that may interfere with T-cell activation. Lipoarabinomannan, a mycobacterial cell wall glycolipid, suppresses T-cell proliferation, blocks transcriptional activation of interferon (IFN)-γ–inducible genes in macrophages cell lines, and might prevent macrophage activation by IFN-γ. A fibronectin-binding protein may be involved in fibronectin depletion, making it unavailable for binding and stimulation of T cells and interfering with the activated macrophage response.

The ability to mount a rapid and effective activated macrophage response determines the outcome of an encounter with *M. tuberculosis*. The immune system effectively contains the infection, and less than 10% of those infected develop disease. In healthy adults exposed to relatively low numbers of mycobacteria, the immune response stops the infection before appreciable damage to the lung, and, although the patient will likely become skin-test positive, symptomatic tuberculosis does not develop. In many cases *M. tuberculosis* is not eradicated but is contained in discrete lesions, and disease may develop through reactivation when resistance is weakened.

The immune response to *M. tuberculosis* is T-cell dependent, but the immune mechanisms of acquired resistance are associated with activation of macrophages by cytokines and direct cytolytic activity. The initial interaction between *M. tuberculosis* and macrophages elicits a T-helper (CD4) cell response; the Th2 subset mediates antibody production that has been repeatedly shown to have no role in protection against or recovery from infection. The main contribution of CD4 T cells is by those of subset Th1, which release IFN-γ, stimulating activation of macrophages, which then ingest and kill mycobacteria. IFN-γ also stimulates endothelial binding and emigration of T cells, allowing them to converge on the infected area; transgenic mice incapable of producing IFN-γ are much more susceptible than the wildtype to *M. tuberculosis* infection. The CD8 response yields cytotoxic T cells that kill and disrupt infected phagocytes. In addition, gamma-delta T cells recognize phospholigands and CD1-restricted T cells recognize glycolipids, both of which are plentiful in the mycobacterial cell wall.

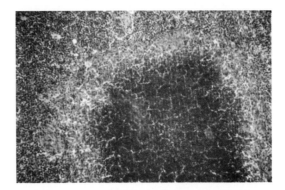

FIGURE 11-3 Hematoxylin and eosin–stained section of a tubercle in a case of bovine tuberculosis. (Courtesy J. Glenn Songer.)

If the immune response is delayed or nonexistent, viable *M. tuberculosis* may reach regional lymph nodes and even pass farther by way of lymphatics and the bloodstream, to distant tissues, nearly always within macrophages. Most bacteria, however, are contained locally, in a specific type of granuloma called a tubercle (Figure 11-3); layers of T cells, neutrophils, macrophages, multinucleated giant cells, and a thick fibrin coat form around growing foci of necrosis and sometimes wall off the lesion. Calcified tubercles appear as lesions in chest radiographs. The walled-off lesions may contain viable bacteria, leaving open the possibility of reactivation tuberculosis.

Mechanisms of tissue destruction in tuberculosis are not fully understood, but certainly involve local and systemic inflammatory responses. Cord factor (trehalose 6,6'-dimycolate), a component of the mycobacterial cell wall, is systemically lethal, inactivates phagocyte mitochondria, and inhibits macrophage chemotaxis. Lung damage may also result from the action of TNF-α, which accumulates in response to mycobacterial cell wall components; injection of TNF-α into lungs causes damage suggestive of tuberculosis, and administration of antibodies against TNF-α reduces lung damage in infected animals without affecting bacterial growth.

Laboratory Diagnosis of Tuberculosis

Diagnosis is based in part on microscopic examination of acid-fast–stained sputum smears. Fluorochrome stains (auramine O-acridine orange) are also useful, and evidence suggests that they are more sensitive than traditional acid-fast stains. Bacteriologic culture of appropriate specimens is imperative, both to confirm the etiology and allow for sensitivity testing. Isolation is facilitated by the resistance of the organism to disinfectants and extremes of pH. Steps in the procedure may include treatment with N-acetyl L-cysteine (to liquefy sputum samples), exposure to high pH, or disinfection with quaternary ammonium compounds. Culture is often on inspissated egg-based media (such as Lowenstein-Jensen), agar-based egg media (such as Herrold's medium), or non-egg media (such as Middlebrook's 7H10), prepared as slants to allow humidity control. Mature colonies become apparent after 14 to 21 days' incubation.

The diagnostic key to rapid surveillance has been the intradermal skin test. Tuberculin (a crude extract of the *M. tuberculosis* cell wall) or purified protein derivative (PPD) injected intradermally stimulates cytokine secretion by preprimed CD4 T-helper cells, which in turn recruits neutrophils, mononuclear cells, and macrophages to the site. If erythema and induration follow, the test is positive. Conversion to positive occurs within about 1 month of exposure to *M. tuberculosis,* and is associated with immunization. Many with active tuberculosis, especially disseminated disease, convert to skin-test negative, in an immune phenomenon that can be specific for reactivity to tuberculin or PPD, rather than a general decrease in immune competence. However, any general decrease in immune competence can convert a positive skin test to negative. The current recommendation is that recent converters take the full course of therapy for tuberculosis.

Immunization Against Human Tuberculosis

Immunization is widely practiced in many countries through the use of the controversial BCG vaccine. It is based on the attenuated Bacillus of Calmette and Guérin strain of *M. bovis;* given orally, it is safe even for infants and is inexpensive enough for use in any setting. However, its effectiveness has been repeatedly questioned because results in field trials have been mixed. It may be more effective in preventing cases following new exposure than at interfering with reactivation.

Treatment of Tuberculosis

Antimicrobial therapy has been accomplished with streptomycin, isonicotinic acid hydrazide (isoniazid, INH), rifampin, ethionamide, pyrazinamide, ethambutol, and para-aminosalicylic acid (PAS), and newer therapies employing fluoroquinolones (such as sparfloxacillin) have been rapidly compromised by the appearance of resistance. Resistance to streptomycin, isoniazid, ethionamide, and rifampin occurs at high frequency and is the basis for the recommendation that treatment never be based on a single antimicrobial. Use of combinations of antimicrobials, such as INH and rifampin, carries a treatment success rate of more than 90%, even in patients with AIDS. When multiply-resistant strains are involved, the case fatality rate approaches 50% in immunologically intact patients and 80% in the immunocompromised.

MYCOBACTERIUM AFRICANUM

Mycobacterium africanum is another member of the tuberculosis complex and a cause of tuberculosis. Current evolutionary thought is that modern *M. tuberculosis* and *M. canettii* strains are more direct descendants of progenitor tubercle bacilli and that *M. africanum,* with *Mycobacterium microti* and *M. bovis,* diverged from this lineage. This apparently supersedes the earlier dogma that *M. tuberculosis* evolved from *M. bovis.*

MYCOBACTERIUM BOVIS

Mycobacterium bovis is best known as the cause of tuberculosis in cattle and other ruminants, but it also infects humans, swine, and other animals. Clinical disease occurs only in a small proportion of cattle that are exposed to *M. bovis* (Figure 11-4); most animals clear the infection, possibly resulting

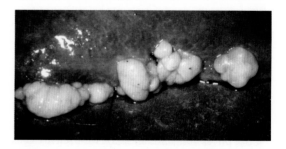

FIGURE 11-4 *Mycobacterium bovis* infection at the margin of a bovine liver. (Courtesy J. Glenn Songer.)

in latency. Molecular epidemiology has a key role to play in furthering our understanding of *M. bovis* and bovine tuberculosis, including addressing issues of transmission (direct, via the inanimate environment, or involving wildlife reservoirs). Strain differences in antigenic makeup and stability, virulence, and transmissibility impact interpretation of field data, and *M. bovis* ssp. *caprae* is of uncertain importance. White-tailed deer are reservoir hosts of bovine tuberculosis. The most likely associated factor is congregation of deer in artificially high numbers at feed sites.

In humans, *M. bovis*–associated disease often begins with infection of cervical and mesenteric lymph nodes, with systemic metastases that often affect joints and bones. A popular historical reference is to individuals infected in childhood by consumption of milk from tuberculous cows, who developed, as a result, severe postural abnormalities, illustrated in literature by Victor Hugo in *The Hunchback of Notre Dame*. Infections may also be pulmonary if initiated by inhalation of the organism. In the United States, eradication of bovine tuberculosis was begun in 1917, and is nearly complete. Most states have achieved and maintain tuberculosis-free status, but some have occasional or continual disease incidents.

Vaccination against bovine tuberculosis could be important in areas where *M. bovis* infection persists in wildlife and in countries where a "test and slaughter" program would have devastating economic effects. Results of some field trials with a BCG vaccine have been mainly disappointing, in that animals readily convert to tuberculin skin-test positive but are afforded little, if any, protection. Other experimental studies, with different doses of BCG and with other attenuated strains of *M. bovis*, have been more encouraging and may lead to prevention of spread of the disease in the field.

The apparently identical clinical disease caused by both in humans and the extensive genetic similarities suggest that many virulence factors of *M. bovis* and *M. tuberculosis* coincide. Virulence of *M. bovis* resides in part in its cell wall lipids (mycosides, phospholipids, and sulpholipids) that protect the organism from effects of phagocytosis and glycolipids that mediate the host's granulomatous response and enhance intracellular survival; wax D and various tuberculoproteins induce a delayed hypersensitivity reaction detected in the tuberculin test.

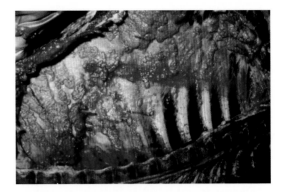

FIGURE 11-5   Advanced bovine tuberculosis, with granulomatous lesions on interior of rib cage. (Courtesy J. Glenn Songer.)

Infection of cattle is usually via the respiratory and intestinal tracts; local multiplication, survival in phagocytes, and transport to regional lymph nodes is followed by entry to systemic circulation by way of the thoracic duct. Cell-mediated immune reactions gradually strengthen the host response; activated macrophages kill some organisms, lesions are encompassed by a fibrous layer, and caseous necrosis at the center becomes calcified (see Figure 11-3). Lymphatic spread is slowed, but infection may continue to disseminate by erosion of bronchi, blood vessels, or visceral organs (Figures 11-4 and 11-5). T-cell–mediated reactions may participate in tissue damage. Hematogenous dissemination leads to miliary tuberculosis, especially in deer, which is characterized by multifocal tubercle formation in organs or on serosal surfaces.

MYCOBACTERIUM AVIUM SSP. AVIUM

Mycobacterium avium is subdivided into subspecies *avium* (*M. avium*), *paratuberculosis* (*Mycobacterium paratuberculosis*), and *silvaticum* (*Mycobacterium silvaticum*). Subspecies *paratuberculosis* can be differentiated from *M. avium* and *M. silvaticum* by its mycobactin-dependent phenotype and by its multiple copies of insertion sequence IS*900*.

Mycobacterium intracellulare is commonly grouped with *M. avium,* in the *Mycobacterium avium-intracellulare* complex (MAC), but it is a genetically distinct species. These organisms are found widely in soil and water, and are not readily distinguishable based on phenotype. Both cause disease in animals and humans, and *M. avium* is a predominant isolate from AIDS patients and from infections in swine and cattle. MAC isolates fall into 28 serovars, with *M. avium* comprising serovars 1 to 6, 8 to 11, and 21, and *M. intracellulare* falling into serovars 7, 12 to 20, and 25. Serovars 22 to 24 and 26 to 28 may be *M. intracellulare, Mycobacterium scrofulaceum,* and others. Serovars 1 through 3 are "typical" avian tubercle bacilli found commonly in tuberculous lesions in birds, but serovars 4 to 21 produce minimal disease, even in response to experimental IV or IP inoculation.

Disease in cattle often involves mesenteric lymph nodes, and may sensitize them to tuberculin; bovine skin testing is done on a comparative basis, examining the reactions to both bovine and avian PPD.

Historically, the primary causative agents of swine mycobacteriosis were *M. bovis* (when bovine tuberculosis was more prominent, and pig-to-cattle contact was common) and *M. tuberculosis* (when human tuberculosis was more prevalent). As early as 1925, however, *M. avium* ssp. *avium* began to appear more frequently in swine with mycobacteriosis. This trend has continued, and today *M. avium* ssp. *avium* is the most important cause of mycobacterial infection in pigs. Infection by *M. avium* ssp. *avium* certainly occurs today, but its impact on the swine industry is greatly diminished by the major changes in production and housing methods of the past 25 years. *Mycobacterium porcinum* and *M. scrofulaceum* have also been associated with lymphadenitis in swine. Porcine *Rhodococcus equi* infections can be confused with *M. avium* ssp. *avium* infection on gross examination, but are readily distinguishable on bacteriologic culture.

By industry preference, this condition is referred to as mycobacteriosis, rather than tuberculosis; granulomatous lesions associated with the disease have, in fact, all the characteristics of a tubercle, but there are important differences in the manifestations of infection in the host and in potential public health impacts. Typical swine mycobacteriosis has no apparent effects on the health of the animal, and there is no evidence for transmission from pigs to humans. However, meat inspection regulations have been promulgated on the lack of evidence that the infection cannot be transmitted, and economic factors are based on the end result of these regulations.

Pigs usually become infected by ingestion. The organism passes through the mucosal epithelium and is transported by macrophages, usually to cervical and mesenteric lymph nodes. Granulomagenesis occurs in these nodes, but infection rarely goes beyond this initial site. The health and condition of the pig remain unaffected in most cases, and it is rarely possible to diagnose porcine mycobacteriosis based on clinical signs. However, lymph node lesions found at slaughter require condemnation of the affected part (heads for cervical lymph node lesions and viscera for mesenteric lymph node lesions) or the entire carcass (for lesions in two discrete locations). Condemned carcasses can be "passed for cooking" if a processing plant is so equipped, but they nonetheless lose most of their economic value.

Pig-to-pig transmission may occur, as a result of shedding of the organism from lesions in the intestinal wall, although this is likely responsible for only a small percentage of cases. Epidemiologic studies have shown that sawdust or wood shavings used for bedding may be a source of infection, and *M. avium* ssp. *avium* can be isolated from these and other wood products. Soil contaminated by tuberculous chickens is another possible reservoir.

Diagnosis can be safely based upon detection of compatible gross and microscopic lesions and isolation of *M. avium* ssp. *avium.* DNA-based methods are now considered the gold standard for detection of MAC serovars. Insertion sequences (IS) in MAC strains include IS*900* in *M. avium* ssp. *paratuberculosis,* IS*902* in *M. avium* ssp. *silvaticum,* IS*901,* IS*1110,* IS*1245,* and IS*1311* in *M. avium,* and IS*1141* in *M. intracellulare,* and their pattern of occurrence has been used for detection of the organisms and for study of relatedness among strains. Skin testing can be accomplished by ID injection of 0.1 ml of the avian tuberculin or PPD in the dorsal surface of the ear, with reactions recorded after 48 hours (Figure 11-6). Positive reactions are of variable size and intensity but usually include swelling and redness. The skin test is useful as a herd test, but its reliability for testing of individual animals is in question.

Prevention and control efforts are based first upon excluding the disease from noninfected herds. Swine and poultry production should not be mixed, and feeding uncooked food waste should be avoided. Some feel strongly that breeding stock should be purchased from mycobacteriosis-free herds, but there is little evidence to support this position. Herds affected by mycobacteriosis can

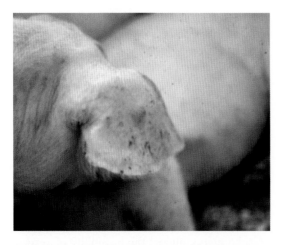

FIGURE 11-6 Positive skin test in a *Mycobacterium avium*–infected pig. (Courtesy J. Glenn Songer.)

be depopulated as a control measure, but unless the source is identified and neutralized, the disease may recur on repopulation. Type of bedding should be examined as a possible source. Concrete surfaces and equipment can be disinfected with a phenol-based disinfectant. Another approach to control is based on the fact that lesions caused by *M. avium* ssp. *avium* usually disappear with age, so gilts that might be passed for cooking or condemned at slaughter can serve a useful function for the producer and perhaps be mycobacteriosis-free when sent to slaughter as retired breeders. Some producers have made heroic efforts to rid their hog lots of wild birds by pyrotechnic or firearm-based methods, but there is little evidence that this accomplishes more than the occasional wildfire or perforated shed roof.

Avian tuberculosis is usually associated with infection by *M. avium* ssp. *avium* serotypes 1, 2, and 3. Domestic and wild birds can become infected, although disease is less common in ducks and geese than in other domestic species. Birds are infected by ingestion of contaminated water or feed, and in ovo transmission has been documented.

Disease develops slowly even in heavily infected flocks, and gross lesions are seldom observed in birds less than 1 year old; indeed, egg producers have dealt quite successfully with avian tuberculosis by maintaining all-pullet flocks. As the disease progresses, birds manifest anorexia and weakness, as well as lameness from bone and joint lesions (Figure 11-7). Granulomas can be found in liver and spleen as multifocal caseous necrosis, and are not uncommon in extravisceral sites (Figure 11-8). Shedding from intestinal lesions begins a few months after exposure and serves as a source of infection for other birds.

Mycobacterium genavense may account for more than 10% of nontuberculous disseminated mycobacterial infections in patients with AIDS, and gut colonization of non–human immunodeficiency virus (HIV)-infected patients can lead to systemic infection following immunosuppressive therapy. It also infects birds, and may in fact be the most common cause of mycobacterial infection in some populations. Lesions include muscular wasting, hepatomegaly, and thickening of the intestinal wall, and granulomas may be found in lung and elsewhere. Acid-fast organisms can usually be found in liver. *M. avium* ssp. *avium* and *M. genavense* produce nearly identical clinical signs, and can be most reliably differentiated by molecular methods based on determination of the sequence of the 16S rRNA gene.

Relatively few cases of *Mycobacterium simiae* infection have been reported during the three decades since its description. Humans and sub-human primates can develop tuberculosis-like disease caused by infection with *M. simiae,* and enteric infection clinically resembling Johne's disease has

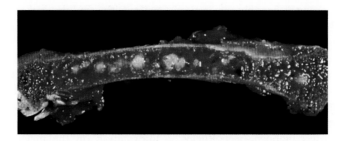

FIGURE 11-7 Bone lesion in *Mycobacterium avium*–infected chicken. (Raymond E. Reed.)

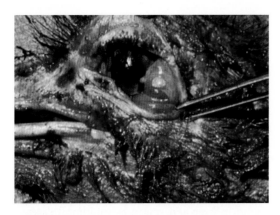

FIGURE 11-8 Conjunctival mycobacteriosis (*Mycobacterium avium*) in an ostrich. (Courtesy J. Glenn Songer.)

been reported in monkeys. This organism is characterized by delayed photochromogenicity and niacin positivity and is resistant to streptomycin, isoniazid, para-aminosalicylate, and rifampin but sensitive to cycloserine. Infection can be transmitted to cagemates, and intrauterine transmission has been reported.

Mycobacterium ulcerans and *Mycobacterium xenopi* are rare causes of atypical mycobacteriosis in cats. Bacteriologic culture usually detects these organisms, setting this type of disease apart from classical feline leprosy.

MYCOBACTERIUM AVIUM SSP. PARATUBERCULOSIS

Mycobacterium avium ssp. *paratuberculosis* is the causative agent of Johne's disease, or paratuberculosis. Paratuberculosis was initially reported in 1894, and *M. avium* ssp. *paratuberculosis* was confirmed as the etiologic agent in 1910. It is a severe form of enteritis, which has major economic impact on the dairy industry worldwide, through reduced production and early culling. Annual losses in the United States alone are estimated at $1.5 billion, but the difficulty in accurately assessing losses in individual herds makes it likely that this figure is too low. A regression model estimated the loss at $40 to $227 per cow inventoried per year.

The ability of *M. avium* ssp. *paratuberculosis* to infect many animal species impacts the effectiveness of control programs. The organism infects many wild and domestic ruminants (such as white-tailed and mule deer, bighorn sheep, Rocky Mountain goats, bison, elk, and red deer) but can

also be isolated from swine and rabbits (wild and domesticated). Infection can sometimes be subclinical, especially in farmed populations, which raises particular concerns regarding reintroduction of animals into wild populations.

Neonatal and juvenile animals are the most prominent risk group for infection by *M. avium* ssp. *paratuberculosis,* and the source of infection is most commonly contaminated milk (or other food) or the environment. Subspecies *paratuberculosis* can be recovered for greater than or equal to 250 days from water and feces, as well as from liquefied cattle waste used as fertilizer. Isolation of *M. avium* ssp. *paratuberculosis* from fetuses, semen, and the uterus suggest the possibility of vertical transmission. Infected animals may not develop clinical disease, but rather remain subclinical, intermittent shedders. Nutritional and hormonal status also influences susceptibility to *M. avium* ssp. *paratuberculosis* infection. In the mouse model, reduced dietary calcium protects against infection, but this is reversed by increased vitamin D in the ration.

Subspecies *paratuberculosis* interacts with mucosa-associated lymphoid tissue (MALT), and has a particular tropism for M cells in ileal Peyer's patches. It is phagocytosed by subepithelial and intraepithelial macrophages, where it interferes with phagosome maturation and multiplies intracellularly. The host immune system responds by rapid deployment of activated gamma-delta T cells, CD4 T cells and cytolytic CD8 T cells, and intestinal granuloma formation is prompted by this cellular immune response. Aggressive interaction of the various T cells with persistently infected macrophages, mediated by a complex network of cytokines, fails to eliminate the organism. Ileum and colon are usually involved, with advancement to the rectum; the continued grappling between the organism and the immune system leads to pronounced intestinal damage, with thickening and corrugation of the tissue and the characteristic malnutrition of Johne's disease. Large numbers of mycobacteria in epithelioid and giant cells in the mucosa are shed in feces. Profuse diarrhea, malabsorption of nutrients, and loss of protein into intestine lead to emaciation and death. Diarrhea is not always seen in sheep and goats.

Intramacrophage survival is, then, the hallmark of *M. avium* ssp. *paratuberculosis* infection. Information on the mechanism by which this occurs is incomplete, but if it follows the pattern of other mycobacteria, it may evade antigen processing in macrophages by inhibiting phagosome-lysosome fusion and acidification. The degree of nitric oxide production by mononuclear phagocytes in response to IFN-γ is probably insufficient to kill intracellular organisms.

Local tissue cytokine production is important in determining the outcome of a mycobacterial infection. IL-1, IL-6, and TNF-α are released when bovine macrophages are stimulated by *M. avium* ssp. *paratuberculosis* antigens, and these cytokines are associated with granulomagenesis (and protection) in other syndromes. IL-1 is particularly protective of mice experimentally infected with *M. avium* ssp. *paratuberculosis* infection. Some cytokines may promote limitation of bacterial growth by causing macrophages to actively limit their intracellular iron concentration. Most mycobacteria produce the mycobactin and exochelin, siderophores that aid in iron acquisition, and may thus be considered virulence attributes. Subspecies *paratuberculosis* synthesizes exochelin, but is a mycobactin auxotroph; the mechanism by which the organism multiplies intracellularly (but not in vitro) despite its inability to produce mycobactin is unknown.

Diagnosis of paratuberculosis involves bacteriologic culture, application of molecular methods for detection and identification of the organism, and assessment of the cellular and humoral immune responses. Bacteriologic culture is still the gold standard for diagnosis of Johne's disease. Specimens disinfected with benzalkonium chloride are inoculated onto Herrold's egg yolk medium with mycobactin; automated rapid methods use media with radiolabeled substrates to allow detection of mycobacterial growth by release of labeled CO_2. It is often necessary to extend incubation through 5 months, and identification is confirmed by mycobactin dependency, acid fastness, and a requirement for 3 weeks of incubation to produce visible colonies with compatible morphology (colorless to white and translucent). Presumptive positives in automated methods can be detected much earlier, and are usually confirmed by a polymerase chain reaction (PCR)–based method. Subspecies *paratuberculosis* is often not cultivable from Johne's disease cases in small ruminants.

PCR-based methods for detection and identification target the 16S rRNA gene or the insertion element IS*900*. In general, PCR assays are less sensitive than fecal culture for detection of small numbers of bacteria, perhaps due to inhibitory substances in feces. However, IS*900*-based PCR is valuable for differentiating subspecies of *M. avium,* particularly in distinguishing *M. paratuberculosis* from *M. avium* and *M. silvaticum*

As noted, infection by *M. avium* ssp. *paratuberculosis* produces granulomatous inflammatory lesions that range in severity from discrete to diffuse. In the discrete form, CD4 Th1 cells, CD8 cells, and monocytes proliferate and secrete IFN-gamma, which can be detected serologically. In the later, diffuse, stage of paratuberculosis, the B-cell response becomes dominant, with high antibody titers. The IFN-γ test is subject to false positives, but it is capable of distinguishing animals in the initial stages of infection. The sensitivity of antibody tests is highest for animals with diffuse lesions, specifically those with clinical symptoms and shedding large numbers of organisms. Enzyme-linked immunosorbent assay (ELISA) is more sensitive than either agar gel immunodiffusion or complement fixation tests, on samples from cattle, sheep, and goats, and it can be used to advantage on either milk or serum samples. The false-positive rate is low with all of these tests, but their major limitation is their failure to identify infected animals early in the clinical course. None of the antibody detection tests identifies all infected animals, possibly due to failure to include the entire range of antigens.

Management, tailored to the conditions in individual herds and based upon good animal husbandry, is the key to controlling paratuberculosis in domestic livestock. Overall environmental cleanliness, manure handling, newborn calf care, and restriction of contact between calves and mature animals are particularly important, but breed of cattle (Guernsey and Jersey cattle are particularly susceptible), proximity of farmed deer, and acidic soils are also risk factors.

Culling of infected animals reduces intraherd exposure, so herd testing is critical. Use of two different tests (most commonly ELISA serology and fecal culture) is more likely to detect infected animals than reliance on a single approach, but testing large numbers of animals in a given herd often reveals the poor positive predictive value of currently available tests; false-positive results are common.

Antibiotic therapy of Johne's disease is limited to extralabel use of antimicrobial agents. However, treatment is aimed only at prolonging life of exceptional breeding animals and most often employs isoniazid with rifabutin or ethambutol, with isoniazid then given daily for life. Curiously, *M. avium* ssp. *paratuberculosis* is resistant to isoniazid in vitro.

Vaccination interferes with diagnosis and elicits granuloma formation at the vaccination site. It is also a potential danger to veterinarians, in that reactions to accidental self-injection can be severe. Experimental evaluation of paratuberculosis vaccines suggest that vaccination reduces the incidence of intestinal lesions and clinical symptoms, as well as shedding of *M. avium* ssp. *paratuberculosis*. Field studies, on the other hand, have been compromised by design flaws. Nonetheless, vaccines apparently protect in part against naturally occurring disease. They reduce the number of clinically affected animals, the number of animals testing positive, and the number of fecal shedders. Booster vaccination does not enhance resistance.

The pathology of Johne's disease superficially resembles that of human Crohn's disease, a chronic debilitating inflammatory bowel condition of unknown etiology. *Mycobacterium avium* ssp. *paratuberculosis* has been demonstrated in intestinal tissue of some Crohn's disease patients, but not in others, and treatment with antimycobacterial agents has yielded mixed results. However, food safety issues have been raised, and there is some sentiment in the dairy industry that these concerns may be fueled illegitimately by the press. This situation is exacerbated by the finding that *M. avium* ssp. *paratuberculosis* may be somewhat more resistant to pasteurization than the reference organisms, *M. bovis* and *Coxiella burnetii*. It is imperative, for political as well as medical reasons, that this be studied further.

MYCOBACTERIUM LEPRAE

The approximately 11 million active cases of leprosy in the world today are found mainly in the tropics. The disease occurs in two forms, the less serious of which is tuberculoid leprosy; the organisms are well contained in granulomatous lesions and progression results in relatively little disfigurement. Lepromatous leprosy, on the other hand, is more serious, with disfigurement resulting from the proliferation of nodular swellings in tissue. Fibrosis of peripheral nerves results in anesthesia, which is followed by spontaneous amputation of toes and fingers in response to unfelt trauma.

Mycobacterium leprae is cultivated experimentally in mouse footpads and in the nine-banded armadillo, but has never been cultivated in vitro. Comparison of the *M. leprae* genome with that of *M. tuberculosis* has revealed extreme reductive evolution in the former, in that inactivated or pseudogenes are abundant, but less than half of the genome contains functional genes. Entire metabolic pathways have been eliminated by gene decay and genome downsizing, and this may explain both the lengthy generation time in vivo and failed attempts to culture the organism in vitro.

Diagnosis of leprosy is based primarily on clinical signs, but skin testing is also possible. The skin test reagent, lepromin, is extracted from leprous tissue. Therapy is often with diaminodiphenylsulfone (dapsone), administered long term, often for several years.

MYCOBACTERIUM LEPRAEMURIUM

Cutaneous mycobacteriosis in cats takes three forms, the most common of which is feline leprosy, a granulomatous nodular disease believed to be caused by *M. lepraemurium*. Firm to soft, intact nodules in the skin or subcutis of the head, limbs, and trunk are subject to nonhealing ulceration, and superficial lymphadenopathy is common. Diagnosis is frequently based on the lack of growth on routine culture medium for acid-fast organisms. Atypical mycobacteriosis, caused by rapidly growing mycobacteria, and cutaneous tuberculosis, associated with infection by *M. tuberculosis* or *M. bovis,* are other forms of feline infection.

MYCOBACTERIUM KANSASII

Mycobacterium kansasii is an opportunistic pathogen of humans, causing mainly respiratory infections and lymphadenitis in individuals with predisposing immunosuppressive problems. It is the nontuberculous mycobacterium most likely to infect humans, other than *M. avium* ssp. *avium* in patients with AIDS. It has been rarely associated with mesenteric lymphadenitis in calves and occasionally with other infections in cattle, in which it mainly provokes hypersensitivity to bovine and avian tuberculin. It is perhaps even more rare as a cause of infections in dogs, with at least one reported isolation from a treatment-resistant pleural effusion. *Mycobacterium kansasii* has also been isolated from bronchial lymph nodes of squirrel monkeys, which converted to tuberculin positive in the absence of

M. tuberculosis infection. This organism is recognizable in culture by its photochromogenicity, with production of striking yellow to orange pigment.

MYCOBACTERIUM MARINUM

Mycobacterium marinum infection in humans often takes the form of so-called swimming pool granuloma, a chronic but superficial infection, usually of the extremities. Optimal growth at 33° C is probably a major factor in restricting growth of *M. marinum* to the cooler surfaces of the body, but fatal systemic infections are common in poikilotherms (Figure 11-9). Infection has been reported in more than 150 species of fish, and granulomas may be found in any internal organ. *Mycobacterium marinum* produces brilliant yellow colonies when cultivated in vitro (see Figure 11-1).

Phylogenetic analysis revealed that *M. marinum* is most closely related to members of the *M. tuberculosis* complex; examination of 16S rRNA sequences revealed 99.4% sequence homology between *M. marinum* and *M. tuberculosis*. Significant genotypic and phenotypic similarities, including manifestation in *M. marinum* infection of granulomagenesis and many other pathologic features of tuberculosis, have suggested this organism as a model for study of the pathogenesis of *M. tuberculosis* infection. It survives and multiplies in host macrophages, preventing phagosome maturation, and offers advantages of more rapid growth (generation time 4 hours, compared with 20 hours for *M. tuberculosis*) and safer handling in the laboratory.

RAPIDLY GROWING MYCOBACTERIA

Rapid growers include the *Mycobacterium fortuitum* group, the *Mycobacterium chelonae/abscessus*

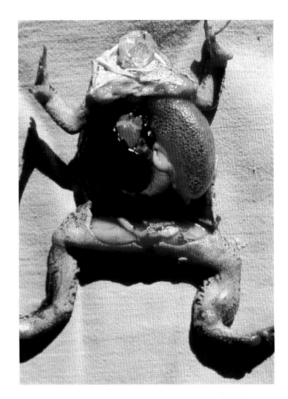

FIGURE 11-9 Systemic *Mycobacterium marinum* infection in a frog. (Courtesy Raymond E. Reed.)

group, and the *Mycobacterium smegmatis* group (Table 11-3). Fundamental characteristics of these groups are appearance of readily visible colonies within 7 days on primary isolation, arylsulfatase activity, and the absence or slow appearance of pigments. In humans, they are often found in surgical wound infections, postinjection abscesses, and localized cutaneous infections. Members of the *M. fortuitum* group are lung pathogens, but

TABLE **11-3** Phenotypic Properties of Rapidly Growing Mycobacteria Encountered in Veterinary Clinical Specimens

| Species | Utilization | | | | 3-Day Arylsulfatase | Nitrate Reduction | Iron Uptake | 5% NaCl |
	Mannitol	Inositol	Citrate	Sorbitol				
M. abscessus	Neg	Neg	Neg	Neg	Pos	Neg	Neg	Pos
M. chelonae	Neg	Neg	Pos	Neg	Pos	Neg	Neg	Neg
M. fortuitum	Neg	Neg	Neg	Neg	Pos	Pos	Pos	Pos
M. peregrinum	Pos	Neg	Neg	Neg	Pos	Pos	Pos	Pos
M. smegmatis*	Pos	Pos	Pos/Neg	Pos	Neg	Pos	Pos	Pos

*May be pigmented.
Neg, Negative; *Pos,* positive.

most often in association with chronic aspiration secondary to gastroesophageal disease. Rapid growers in general have also been associated with cervical lymphadenitis, mastoiditis, and meningitis, and *M. chelonae* and *M. abscessus* cause rare disseminated disease. Infection of humans and animals by rapidly growing mycobacteria occurs worldwide although clustering of outbreaks is common (e.g., in the southern United States). Members of this group are quite robust, especially regarding survival and propagation in water; acid-fast organisms can be found in up to 90% of biofilms. Municipal tapwater is commonly infected, and nosocomial outbreaks in humans have been linked to the organism in hospital water systems.

Mycobacterium fortuitum and *Mycobacterium peregrinum* (formerly known as biovars of *M. fortuitum*) are the important species in the *M. fortuitum* group. The former is associated with granulomatous disease in cattle (mastitis), fish, dogs (lung and skin), and pigs (joint and lung disease). Opportunistic mycobacterial granulomatous disease in cats is identified by chronic fistulous tracts, fasciitis, and ulcerative nodules, with lesions on the ventral abdomen. Most of these yield cultures of *M. fortuitum,* but this condition is also associated with *Mycobacterium phlei, M. smegmatis,* and *M. chelonae.* In humans, *M. fortuitum* is found in soft tissue abscesses, osteomyelitis, implanted heart valves, and occasional disseminated disease. *Mycobacterium peregrinum* has been recovered from feline pyogranulomatous panniculitis. It has also been isolated from multifocal, black, melanized lesions in the carapace of the Pacific white shrimp (*Penaeus vannamei),* which also had microscopic granulomas in the lymphoid organ, heart, and intertubular connective tissue in the hepatopancreas. It is associated also with a very small number of cases of human chronic lung disease and nodular skin infections.

Mycobacterium chelonae and *M. abscessus* (formerly *M. chelonae* ssp. *chelonae* and *M. chelonae* ssp. *abscessus*, respectively) comprise a major portion of the *M. chelonae/abscessus* group. Members of this group are found in soil and water worldwide, and in the United States outbreaks are most common in southern coastal states. The general phenotype of members of the group includes rapid arylsulfatase positivity, lack of pigmentation, preference for incubation at 30° C, inability to reduce nitrate, lack of iron uptake, and resistance to most antimicrobials other than amikacin and clarithromycin. These organisms are well known for their resistance to organomercurials, chlorine, and alkaline glutaraldehyde. *Mycobacterium chelonae* is not a common pathogen of domestic animals, but can be isolated from various lesions in turtles (Figure 11-10). The organisms cause chronic lung disease in humans, especially in patients with bronchiectasis or cystic fibrosis, and are occasionally recovered from cases of cellulitis, osteomyelitis, and small-joint arthritis. These two species among the rapid growers are responsible for nearly 100% of disseminated cutaneous infections in humans, a condition characterized by many draining abscesses, usually on the arms and legs. Most of these cases are caused by *M. chelonae,* but when it occurs, disseminated *M. abscessus* disease is quite serious; most cases occur in chronically immunosuppressed individuals, and disease manifests as fistulous nodules on the legs. *Mycobacterium abscessus* and *Mycobacterium chelonae* are likely the most antibiotic resistant of the rapid growers.

The *M. smegmatis* group comprises *M. smegmatis, Mycobacterium goodii,* and *M. wolinskyi,* the first of which is by far the most important. It can be

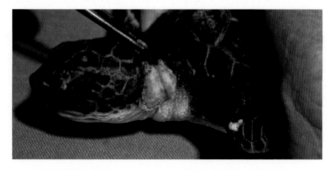

FIGURE 11-10 Cutaneous *Mycobacterium chelonae* infection in a turtle. (Courtesy Raymond E. Reed.)

recovered from cases of lymphadenitis, traumatic and nontraumatic cellulitis, and osteomyelitis in humans. In animals it is perhaps most common as a cause of acute bovine mastitis, especially in cows recently treated with antimicrobials for other forms of mastitis. Moderate hypertrophy, which may persist for several months, occurs in affected quarters and small clots may be found in milk for several weeks following infection. Mean cell counts for affected quarters may approximate 5×10^6 per ml in the acute stage and remain as high as 6×10^5 per ml after 12 months. Estimated production losses range from 10% to 30%, and many affected cows are eventually culled due to poor yield. A phenotypic feature of *M. smegmatis* that contrasts with most other rapidly growing mycobacteria is lack of susceptibility of human isolates to many newer macrolides, including clarithromycin.

Mycobacterium senegalense has never been isolated outside Africa, where it has been known for 30 years as a relative of *Mycobacterium farcinogenes*. Both are etiologic agents of farcy, an economically devastating disease of skin and superficial lymphatics. This chronic infectious disease, which specifically affects zebu cattle, is endemic in Chad, Nigeria, Senegal, Somalia, the Sudan, and throughout east and central Africa. *Mycobacterium farcinogenes, M. senegalense,* and a biovariant of *M. fortuitum* have identical 16S rDNA sequences, and are very similar in chemotaxonomic, numerical taxonomic, and serotaxonomic analyses, but these same data confirm their status as separate species.

Diagnosis is based on traditional methods of bacteriologic culture and identification of phenotype; growth rate, biochemical tests, pigmentation, and colony morphology are key properties. As noted, colonies of rapidly growing mycobacteria mature in less than or equal to 7 days. Members of the *Mycobacterium fortuitum* and *M. chelonae/abscessus* groups are strongly arylsulfatase positive after 3 days' incubation; *M. smegmatis* is arylsulfatase negative at 3 days, but stands alone as a pigment producer (yellow-orange with extended incubation) among the rapid growers (see Table 11-3).

Patterns of antimicrobial therapy for diseases caused by rapidly growing mycobacteria can be quite different from those applied to infections by slowly growing mycobacteria. Most notable is the frequent sufficiency of single-drug therapy for minor infections, which is possible due to the minimal risk of development of antimicrobial resistance. More extensive and serious infections (disseminated cutaneous or pulmonary disease in humans) are usually treated with multiple antimicrobials. *Mycobacterium fortuitum* and its relatives are much less likely to be drug resistant than *M. abscessus* and *M. chelonae,* so treatment is usually more effective. *Mycobacterium smegmatis* infections can be treated with doxycycline and trimethoprim-sulfamethoxazole, but all organisms in the group are susceptible to sulfonamides, doxycycline, imipenem, and amikacin.

SUGGESTED READINGS

Bercovier H, Vincent V: Mycobacterial infections in domestic and wild animals due to *Mycobacterium marinum, M. fortuitum, M. chelonae, M. porcinum, M. farcinogenes, M. smegmatis, M. scrofulaceum, M. xenopi, M. kansasii, M. simiae* and *M. genavense, Rev Sci Tech* 20:265-290, 2001.

Cocito C, Gilot P, Coene M, et al: Paratuberculosis, *Clin Microbiol Rev* 7:328-345, 1994.

Eiglmeier K, Parkhill J, Honore N, et al: The decaying genome of *Mycobacterium leprae, Lepr Rev* 72: 387-398, 2001.

Harris NB, Barletta RG: *Mycobacterium avium* subsp. *paratuberculosis* in veterinary medicine, *Clin Microbiol Rev* 14:489-512, 2001.

Mendenhall MK, SL Ford, CL Emerson, et al: Detection and differentiation of *Mycobacterium avium* and *Mycobacterium genavense* by polymerase chain reaction and restriction enzyme digestion analysis, *J Vet Diagn Invest* 12:57-60, 2000.

Roberts GD, Koneman EW, Kim YK: Mycobacterium. In Balows A, ed: *Manual of clinical microbiology,* ed 7, Washington, DC, 1991, American Society for Microbiology.

Schultze W, Brasso WB: Characterization of *Mycobacterium smegmatis* in bovine mastitis, *Am J Vet Res* 48:739-742, 1987.

Tell LA, Woods L, Cromie RL: Mycobacteriosis in birds, *Rev Sci Tech* 20:180-203, 2001.

Chapter 12

The Genus *Rhodococcus*

The genus *Rhodococcus* is part of a distinctive actinomycete taxonomic group that includes the genera *Corynebacterium, Mycobacterium,* and *Nocardia.* This taxonomic group is defined by the presence of unique lipid-rich cell envelope structures rich in mycolic acids that promote intramacrophage survival and granuloma formation. The only pathogenic *Rhodococcus* is *Rhodococcus equi,* a cause of granulomatous pneumonia in foals and immunosuppressed humans.

Rhodococcus (Corynebacterium) equi is an aerobic, gram-positive, pleomorphic coccobacillus that may be partially acid fast at some stage of growth. It produces a characteristically mucoid colony on blood agar. On extended incubation, the salmon pink color of these colonies becomes deeper red. *Rhodococcus equi* is catalase positive, with oxidative metabolism, and its cholesterol oxidase produces synergistic hemolysis with products of *Staphylococcus aureus* and *Corynebacterium pseudotuberculosis.*

Disease and Epidemiology

The simple growth requirements of *R. equi* are provided by nutrients in herbivore manure and high environmental temperatures. Sandy acid soils in paddocks continually used for breeding mares are likely sites for infection of foals, which inhale the organism with blowing dust. The resulting disease is a pyogranulomatous bronchopneumonia (Figure 12-1), with cranioventral abscesses a reflection of inhalation of organisms. Swallowing of infected sputum gives rise to ulcerative colitis and mesenteric lymphadenitis (Figure 12-2), with diarrhea. Hematogenous dissemination may result in osteomyelitis in long bones or vertebrae. Affected foals are typically about 6 weeks of age, but age at onset ranges from 1 to 6 months.

Rhodococcus equi infection in pigs causes cervical lymphadenitis, and the resulting granulomatous lesions resemble mycobacterial infection. As such, they may result in condemnation of parts or carcasses at slaughter. Isolation of *R. equi* from other animal species is rare, but when infection occurs it usually takes the form of pyogranulomatous pneumonia, hepatic abscesses, or lymphadenitis.

Infection by *R. equi* is frequently isolated from immunosuppressed humans, particularly from

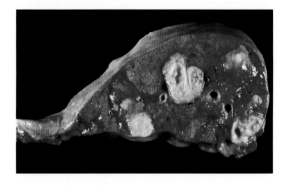

FIGURE 12-1 Multifocal pyogranulomatous pneumonia in an Arabian foal. (Courtesy M. Kevin Keel.)

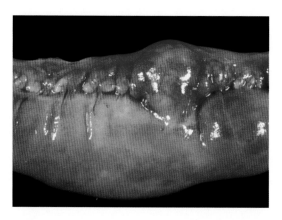

FIGURE 12-2 Chronic suppurative colitis in a 3-month-old Thoroughbred foal. (Courtesy M. Kevin Keel.)

cases of pyogranulomatous pneumonia in patients with acquired immunodeficiency syndrome (AIDS). If isolates from patients with AIDS have the virulence plasmid, it is usually of the porcine type, although a small proportion possess the foal type. Thus *R. equi* probably has little zoonotic significance.

Other types of *R. equi* infection are equine mastitis and wound infections, bovine ulcerative lymphangitis, lymphadenitis and abscesses in cats, caprine and ovine pneumonia and internal abscesses, canine pyogranulomatous hepatitis and osteomyelitis, septicemia in alligators and crocodiles, and lung abscesses in seals.

Pathogenesis

Virulence of *R. equi* from foals is associated with an 85 kb pair plasmid that encodes a surface-expressed, virulence-associated protein known as VapA. Its production is temperature regulated, being expressed at or near foal body temperature. Virulence of pig strains is also associated with a large plasmid, but these strains do not produce VapA; isolates from patients with AIDS usually do not possess virulence plasmids. Both pig and human strains are of low mouse virulence.

Chain length of cell wall mycolic acids may determine resistance to intracellular killing and, indeed, pathogenesis of *R. equi* infection relates to the ability of the organism to persist in macrophages. It is apparently specifically targeted to macrophages by the complement receptor, CR3; this mode of cell entry may reduce oxidative killing of the organism, whereas antibody-mediated entry (via the Fc receptor) may be more likely to result in intracellular killing. Neutrophil infiltration follows death of macrophages, and abscess formation can be extensive and life threatening.

Infection occurs with heavy environmental challenge in foals with low levels of maternally derived antibodies, and may be associated with infection by equine herpesvirus 4. Although immunosuppression is a major factor in human *R. equi* infection, this has not been demonstrated in foals.

CD4+ T-lymphocytes (particularly Th1 lymphocytes) mediate immunity to experimental murine infection with *R. equi;* Th2 responses do not prevent lung lesions. However, hyperimmune plasma is effective in controlling infection in foals, so it seems likely that the humoral response plays a role in protection or recovery.

Diagnosis

Transtracheal aspirates or bronchoalveolar lavage samples are examined by Gram stain and bacteriologic culture. After 48 hours' incubation, colonies are 2 to 4 mm diameter, irregular to round, smooth, semiopaque, and glistening. Most strains are mucoid, and some are extremely so. Cultures may also have a slight earthy smell. Pigment production occurs after 4 to 7 days' incubation on nonselective media; most are salmon-pink, but yellow, fawn-colored, and nonpigmented strains may occur.

Rhodococcus equi is a catalase-positive coccobacillus that produces synergistic hemolysis (CAMP reaction) with *Staphylococcus aureus* β-toxin or *Corynebacterium pseudotuberculosis* phospholipase D (Table 12-1). Serologic diagnostic tests (including agar gel immunodiffusion, enzyme-linked immunosorbent assay (ELISA), and synergistic hemolysis inhibition) have been developed, but their sensitivity and specificity are not known. Polymerase chain reaction (PCR) diagnosis is also available but is not widely used.

Control and Prevention

On farms where infection is sporadic, sick foals should be isolated and treated, and manure composted. A definitive diagnosis of *R. equi* infection should be made, in every case, by bronchoalveolar lavage and culture because certain other causes of pneumonia do not require persistent treatment with antibacterial drugs. Passive immunoprophylaxis can be achieved by administration of 1000 ml of hyperimmune plasma, at about 2 to 3 weeks of age, to foals on farms where the disease is enzootic.

TABLE **12-1** Characteristics of *Rhodococcus equi*

Characteristic	Reaction	Percent Positive
Catalase	Pos	100
Cytochrome c oxidase	Neg	1-5
Carbohydrate fermentation	Neg	100
Gelatin hydrolysis	Neg	100
Indole	Neg	100
Hydrogen sulfide	Var	32-62
Urease	Pos	95
Hippurate hydrolysis	Neg	1
Esculin hydrolysis	Neg	4
Nitrate reduction	Pos	88
Lipase	Pos	100
CAMP *(Staphylococcus aureus/* *Corynebacterium pseudotuberculosis)*	Pos	100

Neg, Negative; *Pos,* positive; *Var,* variable.

Antimicrobial therapy of *R. equi* infection is with a combination of erythromycin and rifampin. These drugs penetrate macrophages well, can be administered orally, and have low minimum inhibitory concentrations for the organism. It is important to use them in combination, to discourage the development of bacterial resistance, which is emerging due to extensive use on some farms. Alternative drugs are trimethoprim-sulfamethoxazole, administered orally early in the infection. Drugs are administered until there is clinical and radiographic evidence of cure. Vancomycin and imipenem have been useful in treating human infections.

Immunization has produced mixed results; there have been claims of reduced incidence following use of bacterins enriched with supernatant fluids, but disease enhancement in others.

SUGGESTED READINGS

Cornish N, Washington JA: Rhodococcus equi infections: clinical features and laboratory diagnosis, *Curr Clin Top Infect Dis* 19:198-215, 1999.

Giguere S, Prescott JF: Clinical manifestations, diagnosis, treatment, and prevention of *Rhodococcus equi* infections in foals, *Vet Microbiol* 56:313-334, 1997.

Hines SA, Kanaly ST, Byrne BA, Palmer GH: Immunity to *Rhodococcus equi, Vet Microbiol* 56:177-186, 1997.

Kedlaya I, Ing MB, Wong SS: *Rhodococcus equi* infections in immunocompetent hosts: case report and review, *Clin Infect Dis* 32:E39-E46, 2001.

Takai S: Epidemiology of *Rhodococcus equi* infections: a review, *Vet Microbiol* 56:167-176, 1997.

Gram-Negative Bacteria

Enterobacteriaceae

Chapter **13**

The Genera *Escherichia* and *Shigella*

The genera *Escherichia* and *Shigella* are class γ-proteobacteria, in the order Enterobacteriales and family Enterobacteriaceae.

THE GENUS *ESCHERICHIA*

The genus *Escherichia* was named in honor of German pediatrician Theodor Escherich, who first isolated the type species, *Escherichia coli*. Five additional species within the genus are *Escherichia albertii*, *Escherichia blattae*, *Escherichia fergusonii*, *Escherichia hermannii,* and *Escherichia vulneris,* but *E. coli* is the most significant pathogen. Escherichiae are straight gram-negative medium to long rods ranging from 0.4 to 0.7 μm by 1 to 3 μm, and occurring singly or in pairs. They have both oxidative and fermentative metabolism and are oxidase negative and catalase positive. Acid and gas are produced from D-glucose and most species are motile.

Diseases and Epidemiology

Escherichia coli inhabits the lower ileum and large intestine of most vertebrates, with colonization of the neonatal gastrointestinal tract occurring within hours of birth. At about 10^8 organisms per gram, it is the predominant facultatively anaerobic bacterium isolated from the feces. Survival and multiplication of *E. coli* in the environment makes "coliform" counts valuable indices of fecal contamination, especially in testing water for potability.

Most strains of *E. coli* are of low virulence and associated with opportunistic infections, whereas others are highly virulent. Different strains cause different types of disease, so it is important to discriminate between pathogenic and nonpathogenic strains. Serologic classification, based on seroreactivity of *E. coli* surface molecules, was developed for this purpose. It is especially useful for identifying strains that cause intestinal disease and has been used extensively for epidemiologic purposes. Two *E. coli* surface components that are the basis for serologic classification are the O antigen of the lipopolysaccharide and the H antigen of the flagellum. The O antigen determines the serogroup and the H antigen the serotype. A capsular antigen (K) may also be used for classification.

Escherichia coli are primary pathogens causing enteritis and septicemia in a variety of domestic species, including poultry, pigs, ruminants, dogs, cats, horses, and rabbits. Other important diseases are ruminant mastitis, canine pyometra and cystitis,

TABLE **13-1** *Escherichia coli* Pathotypes Associated with Gastrointestinal Disease in Animals

Pathotype	Site of Action	Disease	Pathogenesis	Virulence Factors
Enterotoxigenic *E. coli* (ETEC)	Small intestine	Neonatal diarrhea in all mammals	Enterocyte adherence via fimbriae; elaborated enterotoxins cause secretory diarrhea	K88, K99, 987P, F41, F1845, STa, STb, LT
Enteropathogenic *E. coli* (EPEC)	Small, large intestine	Calf, pig, rabbit, and puppy diarrhea	Microvillus effacement, intimate adherence of bacteria to epithelial cell membranes (attaching and effacing lesions); diarrhea associated with malabsorption	Unknown toxins? Adherence to HEp-2 cells
Enterohemorrhagic *E. coli* (EHEC)	Large intestine	Calf hemorrhagic colitis	Attaching and effacing lesions; microvillous destruction; Shiga toxin causes hemorrhage, edema	Shiga toxins 1 and 2
Necrotoxigenic *E. coli* (NTEC)	Small intestine	Calf and pig diarrhea	Intestinal colonization; cytotoxic necrotizing factors damage enterocyte cytoskeleton	Invasin, fimbrial and afimbrial adhesins, cytotoxic necrotizing factors 1 and 2

LT, Heat labile; *HEp-2,* human epithelial cells; *STa,* heat-stable enterotoxin A; *STb,* heat-stable enterotoxin B.

and oomphalitis in young chicks. Infections may be endogenous or exogenous in nature. Extraintestinal disease is generally caused by the animal's normal microbial flora, whereas strains causing gastroenteritis are usually from an exogenous source.

Strains of *E. coli* associated with disease in the gastrointestinal tract are classified based on virulence properties (Table 13-1). At least six different groups or pathotypes are recognized, including enterotoxigenic (ETEC), enteropathogenic (EPEC), enterohemorrhagic (EHEC), necrotoxigenic (NTEC), enteroinvasive (EIEC), and enteroaggregative (EAggEC). EAggEC and EIEC strains have not been reported from domestic animals. The former is associated with persistent diarrhea in humans in developing countries. Food- or water-borne outbreaks of human diarrhea have been attributed to EIEC.

ETEC strains are generally species specific (Figure 13-1). They adhere via fimbriae and elaborate cytotoxins. In neonatal mammals they cause acute, watery diarrhea that may be followed by terminal bacteremia and remain an important cause of economic loss for cattle and swine producers. Clinical signs include white, yellow, or gray scours that occur during the first week of life,

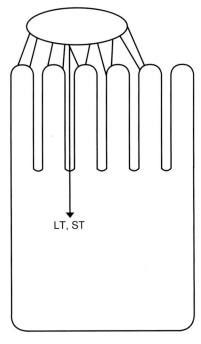

FIGURE 13-1 Enterotoxigenic *Escherichia coli* bind by way of fimbriae and produce one or more enterotoxins. Their intracellular effects result in an outpouring of fluid that manifests clinically as diarrhea. There is little or no gross or microscopic damage to enterocytes. *LT,* Heat-labile enterotoxin; *ST,* heat-stable enterotoxin. (Courtesy Ashley E. Harmon.)

and microscopic examination of distal jejunum and proximal ileum reveals bacterial colonization of the mucosal epithelium, without villus atrophy. Some ETEC strains express K88 or F18 fimbriae, colonizing small intestine and producing diarrhea in recently weaned pigs. The common fimbrial adhesins and serogroups associated with disease are in Table 13-2.

EPECs (Figure 13-2) are isolated from humans and farm animals, as well as dogs, cats, and rabbits,

TABLE **13-2** Fimbrial Adhesins and Serogroups Associated with ETEC in Domestic Animals

Fimbrial Adhesin	Animal Host	Serogroups
K88 (F4)	Pig	O8, O141, O147, O149
K99 (F5)	Pig, calf, lamb	O8, O9, O20, O107
987P (F6)	Pig	O9, O20, O141
F41	Pig, calf	O9, O101
F18	Pig	O138, O139, O141
F1845	Calf	O101
F17	Calf, lamb, kid	

in all of which they produce attaching and effacing lesions. Strains are emerging as important causes of diarrhea in puppies and in other animals, and are associated with "failure to thrive" syndrome. Diarrhea is often mucoid and chronic, as opposed to the watery diarrhea associated with ETEC. Histologically, attaching-effacing lesions are the hallmark of disease.

Many EHEC strains (Figure 13-3) produce Shiga toxin, which is similar to the cytotoxin of *Shigella dysenteriae* O1. These strains are often referred to as Shiga toxigenic *E. coli* (STEC) or verotoxigenic *E. coli* (VTEC), with the latter name derived from toxin effects on vero cells in culture. EHEC and STEC are important causes of diarrhea in calves less than 8 weeks of age. Affected animals exhibit mucoid to bloody diarrhea that is rarely fatal, but leaves calves dehydrated, weak, and stunted.

Edema disease, also known as "gut edema" or "bowel edema," is a communicable enterotoxemia that results in significant death losses in recently weaned pigs. It is caused by EHEC-like bacteria that have acquired the genes for production of a Shiga toxin variant called Stx2e. Strains carrying the F18ab fimbrial type, originally described as F107,

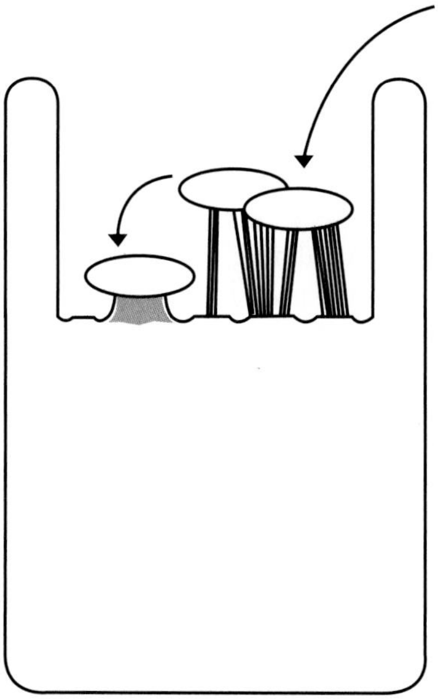

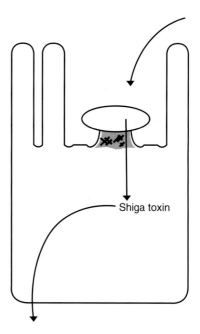

FIGURE 13-2 Enteropathogenic *Escherichia coli* attach nonintimately and then intimately, and the key factor in the process is intimin. Signaling proteins produced by the bacteria and injected into host cells mediate production of a pedestal-like matte of actin filaments on which the organism settles. Microvilli are effaced. (Courtesy Ashley E. Harmon.)

FIGURE 13-3 Enterohemorrhagic *Escherichia coli* bind and efface microvilli in much the same manner as enteropathogenic *E. coli*, but also produce Shiga toxin, which damages the adjacent cell and enters circulation to cause systemic effects. (Courtesy Ashley E. Harmon.)

are most often associated with this condition. Unweaned pigs may acquire infection in the farrowing house, but lack of full expression of the F18 receptor in piglets younger than 20 days of age augurs against disease in neonates. Clinical signs include ataxia, paddling, confusion, palpebral edema, and sudden death. Postmortem examination reveals edema in colonic mesentery, submucosa of the glandular cardiac portion of the stomach, gallbladder and small intestine, and areas of cerebellar hemorrhage. Adherent gram-negative rods are seen in small intestine, and degenerative angiopathy in small arteries and arterioles, swelling of endothelial cells, and focal encephalomalacia in brainstem are common.

Escherichia coli O157:H7 is the most common EHEC serotype implicated in cases of human diarrhea and hemorrhagic colitis. Hemolytic-uremic syndrome (HUS) is a complication of EHEC infection, characterized by acquired nonimmune hemolytic anemia, thrombocytopenia, and acute renal failure. Infection with O157:H7 is zoonotic. As many as one third of domestic ruminants are asymptomatic carriers and represent the principal reservoir for human infection. Fecal shedding is transient, often lasting 1 to 3 months. Swine, horses, and deer can also be carriers of *E. coli* O157:H7, but do not appear to be major sources. Transmission occurs through consumption of undercooked meat, unpasteurized dairy products, and vegetables or water contaminated by feces of carrier animals. Epidemiologic investigations have clearly linked human infection to consumption of contaminated and improperly cooked beef. On occasion, O157:H7 has been associated with hemolytic-uremic syndrome in racing greyhounds fed undercooked or raw ground beef.

Cytotoxic necrotizing factors 1 and 2 are elaborated by NTEC. NTEC 1 strains have been recovered from humans, cattle, piglets, dogs, cats, and horses in association with diarrhea, urinary tract infection, and septicemia. NTEC 2 strains have been isolated from diarrheic and septicemic cattle and sheep.

Several fimbriated strains of *E. coli* are associated with intestinal, as well as extraintestinal disease. The F17 group of fimbriae has three epitopes. F17a fimbriae are isolated from bovine ETEC strains, septicemia in lambs and calves is associated with the F17b type, and F17c strains are recovered from septicemic and diarrheic cattle. The last are also associated with lamb nephrosis syndrome.

F18 strains producing Shiga-like toxins cause swine edema disease.

Colibacillosis or colisepticemia of poultry is a common systemic disease with significant economic impact. Bacteremia follows intestinal infection or respiratory exposure to high numbers of organisms in the environment. The infection is characterized by acute septicemia or subacute airsacculitis and polyserositis in poults and young broilers. Adverse environmental conditions or concurrent infectious diseases predispose to clinical disease. Signs are nonspecific and age of affected birds, duration of illness, and affected organs vary from case to case. In 4- to 8-week-old birds, acute death may be preceded by anorexia and lethargy. Postmortem lesions include hepatitis and splenitis, with increased fluid accumulations in the thoracic and abdominal cavities. Survivors of acute septicemia usually develop pericarditis, perihepatitis, and fibrinopurulent airsacculitis, and the latter is the hallmark of colibacillosis. Other less common disease manifestations are pneumonia, salpingitis, arthritis, and osteomyelitis.

Peracute bovine mastitis most frequently results from a coliform infection, with *E. coli* being the most commonly recovered pathogen. Disease is characterized by rapid onset of fulminating infection, with painful swelling of the udder, production of milk with a serumlike consistency, lethargy, anorexia, and signs of endotoxemia (including fever, cold extremities, brick-colored mucous membranes, shock, and sudden death). Mastitis typically occurs during the early postpartum or peak production period and is reflective of heavy fecal contamination of the environment. Disease tends to be confined to cattle housed in restricted space. Predisposing factors may include anatomic abnormalities in the teat or udder, wet or dirty loafing areas, udder trauma, and unsanitary or malfunctioning milking equipment or techniques.

Escherichia coli is the organism recovered most frequently from the infected uterus of dogs and cats. Pyometra occurs more commonly in dogs than in cats. Affected bitches tend to be middle aged or older, whereas younger queens may develop disease. Canine and feline pyometra most often develops during the luteal phase of the cycle or after the administration of progestins. Examination of isolates recovered from cases of pyometra are similar to corresponding fecal isolates, suggesting that fecal contamination of the vaginal vault may be a predisposing factor. Clinical signs in bitches may include vaginal discharge, anorexia, lethargy, polyuria, polydipsia, and vomiting. Vaginal discharge and abdominal bloating are the most common signs in cats. Septicemia and endotoxemia may be sequelae in untreated animals.

The organism is also a common cause of canine cystitis. As with pyometra, affected animals are likely to harbor the same strain in their intestinal tracts, vagina, or prepuce, and infections are typically ascending. Predisposing factors include urolithiasis, anatomic or neurologic abnormalities of the urinary tract, neoplasia, indwelling urinary catheters, or prolonged antimicrobial therapy. Clinical signs include dysuria, polyuria, hematuria, and production of foul-smelling cloudy urine. In many instances cystitis is asymptomatic, manifesting simply as bacteriuria. Untreated disease can progress to pyelonephritis.

The spread of virulent strains of *E. coli* in the farm environment is presumed to occur through feed, aerosols, fomites, and carrier animals. Factors that predispose to disease include failed passive transfer in neonates, intensive husbandry practices, poor sanitation, and stressors such as dietary changes, cold weather, and commingling of animals from different sources. Neonates less than 1 week of age are especially prone to infection due to their lack of a fully developed immune response and established intestinal microflora. In addition, receptors for certain *E. coli* adhesins are present only for the first few days or weeks of life. Sudden dietary changes at weaning, including increased protein and decreased fiber levels, can result in a massive overgrowth of enterotoxigenic or Shiga toxin–producing strains. Inheritance of an autosomal recessive gene in large white breeds such as Yorkshire and Landrace is correlated with genetic predisposition to edema disease.

Pathogenesis

Escherichia coli, once considered solely as an opportunist, has become recognized as an extremely versatile frank pathogen. Certain serotypes have become adapted to cause severe disease in specific hosts by differing mechanisms. The organism accommodates plasmids, temperate bacteriophages, and other mobile elements that carry genes encoding virulence attributes or antimicrobial resistance. The full range of virulence is yet to be elucidated.

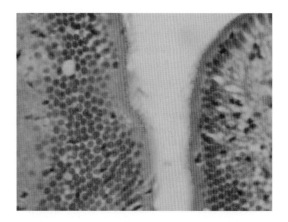

FIGURE 13-4 Adherence of F18 *Escherichia coli* to porcine small intestinal epithelium. (Courtesy Peter Moisan.)

After ingestion, ETEC strains colonize the small intestinal epithelium via fimbrial adhesins. They produce enterotoxins, causing fluid secretion (Figure 13-4, see also Figure 13-1) and manifesting as severe, watery diarrhea. Host species lacking specific receptors are refractory to infection. Receptors may be present only at certain ages, limiting susceptibility to that time interval. Two major toxins produced by ETEC are heat-stable (ST) and heat-labile (LT) enterotoxins. ST occurs as types A (STa) and B (STb). Binding and entry of STa lead to production of increased intraenterocyte levels of cyclic guanosine monophosphate (cGMP), stimulating chloride secretion and/or inhibiting sodium and chloride absorption and resulting in secretory diarrhea. STb directly damages the intestinal epithelium, causing loss of epithelial cells and villous atrophy, as a result of hypovolemia, ischemia, and circulatory collapse. It also stimulates secretion of bicarbonate from enterocytes and causes release of prostaglandins and serotonin. LT dysregulates enterocyte adenylate cyclase, leading to increased cAMP production. Chloride ion and water secretion follows, manifesting as watery diarrhea.

EPEC infections (see Figure 13-2) are characterized by effacement of intestinal microvilli and adherence between bacteria and epithelial cell membranes. The infection process begins with adherence and formation of bacterial microcolonies. This adherence is attributed to intimin, a bacterial outer membrane protein encoded by *eae,* and Tir, a bacterial protein that is inserted into the enterocyte membrane and serves as the receptor for intimin. The attaching and effacing lesion results from both bacterial attachment to entero-cytes and disruption of brush border microvilli. Communication between bacteria and host cells results in accumulation of highly organized cytoskeletal components (actin, myosin, talin, ezrin) in epithelial cells beneath adherent bacteria, leading to formation of pedestal-like structures. EPEC attachment is also associated with increases in intraenterocyte calcium ion levels. These changes inhibit sodium and chloride absorption, and stimulate chloride secretion by enterocytes. EPEC strains apparently do not produce toxins.

EHEC strains also adhere via an intimin-mediated process, but have Shiga toxin genes, on a plasmid that also carries a hemolysin gene and the locus for enterocyte effacement (LEE). The latter is a cluster of genes that are responsible for the attachment of the bacterium to the enterocyte apical membrane and subsequent destruction of microvilli. Shiga toxins occur in multiple forms, called Stx1 and Stx2. A variant within Stx2, called Stx2e, is associated with edema disease in swine.

Pathogenesis of swine edema disease has remained largely unexplored. K88 or F18 fimbriae mediate binding to enterocyte receptors in small intestine of susceptible individuals. Receptor avail-ability can be modulated by feed lectins, especially from leguminous plants. After colonization and multiplication, Shiga-like toxins are elaborated and then absorbed into the bloodstream, where they bind to erythrocytes and are distributed throughout the body. Toxin causes damage to vascular endothelium, leading to edema in target tissues. The consequences of toxin action in brain are neurologic abnormalities and sudden death.

Cytotoxic necrotizing factors type 1 (CNF1) and type 2 (CNF2) are dermonecrotic protein toxins produced by NTEC. They induce enlargement and multinucleation of vero and HeLa cells, cause necrosis in rabbit skin, and are lethal for mice. In addition, CNF2 induces moderate fluid accumula-tion in rabbit ileal loops, and CNF1 can trigger entry of noninvasive bacteria into HEp-2 cells. The gene encoding CNF1 is located on a pathogenicity island that also carries genes for α-hemolysin and P-fimbriae. The necrotic and lethal properties of these toxins, coupled with their ability to alter the cytoskeleton, are fundamental to virulence.

Escherichia coli septicemia occurs primarily in neonatal animals that are not fully immunocom-petent. The umbilicus is a common route of entry.

Virulence factors in this type of infection are serum resistance and production of CNF2 and the CS31A antigen. Ovine septicemia strains harbor a transmissible plasmid encoding CNF2 and the col-icin V plasmid, which is associated with survival of *E. coli* in host serum. Most F17c bovine strains also express the CS31A antigen. Disease has been reproduced experimentally with strains producing this capsulelike antigen, which is also encoded by a plasmid-borne gene.

Bovine mastitis is caused by serum-resistant strains of *E. coli*. Inflammation and death are primarily attributed to endotoxin activity, which is released at bacterial cell lysis. The systemic manifestations of endotoxemia are complement activation, cytokine release, thrombocytopenia, fever, decreased peripheral circulation, dissemi-nated intravascular coagulopathy, shock, and death resulting from circulatory collapse.

Canine pyometra typically occurs during diestrus, when progesterone levels are highest. Cystic endometrial hyperplasia, fluid accumulation, and decreased myometrial activity are conducive to an ascending infection from vagina to uterus. *Escherichia coli* adhere to the endometrial cells during the luteal phase of the estrous cycle.

Uropathogenic *E. coli* colonizes the urethra from the colon, prepuce, or vaginal tract. In the bladder, bacteria adhere (via type 1 fimbriae) to and invade uroepithelial cells. The organisms may activate signal transduction pathways within the cells, causing them to slough. Cystitis results from the local inflammatory response to lipopoly-saccharide and the production of exotoxins such as α-hemolysin and CNF1. α-Hemolysin belongs to the RTX family of pore-forming toxins that cause cellular lysis and stimulate production of cytokines and superoxides. CNF1 is also cytolethal. A certain percentage of cystitis cases progress to kidney infections. P fimbriae, adhesins found mainly in strains that cause human pyelonephritis, are important factors for colonization of the ureters.

Diagnosis

Escherichia coli in the intestinal tract invades tissues within hours of death, so care should be exercised to collect specimens only from fresh carcasses. Aseptic culture of heart blood, bone marrow, and parenchymatous organs is useful in diagnosis of septicemic disease. The organism is easily recovered from intestinal contents, urine,

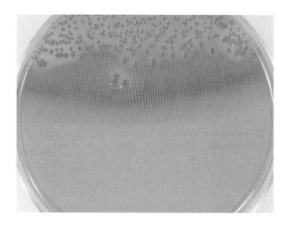

FIGURE 13-5 Colonies of *Escherichia coli* on MacConkey agar, surrounded by precipitated bile. (Courtesy Karen W. Post.)

milk, and vaginal exudates and grows readily on most simple media. Tryptose blood agar and MacConkey agar are routinely used for isolation. After 24-hour aerobic incubation at 37° C on blood agar, *E. coli* colonies may be smooth or rough, and are usually 2 to 3 mm in diameter, low convex, moist, shiny, entire, and gray. Hemolysis is variable and strain dependent. Most isolates (90%) are lactose positive on MacConkey agar and are usually surrounded by a zone of precipitated bile (Figure 13-5). They can be identified by classical tube biochemical or commercial strip tests. Spot indole and MUG (4-methylumbelliferyl beta-D-glucuronidase) tests are widely used for rapid presumptive identification. Ninety-nine percent of *E. coli* are indole and MUG positive.

Several methods allow diagnosticians to distinguish virulent isolates from those that are avirulent. Serotypic markers correlate well with specific categories of diarrheagenic *E. coli*. Latex agglutination kits, enzyme immunoassays, and antisera are commercially available for identifying K88, K99, F41, and 987P fimbrial antigens. The second and more commonly used method is molecular detection. Deoxyribonucleic acid (DNA) probes and polymerase chain reaction (PCR) assays have been developed to detect virulence factor genes.

Histologic examination of the intestine is often useful in diagnosis. Molecular detection of fimbrial adhesin or toxin genes, or *eae* in the absence of Shiga toxin genes, could confirm the involvement of a specific virotype in a pathogenic process. Laboratory diagnosis of edema disease is based

upon compatible clinical signs, gross and histologic lesions, and recovery of β-hemolytic Shiga toxigenic *E. coli* from the midjejunum or ileum.

Treatment and Control

Prevention of *E. coli* infection can be achieved by ensuring adequate colostral intake by neonates, improving farm sanitation procedures and husbandry, decreasing stocking density, and using commercial vaccines in dams to improve colostral immunity. K88, K99, 987P, and F41 pili are contained in most commercial swine or bovine vaccines. Antimicrobial therapy has met with variable success because of multiple resistance in many strains.

In the case of edema disease, dietary management measures, such as increasing zinc in the ration from 1800 to 3000 ppm, reducing protein levels by 50% in starter rations of recently placed pigs, and increasing fiber levels to 15% to 20% have met with some success in preventing and controlling outbreaks. Recently developed genetically resistant pigs may prove to be the most effective means of preventing edema disease. Commercial vaccines are not yet available for the prevention and control of edema disease. Experimental toxoids and a genetically modified Shiga toxin mutant have been used successfully.

The J5 strain of *E. coli* in a commercial vaccine is used for parenteral immunization of dairy cattle against coliform mastitis through its effect against endotoxin. The vaccine utilizes a rough strain of *E. coli* that lacks the repeating polysaccharide subunits of the O antigen.

In dogs and cats, treatment of pyometritis and cystitis is by prompt antimicrobial therapy and evacuation of uterine or bladder contents. Supportive therapy with fluids may be indicated. Predisposing factors should be elucidated and eliminated.

THE GENUS *SHIGELLA*

The four species in the genus *Shigella*, *Shigella boydii*, *Shigella dysenteriae*, *Shigella flexneri*, and *Shigella sonnei*, are usually associated with disease in humans and nonhuman primates. *Shigella sonnei* is the most common cause of shigellosis in developed countries, whereas *S. flexneri* is more common in Third World nations. Gastroenteritis of children is the most common manifestation of disease. *Shigella dysenteriae* causes severe watery diarrhea or dysentery. More rarely, hemolytic colitis and hemolytic uremic syndrome may result. The organism produces disease through the production of Shiga toxin, which that disrupts cellular protein synthesis and causes endothelial damage.

Humans are the sole reservoir of shigellae, and symptomatic carriers are not uncommon. Disease is spread by the fecal-oral route and is highly infectious in that the infectious dose is only a few organisms.

SUGGESTED READINGS

DebRoy C, Maddox CW: Identification of virulence attributes of gastrointestinal *Escherichia coli* isolates of veterinary significance, *Anim Health Res Rev* 1:129-140, 2001.

Nataro JP, Kaper JB: Diarrheagenic *E. coli, Clin Microbiol Rev* 11:142-201, 1998.

Sanchez S, Lee MD, Harmon BG, et al: Animal issues associated with *Escherichia coli* O157:H7, *J Am Vet Med Assoc* 221:1122-1126, 2002.

Chapter 14

Miscellaneous Coliforms: The Genera *Klebsiella, Enterobacter,* and *Citrobacter*

Members of the family Enterobacteri-aceae ferment lactose, producing acid and gas, with the former evidenced in the pink colonies they produce on MacConkey agar (Figure 14-1). Colonies of *Klebsiella, Enterobacter,* and *Citrobacter* on blood agar are nonhemolytic, shiny, round, gray with entire margins, and 2 to 3 mm diameter after 24-hour incubation at 37° C. All are facultatively anaerobic, oxidase-negative, gram-negative rods. Infections associated with these organisms are opportunistic.

THE GENUS *KLEBSIELLA*

The genus *Klebsiella* contains nonmotile encapsu-lated organisms that are Voges-Proskauer positive,

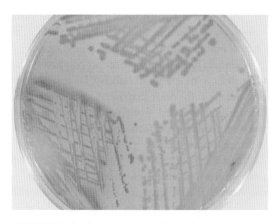

FIGURE 14-1 Lactose-fermenting colonies on MacConkey agar. *Klebsiella, Enterobacter,* and *Citrobacter* spp. (Courtesy Karen W. Post.)

hydrolyze urea, ferment inositol, and utilize citrate, but fail to produce ornithine decarboxylase or hydrogen sulfide (Table 14-1). The three species currently in the genus are *Klebsiella pneumoniae, Klebsiella oxytoca,* and *Klebsiella granulomatis. Klebsiella pneumoniae* is divided into subspecies *ozaenae, pneumoniae,* and *rhinoscleromatis.* The animal pathogenic species are *K. pneumoniae* ssp. *pneumoniae* and *K. oxytoca.*

Diseases and Epidemiology

Klebsiella spp. are common in nature, where they are found in surface water, sewage, soil, and on plant material. Klebsiellae are commensals of the mammalian intestinal tract. *Klebsiella pneumoniae* ssp. *pneumoniae* has been associated with a variety of infectious processes in animals, including bovine mastitis, equine metritis, navel ill/joint ill, and neonatal septicemia in foals, calves, and kids, and is a cause of various infections in dogs, pet birds, poultry, and captive reptiles.

Bovine mastitis attributed to *K. pneumoniae* ssp. *pneumoniae* is economically significant, occurring as peracute disease in individual animals or as outbreaks of acute disease. Case fatality rates may be as high as 80%. Sawdust and shavings are major reservoirs of klebsiellae, and disease is most common in dairy cattle housed during the winter months on sawdust bedding. It is also diagnosed in animals kept in confinement on dry lots. Mastitis is associated with gross contamination of udder and teats with feces and bedding, and is

TABLE **14-1**   Biochemical Differentiation Among Genera *Klebsiella, Enterobacter,* and *Citrobacter*

Characteristic	Klebsiella	Enterobacter	Citrobacter
Motility	Neg	Pos	(Pos)
Voges-Proskauer	Pos	Pos	Neg
Methyl red	(Neg)	Neg	Pos
Citrate	(Pos)	(Pos)	(Pos)
Urease	(Pos)	Var	Var
Hydrogen sulfide in TSI agar slants	Neg	Neg	(Pos)
Ornithine decarboxylase	Neg	Pos	(Pos)

Neg, Negative; *(Neg),* most negative; *Pos,* positive; *(Pos),* most positive; *TSI,* triple-sugar iron; *Var,* variable.

frequently seen within a few days of calving. Moist bedding promotes environmental replication of the organism, and trauma induced by improperly functioning milking machines predisposes the udder to infection. Sporadic cases of caprine and porcine mastitis caused by *K. pneumoniae* have also been reported (Figure 14-2).

Klebsiella pneumoniae and *K. oxytoca* are opportunistic pathogens of the equine reproductive tract. The clitoris, urethra, and vestibule of mares may become colonized, and vaginitis, infertility, metritis, and abortion occur in some of these individuals. Stallions acquire the infection during coitus and transmit it to other mares during natural service. However, stallions are not considered to be important reservoirs of infection, as klebsiellae are usually cleared from the male reproductive tract within 2 weeks. Fomites, such as vaginal speculums and biopsy equipment, can also serve to transmit infection.

The acute neonatal infection known as navel ill can be caused by a variety of bacteria, but coliforms are commonly involved. It is more common in animals with failed passive transfer resulting from ingestion of inadequate amounts of colostrum. Disease manifests as septicemia, often with a purulent focus in umbilicus, joints, lungs, or kidney, resulting in omphalitis, septic arthritis, pneumonia, and pyelonephritis.

Klebsiella pneumoniae has been recovered from a wide range of canine infections. Disease manifestations include pyometra, cystitis, prostatitis, pneumonia, meningoencephalitis, enteritis, mastitis, neonatal septicemia, hepatic abscessation, and otitis externa. The ability of *Klebsiella* to acquire extended-spectrum β-lactamase resistance and to spread within the hospital environment has resulted in its emergence as an important nosocomial pathogen of hospitalized animals. Canine nosocomial infections are primarily associated with surgical wounds, the urinary tract, and septicemia.

Klebsiella pneumoniae and *K. oxytoca* are important pathogens of companion birds. These organisms are contaminants of birdseed, fruits, and vegetables. Birds are easily colonized, and the organisms are frequently isolated from the cloaca and choana of clinically normal birds. Respiratory infections, septicemia, and diarrhea are common disease manifestations in compromised hosts.

Klebsiella pneumoniae is occasionally associated with embryo mortality in poultry. Disease is often associated with poor hatchery sanitation. The organism is isolated from various reptiles with pneumonia and hypopyon, and from osteomyelitis in snakes and iguanids.

Klebsiella spp. account for 3% to 7% of all nosocomial bacterial infections of humans in the United States. The urinary tract is the most common site of infection. In pediatric wards, *Klebsiella* spp. are often associated with neonatal septicemia. *K. granulomatis* is the etiologic agent of granuloma inguinale, a sexually transmitted

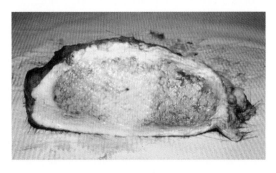

FIGURE 14-2   Porcine mastitis caused by *Klebsiella pneumoniae.* (Courtesy J. Glenn Songer.)

disease characterized by anogenital granulomatous lesions.

Pathogenesis

Virulence factors may include capsule, endotoxin, enterotoxin, adhesins, and siderophores. The capsule is essential to virulence, enabling binding to epithelial cells in urinary and respiratory tracts. It has antiphagocytic properties and prevents killing by bactericidal factors in serum. Endotoxin is responsible for fever, neutropenia, petechiae and ecchymoses, shock, pulmonary edema, and vascular collapse in coliform septicemia. Some strains of *K. pneumoniae* produce an enterotoxin, similar to the heat-stable toxin of *Escherichia coli,* which stimulates the hypersecretion by dysregulation of host cell guanylate cyclase. Several adhesins (type 1 pili, KPF-28 fimbriae, CF29K, and aggregative adhesin) have been described. Siderophores aerobactin and enterobactin are found in strains of *K. pneumoniae.*

Diagnosis

Klebsiellae are easily isolated by bacteriologic culture, producing large mucoid viscous colonies on blood agar (Figure 14-3). Mucoid colonies indicative of capsule production distinguish *Klebsiella* spp. from other enterobacteriaceae. Commercially available systems are adequate for identification of

TABLE **14-2** Differentiation Between *Klebsiella* spp. Most Frequently Recovered from Veterinary Clinical Specimens

Characteristic	*K. pneumoniae*	*K. oxytoca*
Indole	Neg	Pos
Growth at 10° C	Neg	Pos

Neg, Negative; *Pos,* positive.

Klebsiella spp., and differentiation can be achieved by biochemical characterization (Table 14-2).

Prevention and Control

It is inadvisable to bed animals on sawdust or wood shavings. Nosocomial infections can be prevented by improved handwashing, sterilization procedures, closed-system urinary drainage, and reduced prophylactic use of antimicrobials. Resistance among *Klebsiella* spp. has been on a steady increase, especially in the form of organisms that harbor resistance to extended-spectrum β-lactamases. They are uniformly resistant to ampicillin and ticarcillin, and variably susceptible to aminoglycosides, fluoroquinolones, and tetracyclines.

THE GENUS *ENTEROBACTER*

Enterobacter spp. are motile and most are Voges-Proskauer positive. They hydrolyze gelatin slowly and utilize citrate, but do not produce hydrogen sulfide. *Enterobacter aerogenes* and *Enterobacter cloacae* are the opportunistic veterinary pathogens among the 12 currently valid species.

Enterobacter spp. are recovered from cases of bovine mastitis, navel ill/neonatal septicemia, equine uterine infections, canine urinary tract infections, and wound infections in many animal species. They are fairly common disease agents in companion birds and are also isolated from seeds. In humans, *Enterobacter* spp. cause significant nosocomial infections associated with the urinary tract; cardiovascular system; and ear, nose, and throat.

Clinical disease usually occurs in compromised hosts. Little is known about pathogenesis and virulence, other than effects of endotoxin. A cytolytic toxin was discovered recently, but its role in pathogenesis remains to be elucidated.

Diagnosis is based on recovery of the agent from clinical materials and identification by

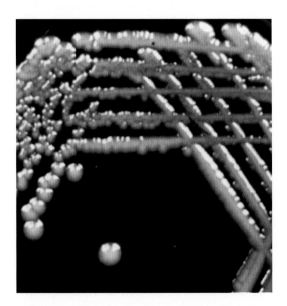

FIGURE 14-3 Large mucoid viscous colonies of *Klebsiella pneumoniae* growing on blood agar. (Courtesy J. Glenn Songer.)

TABLE **14-3** Differentiation Between the *Enterobacter* Species Most Frequently Recovered from Veterinary Clinical Specimens

Characteristic	E. aerogenes	E. cloacae
Arginine dihydrolase	Neg	Pos
Lysine decarboxylase	Pos	Neg
D-sorbitol fermentation	Pos	Neg

Neg, Negative; *Pos*, positive.

either tube biochemical tests or use of commercial microbial identification systems (Table 14-3).

These organisms are innately resistant to most of the older antimicrobials and have the genetic machinery to rapidly develop resistance to newer agents. *Enterobacter aerogenes* and *E. cloacae* are resistant to ampicillin, cephalothin, and tetracyclines. Drugs that are most active against *Enterobacter* spp. include aminoglycosides, fluoroquinolones, and carbapenems (imipenem and meropenem). In addition, many *Enterobacter* spp. are not susceptible to common disinfectants.

THE GENUS *CITROBACTER*

The genus *Citrobacter* has recently been reclassified based on DNA relatedness and now includes 11 species. These organisms are widely distributed in the environment, and are frequently recovered from soil, water, sewage, and food. They are also intestinal tract inhabitants of cold- and warm-blooded animals. *Citrobacter* spp. are opportunistic pathogens associated with a variety of extraintestinal infections, including mastitis, wound infections, septicemia, and pneumonia, in a wide range of animals. The most important animal disease is transmissible murine colonic hyperplasia.

Transmissible murine colonic hyperplasia occurs naturally in laboratory mice and, more rarely, in gerbils and guinea pigs. Disease is characterized by epithelial cell hyperproliferation in the descending colon. The etiologic agent, *Citrobacter rodentium,* was first identified as an atypical strain of *Citrobacter freundii* biotype 4280. The organism has been isolated solely from rodents and is transmitted by the fecal-oral route.

Fomites have also been incriminated in the spread of disease within rodent colonies. Disease susceptibility is known to be influenced by age and genetic background, as well as sudden dietary changes. Infection in most adult mice is self-limiting, with low morbidity and mortality. Some inbred and transgenic lines, and suckling mice of any genotype, are much more susceptible than others, developing diarrhea, growth retardation, and rectal prolapse. Mortality may be high. At necropsy, affected animals have a grossly thickened distal colon that is devoid of feces. Microscopic lesions are morphologically indistinguishable from the histopathologic changes caused by enteropathogenic *E. coli.* Layers of adherent gram-negative rods line the surface mucosa and the superficial portion of the glands. Effacement of the normal brush border, with pedestal-like extensions of the epithelial cells beneath the adherent bacteria, is commonly observed.

Citrobacter rodentium has a homolog of the enterocyte effacement pathogenicity island (locus of enterocyte effacement [LEE]), which contains the genes required for production of the attaching and effacing lesions. A translocated intimin receptor is an essential virulence factor for intestinal colonization. Translocation of this receptor into the host cytoplasmic membrane serves as a point of attachment for bacterial intimin.

Immune suppression may be involved in pathogenesis. *C. rodentium* has a gene that is homologous to that for a toxin produced by enterotoxigenic *E. coli* that mediates suppression of cytokine production and release. Epithelial cell damage via formation of attaching and effacing lesions and disruption of the cytoskeleton appears to be responsible for mucosal hyperplasia.

Laboratory diagnosis has traditionally been based on the characteristic gross lesions, and isolation of the organism from affected animals. The agent is readily cultured and has unique biochemical properties (Table 14-4). *Citrobacter* spp. are motile, and most utilize citrate. They do not decarboxylate lysine and are negative in the Voges-Proskauer test. Citrobacteria may or may not ferment lactose quickly, but nearly always produce β-galactosidase, an enzyme that reveals a genetic capability to attack lactose. Most strains produce hydrogen sulfide in the butt of triple sugar iron agar slants. Databases accompanying commercial bacterial identification systems do not contain

TABLE **14-4** Biochemical Properties of *Citrobacter rodentium*

Reaction	Result
Hydrogen sulfide in TSI slant	Neg
Indole	Neg
Citrate	Neg
Motility	Neg
Malonate	Pos
Ornithine decarboxylase	Pos
Acid production from adonitol	Neg
Acid production from dulcitol	Neg
Acid production from glycerol	Neg
Acid production from melibiose	Neg
Acid production from sucrose	Neg

Neg, Negative; *Pos,* positive; *TSI,* triple-sugar iron.

C. rodentium, so identification is accomplished through traditional biochemical testing. Polymerase chain reaction (PCR) assays, which are more sensitive than bacteriologic culture, detect *C. rodentium* in mouse feces.

Disease prevention is based on proper husbandry and sanitation. Oral solutions of neomycin, tetracycline, or sulfamethazine have been used successfully to reduce clinical disease

SUGGESTED READINGS

Luperchio SA, Schauer DB: Molecular pathogenesis of *Citrobacter rodentium* and transmissible murine colonic hyperplasia, *Microbes Infect* 3:333-340, 2001.

Podschun R, Ullmann U: *Klebsiella* spp. as nosocomial pathogens: epidemiology, taxonomy, typing methods, and pathogenicity factors, *Clin Microbiol Rev* 11:589-603, 1998.

Roberts DE, McClain HM, Hansen DS, et al: An outbreak of *Klebsiella pneumoniae* infection in dogs with severe enteritis and septicemia, *J Vet Diagn Invest* 12:168-273, 2000.

Sanders WE, Sanders CC: *Enterobacter* spp.: pathogens poised to flourish at the turn of the century, *Clin Microbiol Rev* 10:220-241, 1997.

Chapter 15

The Genera *Proteus, Morganella,* and *Edwardsiella*

Members of these genera are facultatively anaerobic, non–lactose-fermenting, small, straight, gram-negative rods in the family Enterobacteriaceae. Colorless or whitish colonies are formed on MacConkey agar (Figure 15-1). Nitrate is reduced to nitrite, and the oxidase tests are negative. They are usually considered to be opportunists.

THE GENUS *PROTEUS*

The genus was named for Proteus, a Homeric character who was able to change forms. *Proteus* spp. produce swarmer cells with peritrichous flagella, and these are responsible for the swarming motility of these organisms over moist agar surfaces (Table 15-1). They hydrolyze urea, produce hydrogen sulfide, and are distinguished from other members of the Enterobacteriaceae by their ability to oxidatively deaminate phenylalanine and tryptophan. The five current species are *Proteus hauseri, Proteus mirabilis, Proteus myxofaciens, Proteus penneri,* and *Proteus vulgaris.* The species of medical significance are *P. mirabilis* and *P. vulgaris.*

Diseases and Epidemiology

Proteus spp. are ubiquitous in the environment, and are commonly recovered from soil, polluted water, and the intestinal tracts of birds, cold-blooded animals, and mammals, including humans. *Proteus mirabilis* and *P. vulgaris* have also been isolated from urinary tract infections, otitis externa, wound infections, prostatitis, nosocomial bacteremia, and occasionally from cases of neonatal enteritis in humans and other animals.

Proteus mirabilis and *P. vulgaris* are isolated most frequently from canine infections such as cystitis, pyelonephritis, prostatitis, wounds, and otitis externa. Equine urinary tract infections as a result of *Proteus* spp. have been reported. Diarrhea in neonatal ruminants, mink, and puppies attributed to *P. mirabilis* has also been described. In calves, prolonged treatment with antimicrobials predisposes to *Proteus* enteritis. *Proteus* spp. are occasionally encountered as reptile pathogens in association with abscesses and bite wounds.

Pathogenesis

Potential virulence factors include urease, endotoxin, IgA protease, swarming motility, fimbriae, hemolysins, and iron-binding siderophores.

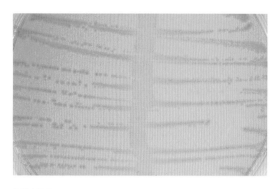

FIGURE 15-1 Non–lactose-fermenting colonies on MacConkey agar plate. (Courtesy Karen W. Post.)

TABLE **15-1** Differentiation Among the Genera *Proteus, Morganella,* and *Edwardsiella*

Biochemical Test	Proteus	Morganella	Edwardsiella
H$_2$S in TSI	Pos	Var	Var
Urea hydrolysis	Pos	Pos	Neg
Citrate utilization	Var	Neg	Neg
Swarming on blood agar	(Pos)	Neg	Neg
Gelatinase (22° C)	Pos	Neg	Neg
D-mannose fermentation	Neg	Pos	Pos

Neg, Negative; *Pos,* positive; *(Pos),* most positive; *TSI,* triple-sugar iron; *Var,* variable.

The organism hydrolyzes urea in the urine to ammonia and CO_2. The urinary epithelial cells become damaged because ammonia is a toxin. The change in urinary pH also leads to precipitation of soluble ions, which results in formation of urinary calculi in the form of struvite or apatite crystals. Urolithiasis is the hallmark of *Proteus* infection. Lipopolysaccharide enhances or inhibits crystallization of struvite and apatite, depending on its chemical structure and ability to bind cations. Stone formation protects the bacterium from the host immune response and the action of antimicrobials because *Proteus* is sequestered in the interstices of the urolith, but continues to replicate.

Proteus mirabilis secretes a metalloprotease, ZapA, that may be a virulence factor because of its ability to degrade IgA. Swarming is a form of multicellular behavior that involves a cyclical differentiation of short vegetative rods called swimmer cells into filamentous hyperflagellated swarmer cells. The result is a coordinated population migration across surfaces.

Proteus mirabilis expresses different types of fimbriae simultaneously. These are involved in bacterial colonization of the bladder and the kidney. *Proteus* hemolysin is pore forming and causes efflux of sodium ions from eukaryotic cells. It may play a role in dissemination from bladder to kidneys. An amino acid deaminase produced by *P. mirabilis* catalyzes the deamination of amino acids to α-keto acids, which bind iron and may serve a siderophore-like function.

Most of what is known about the pathogenesis of *Proteus* is from investigations of urinary tract infections. Organisms gain entry into the urethra by periurethral fecal contamination. Flagella play a significant role in allowing the bacteria to ascend into the bladder. Bacteria adhere to bladder epithelial cells via fimbriae and adhesins, and the activity of urease causes tissue damage, leading to cystitis. If stones block the drainage of urine into ureters, the ammonia buildup further damages host tissues. From the bladder, *Proteus* ascends the ureter and colonizes the kidney, causing pyelonephritis. Hematogenous dissemination may occur.

Diagnosis

Bacterial culture from clinical materials is the method for diagnosis. *Proteus* grows well on a variety of routine media such as MacConkey agar and blood agar. Colonies of *P. mirabilis* swarm on nonselective agar media, producing a surface film (Figure 15-2). The organism also has a characteristic strong odor that has been likened to "burned chocolate." On MacConkey agar plates, clear colonies are produced in 24 hours. *Proteus* colonies may be confused with those of *Salmonella* on selective media, in that they share a similar

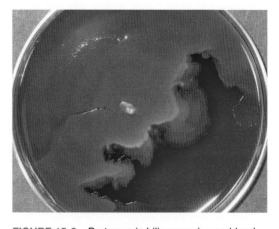

FIGURE 15-2 *Proteus mirabilis* swarming on blood agar plate. (Courtesy Karen W. Post.)

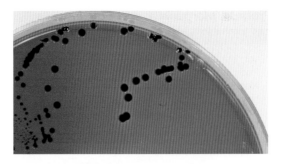

FIGURE 15-3 XLT4 agar plate with hydrogen sulfide–producing colonies, typical of *Proteus, Salmonella,* or *Edwardsiella tarda.* (Courtesy Karen W. Post.)

colony morphology (Figure 15-3). *Proteus* can be rapidly identified in the laboratory with minimal testing, including demonstration of swarming on blood agar and results of spot or tube biochemical tests (Table 15-2). The accuracy of commercial systems in the identification of *Proteus* spp. approaches 100%.

Prevention and Control

Proteus mirabilis is usually susceptible in vitro to ampicillin, cephalosporins, chloramphenicol, fluoroquinolones, and aminoglycosides. *Proteus vulgaris* is often resistant to ampicillin and cephalosporins. Both species carry plasmid-encoded resistance to tetracyclines. Recently a progressive increase of β-lactam resistance, mediated by the production of acquired β-lactamases, has been reported.

THE GENUS *MORGANELLA*

Morganella morganii ssp. *morganii* and *M. morganii* ssp. *sibonii* were previously named *Proteus morganii,* but were placed as the sole species in a new genus, based on DNA–DNA hybridization studies. Morganellae are motile, produce urease and indole, and deaminate phenylalanine. Unlike *Proteus* spp. they do not swarm over agar surfaces.

They are normal inhabitants of the gastrointestinal tract of humans, other mammals, and reptiles, and are found widely in the environment. *Morganella morganii* was originally isolated from infants with diarrhea and is infrequently encountered as an animal pathogen. Otitis externa and cystitis in dogs have been reported. The organism has been isolated in pure culture from pneumonic lungs of a piglet and a captive jaguar. Cutaneous abscesses, septic arthritis, and septicemia have been described in reptiles.

There is a paucity of information in the literature regarding pathogenesis and virulence factors of *M. morganii,* but they are postulated to be similar to those of *Proteus* spp.

Commercial identification systems may be used to confirm the identity of these organisms, but most cannot discriminate between the subspecies. *Morganella morganii* ssp. *sibonii* ferments trehalose and *M. morganii* ssp. *morganii* does not.

Morganella morganii is susceptible to many antimicrobials, including third-generation cephalosporins, fluoroquinolones, aminoglycosides, and imipenem.

THE GENUS *EDWARDSIELLA*

Edwardsiellae are fastidious when compared with many taxa in the Enterobacteriaceae family, requiring vitamins and amino acids for their growth. Three species in the genus include *Edwardsiella tarda, Edwardsiella ictaluri,* and *Edwardsiella hoshinae,* and the first two are associated with animal infections. *Edwardsiella hoshinae* has been recovered from reptiles and birds, but not in association with disease.

Diseases and Epidemiology

Edwardsiella spp. inhabit freshwater environments and the intestinal tracts of cold-blooded animals. They are recognized pathogens of fish, eels, and some higher vertebrates. The main source of

TABLE **15-2** Differentiation Among *Proteus mirabilis, Proteus penneri,* and *Proteus vulgaris*

Property	P. mirabilis	P. penneri	P. vulgaris
Swarming	Pos	Var	Rare
Oxidase	Neg	Neg	Neg
Indole production	Neg	Neg	Pos
Ornithine decarboxylase	Pos	Neg	Neg

Neg, Negative; *Pos,* positive; *Var,* variable.

infection appears to be the intestinal contents of carrier aquatic animals, although *E. tarda* may also be isolated from mud and pond sediment. High water temperatures, increased stocking density, and poor water quality are predisposing factors for disease.

Edwardsiella tarda is most often isolated from warm-water fish in association with localized cutaneous lesions and septicemia. The skin sores eventually progress to ulcers that emit an objectionable odor. Disease is more prevalent in the Far East than in the United States. *Edwardsiella tarda* is the etiologic agent of "red disease" of cultured eels. Infected eels are lethargic and develop ventral and perineal petechial hemorrhages. Affected eels succumb to hepatitis and nephritis. The organism has been recovered from the intestines of apparently healthy fish-eating birds, marine mammals, and, occasionally, cattle, pigs, and dogs. However, mild enteritis has occasionally been reported in penguins, turtles, piglets, puppies, and calves.

Edwardsiella ictaluri was first described 20 years ago as the cause of enteric septicemia in catfish, commonly known as "hole in the head" disease. Enteric septicemia is one of the most important bacterial diseases in aquaculture, with mortalities up to 50% and annual losses totaling millions of dollars. Handling of fish and low oxygen levels increase mortality. Channel catfish are much more susceptible than other ictalurids, and all ages are affected. Disease is most prevalent in the southeastern United States, but cases have occasionally been reported from other states and even other countries (Australia and Thailand). Outbreaks occur when water temperatures rise above 65° F. *Edwardsiella ictaluri* causes a chronic to subacute disease with pathognomonic clinical signs in which affected fish hang in a vertical position at the pond surface and may spin rapidly in circles. External necropsy findings include pale gills, exophthalmia, petechial hemorrhages on the skin in the mouth or throat regions, areas of depigmentation of the scales along the sides and back, shallow skin ulcers, and distended abdomens. In chronic infections, open lesions are found on the head, especially on the frontal bone of the skull between the eyes, hence the name hole in the head disease (Figure 15-4).

Edwardsiella tarda is the only species associated with human disease, in which it may cause gastroenteritis or rare septicemia.

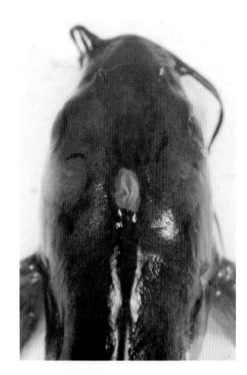

FIGURE 15-4   Catfish with cephalic lesion of *Edwardsiella ictaluri.* (Courtesy Donald V. Lightener.)

Pathogenesis

Virulence factors of *Edwardsiella* spp. include invasins, siderophores, and hemolysins. Bacteria invade human epithelial (HEp)–2 cells in vitro, although by an unknown mechanism. Siderophores, produced by *E. tarda,* facilitate iron acquisition. Hemolysins may provide iron by releasing hemoglobin from lysed red blood cells. Hemolysins may also damage intestinal epithelial cells, leading to villus disruption and diarrhea. *Edwardsiella* spp. are readily phagocytized by host immune cells, but experimental evidence suggests that they are not destroyed.

Diagnosis

Bacterial isolation from affected tissues is the primary method of diagnosis. These organisms grow readily on brain heart infusion or blood agar. A selective or differential *Edwardsiella* isolation medium is used in fish diagnostic laboratories to distinguish the slowly growing *E. ictaluri* and *E. tarda* from more rapidly growing bacteria, such as *Pseudomonas* and *Aeromonas* spp. With incubation at 25° C for 48 hours on nonselective

TABLE **15-3** Differentiation Between *Edwardsiella tarda* and *Edwardsiella ictaluri*

Biochemical Test	E. tarda	E. ictaluri
H₂S in TSI	Pos	Neg
Methyl red production	Pos	Neg
Indole production	Pos	Neg
Motility	Pos	Neg
Growth at 42° C	Pos	Neg

Neg, Negative; *Pos,* positive; *TSI,* triple-sugar iron.

media, *E. ictaluri* forms smooth, circular, convex, entire-edged nonpigmented colonies that are 2 mm in diameter. Colonies of *E. tarda* also develop in 48 hours at 25° C and are small (0.5 mm diameter), round, transparent, and raised. Morphology in Gram-stained smears is similar for both species, revealing regular short rods, 0.8 μm wide by 1 to 3 μm long. Biochemical tests for identification should be incubated at 25° C (Table 15-3). Because *E. tarda* is lactose negative and produces hydrogen sulfide, it may be indistinguishable from salmonellae on enteric plating media (see Figure 15-4). Positive identification of *E. tarda* and *E. ictaluri* can be achieved by specific serum agglutination or fluorescent antibody tests performed on live cultures.

Serologic methods, including fluorescent antibody and enzyme immunoassays, allow antemortem diagnosis of *E. ictaluri* infection. Molecular-based diagnostic tests are available only in aquatic specialty laboratories.

Prevention and Control

Dead fish are a source of large numbers of bacteria, and their removal from ponds can significantly reduce transmission. Aquatic birds are porters of edwardsiellae, and programs to control them should be instituted. Dietary modifications, such as supplementation with zinc (15-30 mg/day), may decrease fish susceptibility to disease. Addition of vitamin E appears to enhance the ability of macrophages to phagocytose edwardsiellae. Outbreaks of disease have been controlled using feed containing oxytetracycline and trimethoprim-sulfamethoxazole.

SUGGESTED READINGS

Coker C, Poore CA, Li X, Mobley HLT: Pathogenesis of *Proteus mirabilis* urinary tract infection, *Microbes Infect* 2:1497-1505, 2000.

Janda JM, Abbott SL, Kroske-Bystrom S, et al: Pathogenic properties of *Edwardsiella* species, *J Clin Microbiol* 29:1997-2001, 1991.

O'Hara CM, Brenner FW, Miller JM: Classification, identification, and clinical significance of *Proteus, Providencia,* and *Morganella, Clin Microbiol Rev* 13:534-546, 2000.

Plumb JA: *Health maintenance and principal microbial disease of cultured fishes,* Ames, Iowa, 1999, Iowa State University Press.

Chapter 16

The Genus *Salmonella*

Members of the genus *Salmonella* colonize vertebrate hosts, with outcomes ranging from subclinical to systemic infection with high mortality. Animal infection has direct economic consequences, but asymptomatic carriage, leading to direct or indirect transmission to humans, may be even more important.

The genus comprises nearly 2500 serovars, traditionally based on the Kauffman-White scheme in which H (flagellar) and O (somatic) antigens determine the serovar. However, multilocus enzyme electrophoresis and DNA–DNA hybridization analysis revealed that the genus can be divided into two species, *Salmonella enterica* (2443 serovars) and *Salmonella bongori* (20 serovars). *Salmonella enterica* is divided into subspecies *salamae, arizonae, diarizonae, houtenae, indica,* and *enterica*. The last contains most of the approximately 50 serovars that cause most disease cases. *Salmonella bongori* serovars lack *Salmonella* pathogenicity island–2 (SPI-2) (see p. 134). The type species remains officially *Salmonella choleraesuis,* but the two-species concept, with *S. enterica* as the type species, is increasingly accepted. Nonitalicized serovar names are retained.

Serovar-to-serovar variations in virulence and epidemiology are common in *S. enterica,* despite close genetic relationships. Most serovars cause gastroenteritis, but a specific few (serovars Typhi, Paratyphi A and C, and Sendai) cause systemic disease originating in the gastrointestinal tract and others (serovars Choleraesuis and Dublin) are frequently associated with bacteremia and less commonly with diarrhea. Host adaptation also varies widely, from the strong host preferences of Typhi (humans), Pullorum (poultry), Choleraesuis (swine), Abortus-ovis (sheep), and Dublin (cattle) to the relative promiscuity of serovar Typhimurium.

Genetic mechanisms underlying the diverse phenotypes in the genus are based in part on polymorphisms in genes encoding surface structures (lipopolysaccharides [LPS], flagella, and fimbriae), which are often virulence factors and thus targets of nonspecific and induced host defenses. Therefore there is selective pressure toward genetic polymorphism, which results in antigenic diversity. Transfer of virulence determinants on pathogenicity islands, plasmids, or phage augurs toward increased diversity in virulence phenotypes.

DISEASES AND EPIDEMIOLOGY

Disease occurs as peracute septicemia and acute, subacute, or chronic enteritis. Acute disease caused by some serovars (such as *Salmonella* Typhimurium) is characterized by high morbidity, and low mortality, manifesting as depression, diarrhea, and fever. Dehydration and electrolyte imbalance may be sufficiently severe, especially when accompanied by septicemia, to be fatal in infection by other serovars (*Salmonella* Dublin in calves and *Salmonella* Choleraesuis in piglets). Young animals are often more severely affected than adults, and shipping, concurrent infections, treatment with immunosuppressive drugs, and oral antibiotics are risk factors.

Outbreaks of disease in animals and humans have been associated with *Salmonella* Newport since the 1970s. The organism has emerged as an important cause of diarrhea outbreaks in horses and dairy cattle, with high mortality in periparturient and neonatal animals. The serovar has consistently been ranked among the 10 salmonellae most commonly isolated from human food-borne infections, having been recovered from hamburger, chicken, roast beef, potato salad, pork, alfalfa sprouts, and seafood. Multidrug resistance is a major problem, with resistance described to chloramphenicol, sulfamethoxazole, tetracycline, streptomycin, and most recently to cephalosporins.

Serovars commonly affecting swine are Typhimurium, Copenhagen, Derby, Newport, Agona, and Choleraesuis var. Kunzendorf. Typhimurium causes enteritis, whereas Choleraesuis is swine adapted, causing systemic disease with high mortality and low morbidity in young pigs. Asymptomatic carriage and sometimes sporadic shedding by recovered or subclinically affected animals maintains the infection in herds. A classic experimental epidemiologic study examined *Salmonella* shedding in "joyriding pigs"; the authors demonstrated that culture-negative pigs, loaded onto a truck and driven a few hundred miles, were then detected as shedders. It is also not uncommon for pigs to develop severe enteritis during shipping, creating challenges for shippers and packers, through contamination of equipment and pens and transmission to previously uninfected animals.

Calves 1 to 2 weeks of age usually develop enteric symptoms when infected with S. Typhimurium and septicemia with S. Dublin. Most calves recover and become carriers, but dehydration and severe pneumonia contribute to mortality; some calves experience polyarthritis, osteomyelitis, or meningoencephalitis. Salmonellosis is rarely life threatening in adult cattle, but short- or long-term recovered carriers may expose others in the herd and contaminate milk. *Salmonella* Typhimurium and *Salmonella* Dublin are the leading entries on an extensive list of infecting serovars. *Salmonella* Dublin and *Salmonella* Muenster also cause abortion in dairy cattle.

Salmonella Gallinarum and *Salmonella* Pullorum cause septicemic disease in turkeys (fowl typhoid) and chickens, respectively, but these birds are infected with a wide variety of serovars. Young chicks often develop fatal septicemia (Figure 16-1), and *Salmonella* Enteritidis phage type 4 causes a lethal infection in older chickens (Figure 16-2). *Salmonella enterica* ssp. *arizonae* is a common problem in turkeys. Even where the traditional avian pathogens S. Gallinarum and S. Pullorum have been eliminated, poultry are frequently colonized with one or more serovars, including Typhimurium, Enteritidis, Heidelberg, Infantis, Montevideo, and Anatum, any of which may be transmitted to humans. Vertical transmission, especially of S. Enteritidis, S. Typhimurium, and *Salmonella* Heidelberg, makes eggs a common vehicle for human infection.

Equine salmonellosis is an uncommon but nonetheless important problem, especially as a nosocomial infection in veterinary teaching hospitals. Many strains isolated from this setting are resistant to multiple antimicrobials. The infectious dose is apparently quite small in horses that have been exposed to the stress of transportation and are affected by underlying illness. *Salmonella* Typhimurium is encountered most frequently,

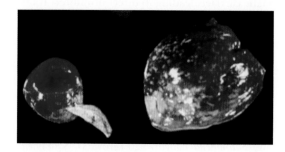

FIGURE 16-1 Systemic lesions of *Salmonella* infection in a cockatiel. (Courtesy Raymond E. Reed.)

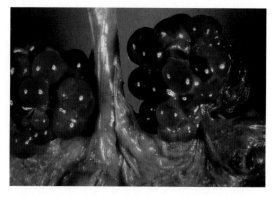

FIGURE 16-2 Avian salpingitis as a result of *Salmonella* infection. (Courtesy Raymond E. Reed.)

but others implicated in disease include Agona, Krefeld, Anatum, and Saint-Paul. Foals are more susceptible than adults, often developing septicemic disease.

Clinical salmonellosis is a common problem in companion animals. The likelihood that a dog will be a carrier is higher in dogs from contaminated environments (such as dogs working cattle). Frequent infection of racing greyhounds is apparently related to contaminated meat used as food.

Salmonella enterica ssp. *arizonae* occasionally causes fatal infections in chicks, turkey poults, humans, dogs, and cats, and is found frequently in snakes and lizards.

Abortion is a manifestation of *Salmonella* infection in several species. *Salmonella* Abortusovis is commonly associated with ovine abortion (without enteritis) and *S.* Dublin may also be isolated (usually from animals with enteritis). *Salmonella* Abortusequi infection causes equine abortion.

Salmonellae reside in the normal vertebrate gastrointestinal tract, and asymptomatic carriers among domestic and wild animals and birds introduce the infection to and maintain it in herds and flocks (Figure 16-3). Feeds of animal origin (fish meal, bone meal, and meat meal) and contaminated water are also common sources of infection. Long-term survival in manure, soil, and other aspects of the environment facilitate transmission. Turtles, lizards, and snakes, as well as sick and recovering humans may shed organisms. Other sources are whole eggs (duck eggs may have a higher prevalence of infection) and egg products, meat and meat products, contaminated water, contaminated equipment and utensils, fertilizers, and animal feeds prepared from bones, fish meal, and meat. Biosecurity is also often compromised by *Salmonella*-carrying rodents and wild birds.

Host adaptation is an important epidemiologic feature of some *Salmonella* infections (Table 16-1). These cause severe, systemic disease in young and old alike. However, most serovars show no host adaptation and, perhaps due to lack of ability to deal with the mature immune system, cause enteric disease primarily in the young. Serovars Typhimurium and Enteritidis are perhaps the most promiscuous, being isolated from many vertebrates with and without clinical disease. Transmissibility and high virulence may be linked in the evolution of host adaptation, and gene deletion may drive (or accompany) the focusing of a serovar's attention on a specific host.

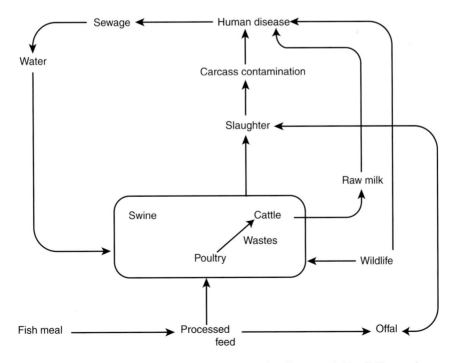

FIGURE 16-3 Movement of *Salmonella* serovars among reservoirs. (Courtesy Ashley E. Harmon.)

TABLE **16-1** Host-Adapted Serovars of *Salmonella enterica*

S. enterica Serovar	Preferred Host
Typhi	Humans (exclusively)
Paratyphi A, Sendai	Humans
Dublin	Cattle
Choleraesuis	Swine
Pullorum, Gallinarum	Poultry
Abortusequi	Horses
Abortusovis	Sheep
Arizona	Reptiles

PATHOGENESIS

Salmonella diverged from *Escherichia coli* approximately 100 million years ago. In the intervening years, clusters of conserved virulence genes retained by *Salmonella* spp. have been lost from avirulent strains of *E. coli*. These chromosomal regions, called *Salmonella* pathogenicity islands (SPIs), have lower G + C content than in flanking DNA, intimating acquisition through horizontal transfer. Five pathogenicity islands in *S.* Typhimurium and *Salmonella* Typhi are in or near tRNA genes, which are anchor points for temperate phage insertion. There is clear evidence of crosstalk between genes in different pathogenicity islands.

SPI-1 is found in all *Salmonella* spp. It encodes a secretion apparatus, transcriptional regulators, and effector proteins that facilitate uptake of *Salmonella* by enterocytes. SPI-1 invasion genes are regulated by environmental stimuli in the intestinal tract, and the regulatory molecules are encoded inside *or* outside SPI-1. Effector proteins delivered to the host cell cytoplasm coordinate intracellular changes that result in uptake of the organism. Mutants are avirulent by the oral route but virulent by IP or IV routes.

Intramacrophage survival of *Salmonella* spp. is not possible without the contribution of SPI-2 and mutants are profoundly attenuated for virulence by oral or IP routes and cannot proliferate in spleen or liver of infected mice. SPI-2 gene products may interfere with trafficking of NADPH oxidase to *Salmonella*-containing phagosomes, thereby preventing oxidative killing. SPI-2–deficient mutants of *S.* Typhimurium are 1 million-fold attenuated in mice. SPI-3 genes are required for growth in Mg^{+2}-limiting conditions and for intramacrophage survival. SPI-4 may play a role in

invasion. SPI-5 was first identified in *S.* Dublin and is required for enteric but not systemic salmonellosis.

Host-adapted *Salmonella* serovars that cause severe systemic disease (e.g., Dublin, Pullorum, Gallinarum, Choleraesuis, Abortusovis, and some strains of Typhimurium and Enteritidis, but not *S.* Typhi) harbor virulence plasmids. In *S.* Typhimurium, an 8 kb region of the virulence plasmid encodes the *spv* (*Salmonella* plasmid virulence) genes, which affect bacterial growth during systemic infection. They are expressed during intracellular residence and increase virulence by 10- to 10,000-fold. Spv proteins may attract macrophages to sites of infection as a source of cells permissive for intracellular growth.

Salmonellae often enter the host by ingestion, and even with several systems to mediate acid resistance, few survive the stomach and move into the small intestine. Normal flora protect against colonization and administration of oral antibiotics facilitates establishment of infection.

Salmonellae must adhere to and invade enterocytes in order to cause enteritis or systemic disease. Fimbriae and an outer membrane protein involved in enterocyte invasion are encoded by virulence plasmid-associated genes in *S.* Typhimurium. Numerous fimbrial operons in *S.* Typhi may encode adhesins mediating attachment to different cell types, but a role for fimbriae in domestic animal infections has not been documented. Most pathogenic salmonellae switch between flagellar phases by inversion of a genetic element, and this may be another means of evading the immune system. Flagella contribute to intestinal invasiveness of *Salmonella* spp., neutrophil recruitment (through stimulation of interleukins (IL)-8 production), and fluid secretion in calves.

Entry of salmonellae usually occurs without mucosal damage in systemic infections, but enteric infection is characterized by local damage without septicemia. *Salmonella* interaction with M cells in Peyer's patches is facilitated by fimbrial adhesins. This is followed by ruffling of the target cell membrane, which results in internalization of bacteria in membrane-bound vacuoles. Invasion of enterocytes is also important and is, in fact, the major event in disease in some domestic animals (e.g., calves). Enterocyte microvilli and tight junctions undergo morphologic changes when *Salmonella* approaches the mucosa, due to profound rearrangement of the actin cytoskeleton.

Interestingly, these morphologic changes are reversed as *Salmonella*-containing vesicles move toward the basolateral aspect of the enterocyte.

Invasion is followed by inflammation, with a notable profusion of neutrophils as a result of production of IL-8 at the basolateral surface and of an epithelial chemoattractant at the apical border. Neutrophils migrate into lamina propria and then to the lumen. Disruption of tight junctions permits access to receptors on the basolateral surface, increasing production of proinflammatory cytokines. Dogma has held that *Salmonella* infection induces secretory diarrhea. The diarrheagenic mechanism apparently does not involve a toxin, in that none have been demonstrated by direct examination of cultures and no toxinlike genes have been found in complete genome sequences of serovars Typhimurium, Typhi, Dublin, and Choleraesuis.

Cell death and sloughing allow bacterial invasion of the submucosal tissues. M cell transcytosis brings the organisms into contact with host phagocytes. Some macrophages are killed rapidly, in a process that shares features of apoptosis and necrosis. Intraphagosomal survival is required for establishment of *Salmonella* spp. in the intestine and for systemic spread. The PhoP/PhoQ regulon plays a major role in resistance to oxygen-dependent and oxygen-independent killing. PhoP-activated genes encode proteins that change the composition of LPS and the outer membrane and reduce the charge of the bacterial surface, with decreased permeability and greater resistance to antimicrobial peptides. Oxidative stress resistance in *S.* Typhimurium involves more than 60 genes, although not all of these are required for intramacrophage survival. Catalase mutants are sensitive in vitro to oxidative stress, but remain fully virulent. DNA repair mutants replicate in murine macrophages unable to generate a respiratory burst, but are killed in burst-competent macrophages. Inhibition of phagosome-lysosome fusion is mediated by products of SPI-2 genes.

Survival and replication in phagocytes, and subsequently in lymph nodes, can lead to extraintestinal dissemination. Bacteria delivered to circulation are removed by cells of the reticuloendothelial system, particularly in liver and spleen. Toxic effects of LPS result in overstimulation of the host cytokine response, and the ultimate effects include inflammation, shock, fever, and death. Extensive growth of lipid A mutants in liver and spleen does not result in death, whereas growth of wildtype strains is lethal at 3 logs lower. Rough mutants (lacking normal LPS) are sensitive to complement, antimicrobial peptides, and detergents, and are killed more efficiently by phagocytes.

DIAGNOSIS

Salmonellae are facultatively anaerobic and non–spore forming, growing optimally at 37° C. All serovars (except Pullorum and Gallinarum) are motile by means of peritrichous flagella. It is common practice to plate highly contaminated specimens directly on selective and differential agar media and after enrichment in selective broth (e.g., Rappaport-Vassiliadis medium or tetrathionate broth). Solid media include xylose lysine deoxycholate (XLD) and Hektoen enteric (HE) agars, followed by incubation at 37° C for at least 12 hours. On XLD, salmonellae produce pink colonies with black centers (caused by H_2S production). Some colonies may appear completely black with a small pink margin, depending on the level of H_2S production. On HE agar, colonies are blue-green or blue, with or without black centers. Polymerase chain reaction (PCR) methods targeting *Salmonella*-specific genes facilitate identification. O-grouping by serologic methods is done in many routine diagnostic laboratories, but serotyping is limited to reference laboratories. Biochemical characteristics are useful in differentiating species and subspecies. Salmonellae are non–lactose fermenting, except for *S. enterica* ssp. *arizonae* and *S. enterica* ssp. *diarizonae*, and do not produce indole or urease. They are also Voges-Proskauer negative, but are positive in methyl red, citrate utilization, H_2S production, and lysine and ornithine decarboxylase tests. Most are catalase positive and all are resistant to bile salts. Salmonellae other than serovars Typhi and Paratyphi produce a red butt (indicative of acid fermentation) and a black stab (revealing H_2S production) in triple-sugar iron (TSI) or lysine-iron agar (LIA) slants. Somatic (O) and flagellar (H) antigens can be detected by immunoassays, and serovar-specific sera are commercially available. Reference laboratories identify *Salmonella* to serovar and phage group.

PREVENTION AND CONTROL

Salmonella control based on vaccination and antibiotic treatment has been largely unsuccessful. Competitive exclusion by adult chicken cecal flora has been somewhat more useful; effects vary between groups and among flocks, and the mechanism of exclusion is not understood.

Therapy of *Salmonella* spp. infections is increasingly hampered by resistance to antimicrobial agents. More than 90% of isolates, especially of serovar Typhimurium, from domestic animals have exhibited resistance to an expanding collection of antimicrobials. Multiple resistance is less common in isolates from humans, occurring in 26% of all isolates and in 50% of serovar Typhimurium. Resistance can occur in distinct patterns, but usually includes tetracycline, sulfamethoxazole, streptomycin, ampicillin, and chloramphenicol or kanamycin. Susceptibility to ciprofloxacin and ceftriaxone, which are used to treat human salmonellosis, is decreasing. Antimicrobial resistance in phage type DT104, a highly publicized human pathogen, arises from chromosomal genes that are physically linked. In phage type DT193, resistance factors are on conjugative plasmids, which are readily transferred.

Innate immune responses are important in controlling the early phases of infection with *Salmonella* spp. Neutrophils ingest and kill *Salmonella*, but until activated as part of the specific immune response, macrophages are permissive for growth of the organisms and even participate in dissemination of infection. To a small extent in naive macrophages and to a much greater degree in specifically activated macrophages, *Salmonella* antigens are presented on MHC-I and MHC-II. Dendritic cells also participate in antigen presentation, and in either case, cell-mediated immunity (CMI) and humoral responses result. The former is widely acknowledged to be of greatest importance, because of the intracellular nature of *Salmonella* interaction with the host. Transfer of sensitized T cells protects the recipient, but transfer of macrophages, B cells, or hyperimmune serum has no such effect. Extent of protection is directly proportional to the degree of cell-mediated immunity.

However, calves can be protected by oral administration of attenuated strains, even though they lack an obvious CMI response. Taking into account the facts that normally suckled neonatal calves are seldom infected and that serum antibody levels are unrelated to protection, one might conclude that specific secretory immunoglobulin (sIgA) produced at the mucosa may provide protection, perhaps by interfering with M cell uptake of organisms.

These responses occur as a matter of course in natural, nonfatal infections, but have also been the subject of extensive efforts aimed at development of effective vaccines. Live, orally administered vaccines present a population of antigens similar to that to which the host is exposed in a mild infection and induce CMI and both systemic and mucosal antibodies. Protection across serovars and across species has been achieved. Duration of immunity is a major concern with many commercial products.

Rational attenuation of *Salmonella* for vaccine development has been based on inactivation of genes for a crucial requirement that can be filled in vitro but which will result in gradual decline of the population in vivo. It is common practice to include at least two attenuating mutations, to decrease the risk of reversions to virulence. Such products are more effective against host-adapted than nonadapted serovars, suggesting that they may elicit better responses against systemic disease than against enteric infection. Vaccines based on rough mutants of serovar Gallinarum have been widely used for many years.

SUGGESTED READINGS

Fierer J, Krause M, Tauxe R, Guiney DG: *Salmonella typhimurium* bacteremia: association with the virulence plasmid, *J Infect Dis* 166:639-642, 1992.

Fierer J, Swancutt M: Non-typhoid *Salmonella*: a review, *Curr Clin Top Infect Dis* 20:134-157, 2000.

Libby SJ, Adams LG, Ficht TA, et al: The spv genes on the *Salmonella dublin* virulence plasmid are required for severe enteritis and systemic infection in the natural host, *Infect Immun* 65:1786-1792, 1997.

Lu S, Manges AR, Xu Y, et al: Analysis of virulence of clinical isolates of *Salmonella enteritidis* in vivo and in vitro, *Infect Immun* 67:5651-5657, 1999.

Mittrücker H-W, Kaufmann SHE: Immune response to infection with *Salmonella typhimurium* in mice, *J Leukoc Biol* 67:457-463, 2000.

Ochman H, Soncini FC, Solomon F, Groisman EA: Identification of a pathogenicity island required for *Salmonella* survival in host cells, *Proc Natl Acad Sci U S A* 93:7800-7804, 1996.

Tsolis RM, Adams LG, Ficht TA, Baumler AJ: Contribution of *Salmonella typhimurium* virulence factors to diarrheal disease in calves, *Infect Immun* 67:4879-4885, 1999.

Vassiloyanakopoulos AP, Okamoto S, Fierer J: The crucial role of polymorphonuclear leukocytes in resistance to *Salmonella dublin* infections in genetically susceptible and resistant mice, *Proc Natl Acad Sci U S A* 95:7676-7681, 1998.

Chapter 17

The Genus *Yersinia*

Yersiniae are oxidase-negative, facultatively anaerobic, catalase-positive, gram-negative rods, members of the family Enterobacteriaceae. The genus contains seven species, including *Yersinia pestis*, the causative agent of plague. The organisms can be readily cultivated on standard bacteriologic media, and pathogens or potential pathogens can be distinguished based on phenotype (Table 17-1).

Yersinia pestis, the causative agent of plague, is nonmotile and resembles a safety pin when stained with Wright's, Giemsa, or Wayson stains (Figure 17-1). It participates in a flea-rodent-flea life cycle, occasionally breaking out to cause plague, an often fatal zoonosis. The organism killed more than one quarter of the European population during the fourteenth century, and at least 10 million people in Asia as recently as the first half of the twentieth century. The extent of its devastation of societies has been unequaled by any other infectious agent. *Yersinia pestis* infection is endemic in the western United States, causing several human cases annually. Transmission can occur via fleas acquired by dogs and cats from infected rodents, but plague is not ordinarily considered a significant occupational hazard for veterinarians.

The 10 serotypes of *Yersinia pseudotuberculosis* cause less severe systemic disease in humans and other animals, whereas *Yersinia enterocolitica* causes enteritis mainly in humans and is less likely to become systemic. The latter organism is divided into five biotypes and more than 30 serotypes. Serotype O:8 strains, which are common in North America, are atypically invasive in humans as well as animals.

Yersinia ruckeri is responsible for red-mouth (pink mouth, pink or red throat) of salmon and trout. *Yersinia intermedia, Yersinia kristensenii,* and *Yersinia frederiksenii* are occasional opportunistic pathogens.

TABLE **17-1**   Differential Characteristics of Animal Pathogens in the Genus *Yersinia*

Yersinia Species	Indole	Ornithine Decarboxylase	Urease	Sucrose	Mannitol	Glucose (Gas)	Sorbitol	Rhamnose
Y. enterocolitica	(Neg)	Pos	(Pos)	Pos	Pos	Neg	Pos	Neg
Y. pestis	Neg	Neg	Neg	Neg	Pos	Neg	Neg	Neg
Y. pseudotuberculosis	Neg	Neg	Pos	Neg	Pos	Neg	Neg	Pos

Neg, Negative; *(Neg),* most negative; *Pos,* positive; *(Pos),* most positive.

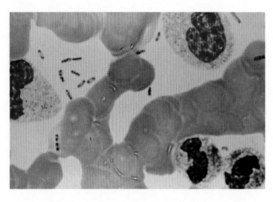

FIGURE 17-1 Dark-staining ends demonstrate the safety pin morphology of *Yersinia pestis* in this Wright's-stained blood smear. (Courtesy Public Health Image Library, PHIL #2050, Atlanta, 1993, Centers for Disease Control and Prevention.)

YERSINIA PESTIS

Disease

Numerous references to plagues that may have been caused by *Y. pestis* appear in ancient literature, including the Old Testament. The first documented plague epidemic occurred in Athens in 430 BC; it resulted in the death of one third of the population and precipitated the downfall of classical Greece. Outbreaks between AD 541 and 750 comprise the Justinian pandemic, beginning in Ethiopia and spreading from Egypt through the Middle East and into Mediterranean Europe. Epidemics occurred between AD 558 and 654 in 8- to 12-year cycles in North Africa, Europe, and Asia, with mortality rates approaching 50%. The so-called second pandemic (1330-1346) originated in central Asia; Mongolian plague victims were catapulted over the city walls of Caffa in 1346. Plague spread westward along trade routes, mediated by sales of furs from animals dead of plague, and entered Europe by way of Messina, Genoa, and Marseilles in 1347. It was during these epidemics that plague came to be known as the Black Death, killing as many as 28 million (40% of the population). The disease recurred in regular cycles until the early 1700s. Cases arrived in southern France from Syria and Lebanon in early 1720, and the ensuing epidemic killed 50,000 people in Marseilles. Examination of the graves from this period provided the first evidence that bronze pins were driven into the toes to verify death. The third pandemic began in 1855 in China, progressing rapidly to Hong Kong and beyond, including Hawaii and then North America.

Alexandre Yersin, a protégé of Louis Pasteur sent to Hong Kong to study the plague, and the Japanese scientist Shibasaburo Kitasato independently isolated the plague bacillus within a few days of each other, and the organism was originally named *Pasteurella pestis* in honor of Pasteur. Yersin described a connection between rats and plague, and Paul Louis Simon discovered the role of the rat flea in transmission. Enzootic foci of plague are found today on every continent except Australia, and the World Health Organization now classifies it as a reemerging infectious disease.

Molecular analysis has revealed that *Y. pestis* is a subspecies of *Y. pseudotuberculosis*, although the name has been retained. *Yersinia pestis* is thought to have emerged as a separate clone within *Y. pseudotuberculosis* shortly before the first pandemics. Biotypes of *Y. pestis* are distinguished by their differential ability to reduce nitrate and to ferment glycerol and melibiose. Biovar Antiqua probably spread from central Asia to central Africa to cause the first pandemic. Biovar Medievalis (similar genetically, but unable to reduce nitrate) later emerged (also in central Asia), spreading to Crimea and causing the second pandemic. Later still, biovar Orientalis emerged to cause the third pandemic.

Fleas ingest *Y. pestis* in blood meals from septicemic animals, and in most cases the organism proliferates in the normally sterile flea midgut (Figure 17-2). The proventriculus is a spine-lined organ that lies between the esophagus and midgut. In addition to mechanically disrupting blood cells, it serves as a valve, permitting entry of blood to the midgut while precluding escape of ingested blood. *Yersinia pestis* attaches in aggregates to the proventricular surface and, with continued multiplication, causes blockage and, in effect, starvation of the flea (Figure 17-3). In response, fleas attempt to feed more often. Blood enters the esophagus, becomes infected with *Y. pestis*, and is pumped back into the bite wound. Fleas do not block at higher temperatures, and dogma is that bubonic plague epidemics end with the onset of warmer temperatures. The temperature-sensitive activity of plasminogen activator in allowing or prohibiting flea blockage may be related to this phenomenon.

Sylvatic plague is generally transmitted by the bite of an arthropod, and symptoms appear after

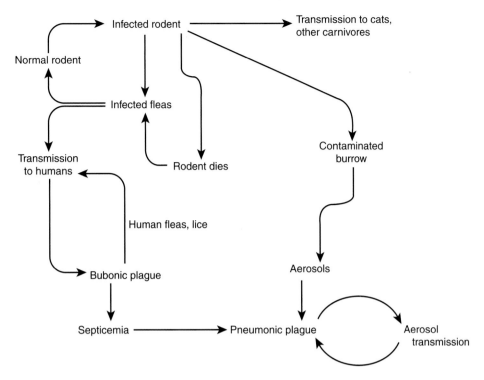

Infected rodent

Normal rodent

Transmission to cats, other carnivores

Infected fleas

Transmission to humans

Rodent dies

Contaminated burrow

Human fleas, lice

Bubonic plague

Aerosols

Septicemia ⟶ Pneumonic plague

Aerosol transmission

FIGURE 17-2 Transmission cycle of *Yersinia pestis*. (Courtesy Ashley E. Harmon.)

an incubation period of 2 to 6 days. It proliferates to some degree at the site of the bite. The organism is carried to regional lymph nodes, where proliferation occurs with enthusiasm. Inflammation, necrosis, and swelling in the lymph node lead to formation of the bubo, a classic gross lesion from which bubonic plague derives its name. Invasion may be contained by the antibacterial effects

of lymph node residence, but the organism is also likely to escape, eventually entering circulation and causing massive septicemia (Figure 17-4). Additional foci of infection develop in liver, spleen,

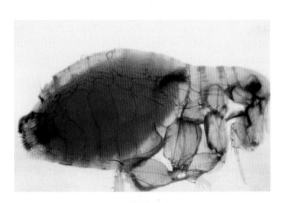

FIGURE 17-3 *Xenopsylla cheopis,* the Oriental rat flea, with a proventricular plague mass. (Courtesy Public Health Image Library, PHIL #2025, Atlanta, date unknown, Centers for Disease Control and Prevention.)

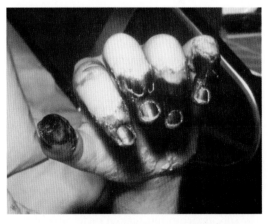

FIGURE 17-4 Plague-associated gangrene as a consequence of disseminated *Yersinia pestis* infection. This clinical presentation likely gave rise to Black Death as a common name for plague. (Courtesy Public Health Image Library, PHIL #4091, J. Poland, Atlanta, 1975, Centers for Disease Control and Prevention.)

and lungs, the last often resulting in airborne spread and the development of primary pneumonic cases of urban plague. There is a strong correlation between substantive bacteremia and subsequent mortality, and in any case, untreated pneumonic plague rarely has a clinical course longer than 3 days. Primary pneumonic plague, without the bubonic form as a precursor, is most common among plague cases in the United States today.

In addition to rodents, a number of mammalian species have been found to be naturally infected with Y. pestis, including lagomorphs, felids, canids, mustelids, and some ungulates.

Pathologic changes in feline plague are akin to those in humans. After introduction by fleabite or contact with infected material, Y. pestis multiplies locally and is transferred via lymphatics to regional lymph nodes. Nodal necrosis and suppuration, with hemorrhage, edema, fibrin, and acute necrotizing inflammation, are common. Large numbers of Y. pestis are in evidence in blood and lymphatic vessels associated with lymph nodes. Dissemination beyond regional lymph nodes to circulation eventually involves spleen, liver, heart, lungs, and other organs. Pneumonic plague may result, or may be the primary clinical presentation, through inhalation of infectious aerosols. Pulmonary lesions in cats include diffuse interstitial pneumonia and devastation of lung architecture by coalescing necrotic areas of necrosis. Lung abscesses are uncommon.

The clinical presentation of feline plague is rapidly progressing febrile illness with an incubation period of 1 to 4 days. Cats with primary septicemia are lethargic and anorexic, with signs of sepsis including vomiting, diarrhea, weak pulse and tachycardia, cold extremities, and disseminated intravascular coagulopathy (DIC). The bubonic form is most common, and one or more enlarged, abscessed, or draining lymph nodes are painful on palpation. Some infected individuals do not develop classic signs, so plague should be part of the differential diagnosis in cats with a suggestive history and a systemic infectious process.

Most cats exposed experimentally to Y. pestis (by subcutaneous inoculation or feeding of mice dead of plague) develop infection. In affected cats, rectal temperature peaked at 40.5° to 41.1° C on the third days after inoculation. Nearly two thirds of clinically ill cats developed enlarged cervical or cranial lymph nodes in the head and neck region within 4 to 6 days, and half died. Oral exposure is more likely to result in bubo formation. In natural cases, lymphadenopathy is most likely to be unilateral and submandibular. Oral and lingual ulcers or abscesses have also been reported.

Dogs are less likely to develop severe clinical illness following natural or experimental exposure. Fever, lethargy, submandibular lymphadenitis, suppurative intermandibular lymphadenitis, oral lesions, and cough have been documented in naturally infected dogs. Antibodies suggestive of plague exposure have been found unexpectedly in dogs in areas with low elevation and high average temperatures. This, and their relative resistance to clinical disease, suggests that dogs may be useful as sentinels.

Cattle, horses, sheep, and pigs are apparently not susceptible to clinical manifestations of plague. Goats and camels, on the other hand, are susceptible and human plague has been associated with ingestion of Y. pestis–infected camel meat in the Middle East. Disease has also been reported in a llama, mule deer, and antelope, and effects in mountain lions and bobcats may be similar to those in domestic cats. Foxes, raccoons, skunks, bears, and coyotes are apparently resistant, and the last two species are often used as natural sentinels.

Yersinia pestis is widely acknowledged to have been weaponized in modern times for use in biological warfare and bioterrorism. The United States and the former Soviet Union investigated the use of plague as a biological weapon during the cold war. A plague-based weapon delivered by aerosol would likely cause signs consistent with severe community-acquired pneumonia, and confusion with more common respiratory illnesses (e.g., legionnaires' disease) may delay recognition. True Y. pestis pulmonary infections may thus progress rapidly to septic shock and death without early treatment. The organism is a Category A Critical Biological Agent.

Epidemiology

Yersinia pestis is maintained in a cycle that forces infected fleas to abandon one host (which is dying and thus no longer a source of blood) in search of another. The cycle is sustained by selection for high virulence and relieves Y. pestis of the need to compete in the environment. In this aspect, its life is substantially different from that of Y. pseudotuberculosis and Y. enterocolitica.

The Oriental rat flea, Xenopsylla cheopis, is generally accepted as the main vector of Y. pestis, at least during the most recent pandemic. Fleas transmit *Y. pestis* among natural North American hosts (including ground squirrels, prairie dogs, woodrats, kangaroo rats, chipmunks, and other rodents). High rates of morbidity and mortality in rodents lead to direct (via contact with infected animals or through exposure to infectious aerosols from dens) or indirect (after transfer of fleas to urban rodents) exposure of humans. Fleas can survive for several months in abandoned rodent burrows, serving as a source of infection for potential hosts, including domestic animals.

Infection can be transmitted to humans, via aerosol or fleabite, from cats with plague. About 25% of those infected are veterinarians or staff, and more than one case in five is fatal. Three quarters of cases of cat-associated human plague have been bubonic, and most of the remaining cases are pneumonic.

In medieval Europe, the predominant rat flea is more likely to have been *Nosopsyllus fasciatus,* which rarely feeds on humans. This, combined with the grouping of cases in households, the putative role of clothing and bedding in transmission during the second and third pandemics, and modern experience with plague transmission in cold climates, stands as evidence for an important role in transmission for the human flea, *Pulex irritans.* Dog and cat fleas (*Ctenocephalides* spp.) are not efficient vectors of *Y. pestis.*

Human plague in the United States occurs at a rate of slightly more than 12 cases per year. On average, more than half of cases are from New Mexico, but substantial numbers also occur in Arizona, Colorado, and California. Disease has also been reported in Idaho, Nevada, Oklahoma, Oregon, Texas, Utah, Washington, and Wyoming. Most human cases occur between March and October, and even with generally effective antimicrobial therapy, the case fatality rate is about 15%. *Yersinia pestis* is endemic in the western United States, and its range has extended east to central Texas and western Kansas, Nebraska, Oklahoma, and South Dakota.

Domestic animals such as dogs and cats are most likely to be exposed to *Y. pestis* by contact with an infected rodent or rabbit or by the bite of an infected flea. Perhaps the most important risk factors for infection of dogs, cats, and probably other domestic animals is residence in (or visiting of) a rural endemic area. Rodent fleas will briefly parasitize a nonpreferred host species, so detection of fleas on normally flea-free pets in these areas is noteworthy.

YERSINIA PSEUDOTUBERCULOSIS
Disease

Disease in humans is characterized by abdominal pain (without diarrhea), reminiscent of acute appendicitis, but with only inflamed mesenteric lymph nodes in evidence at laparotomy. The course of disease associated with *Y. pseudotuberculosis* infection in experimental animals is similar to that of plague. The organism is (like *Y. pestis*) primarily a rodent pathogen, causing diarrhea and death as a result of septicemia.

Yersinia pseudotuberculosis causes pseudotuberculosis in rodents, guinea pigs, cats, and turkeys. It has been associated with bovine and caprine abortion, epididymitis and orchitis in rams, ulcerative typhlocolitis in pigs, and occasional infections in bison, sheep, deer, and wild birds. An epornitic of *Y. pseudotuberculosis* infection in a wildlife park may have initiated an epizootic in captive ruminants. Pseudotuberculosis in small animals begins as caseous abscesses in mesenteric lymph nodes, spreading to liver, spleen, and other tissues.

Epidemiology

Starlings, grackles, and other birds are reservoirs of *Y. pseudotuberculosis,* and dogs and cats can become infected through predation. Consumption of feed contaminated with bird feces or even consumption of moribund birds themselves, has been associated with outbreaks of *Y. pseudotuberculosis* infection in pigs.

YERSINIA ENTEROCOLITICA
Disease

Human disease caused by *Y. enterocolitica* is similar in some respects to that associated with *Y. pseudotuberculosis* infection. The clinical picture is often limited to mild diarrhea, and asymptomatic infections with mild bacteremia are common. However, symptoms may also include terminal ileitis with mesenteric lymphadenitis, resembling appendicitis. *Yersinia enterocolitica* strains pathogenic for humans are of either high or low virulence. The former cause systemic infection in humans and have a low minimum infectious dose for mice, whereas the latter cause mild disease in humans and are nonlethal for mice. It is not uncommon for large numbers of organisms to be recovered from stools. *Yersinia enterocolitica* is psychrophilic, a property that has mediated infection via transfusion of contaminated blood.

Ileitis, gastroenteritis, and mesenteric adenitis are the common disease processes in animals, resembling infections by *Y. pseudotuberculosis. Yersinia enterocolitica* has been isolated from rabbits and hares, dogs, pigs, horses, mink and other fur bearers, birds, and wild and domestic ruminants.

Ingested bacteria transit the stomach, perhaps aided by production of urease, and then colonize the small intestinal epithelial mucosa. Diarrhea may be caused by production of a heat-stable toxin, *Yersinia* heat-stable toxin (YST) (see p. 143). Epithelial cells are invaded in a complex, thermo-regulated process. Penetration of M cells, facilitated by *Yersinia* adhesin A (YadA) and the products of *inv* and *ail* (see below), is followed by multiplica-tion in Peyer's patches. *Yersinia* outer proteins (Yops) (see p. 143) and other surface components facilitate survival of phagocytosis and effects of complement. Inflammation, microabscessation, and mucosal ulceration follow, and bacteria escaping the draining mesenteric lymph nodes enter circulation. Invasin mutants (see p. 143) are limited in their ability to colonize mesenteric lymph nodes, but colonize deeper tissues to the same degree as wildtype strains, suggesting two possible routes of dissemination.

Epidemiology

Yersinia enterocolitica causes several thousand cases of food-borne disease annually in the United States, in many countries at rates compara-ble to *Campylobacter-* and *Shigella*-associated dis-ease. The source of infection may be contaminated milk or water, and cases have been associated with eating tofu and bean sprouts. The organism's psychrophilic nature has favored its transmission by way of transfusion of contaminated blood. The organism is found in aquatic environments, but normal swine are the only known animal reservoirs of human pathogenic *Y. enterocolitica.* It can be isolated from feces, tongues, tonsils, and carcasses at slaughter, and outbreaks have been associated with consumption of chitterlings. *Yersinia enterocolitica* survives for lengthy periods in sewage or contaminated soil or water.

Swine are documented oral (rather than intestinal) carriers of human virulent serotypes

O:3 and O:9. In North America the epidemiology of the highly invasive O:8 serotype remains largely unknown. Avirulent serotypes of *Y. enterocolitica* are found in a variety of wild animals and natural environments.

YERSINIA RUCKERI

Yersinia ruckeri, the etiologic agent of red-mouth (pink mouth, pink or red throat) of salmon and trout, is the oldest *Y. enterocolitica*–like species. It was first described in North America, but is commonly found in Australia, South Africa, and Europe. This organism may also be responsible for fatal piscine septicemia. It survives in water for months after an outbreak.

There is an association in *Y. ruckeri* between virulence and serum resistance. Virulent organ-isms are serum resistant, whereas those that are avirulent are mainly serum sensitive. However, serum resistance in some avirulent strains sug-gests that other factors may be required for full virulence. A lipid "heat-sensitive factor" from vir-ulent strains may also be a virulence determinant.

Yersinia intermedia, Y. kristensenii, and *Y. fred-eriksenii* are apparent normal inhabitants of uncontaminated running water.

PATHOGENESIS OF *YERSINIA* SPP. INFECTIONS

Yersiniae are facultative intracellular parasites that localize in and destroy macrophages. Septicemia may follow, but proliferation occurs primarily within host cells and interstitial spaces. They resist oxidative and nonoxidative killing mechanisms, multiplying extensively in phagolysosomes.

The adhesion protein YadA (Figure 17-5) is encoded by a gene on virulence plasmid pYV,

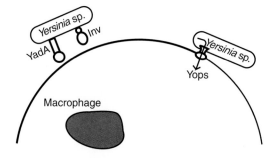

FIGURE 17-5 Diagrammatic representation of the role of YadA, the *inv* gene product, and Yops in interaction of *Yersinia* spp. with host cells. (Courtesy Ashley E. Harmon.)

found in *Y. pestis, Y. pseudotuberculosis,* and *Y. enterocolitica.* YadA is a virulence factor for *Y. enterocolitica,* but seems to have little impact on virulence of *Y. pseudotuberculosis (yadA* in *Y. pestis* is silent). YadA is anchored to the outer membrane via the C-termini of its subunits. The N-termini form a globular arrangement, and the lollipop-shaped YadA structures cover the bacterial surface and convey hydrophobic properties. *yadA* expression is induced at 37° C and mediates binding to collagen, laminin, fibronectin, intestinal mucosa, and submucosal tissue. It inhibits classical pathway activation of complement, thus providing serum resistance. *Yersinia enterocolitica* may require YadA-mediated collagen binding to induce joint disease.

YST is a heat-stable enterotoxin that is structurally and functionally similar to the heat-stable toxin of *Escherichia coli.* It may be involved in pathogenesis of diarrhea in *Y. enterocolitica* infection.

pH6 antigen is a fibrillar adhesin structure, loss of which leads to a 200-fold increase in the mouse intravenous LD_{50} of *Y. pestis.* Homologous genes in *Y. pseudotuberculosis* (called *psaA*) and *Y. enterocolitica* (called *myfA*) may also have products that are involved in virulence.

The product of *ail* is involved in attachment and invasion and is required for resistance to killing by human serum. This phenotype is not required for virulence in mice because *Y. enterocolitica* is not killed by mouse serum. *ail* is found in pathogenic *Y. enterocolitica* but not in nonpathogenic strains or in nonpathogenic members of the genus. *ail* in *Y. pseudotuberculosis* does not mediate attachment and invasion, but does promote serum resistance.

Yersinia pseudotuberculosis and *Y. enterocolitica* make a functional invasin protein, the primary factor by which *Y. enterocolitica* invades cultured cells and translocates across intestinal epithelium in mice. The *Y. pseudotuberculosis* invasin binds to integrins on the apical surface of antigen-sampling M cells. The oral LD_{50} of *Y. enterocolitica* knockout mutants is no greater than parent strains, and liver and spleen are efficiently colonized; however, mutants are less able to colonize Peyer's patches early in infection and do not colonize mesenteric lymph nodes as frequently as wildtype.

Yersinia pestis, Y. pseudotuberculosis, and *Y. enterocolitica* share the so-called Yop virulon, by which yersiniae anchored to host cells inject Yops (Table 17-2; see Figure 17-5). Yops disrupt the

TABLE **17-2** Yops and Their Actions

Yop	Action
YopE	Cytotoxin, disrupts microfilament structure; blocks phagocytosis (with YopH)
YopH	Tyrosine phosphatase; inhibits phagocytosis by PMNs (mediated by complement receptors) and macrophage (mediated by Fc receptors)
YopM	Target and action unknown
YopO/YpkA	Protein kinase, causes cell rounding in vitro; target protein unknown
YopP/YopJ	Induces macrophage apoptosis, reduces TNF-α release
YopT	HeLa cell toxicity, actin filament disruption, alteration of cytoskeleton

PMN, Polymorphonuclear neutrophils; *TNF,* tumor necrosis factor.

cytoskeleton and abolish production of proinflammatory cytokines, protecting the organism from phagocytosis and abrogating early onset of inflammation. The Yop virulon is the paradigm of so-called type III secretion virulence mechanisms identified in many other pathogens.

The Yop virulon is carried on a 70 kb virulence plasmid, pYV, which is necessary, but not sufficient for virulence. Translocator Yops (YopB, YopD, LcrV) form a pore in the eukaryotic cell membrane, through which effector Yops (YopE, YopH, YpkA/YopO, YopP/YopJ, YopM, and YopT) are chaperoned into the cytoplasm. YopH is a phosphotyrosine phosphatase that is antiphagocytic through dephosphorylation of focal adhesion proteins. YopsE and T contribute further antiphagocytic effects by inactivation of GTPases controlling cytoskeleton dynamics. YopP/YopJ is antiinflammatory and induces macrophage apoptosis.

Virulence in the genus *Yersinia* also depends upon iron acquisition in vivo. The most virulent species are those that reach fixed macrophages, where iron is amply available, from peripheral sites of initial infection. All species are highly virulent when injected IV (providing rapid contact with fixed macrophages). Minimally virulent strains of *Y. enterocolitica* (biotypes 2 and 4) usually cause moderate intestinal symptoms, but systemic infections result in patients who are iron overloaded (e.g., those with hemochromatosis).

Siderophore-deficient strains of *Y. pestis* are virulent only if administered subsequent to iron injection.

Biosynthetic machinery for the siderophore yersiniabactin is found in a 36 to 43 kb chromosomal region called the high-pathogenicity island (HPI). It incorporates several repeat sequences and a mobility gene, and the G + C content of the open reading frames is 10% to 15% higher than the average for the organism as a whole. The HPI has never been detected in low-pathogenicity or avirulent strains.

A small *Y. pestis* plasmid carries genes for the bacteriocin pesticin, a lytic antibacterial enzyme active against *Y. pseudotuberculosis* and *Y. enterocolitica*, plus coagulase and fibrinolytic activities. Plasmid loss converts the organisms to a virulence phenotype similar to that of *Y. pseudotuberculosis* or *Y. enterocolitica*.

Another plasmid exists in all three pathogenic species, and its loss results in avirulence. It carries genes involved in expression of V antigen. Monospecific antibodies against this structure passively protect against infection by *Y. pestis*, *Y. pseudotuberculosis*, and invasive *Y. enterocolitica*. Expression of adhesins that facilitate colonization via the oral route is also mediated by genes on this plasmid, and *Y. enterocolitica* strains lacking the plasmid are serum sensitive.

Flea-plague interactions are nearly as complex as plague-mammalian host interactions. Two bacterial factors playing important roles in *Y. pestis*–infected fleas are *Yersinia* murine toxin (Ymt), a cytoplasmic phospholipase D (PLD), and the hemin storage (Hms) phenotype. Toxicity of Ymt manifests as hypotension and vascular collapse when this molecule is released from lysing bacteria at the terminal stage of septicemic plague in mice. *ymt* is on the 100 kb plasmid pFra, which is unique to *Y. pestis*. Ymt is highly lethal for mice, but selective mutation of the gene does not reduce virulence of *Y. pestis*. However, Ymt is required for survival in the flea. An agent in the flea midgut that induces spheroplast formation and lysis of Ymt mutants is apparently inactive in the presence of Ymt-positive cells. A *Y. pestis* hemin adsorption system (Hms) may have a similar role. Hms-positive strains colonize and eventually block the proventriculus of the flea, whereas Hms-negative strains infect the midgut without colonizing or blocking. Thus introduction of Ymt and Hms was probably a decisive step in the evolutionary of *Y. pestis* to arthropod-borne transmission, which

is apparently unique among enteric bacteria. This mode of transmission may have favored selection of strains producing high-density septicemia, completing the transmission cycle and resulting in the emergence of plague.

Diagnosis

Yersinia pestis infections. History is important in a diagnosis of plague, so pet owners should be queried about the presence or recent disappearance of rodent populations in the animal's environment. Differential diagnoses for plague include tularemia, injuries resulting in abscess formation, other causes of cutaneous infection (*Staphylococcus* spp., *Streptococcus* spp.), pneumonia, or oral lesions.

Definitive diagnosis of plague begins with a Gram stain of exudate from an abscess, which reveals a homogeneous population of gram-negative bipolar coccobacilli (see Figure 17-1). Detection of *Y. pestis* antigen may be the most valuable diagnostic approach in acute disease. Lymph node aspirates, material from draining lesions, or swabs from the oral cavity or pharynx, collected before antimicrobials are administered, should be shipped overnight on ice. It may be necessary to inject saline into a bubo to facilitate collection of an aspirate. Blood culture may also be useful. Liver, spleen, lung, and affected lymph nodes should be collected from animals dying of plague. Initial antigen detection is based upon a fluorescent antibody test for the *Y. pestis* F1 antigen (Figure 17-6), which presents the best combination of sensitivity, specificity, and rapidity. Serologic detection of anti-F1 is by enzyme-linked immunosorbent assay (ELISA) or passive hemagglutination. Results of serologic tests are often negative early on, so paired samples should be examined for a fourfold increase in titer 2 to 3 weeks after onset. A titer greater than or equal to 1:32 in a single sample from an animal with signs consistent with plague is supportive.

Yersinia pestis grows slowly, even at its 28° C optimum, so false negatives may be avoided by extended incubation. Small (1-2 mm) gray colonies are nonmucoid and have a hammered-copper appearance on selective and nonselective media (Figure 17-7). An interesting historical note is the detection of *Y. pestis* by polymerase chain reaction (PCR) and deoxyribonucleic acid (DNA) sequencing in skeletal materials buried more than 400 years ago. These findings confirmed that the so-called Black Death (the second pandemic) was, indeed, plague.

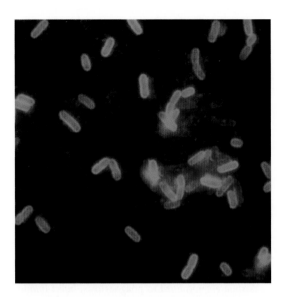

FIGURE 17-6 Direct fluorescent antibody stain of *Yersinia pestis,* with antibody specific for capsular antigen. (Courtesy Public Health Image Library, PHIL #1919, Atlanta, 2002, Centers for Disease Control and Prevention, Larry Stauffer, Oregon State Public Health Laboratory.)

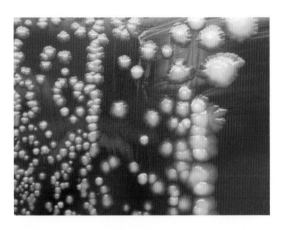

FIGURE 17-7 *Yersinia pestis* on sheep blood agar after 72 hours' incubation. Gray-white to slightly yellow opaque colonies, with raised irregular fried-egg morphology. (Courtesy Public Health Image Library, PHIL #1921, Atlanta, 2002, Centers for Disease Control and Prevention, Larry Stauffer, Oregon State Public Health Laboratory.)

Infection by other yersiniae. Cefsulodin irgasan novobiocin (CIN) agar is selective for yersiniae, and takes advantage of the pH change associated with mannitol fermentation, causing *Y. enterocolitica* to produce bull's-eye colonies with deep red centers and transparent borders. Cefsulodin, irgasan, crystal violet, sodium deoxycholate, and novobiocin selectively inhibit gram-positive and many gram-negative organisms. Identification is based on morphologic, cultural, and biochemical characteristics (see Table 17-1), and is best achieved on organisms grown at 25° C rather than at 37° C. Cold enrichment (several days' incubation at 4° C in buffer or broth) increases recovery of *Y. enterocolitica* from stool specimens, but may favor growth of nonpathogenic strains.

Pathogenic strains are linked with specific biogroups and serogroups, such as biogroup 1B, serogroups O:8, O:13a,13b, and O:20, and biogroup 2 serogroups O:3, O:5,27, and O:9. Over the past 20 years, serogroup O:3 has replaced O:8 as the predominant serotype in the United States.

Yersinia enterocolitica may be identified by PCR amplification and colony blot hybridization, but these methods are not widely used in clinical laboratories. Real-time PCR is apparently more sensitive than either multiplex PCR or traditional culture methods.

Prevention and Control

Yersinia pestis infections. Plague deaths are often the result of misdiagnosis or lack of urgency on the part of family or caregivers, both of which delay initiation of treatment. Rapid implementation of antimicrobial therapy is a key element, and this should precede definitive diagnosis. Streptomycin is used for treatment of human plague, but is not available for veterinary use; gentamicin is a good alternative, and doxycycline can be used in less severe cases. Tetracycline, chloramphenicol, and sulfonamides may also be useful. *Yersinia pestis* is susceptible to penicillins in vitro but not in vivo. Fluoroquinolones are as effective as streptomycin in experimentally infected mice. Treatment is continued for 10 to 21 days, and clinical improvement should be evident in less than or equal to 72 hours. Strains resistant to streptomycin, gentamicin, tetracycline, chloramphenicol, and sulfonamides have been reported.

Care should be taken to minimize further risk of transmission of plague from pets to owners. When possible, affected (especially pneumonic) animals should be hospitalized. Human plague cases have been attributed to contact occurring while administering oral medication to plague-affected animals. It should go without saying that protection of caregivers against infection is of paramount importance. Precautions against exposure by way of respiratory and conjunctival routes should be implemented until treatment has been in progress for 72 hours and clinical improvement is evident. Public health officials should be notified.

To the extent that it is possible, pet owners in endemic areas should supervise pets' roaming and hunting enterprises. Flea control is equally important because pets may bring infected rodent fleas into the household.

Killed whole-cell vaccines for plague used for more than 100 years protect against the bubonic form of the disease. However, protection against the pneumonic form has been limited. A live attenuated vaccine had questionable efficacy and produced severe side effects. A fully recombinant subunit vaccine comprising F1 and V antigens is efficacious against both bubonic and pneumonic plague in animal models. Protection is principally antibody mediated.

Infection by other yersiniae. Cleaning and cooking raw pork intestines to prepare chitterlings is a risk factor for both the preparers and innocent bystanders (including infants). Public education in better methods of preparation has not prevented chitterling-associated outbreaks of *Y. enterocolitica*–induced disease, but is the key to decreasing incidence.

Yersinia pseudotuberculosis and *Y. enterocolitica* are susceptible to tetracyclines, trimethoprim-sulfamethoxazole, aminoglycosides, and chloramphenicol. Intracellular residence should be taken into account when developing treatment strategies.

SUGGESTED READINGS

Cornelis GR: Molecular and cell biology aspects of plague, *Proc Natl Acad Sci U S A* 97:8778-8783, 2000.

Eidson M, Thilsted JE, Rallag OJ: Clinical, clinico-pathologic, and pathologic features of plague in cats: 119 cases (1977-1988), *J Am Vet Med Assoc* 199:1191-1197, 1991.

Gage KL, Dennis DT, Orloski KA, et al: Cases of cat-associated human plague in the western US, 1977-1998, *Clin Infect Dis* 30:893-900, 2000.

Grosdent N, Maridonneau-Parini I, Sory MP, Cornelis GR: Role of the Yops and adhesins in resistance of *Yersinia enterocolitica* to phagocytosis, *Infect Immun* 70:4165-4176, 2002.

Gross L: How the plague bacillus and its transmission through fleas were discovered: reminiscences from my years at the Pasteur Institute in Paris, *Proc Natl Acad Sci U S A* 92:7609-7611, 1995.

Hinnebusch BJ: Bubonic plague: a molecular genetic case history of the emergence of an infectious disease, *J Mol Med* 75:645-652, 1997.

Orloski KA, Eidson M: *Yersinia pestis* infection in three dogs, *J Am Vet Med Assoc* 207:316-318, 1995.

Perry RD, Fetherston JD: Yersinia pestis—etiologic agent of plague, *Clin Microbiol Rev* 10:35-66, 1997.

Williamson ED, Eley SM, Stagg AJ, et al: A single dose subunit vaccine protects against pneumonic plague, *Vaccine* 19:566-571, 2001.

Chapter 18

The Genus *Bordetella*

The genus *Bordetella* is taxonomically assigned to the family Alcaligenaceae within the β-*Proteobacteria* and is most closely related to the genera *Achromobacter* and *Alcaligenes*. These small gram-negative rods were named for Jules Bordet, who first cultivated the type species, *Bordetella pertussis*. The seven additional species are *Bordetella parapertussis, Bordetella bronchiseptica, Bordetella avium, Bordetella hinzii, Bordetella holmesii, Bordetella trematum,* and the recently characterized *Bordetella petri* (Table 18-1). Most *Bordetella* spp. occur exclusively in close association with mammals and birds. All are catalase positive and asaccharolytic. Optimal growth is at 35° to 37° C, under aerobic or facultatively anaerobic, nonfermentative conditions.

DISEASE AND EPIDEMIOLOGY

The natural habitat of *Bordetella* spp., except for the environmental organism *B. petri*, is the upper respiratory tract of mammals and birds. Bacteria are transmitted from host to host by aerosol. *Bordetella bronchiseptica, B. avium, B. pertussis,* and *B. parapertussis* are the primary pathogenic species, and they cause disease worldwide.

Bordetella bronchiseptica was originally named *Bacillus bronchicanis* because the organism was initially recovered from dogs with respiratory disease. The name was changed when it became evident that this organism infected other animals, and the literal meaning of the specific epithet is "with an infected bronchus." In addition to canine disease, *B. bronchiseptica* causes respiratory infections in cats, rodents, horses, pigs, nonhuman primates, sea mammals, koalas, and rarely in humans. Most human cases have been associated with underlying immunosuppression and typically present as respiratory tract infections, ranging from sinusitis to pneumonia. However, more serious conditions, such as endocarditis, meningitis, and peritonitis, have been reported. A non–life-threatening whooping cough–like syndrome has been described in immunocompetent children.

Bordetella bronchiseptica is one of the agents involved in the infectious canine tracheobronchitis or "kennel cough" complex of young dogs. Older naïve animals are also susceptible. The organism is an important secondary invader following distemper virus infection, where it is often responsible for a fatal bronchopneumonia. The incubation

TABLE **18-1**   Phenotypic Properties of Members of the Genus *Bordetella*

Feature	B. pertussis	B. parapertussis	B. bronchiseptica	B. avium*	B. hinzii	B. holmesii	B. trematum	B. petri
Host	Humans	Humans, sheep	Mammals	Birds	Birds, humans	Humans?	Humans?	Environment
Disease	Whooping cough	Mild whooping cough, chronic pneumonia	Various respiratory diseases (atrophic rhinitis in pigs, kennel cough in dogs, etc.)	Turkey coryza	Commensal in birds, septicemia in immunocompromised humans	Respiratory disease septicemia	Wound and ear infections	Unknown
Site of isolation	Respiratory tract	Respiratory tract	Respiratory tract	Respiratory tract	Respiratory tract, blood	Respiratory tract, blood	Wound and ear infections	Bioreactor sediment
Growth on blood agar	Neg	Pos	Pos	Pos	Pos	Pos	Pos	Pos
Growth on MacConkey's agar	Neg	Var (delayed)	Pos	Pos	Pos	Pos (delayed)	Pos	Pos
Oxidase	Pos	Neg	Pos	Pos	Pos	Neg	Neg	Pos
Urease	Neg	Pos (24 hr)	Pos (4 hr)	Neg	Neg	Neg	Neg	Neg
Citrate utilization	Pos	Pos	Pos	Pos	Pos	Pos	Pos	ND
Nitrate reduction	Neg	Neg	Pos	Neg	Neg	Neg	Var	Neg
Motility	Neg	Neg	Pos	Pos	Pos	Neg	Pos	Neg

*To further differentiate *B. avium* from *B. hinzii*, use malonate utilization; the former is negative, where as the latter is positive.
ND, Not determined; *Neg,* negative; *Pos,* positive; *Var,* variable.

period for kennel cough is 5 to 10 days, followed by acute onset of a harsh, dry, "honking" cough that is aggravated by excitement or activity. Coughing episodes are often followed by gagging and retching, in attempts to clear mucus from the trachea. The cough can be easily elicited by tracheal palpation. The disease spreads rapidly among closely confined animals, as in boarding kennels or animal hospitals, and the primary infection is often self-limiting. Puppies may shed *B. bronchiseptica* for up to 3 months after infection, and relapses may follow stress and exposure to adverse environmental conditions.

Bordetella bronchiseptica is one of the etiologic agents of atrophic rhinitis and bronchopneumonia in swine, diseases that are associated with intensive rearing conditions. Nearly all herds of swine, including those that are apparently normal, are infected with this organism, and primary introduction is by carrier pigs. The sow is the most common source of infection for piglets, and poor ventilation and overstocking are risk factors. Atrophic rhinitis is characterized by sneezing, nasal discharge, and bony deformity of the nose. Upper respiratory signs may occur in piglets as young as 1 week of age, but more frequently occur at 3 to 4 weeks of age. The characteristic lesion is atrophy of the nasal turbinates, which may be evident only at slaughter, in snouts sectioned at the level of the second premolar tooth. The ventral scroll of the ventral turbinate is the region most commonly affected. *Bordetella bronchiseptica* by itself is responsible for the less severe, transient, self-limiting form of atrophic rhinitis, usually without significant snout deviations. A more severe, progressive form of the disease is caused by toxigenic strains of *Pasteurella multocida* in combination with *B. bronchiseptica*. Histopathologic changes associated with atrophic rhinitis include mucosal infiltration by neutrophils, loss of cilia, metaplasia of the epithelium, and bone resorption with fibrous tissue replacement.

Primary bronchopneumonia in 3- to 4-day-old piglets is a more severe manifestation of infection that usually occurs in the winter months. Coughing is the major clinical sign, and may be accompanied by dyspnea and whooping. Morbidity and mortality may be high.

Tracheobronchitis, conjunctivitis, and pneumonia have been associated with *B. bronchiseptica* infection in cats. Disease not complicated by infection with other agents (such as feline calicivirus and feline herpesvirus) is mild, and signs disappear within 10 days. However, life-threatening bronchopneumonia may develop, particularly in kittens. Clinical signs in experimental infections include sneezing, nasal discharge, rales, fever, and submandibular lymphadenopathy. Coughing is reported occasionally, but does not seem to be a characteristic feature, as in canine disease. Some cats become long-term carriers on recovery, and shedding for at least 19 weeks postexposure has been documented.

Bordetella bronchiseptica is responsible for outbreaks of pneumonia in laboratory rodents and rabbits. Epizootic respiratory disease can have disastrous consequences in guinea pig colonies, resulting in high mortality and abortions or stillbirths. Affected animals are anorectic, dyspneic, and exhibit oculonasal discharge. Acute disease has a sudden onset and lasts 2 to 3 days. Many outbreaks are precipitated by stressors, such as improper diet, temperature fluctuations, and overcrowding. Young, old, or pregnant individuals are particularly susceptible. Subclinical infections and carrier animals are common.

Bordetella avium is responsible for a highly contagious upper respiratory disease known as avian bordetellosis or turkey coryza. Clinical disease is of greatest economic importance in young turkeys, but *B. avium* also infects chickens and several other species of birds. Disease may be exacerbated by environmental stressors and other respiratory pathogens.

The organism exhibits a strong tropism for the ciliated epithelium of the upper respiratory tract. Turkey poults 1 to 6 weeks old experience an acute onset of sneezing, accompanied by open-mouth breathing, conjunctivitis, nasal discharge, moist rales, anorexia, and altered voice. Stunted growth, tracheal collapse (Figure 18-1), and predisposition to other diseases may result. Morbidity may approach 100%, but mortality is usually low in the absence of secondary infections. In older turkeys and chickens, clinical signs are less severe. The most significant necropsy finding in severely affected birds is dorsoventral collapse of tracheal rings with accumulation of a mucopurulent exudate in the tracheal lumen (see Figure 18-1).

Bordetella hinzii, formerly known as *B. avium* type 2, is primarily found as a commensal of poultry respiratory tracts, and is considered to be avirulent for birds. It must be differentiated from *B. avium* in cultures. *Bordetella hinzii* has been

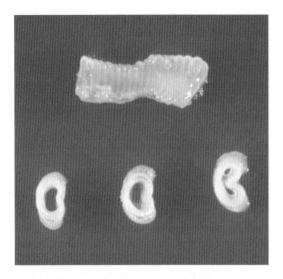

FIGURE 18-1 Flattening of tracheal rings, associated with *Bordetella avium* infection in turkey poults. (Courtesy J. Glenn Songer.)

associated with fatal septicemia in immunocompromised humans.

Bordetella pertussis is the major cause of whooping cough and is considered to be an obligate human pathogen. Rare cases of whooping cough–like illness have been reported in captive chimpanzees. *Bordetella parapertussis* is the etiologic agent of a mild form of human whooping cough, although distinct strains are also found in sheep with chronic pneumonia.

PATHOGENESIS

The principal pathogenic species cause respiratory tract infections in mammals and birds, which usually involves attachment to ciliated respiratory epithelial cells, resulting in ciliostasis. Subsequent death of the ciliated cells, accompanied by accumulation of mucus in the respiratory tract, probably contributes to the clinical signs of coughing and nasal discharge.

Virulence factors of *Bordetella* spp. include toxins (pertussis toxin, adenylate cyclase-hemolysin, dermonecrotic toxin, osteotoxin, and tracheal cytotoxin), adhesins (fimbriae, filamentous hemagglutinin, and pertactin) and lipopolysaccharide (LPS) (Table 18-2).

Pertussis toxin causes increased secretion by the respiratory mucosa and mucus production characteristic of the paroxysmal stage of whooping cough. Adenylate cyclase-hemolysin inhibits

phagocytosis and induces phagocyte apoptosis, protecting bacteria during the early stages of infection. Dermonecrotic toxin causes vasoconstriction of peripheral blood vessels, with localized ischemia and hemorrhage, in mice. Tracheal cytotoxin has a specific affinity for ciliated epithelial cells and causes ciliostasis. It interferes with DNA synthesis and impairs the regeneration of damaged cells, a process that disrupts the normal mucociliary clearance mechanisms of the upper respiratory tract.

A novel cytotoxic protein of *B. avium*, designated osteotoxin, is lethal for osteogenic cells in vitro. Osteotoxin lacks dermonecrotic toxin activity and is apparently antigenically distinct from a dermonecrotic toxin produced by *B. avium*. Osteotoxin is also produced by *B. bronchiseptica*.

Fimbrial proteins play an important role in binding of *Bordetella* spp. to host cells. Filamentous hemagglutinin binds to membrane glycolipids on ciliated epithelial cells. Pertactin, a bacterial surface protein, mediates binding to epithelial cells. A role for LPS in tracheal colonization has been demonstrated, but the exact mechanism remains undetermined. Synergy between LPS and tracheal cytotoxin may cause severe epithelial damage.

Dermonecrotic toxin is probably responsible in large part for the lesions seen in atrophic rhinitis. *Bordetella bronchiseptica* adheres to epithelial cells on turbinates, and cilia become swollen and decreased in number. Swollen mitochondria can be demonstrated in osteoblasts and osteocytes in the underlying bone, and lysis of these cells is common. The accompanying inflammation and fibrosis may be due, in part at least, to the action of cytokines. Dermonecrotic toxin inhibits alkaline phosphatase activity and reduces type 1 collagen formation in vitro, both of which are linked to osteoblastic differentiation. Impairment of differentiation of osteoprogenitor cells may result in decreased bone formation, explaining in part the nasal turbinate atrophy that is characteristic of the disease in pigs.

DIAGNOSIS

Culture provides the definitive diagnosis of bordetellosis, except in the case of atrophic rhinitis, in which diagnosis requires clinical and postmortem observations in addition to bacteriologic culture. Specimens may include transtracheal aspirates, nasal or tracheal swabs, and pneumonic lung tissue.

TABLE **18-2**   Virulence Factors of Pathogenic *Bordetella* Species

	Virulence Factor	Biologic Effect	*B. avium*	*B. bronchiseptica*	*B. parapertussis*	*B. pertussis*
					Bordetella Species	
Adhesins	Filamentous hemagglutinin	Binds to cilia	Neg	Pos	Pos	Pos
	Pertussis toxin	Binds to cilia	Neg	Neg	Neg	Pos
	Fimbriae	Binds to cells	Pos	Pos	Pos	Pos
	Pertactin	Binds to cells	Neg	Pos	Pos	Pos
Toxins	Adenylate cyclase-hemolysin	Inhibits leukocyte chemotaxis, phagocytosis, intracellular killing	Neg	Pos	Pos	Pos
	Dermonectoric toxin	Causes skin lesions and inhibits osteogenesis	Pos	Pos	Pos	Pos
	Osteotoxin	Toxic to osteoblasts	Pos	Pos	Neg	Neg
	LPS	Activates alternate complement pathway, stimulates cytokine release	Pos	Pos	Pos	Pos
	Tracheal cytotoxin	Kills ciliated respiratory cells	Pos	Pos	Pos	Pos

LPS, Lipopolysaccharide; *Neg,* negative; *Pos,* positive.

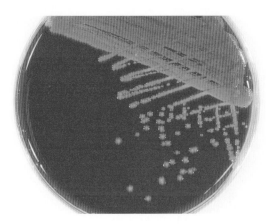

FIGURE 18-2 Colonies of *Bordetella bronchiseptica* (blood agar, 48 hours' incubation). (Courtesy Karen W. Post.)

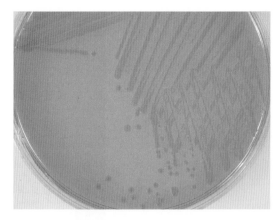

FIGURE 18-3 Colonies of *Bordetella avium* (MacConkey agar, 48 hours' incubation), demonstrating the typical bluish gray color and slightly raised brown-tinged centers. (Courtesy Karen W. Post.)

Most species form characteristic colonies and can be identified antigenically by slide agglutination tests. In addition, species can be distinguished from each other using phenotypic differences such as characteristic growth on blood and MacConkey agars, oxidase production, urease activity, citrate utilization, nitrate reduction, and motility (see Table 18-1). *Bordetella bronchiseptica* and *B. avium* agglutinate sheep and guinea pig erythrocytes, respectively, and this assay is commonly used in identification of *B. avium*.

Bordetella pertussis does not grow on common laboratory media and requires supplementation with charcoal, starch, blood, or albumin. Bordet-Gengou agar (containing 16%-20% blood) is the medium of choice for isolation. It produces minute colonies with 3 to 4 days' incubation, whereas colonies of *B. parapertussis* are larger and appear after 2 to 3 days' incubation. When cultivated on peptone agar, *B. parapertussis* forms characteristic colonies surrounded by a zone of brown, diffusible pigment.

Smith and Baskerville medium selects against interfering respiratory microflora and may be used for recovery of *B. bronchiseptica*. Colonies of *B. bronchiseptica* on bovine blood agar plates after 48 hours' incubation at 35° C are small (0.5-1 mm), circular, glistening or rough with entire edges (Figure 18-2). Some strains are β-hemolytic, and large and small hemolytic and nonhemolytic variants can be present together. Colonies on MacConkey agar are bluish gray and surrounded by small red zones with amber discoloration of the underlying medium.

Colonies of *B. avium* on blood agar plates are similar to those of *B. bronchiseptica;* however, after 48 hours' growth on MacConkey agar, many strains produce bluish gray colonies with slightly raised brown-tinged centers (Figure 18-3). Morphology in Gram-stained smears is similar for all species of *Bordetella;* cells are small (0.2-0.5 × 0.5-1 μm) gram-negative rods with a tendency toward coccobacillary morphology.

Polymerase chain reaction (PCR) assays may also be used to detect and differentiate many *Bordetella* spp. in clinical materials. Serologic methods, including microagglutination and enzyme immunoassays, are also useful, and they are used widely to monitor antibody responses to *B. avium* in turkeys.

PREVENTION, CONTROL, AND TREATMENT

Dogs and cats with mild signs of bordetellosis are usually not treated. However, if clinical signs progress in severity or persist for more than 14 days, antimicrobial therapy may be required.

Affected animals should be isolated immediately. Mechanical transfer on footwear, feeding utensils, or other fomites may be an important means of transmission of *B. bronchiseptica* in kennels, animal shelters, and pet shops, so infected premises should be thoroughly disinfected. *Bordetella bronchiseptica* is susceptible to most commercially available disinfectants. Parenteral and intranasal vaccines have been developed for prevention of canine kennel cough. Most decrease the severity of clinical disease but do not prevent infection.

Management and therapeutic measures are necessary to prevent and control atrophic rhinitis and pneumonia in swine herds. All-in/all-out management systems of pig flow and reduced stocking density decrease the risk of exposure of young piglets to older carrier animals. Use of disease-free replacement stock is recommended, and medicated and segregated early-weaning programs may also be effective in disease prevention. Vaccination of sows reduces the prevalence and severity of disease in suckling and weaned pigs. Sows can be medicated during the final month of gestation with sulfamethazine or oxytetracycline. Sound hygienic practices should be instituted, including maintenance of suitable ventilation rates. Temperature fluctuations and exposure to drafts within houses should be minimized.

Good husbandry, clean stock, and separation of carrier animals from healthy individuals are essential for the prevention of bordetellosis in colonies of laboratory rodents. Entry of new animals should be restricted to those from sources known to be *Bordetella*-free. Use of bacterins

provides protection for 4 to 6 months, and may eliminate the carrier state with prolonged use. Trimethoprim-sulfamethoxazole and chloramphenicol are the antimicrobials of choice, although treatment is often unsuccessful because of the acute nature of the disease.

Prevention and control of turkey coryza involves the use of bacterins or modified live vaccines in susceptible flocks. Use of antimicrobials early in the course of an outbreak may prove beneficial. Cleaning and disinfection of houses after an outbreak is important before restocking birds.

As a general rule, bordetellae are susceptible to aminoglycosides, fluoroquinolones, macrolides, chloramphenicol, trimethoprim-sulfamethoxazole, and tetracyclines. There is widespread resistance to cephalosporins and ampicillin.

SUGGESTED READINGS

Gerlach G, von Wintzingerode F, Middendorf B, Gross R: Evolutionary trends in the genus *Bordetella, Microbes Infect* 3:61-72, 2001.

Woolfrey BF, Moody JA: Human infections associated with *Bordetella bronchiseptica, Clin Microbiol Rev* 4:243-255, 1991.

Chapter 19

The Genera *Pseudomonas* and *Burkholderia*

The genus *Pseudomonas* was described more than a century ago and has been completely revised on multiple occasions because of taxonomic heterogeneity. The nomenclatural arrangements eventually led to creation of the genus *Burkholderia*. Recently proposed taxonomic changes include placement of *Burkholderia* into the class β-Proteobacteria, order Burkholderiales, family Burkholderiaceae. *Pseudomonas* remains in the class γ-Proteobacteria, order Pseudomonadales, family Pseudomonadaceae. Both genera include aerobic, non–spore-forming, oxidase-positive, nonfermentative, gram-negative rods that grow on MacConkey agar. Members of these genera are versatile pathogens (Table 19-1).

THE GENUS *PSEUDOMONAS*

Pseudomonas spp. have worldwide distribution. They are ubiquitous in soil, water, decaying organic matter, and vegetation, but are opportunistic pathogens of animals, plants, and humans. One species, *Pseudomonas aeruginosa,* is commonly

TABLE **19-1**   Diseases and Primary Hosts of the Veterinary Significant Pseudomonadaceae and Burkholderiaceae

Organism	Host(s)	Disease
Pseudomonas aeruginosa	Cattle	Mastitis; abortion
	Dog	Otitis externa
	Horse	Corneal ulcer; metritis
	Mink	Hemorrhagic pneumonia
	Poultry	Embryo mortality
	Sheep	Fleece rot
	Captive snakes	Necrotic stomatitis
	Many animals	Urinary tract infections; septicemia; wound infections; abscesses; granulomas (botryomycosis)
Pseudomonas fluorescens	Cattle	Mastitis
	Fish	Tail/fin rot, septicemia
	Poultry	Embryo mortality
Burkholderia mallei	Mule, donkey	Acute glanders
	Horse	Chronic glanders
	Cat, dog	Acute glanders
Burkholderia pseudomallei	Cat, cattle, dog, horse, marine mammals, pig, ruminants	Melioidosis (chronic nodular form more common than acute septicemia)

encountered as an animal pathogen and is particularly noteworthy for its ability to cause disease in susceptible hosts and its resistance to antibiotics. Another species, *Pseudomonas fluorescens,* is occasionally isolated from veterinary specimens.

DISEASES AND EPIDEMIOLOGY

Unlike many environmental bacteria, pseudomonads have a remarkable capacity to adapt to and thrive in diverse ecological niches. They can utilize a wide range of organic compounds, thus providing exceptional ability to colonize sites where nutrients are limited. The ability to thrive in aqueous environments has become problematic in veterinary hospital settings. *Pseudomonas aeruginosa* and *P. fluorescens* have been found in a variety of aqueous solutions and on equipment, including mastitis preparations, semen extenders, irrigation fluids, antiseptics, hydrotherapy baths, and endotracheal tubes. *Pseudomonas aeruginosa* is found infrequently as part of the microflora of skin, mucous membranes, and gastrointestinal tract of healthy animals.

The organism is the epitome of an opportunistic pathogen because it rarely infects uncompromised tissues, yet there is hardly any tissue that it cannot infect if the host defenses are compromised. Some of the more common *P. aeruginosa*–associated disease conditions in animals are ovine fleecerot, bovine mastitis and abortion, equine metritis and corneal ulcer, canine otitis externa, mink hemorrhagic pneumonia, embryo mortality in poultry, necrotic stomatitis of captive snakes, and botryomycosis, septicemia, urinary tract infections, wound infections, and abscesses in a variety of animals.

Fleece rot of sheep is characterized by superficial inflammation of the skin. It is economically important in sheep-rearing areas because of its effect of downgrading of wool. Predisposing factors are prolonged wetting of the fleece and conditions of high humidity. Animals with long, dense fleece of irregular fiber size are at an increased risk for infection. Initially, a superficial dermatitis develops along the animal's back. Lesions progress to hyperkeratosis, edema, polymorphonuclear cell infiltration, and finally microabscess formation. Clinically, the fleece is bluish green as a result of production of the diffusible pigment pyocyanin. Older lesions develop a putrefactive odor that attracts flies and may result in cutaneous myiasis.

Pseudomonas aeruginosa is a not-infrequent cause of bovine mastitis. Herd epizootics have been traced to the use of contaminated antibiotic preparations for intramammary infusion, teat-dipping solutions, or wash water used for udder preparation. One or all quarters may be affected. Intramammary infections can be acute, but often are chronic and refractory to treatment and end with culling of the affected cow from the herd. In acute outbreaks, animals may die due to endotoxemia. Chronic mastitis is characterized by low-grade inflammation of the mammary gland with recurrent subclinical flare-ups.

Sporadic bovine abortion and equine metritis have been associated with *P. aeruginosa* infection. Cows and mares inseminated naturally or artificially with contaminated semen may develop varying degrees of reproductive tract disease. Mares that repeatedly have been infused with antibiotics before breeding are at an increased risk for disease as a result of the destruction of competing normal microflora.

Pseudomonas aeruginosa is a common invader of the equine cornea. Infection usually follows minor trauma, such as damage caused by sand in the eyes of racehorses. The injured cornea becomes opaque and ulcerated. Loss of vision may occur unless prompt treatment is initiated.

Canine otitis externa caused by *P. aeruginosa* is frequently a complication of atopy, concurrent *Malassezia pachydermatis* or bacterial infections, mange, or trauma. Breeds with long, pendulous ears or those with hair in the external ear canal are predisposed to infection, as are dogs that swim frequently. If the infection is untreated, *P. aeruginosa* may invade the underlying tissues, causing cranial nerve damage, otitis media or interna, and osteomyelitis.

Hemorrhagic pneumonia of mink is a disease of high mortality with worldwide distribution, and outbreaks are most common in fall and winter. Bacteria gain entry to the respiratory tract when kits sniff contaminated food. Illness is acute, and affected animals are anorectic, lethargic, and dyspneic, usually with epistaxis. Lungs are hemorrhagic with focal areas of necrosis.

Pseudomonas aeruginosa is often recovered from dead poultry embryos and newly hatched chicks. Severe disease outbreaks have followed egg injection with contaminated vaccines or egg-dipping in contaminated antimicrobial solutions. Contamination typically results from poor handling of these products rather than from the products themselves.

Pseudomonas aeruginosa is found in the oral cavity and intestinal tract of reptiles. Poor husbandry, including suboptimal environmental temperatures and malnutrition, and trauma can predispose to infection. Necrotic stomatitis, also known as mouth rot or canker mouth, is one of the most common diseases of captive reptiles, and is characterized by ulceration and accumulation of caseous exudates in the oral cavity. The disease may progress to involve teeth sockets and the jawbone, resulting in osteomyelitis. Untreated snakes die from complications such as pneumonia or septicemia.

Botryomycosis is a granulomatous disease of the skin, subcutis, and viscera. The term was used initially because of the histologic resemblance of the lesions to fungal granulomas but is erroneous because the etiology is bacterial rather than mycotic. Most recorded cases of botryomycosis are attributed to *Staphylococcus aureus;* however, *P. aeruginosa* has also occasionally been implicated. Pseudomonal botryomycosis has been described in cattle, laboratory rodents, and man. Trauma is an important prerequisite for inoculation of the bacterium into tissues. In cattle, lesions have been reported on the udder and in the nasopharynx. Pulmonary disease has occurred in guinea pigs. Microscopic examination of lesions reveals pyogranulomas surrounding colonies of gram-negative rods. Granules of eosinophilic material with peripheral, radiating clubs (Splendore-Hoeppli phenomenon) form around the bacterial colonies and are surrounded by neutrophils, eosinophils, and macrophages (Figure 19-1). The granules resemble those of actinomycosis.

Pseudomonas aeruginosa is an opportunistic pathogen of humans, causing urinary tract infections, respiratory system infections, dermatitis, soft-tissue infections, bacteremia, and a variety of systemic infections. These are a particular problem in patients with severe burns, cancer, acquired immunodeficiency syndrome (AIDS), cystic fibrosis, or others who are immunosuppressed.

Pseudomonas fluorescens causes sporadic disease in cattle, poultry, and fish. The organism is an agent of environmentally acquired mastitis. Turkey embryo mortality following dipping of eggs in contaminated disinfectant solutions has been reported. In fish, *P. fluorescens* is associated with fin or tail rot and septicemia.

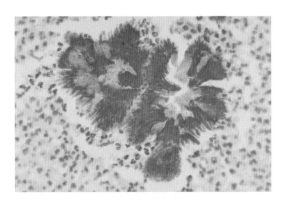

FIGURE 19-1 Botryomycosis lesions in tissue associated with *Pseudomonas aeruginosa.* (Courtesy Public Health Image Library, PHIL #4260, Centers for Disease Control and Prevention, Atlanta, 1973, Lucille K. George.)

PATHOGENESIS

Pseudomonas aeruginosa possesses a wide variety of virulence factors, including pili, capsule, endotoxin, pyocyanin, hemolysins, enzymes, toxins, and an inherent resistance to many antimicrobials. These cause extensive tissue damage at or near the site of infection, cause permanent disruption of host cell membranes, and interfere with immune defense mechanisms. It is difficult to define the specific role for each factor in disease because most investigators believe multiple factors contribute to virulence (Table 19-2).

Because of the opportunistic nature of pseudomonal infections, the first step in pathogenesis in any site is a breach in the host defenses, such as skin trauma, disruption of normal microflora from antimicrobial therapy, or other circumstances. The next step is bacterial adherence to host epithelial cells via pili and capsular polysaccharide. Capsule further protects the organism from phagocytosis by host immune cells. Proteases promote dissemination of *P. aeruginosa* in the tissues. Elastase destroys elastin, disrupting the integrity of host cellular basement membranes and removing physical barriers that would normally inhibit the spread of infection. Elastin is also a major component of lung and vascular tissue. Elastase likely plays a large role in the pathogenesis of mink hemorrhagic pneumonia by damaging lung parenchyma and blood vessels. Toxins and proteases are responsible for edema, hemorrhage, and necrosis that occur in skin wounds. In particular, alkaline protease facilitates the dissemination of bacteria and causes tissue

TABLE **19-2**   Virulence Factors of *Pseudomonas aeruginosa*

Virulence Factors	Biologic Effect(s)
Alkaline protease	Inactivates interferon and tumor necrosis factor; causes tissue damage
Antibiotic resistance	Complicates chemotherapy
Capsule	Protects organism from phagocytosis and antibiotic penetration; functions as an adhesin
Cytotoxin	Inhibits leukocyte function; disrupts pulmonary microcirculation
Elastase	Damages blood vessels, skin, and pulmonary tissue; degrades complement components; inhibits neutrophil chemotaxis
Endotoxin	Mediates biologic effects of sepsis and inflammation
Exotoxin A	Inhibits cellular protein synthesis; causes tissue necrosis; has immunosuppressive effects
Exotoxins S and T	Inhibit cellular protein synthesis; have immunosuppressive effects; facilitate tissue invasion
Phospholipase C	Hemolysin that stimulates inflammation; causes tissue damage
Pili	Mediate adhesion to host cells
Pyocyanin	Pigment that interferes with the mucociliary apparatus; produces toxic oxygen radicals that mediate tissue damage
Rhamnolipid	Hemolysin with lecithinase activity that damages host cell membranes; inhibits the mucociliary apparatus; inhibits macrophage function

damage; phospholipase C degrades cellular membranes by way of its lecithinase activity. The pathogenesis of ulcerative keratitis is mediated by endotoxin, exotoxins, and proteases. Endotoxin attracts and activates polymorphonuclear cells, and corneal inflammation and subsequent tissue damage results from release of oxidative substances by the neutrophils. Pseudomonal exotoxins are also directly responsible for destruction of corneal epithelial cells. Proteases are thought to be crucial for the development of ulcerative keratitis, but their precise role remains to be determined. Pseudomonads have enzymes that are capable of digesting eggshell cuticle in conditions of high humidity, resulting in invasion of the embryo.

The pathogenesis of botryomycosis remains obscure. Disease may require exposure to a large number of organisms, a strain of high virulence, or inoculation of foreign material to provide a nidus for granule formation. A genetic predisposition has been implicated.

Pseudomonas aeruginosa is notorious for its resistance to antibiotics. Natural resistance is often due to permeability barriers afforded by its outer membrane lipopolysaccharide and capsule. Organisms have a tendency to colonize surfaces in a biofilm, which can make the cells impervious to therapeutic concentrations of antibiotics. Because its natural habitat is the soil, living in association with other bacteria and molds, it has developed resistance to a variety of naturally occurring antibiotics. Moreover, *P. aeruginosa* maintains transferable antibiotic resistance. Antibiotics effective against *Pseudomonas* spp. include fluoroquinolones, gentamicin, amikacin, tobramycin, and imipenem, but even these are not effective against all strains.

DIAGNOSIS

Diagnosis is based on isolation of *P. aeruginosa* and *P. fluorescens* from clinical specimens. These pseudomonads are widespread in the environment, so they are frequent contaminants and their recovery is not always significant. *Pseudomonas aeruginosa* and *P. fluorescens* grow well on routine laboratory media, such as trypticase soy agar with or without 5% blood, and MacConkey agar incubated aerobically at 37° C. Cetrimide agar is a commercial formulation that is selective for *P. aeruginosa*. Optimum growth temperature is 37° C, but *P. aeruginosa* is able to grow at temperatures as high as 42° C, which distinguishes it from *P. fluorescens* (Table 19-3).

Pseudomonas aeruginosa is easily recognized on primary isolation media by its colonial morphology, production of pigments, and distinctive odor. Isolates may produce three colony types. Natural isolates from soil or water typically yield small, rough colonies. Clinical samples, in general, yield one or another of two smooth colony types. One type has a fried-egg appearance, large and smooth, with flat edges and elevated center.

TABLE **19-3** Differential Characteristics of *Pseudomonas aeruginosa* and *Pseudomonas fluorescens*

Test	P. aeruginosa	P. fluorescens
Odor	Grapelike	Negative
Growth at 42° C	Positive	Negative
Pyocyanin	Positive	Negative
Kanamycin	Resistant	Susceptible

Another type, frequently obtained from respiratory and urinary tract secretions, can be extraordinarily mucoid, which is attributed to the production of alginate. The diffusible pigments pyocyanin, pyoverdin, pyorubrin, and pyomelanin may be produced in culture. Pyocyanin, a pigment unique to *P. aeruginosa,* is derived from the word "pyocyaneus" in reference to the "blue pus" that may be seen in suppurative infections caused by *P. aeruginosa* (Figure 19-2). Not all strains produce this pigment. Pyoverdin is a yellow pigment that combines with pyocyanin to produce a bright green color that is fluorescent. Pyorubrin (red) and pyomelanin (brown to brownish black) are less frequently produced and may take several weeks to appear. The odor attributed to *P. aeruginosa* has been described as "grapelike," "fruity," or "corn taco–like." *Pseudomonas fluorescens* does not possess a characteristic colonial morphology or odor, but does produce pyoverdin.

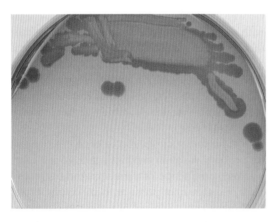

FIGURE **19-2** Pyocyanin production by *Pseudomonas aeruginosa,* cultivated on trypticase soy agar. (Courtesy Karen W. Post.)

TREATMENT, PREVENTION, AND CONTROL

In general, prevention and control of *Pseudomonas* infections are based on identifying predisposing factors and/or eliminating the source of the organism. Reduction of stress and prevention of concurrent bacterial and viral infections will decrease host susceptibility. Antimicrobial therapy for pseudomonal infections is difficult because of inherent resistance. In addition, even susceptible organisms may develop resistance during therapy. Indiscriminate use of antimicrobials should be avoided because it will select for the growth of resistant pseudomonads and suppress the normal microflora. Attempts to eliminate the organism from the hatchery, hospital, or dairy environment have met with variable success. Sound hygienic practices should focus on preventing contamination of sterile equipment and aqueous solutions. Chlorination of well water in dairy or hatchery settings may eliminate contamination.

For prevention and control of fleecerot in sheep, animals should be sheared before a rainy season. Breeds used for wool production should be selected based on hardy skin and suitable fleece. Treatment of sheep through cleaning affected areas followed by topical application of antibiotics and drying agents is often unrewarding. Vaccines may reduce disease severity. Vaccination is also a proven method for prevention and control of hemorrhagic pneumonia in mink.

THE GENUS *BURKHOLDERIA*

The genus *Burkholderia* now comprises more than 30 validly described species, of which only *Burkholderia mallei* and *Burkholderia pseudomallei* are animal pathogens. Both organisms have been classified as Category B select agents because so few organisms are necessary to cause disease, and aerosol infection can occur. *Burkholderia mallei,* in particular, has been weaponized by various bioweapons programs. In World War I, German forces spread the organism among horses to deliberately debilitate enemy cavalries, and in the 1980s the Soviet Union produced more than 2000 tons of the bacterium. Because *B. mallei* and *B. pseudomallei* are so extraordinarily dangerous in a laboratory setting, biosafety level (BSL)-3 precautions should be followed.

DISEASES AND EPIDEMIOLOGY

Burkholderia mallei

Burkholderia mallei is the etiologic agent of glanders, a serious contagious disease of equids. Glanders has historically been a scourge of army horses and mules, and was in fact first described by Hippocrates between 450 BC and 425 BC. The organism is a true parasite because it is unable to survive in nature for extended periods in the absence of its host. Bacteria are unable to maintain viability in infected environments for longer than 2 weeks and are readily killed by most common disinfectants, desiccation, and sunlight. Carnivores may develop acute septicemia if they consume meat from affected animals. Felids are apparently more susceptible than canids, and there have been reports of disease outbreaks in captive felids. Occasional natural infections have been reported in sheep, goats, and camels, but swine and cattle are refractory to infection. Hamsters and guinea pigs are susceptible to experimental infection. The susceptibility of guinea pigs is the basis for the Strauss test, an assay used in diagnosis.

Glanders was once widespread throughout the world, but was eliminated from the United States in the 1940s. Diligent test-and-slaughter methods have resulted in eradication from western and central Europe. Pockets of active disease still exist in North Africa, China, Mongolia, the Middle East, India, the Philippines, southeastern Europe, and Central and South America.

Disease is introduced into equine populations by infected animals. Ingestion of *B. mallei*, which is present in high numbers in secretions of infected individuals, is the most common route of infection. Skin invasion and inhalation are regarded as minor routes of transmission. Transmission is enhanced when horses share common feed buckets or watering troughs.

Glanders may be acute or chronic in nature, and the former is more common in mules and donkeys. These animals have a high fever and exhibit respiratory signs, including swollen nostrils, dyspnea, and pneumonia. Death occurs within a few days.

Glanders usually manifests as a chronic infection in horses, and infected animals may survive for several years. Disease occurs in nasal, cutaneous (farcy), and pulmonary forms, all of which may occur simultaneously in one animal. The prognosis in infected animals is poor, and those that recover

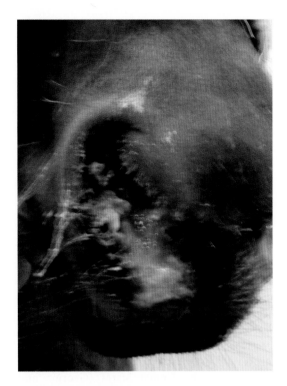

FIGURE 19-3 Bilateral, purulent nasal discharge in a horse inoculated intratracheally with *Burkholderia mallei*. (Courtesy D.E. Woods.)

are not immune to reinfection. These animals remain latently infected and serve as a source of infection for other animals and humans. Clinical signs in affected horses include catarrhal nasal discharge from one or both nostrils (Figure 19-3), gray to yellow nodules on the upper respiratory mucous membranes, submaxillary lymphadenopathy, dyspnea, weight loss, and nodules and/or ulcers along the cutaneous lymphatics. Glanders is a reportable foreign animal disease in the United States.

Glanders is zoonotic, and is transmitted to humans by direct contact with sick animals or infectious materials or through ingestion of glandered meat. Veterinarians, farriers, animal caretakers, abattoir workers, and laboratorians are at increased risk for developing disease. Cases of human-to-human transmission have been reported. The only case of human glanders in the past 50 years in the United States was recently reported in a military research microbiologist. Human disease can manifest as acute localized infection, septicemic illness, acute pulmonary infection, or chronic cutaneous infection.

Symptoms include fever, headache, myalgia, lymphadenopathy, malaise, chest pain, splenomegaly, and pustular skin lesions. Rare cases of human-to-human transmission have been reported. A variety of antimicrobials can be used for therapy, but even with treatment the mortality rate may approach 50%. In untreated humans the case fatality rate is 95% within 3 weeks.

Burkholderia pseudomallei

Burkholderia pseudomallei is the cause of melioidosis or pseudoglanders, a highly fatal disease of humans and other mammals. The organism is a saprophyte, ubiquitous in soil and surface water. Melioidosis has been diagnosed in all domestic species (horses, sheep, goats, cattle, pigs, dogs, cats), and occasionally in marine mammals. Primary disease also occurs in rodents, which have been regarded as a source of infection in endemic tropical and subtropical regions. The highest disease prevalence is in Southeast Asia and northern Australia; however, sporadic cases have been reported in the United States (Georgia and Hawaii), France, China, Africa, India, the Middle East, the Caribbean, and Central and South America. Increased disease incidence often coincides with heavy rainfall. Humans and animals acquire the infection by ingestion of contaminated water, inhalation of dust, and contact with contaminated soil, especially through skin abrasions or wounds. Several cases have been attributed to arthropod bites. Carnivores may become infected by ingesting contaminated carcasses. Although melioidosis occurs in previously healthy individuals, clinical disease is more frequently seen in individuals with impaired host defense mechanisms. To date, zoonotic transmission has not been documented, although rare person-to-person transmission by contact with the blood or body fluids of an infected person has been described.

Animal infections with *B. pseudomallei* are usually systemic and disease manifestations depend on the extent and the distribution of the infection. Melioidosis causes a chronic nodular or purulent inflammatory disease. Nodular lesions may form in any tissue and suppurate. Although most infections are chronic, acute disease with terminal sepsis has been described. The small, caseous, cutaneous nodules eventually rupture, releasing more organisms into the environment or infecting other animals. Melioidosis was an important disease of military dogs stationed in Vietnam.

These animals developed fever, myalgia, dermal abscesses, and epididymitis. Outbreaks of melioidosis have been reported in ruminants and pigs. Arthritis and pneumonia are common clinical findings. Bovine placentitis and endometritis have been described, with multiple abscesses in lungs, regional lymph nodes, spleen, liver, and joints.

Human melioidosis is also called Whitmore's disease. Clinical illness varies greatly in its presentation, ranging from asymptomatic to overwhelming sepsis with rapid fatality. Disease may also present as benign pneumonitis, acute, subacute, or chronic pneumonia, or an acute, subacute, or chronic suppurative process. Long periods of latency and frequent relapses after antimicrobial treatment are characteristic features of melioidosis. During the Vietnam conflict, large numbers of American soldiers became infected with *B. pseudomallei*. Because the organism may remain latent for years, the disease has been dubbed the "Vietnamese time bomb," as cases of melioidosis continue to emerge in veterans.

PATHOGENESIS

After infection, *B. mallei* penetrates the intestinal or pharyngeal mucosa and enters the regional lymphatic vessels, where it passes into the blood via the thoracic duct. The organism disseminates to all parts of the body but colonizes only the lymphatics of the respiratory tract and skin. Nodules may develop in the lymph channels, which thicken and eventually ulcerate to discharge a honeylike exudate containing large numbers of bacteria. Pneumonic lesions may be nodular (reminiscent of tubercles) or diffuse. Primary nodular lesions at the point of entry in the nasal passages and pharynx also ulcerate and discharge sticky, yellow infectious exudates through the nostrils, often leading to airway obstruction. Glanders nodules may occasionally be found in the spleen and liver. Predominance of suppurative or granulomatous lesions is mediated by strain variations in *B. mallei*.

Little is known of virulence factors of *B. mallei*, in large part because of long-term lack of an equine infection model. Recent work has established such a model, and early indications are that capsular polysaccharide is essential for virulence because an acapsular mutant strain of *B. mallei* failed to produce disease. Toxins disrupting host cellular functions include pyocyanin, lecithinase, collagenase, and lipase. Pyocyanin interferes with terminal electron transfer. Lecithinase, collagenase, and lipase mediate cell lysis through membrane degradation.

The pathogenesis of melioidosis is also poorly understood. After phagocytosis, *B. pseudomallei* escapes endocytic vacuoles into host cell cytoplasm and forms membrane protrusions that eventually mediate cell-to-cell spread of the organism. Pyemia is followed by tissue localization, and lymph nodes, spleen, liver, lung, and joints are usually affected. Depending on the infectious dose, acute disease may be associated with suppuration or more indolent disease with chronic abscessation.

Extracellular enzymes include lecithinase, lipase, and dermonecrotic protease. However, their exact role in pathogenesis is currently unknown. Heat-labile components are responsible for cytotoxic and anticoagulant activity. Malleobactin is a siderophore that is involved in iron acquisition. Evasion of complement-mediated killing is probably a key virulence determinant of *B. pseudomallei*. Flagella are apparently necessary virulence determinants of *B. pseudomallei* during intranasal and intraperitoneal infection of mice. The organism likely possesses at least two pilus types that are responsible for epithelial cell adhesion in vitro. The polysaccharide capsule protects against antibiotic penetration. *Burkholderia pseudomallei* is a facultative intracellular pathogen, and this may in part explain aspects of melioidosis such as recrudescence and poor response to antimicrobial therapy.

Environmental isolates, all previously considered to be *B. pseudomallei*, fall into two closely related groups based on their ability to assimilate arabinose. Those that assimilate arabinose have been assigned to a new species, *Burkholderia thailandensis*, and are considered avirulent, whereas those that cannot do so and are associated with melioidosis have been retained within the species *B. pseudomallei*.

DIAGNOSIS

Glanders and melioidosis may be definitively diagnosed through the isolation and identification of the causative agents from blood or tissue. All manipulations of potentially infected material should be performed under conditions of biohazard containment. *Burkholderia mallei* grows well but slowly on most routine laboratory media, such as 5% sheep blood agar, MacConkey agar, and chocolate agar. Its growth may be enhanced by addition of 1% glycerol to agar-based media.

Burkholderia pseudomallei grows more rapidly on routine media.

The use of selective media facilitates the isolation of *B. mallei* and *B. pseudomallei* from specimens with mixed flora. The selective medium for the isolation of *B. mallei* contains polymyxin B, bacitracin, and actidione. Ashdown's medium, effective for the isolation of *B. pseudomallei*, contains gentamicin and crystal violet as selective agents. Plates are incubated aerobically at 37° C for up to 7 days.

Colonial morphology is a useful feature for identifying these agents. Colonies of *B. mallei* are small, round, convex, translucent, moist, viscid and cream to yellow. As colonies age they become dark brown and tough. On glycerol-containing medium, colonies may be confluent and honeylike in appearance. *Burkholderia pseudomallei* grows in 24 to 48 hours on blood agar plates, and forms smooth, small colonies that later become dry and wrinkled (Figure 19-4). On Ashdown's agar, the colonies are deep pink. The organism often produces a characteristic sweet, earthy odor, which is most noticeable on opening the Petri dish.

Morphology in Gram-stained smears differs between these two species. In young cultures, *B. mallei* produces long, slender rods with rounded ends, 2 to 5 μm long and 0.5 μm wide, and often stains irregularly. Older cultures may be quite pleomorphic, with cells varying from coccobacilli to long filaments. Gram stain of *B. pseudomallei*

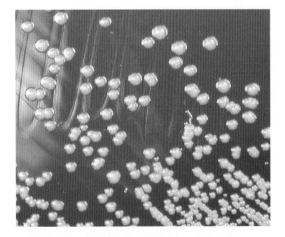

FIGURE 19-4 *Burkholderia pseudomallei* (48-hour incubation on sheep blood agar). (Courtesy Public Health Image Library, PHIL #1926, Centers for Disease Control and Prevention, Atlanta, 2002, Larry Stauffer, Oregon State Public Health Laboratory.)

TABLE **19-4** Differential Characteristics of *Burkholderia mallei* and *Burkholderia pseudomallei*

Test	B. mallei	B. pseudomallei
Oxidase	(Pos)	Pos
Odor	Neg	Earthy
Growth on MacConkey	Pos	Pos
Growth at 42° C	Neg	Pos
Motility	Neg	Pos
Nitrate reduction	Pos	Pos
Reduction of nitrate to gas	Neg	Pos
Arginine dihydrolase	Pos	Pos
Oxidation of glucose	Pos	Pos
Oxidation of maltose	Neg	Pos
Oxidation of mannitol	Neg	Pos

Neg, Negative; *Pos,* positive; *(Pos),* most positive.

cultures reveals small, gram-negative rods with bipolar staining that resemble safety pins. Several phenotypic properties are useful in identification (Table 19-4), and commercial kit systems for bacterial identification may reliably confirm the identity of this organism.

Serology is useful for diagnosis of both glanders and melioidosis. Antibodies can be detected by complement fixation, counterimmunoelectrophoresis, enzyme-linked immunosorbent assay (ELISA), or indirect hemagglutination. The indirect hemagglutination test is most widely available; it is a useful indicator of exposure, but lacks specificity in areas of high prevalence. Many serologic assays may cross-react with *B. pseudomallei.*

For horses being imported into the United States, the official test for glanders is complement fixation. Horses whose sera are anticomplementary must be tested with the mallein test, which is similar in principle to the tuberculin test. Mallein, a glycoprotein extracted from *B. mallei,* is injected intrapalpebrally and the response is read at 24 and 48 hours. Horses infected with *B. mallei* will become allergic and exhibit both local and systemic hypersensitivity reactions. A positive reaction is characterized by marked edema of the eyelid, lacrimation, photophobia, and purulent discharge.

Additional diagnostic tests for *B. mallei* and *B. pseudomallei* include fluorescent antibody assays, polymerase chain reaction (PCR), and immunohistochemistry. The indirect fluorescent antibody test is used on clinical materials. PCR tests can detect organisms from buffy coats or purulent exudates. Immunohistochemical methods have been developed for organism detection in fixed tissue sections or biopsies.

In addition, male guinea pigs injected intraperitoneally with potentially infected clinical material develop orchitis if the inoculum contains *B. mallei,* the so-called Strauss reaction.

PREVENTION AND CONTROL

In endemic areas, control of glanders requires testing suspect clinical cases, screening apparently normal animals, and destroying reactors. Communal feeding and watering of equids should be discouraged, and in outbreaks all contaminated bedding and foodstuffs should be burned or buried. Tack and stalls should be thoroughly disinfected. *Burkholderia mallei* is usually sensitive to tetracyclines, fluoroquinolones, gentamicin, and sulfonamides. Although these agents may be used to treat human infections, treating infected equids is discouraged.

There is no effective method of preventing melioidosis in endemic regions because contact with infected soil or water is so common. Surgical drainage of abscesses, followed by parenteral antimicrobial therapy, may be curative. *Burkholderia pseudomallei* is susceptible to tetracyclines, chloramphenicol, trimethoprim-sulfamethoxazole, imipenem, and amoxicillin-clavulanic acid, but resistant to aminoglycosides and polymyxin B. Several other β-lactam agents, including ceftazidime and ceftriaxone, have demonstrated activity against *B. pseudomallei.* Treatment should be initiated early in the course of disease.

There are currently no commercially available vaccines for glanders or melioidosis.

SUGGESTED READINGS

Dance DAB: Melioidosis: the tip of the iceberg? *Clin Microbiol Rev* 4:52-60, 1991.

Lopez J, Copps J, Wilhelmsen C, et al: Characterization of experimental equine glanders, *Microbes Infect* 5:1125-1131, 2003.

Lyczak JB, Cannon CL, Pier GB: Establishment of *Pseudomonas aeruginosa* infection: lessons from a versatile opportunist, *Microbes Infect* 2:1051-1060, 2000.

Woods DE, DeShazer D, Moore RA, et al: Current studies on the pathogenesis of melioidosis, *Microbes Infect* 2:157-162, 1999.

Chapter 20

The Genera *Aeromonas, Plesiomonas,* and *Vibrio*

The genera *Aeromonas, Plesiomonas,* and *Vibrio* comprise gram-negative, facultatively anaerobic rods in the class γ-Proteobacteria. They ferment glucose and are usually oxidase positive. Recent taxonomic reorganization notwithstanding, they are discussed together because of similarities in epidemiology and associated diseases. All are found in aquatic environments, and most diseases they cause are enteric or septicemic in nature (Table 20-1).

THE GENUS *AEROMONAS*

The genus *Aeromonas* was initially placed in the family Vibrionaceae with the genera *Plesiomonas* and *Vibrio*. Subsequent phylogenetic studies resulted in transfer of *Aeromonas* to the new family Aeromonadaceae, as the sole genus within the order Aeromonadales. There are currently 15 validly published species, which are catalase positive, reduce nitrate to nitrite, and are resistant to the vibriostatic agent O129. Most species possess flagella, although fish strains of *Aeromonas salmonicida* are exceptions.

Aeromonads grow well at temperatures ranging from 10° to 42° C. Most strains pathogenic for fish and shellfish are psychrophilic and seldom grow above 28° C, with optimal growth occurring at 22° to 25° C. Cells are straight, may be coccoid, and range from 1.0 to 3.5 μm long and 0.3 to 1 μm wide (Figure 20-1).

TABLE **20-1** Diseases and Primary Hosts of *Aeromonas, Plesiomonas,* and *Vibrio* Species That Are Significant in Veterinary Medicine

Genus and Species	Host(s)	Diseases
Aeromonas hydrophila	Frogs	Red leg disease
	Eels	Freshwater eel disease
	Reptiles	Necrotic stomatitis
	Cultured warm-water fish	Fin/tail rot and hemorrhagic septicemia
Aeromonas salmonicida ssp. *salmonicida*	Salmonids	Furunculosis
	Carp and goldfish	Erythrodermatitis and ulcer disease
Plesiomonas shigelloides	Cultured tilapia	Septicemia
	Cats	Diarrhea (rare)
Vibrio metschnikovii	Poultry and other young birds	Enteritis
Vibrio ordalii	Salmonids	Hemorrhagic septicemia
Vibrio salmonicida	Cultured Atlantic salmon	Cold-water vibriosis
Vibrio harveyi	Shrimp, fin fish	Vibriosis
Vibrio alginolyticus	Shrimp	Vibriosis

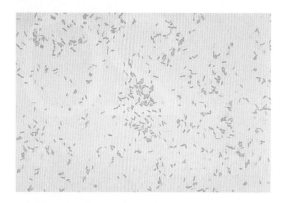

FIGURE 20-1 *Aeromonas hydrophila* Gram stain. (Courtesy Public Health Image Library, PHIL #1255, Centers for Disease Control and Prevention, Atlanta, 1977, W.A. Clark.)

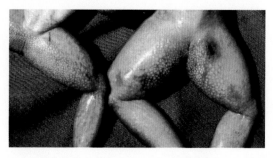

FIGURE 20-2 Frog with lesions of "red leg." (Courtesy Raymond E. Reed.)

DISEASES AND EPIDEMIOLOGY

Aeromonads are found in water, soil, and sewage. Their pathogenicity was first established in poikilothermic animals, in association with massive outbreaks of septicemia, with high mortality in aquatic species. *Aeromonas* spp. inhabit the gastrointestinal tract of many aquatic species, and are important pathogens of reptiles and amphibians. Rare infections have been reported in swine, cattle, birds, and marine mammals.

Aeromonas hydrophila is an opportunistic pathogen associated with hemorrhagic septicemia in cold-blooded animals, including amphibians, reptiles, fish, and shellfish. It is best known as the etiologic agent of "red leg" disease in frogs, so named because of the hemorrhages observed in the leg muscles of affected animals (Figure 20-2). Fish disease has worldwide distribution in warm-water cultured fish such as catfish, carp, and bass. *Aeromonas hydrophila* is also associated with tail or fin rot. Hemorrhagic septicemia, sometimes called motile aeromonad septicemia, is characterized by the presence of small surface lesions that progress to skin sloughing and localized hemorrhages. Necrotic stomatitis of snakes is also attributed to *A. hydrophila* infection.

Aeromonas salmonicida ssp. *salmonicida*, the etiologic agent of furunculosis in salmonid fish, is one of the oldest fish pathogens and is found in most regions of the world. The disease was so named because, in the subacute or chronic form, lesions in the musculature resemble boils or furuncles. Although once considered to be a pathogen of salmonids, the bacterium has increasingly been recovered from other species, such as perch and pike, and may on occasion be associated with disease outbreaks in cultured fish. Infection occurs by fish-to-fish contact either through the skin or by ingestion, and asymptomatic carriers have been implicated in transmission. Risk factors include skin trauma, stress, and presence of concurrent disease. Furunculosis is most prevalent in late spring or summer, when water temperatures are warmest.

Aeromonas spp. have recently emerged as important human pathogens associated with food-borne disease outbreaks and traveler's diarrhea, with *A. hydrophila*, *Aeromonas caviae*, and *Aeromonas veronii* biovar *sobria* being the most frequently isolated species. Infection is generally through consumption of contaminated water and food. Sporadic cases of septicemia, peritonitis, urinary tract infections, and a hemolytic-uremic syndrome have been attributed to *A. hydrophila*. The ability of aeromonads to survive and multiply at a variety of temperatures, over a wide pH range, and at salt concentrations up to 4% have contributed to their ability to cause food-borne illness.

PATHOGENESIS

Aeromonads invade host cells and disseminate to virtually any organ. Death is usually attributed to massive septicemia and toxic extracellular products of the organism, which interfere with host blood supply and result in massive tissue necrosis.

Virulence factors of *Aeromonas* spp. include toxins, surface proteins or structures, and extracellular degradative enzymes. A cytotoxin encoded by a plasmid-based gene is similar to Shiga toxin and may be responsible for gastroenteritis. Distinct hemolysins causing fluid accumulation in ileal loop assays have been detected in β-hemolytic strains of *A. hydrophila*. Aerolysin, another hemolysin, is a pore-forming toxin that causes ion leakage and, ultimately, eukaryotic cell lysis. The cytotoxic enterotoxin, the heat-stable cytotoxic enterotoxin, and the heat-labile cytotoxic enterotoxin all contribute to enteropathogenicity. Certain *Aeromonas* spp. produce polar and lateral flagella; the former mediate swimming, allowing the organisms to reach their target cells, whereas the latter facilitate swarming over surfaces and adhesion to and invasion of host cells. Pili have been described in several *Aeromonas* spp., and type IV pili are known virulence determinants in *A. salmonicida.* An outer-membrane protein in *A. caviae* functions as an adhesin. A capsule, produced by some species, imparts resistance to bacteriolysis and phagocytosis.

Aeromonads produce a wide range of enzymes that cause tissue damage and aid in the establishment of infection by overwhelming host defenses and by providing nutrients for bacterial proliferation. These include serine protease, metalloproteases, aminopeptidases, lipases, and phospholipases. *Aeromonas* spp. produce siderophores to obtain their supply of iron.

DIAGNOSIS

Diagnosis of aeromonad disease is best accomplished through isolation of the organism from clinical specimens and correlation with gross and histologic lesions. These bacteria may be readily recovered from the lesions of affected animals by the use of standard nonselective media like trypticase soy or blood agar and the selective/differential media MacConkey and Rimler-Shotts. *Aeromonas hydrophila* colonies on nonselective media are cream colored, round, shiny, raised, entire, β-hemolytic, 2 to 3 mm in diameter, and develop within 48 hours at 25° C (Figure 20-3). Most strains of *A. salmonicida* produce colonies on trypticase soy agar that are surrounded by a dark

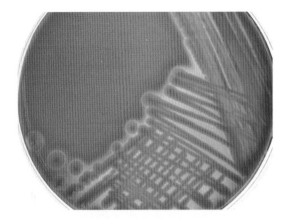

FIGURE 20-3 Colony morphology of *Aeromonas hydrophila* cultivated on blood agar. (Courtesy Karen W. Post.)

brown diffusible pigment after 3 to 4 days' incubation at 25° C. *Aeromonas* colonies are non–lactose-fermenting on MacConkey agar and yellowish orange on Rimler-Shotts medium. *Aeromonas hydrophila* grows at 37° C, whereas *A. salmonicida* does not.

Aeromonads must be differentiated from other oxidase-positive, glucose-fermenting, gram-negative rods, such as *Plesiomonas* spp. and *Vibrio* spp. (Table 20-2). Laboratory identification of aeromonads to the species level is fraught with difficulty, including a complicated taxonomy with numerous biovars and subspecies. Misidentification is a continuing problem.

A major problem in the identification process is lack of defined phenotypic tables for distinguishing the species from each other. This has occurred because only selected biochemical characteristics have been reported when new *Aeromonas* species have been described. Many biochemical schemes

TABLE **20-2** Key Tests for Phenotypic Differentiation of Members of the Genera *Aeromonas, Plesiomonas,* and *Vibrio*

Test	Aeromonas	Plesiomonas	Vibrio
O129 susceptibility (150 µg)	Neg	Pos	Pos
Ornithine decarboxylase	(Neg)	Pos	Pos
Arginine dihydrolase	Pos	Pos	Neg
Inositol fermentation	Neg	Pos	(Neg)
Gas from glucose	Var	Neg	Neg
Growth in nutrient broth without NaCl	Pos	Pos	(Neg)

Neg, Negative; *Pos,* positive; *(Pos),* most positive; *(Neg),* most negative; *Var,* variable.

used in laboratories may predate the description of newer taxa. Strains with biochemical properties atypical for a given species are common. Furthermore, commercial identification test systems do not accurately identify most of the aeromonads and correlate poorly with conventional tube biochemical tests.

In fisheries laboratories, identification of *A. salmonicida* may also be accomplished through serum agglutination, fluorescent antibody tests, enzyme immunoassays, or a specific polymerase chain reaction assay.

PREVENTION AND CONTROL

Fish vaccines are commercially available for prevention and control, but these vaccines offer limited effectiveness, and epizootics are still common in farmed fish. Control of *Aeromonas* infections usually involves chemotherapy and management of environmental factors that precipitate disease outbreaks. Antimicrobial resistance may limit usefulness of ampicillin, sulfonamides, and tetracycline.

THE GENUS *PLESIOMONAS*

The genus *Plesiomonas,* with its single species *Pleisomonas shigelloides* has been reassigned from the family Vibrionaceae to the family Enterobacteriaceae, order Enterobacteriales. The organism is ubiquitous in aquatic environments, being isolated from freshwater, estuarine, and saltwater sources. It has also been recovered from fresh vegetables, shellfish, and the intestines of healthy snakes, monkeys, mice, dogs, cats, swine, goats, raccoons, fish, and ducks.

Plesiomonads have been associated with diarrhea in cats and septicemia of cultured fish, and several reports suggest that *P. shigelloides* might be zoonotic. The organism is emerging as a human enteric pathogen, associated with sporadic episodes and rare outbreaks of diarrheal disease. Infection is acquired through contact with water, exposure to amphibians and reptiles, and consumption of contaminated seafood. Enteritis and dysentery-like syndromes are frequently reported in individuals with a history of travel abroad, particularly to Mexico. Diarrhea is usually self-limiting. An increasing number of extraintestinal infections have been reported, including cellulitis, septicemia, cholecystitis, osteomyelitis, meningitis, and pseudoappendicitis. Factors that predispose to extraintestinal infection are poorly defined, but immunocompromised individuals appear to be more susceptible to infection.

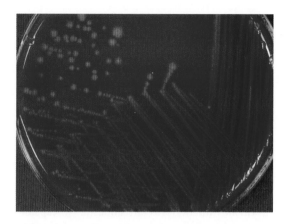

FIGURE 20-4 Colonial morphology of *Plesiomonas shigelloides* cultivated on blood agar. (Courtesy Karen W. Post.)

Lack of experimental infection models has hindered definition of mechanisms of pathogenesis. Reputed virulence factors include a cholera-like toxin, a hemolysin, and a heat-stable enterotoxin. The hemolysin may play a role in iron acquisition in vivo, through lysis of red blood cells, liberating hemoglobin. The heat-stable toxin is toxic for human epithelial (HEp)-2 cells in vitro. About 40% of *Plesiomonas* isolates are serum resistant, and factors encoded by genes on a large plasmid may facilitate the uptake or invasion of *P. shigelloides* in the gastrointestinal tract.

Isolation of the organism from clinical materials is the basis for diagnosis. *Plesiomonas shigelloides* is easily isolated on blood agar, where it produces 2 to 3 mm, convex, opaque colonies (Figure 20-4). It behaves as a nonlactose fermenter on MacConkey agar, and grows well on cefsulodin-irgasan-novobiocin agar (a medium selective for *Yersinia* species), growing as opaque colonies without pink centers. It must be separated from other oxidase-positive organisms, such as aeromonads and vibrios (see Table 20-2).

Resistance to aminoglycosides, β-lactams, tetracycline, and sulfa drugs has been reported. The organism is susceptible in vitro to chloramphenicol, fluoroquinolones, and potentiated sulfa drugs.

THE GENUS *VIBRIO*

The genus *Vibrio* is taxonomically affiliated with the order Vibrionales, family Vibrionaceae. Most species are small, straight, slightly curved to curved motile bacilli that ferment glucose. All species except *Vibrio metschnikovii* are oxidase positive. Growth of vibrios is stimulated by sodium chloride and is for most an absolute requirement. Among more than 30 species presently defined and characterized, 13 have been implicated in fish and shellfish infections and 1 in poultry disease. The most significant veterinary species are *V. metschnikovii, Vibrio ordalii,* and *Vibrio salmonicida.* Twelve species have been reported from human disease, but *Vibrio cholerae, Vibrio parahaemolyticus,* and *Vibrio vulnificus* are the most frequently isolated.

DISEASE AND EPIDEMIOLOGY

Vibrio spp. are common in marine and estuarine environments. They can be isolated from sediment, water, vegetation, shellfish, and the intestinal tracts of marine mammals and fish. Nonhalophilic species can be isolated from brackish freshwater lakes.

Vibrio metschnikovii is recovered from river water, sewage, shellfish, and fish. It has historically been associated with a cholera-like disease of poultry and young birds housed in zoological collections. This infection, which has not been reported in North America, is characterized by a sudden onset of diarrhea and high mortality. Little is known about the epidemiology. A single isolate of unknown clinical significance was obtained from the lung of a dead calf. Isolates have also been recovered from infants with watery diarrhea, and adults with septicemia, cholecystitis, and wound infections.

Vibrio ordalii is the cause of fish "vibriosis," and is another agent of hemorrhagic septicemia. Vibriosis is an extremely widespread problem in eels and in several species of cultured fish, especially salmon and trout. Affected fish exhibit red necrotic lesions in the abdominal musculature and erythema at the base of the fins, vent, and within the oral cavity. They become lethargic and anorexic, and mortality may be high.

Cold-water vibriosis is primarily a disease of farmed Atlantic salmon, but trout and cod are also susceptible. Skin hemorrhages may be present on the base of the fins or abdomen, and infected fish swim on their sides. Transmission is through fish-to-fish contact, and skin trauma may predispose to infection. *Vibrio* spp. enter fish through their gills and disseminate hematogenously. Most disease outbreaks occur during late autumn to winter when water temperatures fall below 4° C.

Vibrio cholerae is the etiologic agent of human cholera, an epidemic disease that has caused millions of acute deaths as a result of massive dehydration. Ingestion of contaminated water is the means of transmission. Members of this species are serotyped based on their somatic O antigens, with more than 200 described serotypes. Serotypes O1 and O139 are responsible for classical cholera epidemics. *Vibrio cholerae* O1 is further subdivided into biotypes El Tor and classical for epidemiologic purposes. Non-O1 strains of *V. cholerae* have been implicated in human gastroenteritis and diarrhea, but they generally lack virulence determinants such as cholera toxin. These strains have been isolated from the nasal cavities of apparently healthy ducks and from the liver of an affected goose. Individuals who have contact with aquatic birds need to be aware of the zoonotic potential. During a recent outbreak of cholera in Peru, *V. cholerae* was isolated from more than 5% of fish from inshore waters, but from less than 2% of mussels and crabs and not at all from frozen shrimp. Marine isolates were mainly nontoxigenic and non-O1.

Vibrio parahaemolyticus is a leading cause of human food poisoning, with disease characterized by vomiting, nausea, intestinal cramping, fever, and chills. Disease is usually self-limiting. Outbreaks have been associated with consumption of raw, contaminated seafood.

Vibrio harveyi is a luminous component of the intestinal microflora of marine animals, but has emerged as a cause of mortality in fish and shellfish over a wide geographic area. It is the main causative agent of luminous vibriosis in cultured shrimp, which causes severe economic losses in Southeast Asia. Significant mortalities have apparently resulted from infection of shrimp by *Vibrio penaeicida* (the etiologic agent of "syndrome 93" in New Caledonia), and *Vibrio alginolyticus* commonly affected cultured shrimp secondary to infection by white spot syndrome virus.

PATHOGENESIS

Virulence factors for *V. cholerae* have been most extensively studied. These include capsular polysaccharide, toxins, lipopolysaccharide, siderophores, and pili. Capsular polysaccharide plays an important role in adherence of *Vibrio* spp. to target cells, and protects the bacteria against attack by the host complement system. Cholera toxin, which is similar to the heat-labile enterotoxin of *Escherichia coli,* is the most important virulence factor. It is a two-component toxin; the B subunit mediates entry of the A subunit, which in turn activates cellular adenylate cyclase, causing cAMP accumulation and the resulting hypersecretion of electrolytes and fluids. Clinical manifestation is watery diarrhea. A *V. cholerae* gene corresponds to the aerolysin structural gene. An RTX toxin gene was recently discovered in *V. cholerae*, but its role in virulence requires further investigation.

The core oligosaccharide portion of the lipopolysaccharide is necessary for survival in the presence of bile. Siderophores allow sequestration of iron, and pili facilitate adherence to mucosal epithelial cells.

Virulence factors for the other *Vibrio* spp. are less well understood. Naupliar mortality of experimentally infected *Artemia* spp. is correlated with production of proteases, phospholipases, or siderophores by *V. harveyi*, but not with lipase or gelatinase production, hydrophobicity, or hemolytic activity.

DIAGNOSIS

Vibriosis is diagnosed by bacteriologic culture of lesions (Figure 20-5). Fish specimens should be inoculated onto brain-heart infusion or trypticase soy agar supplemented with 1% to 4% sodium chloride because many species are halophilic. Growth of *V. ordalii* is enhanced on seawater agar. *Vibrio metschnikovii* grows poorly on MacConkey agar, but well on blood agar. Colonies are small,

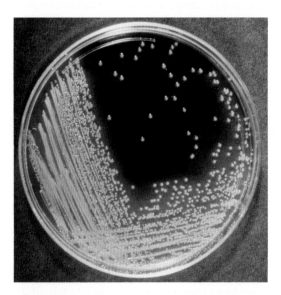

FIGURE 20-5 *Vibrio cholerae* on a differential medium. (Courtesy Public Health Image Library, PHIL #3906, Centers for Disease Control and Prevention, Atlanta, 1971.)

smooth, transparent, nonhemolytic, 2 to 4 mm in diameter after 48 hours' incubation at 37° C. *Vibrio ordalii* produces round, raised, shiny, entire, cream-colored colonies 1 to 2 mm in diameter in 7 days on plated media incubated at 15° to 25° C. *Vibrio salmonicida* grows optimally at 15° to 17° C. Smooth, grayish, opaque raised colonies 1 to 2 mm in diameter are produced after 72 hours' incubation.

Biochemical identification of the fish pathogens is facilitated by use of tables in the book, cited in Suggested Readings, by J. A. Plumb. Enzyme-linked immunosorbent assay (ELISA) and immuno-histochemistry-based tests are used in fish laboratories as adjuncts to bacterial culture for diagnosis of *V. salmonicida* and *V. ordalii* infections.

PREVENTION AND CONTROL

Invertebrates depend on an innate immune system for defense against microbial invaders, and in crustaceans (such as shrimp) the immune response is based on cellular and humoral effects, leading to phagocytosis, encapsulation, coagulation, melanization, and killing of microbial pathogens. Cell wall components of invading microorganisms are identified via plasma recognition molecules, such as lipopolysaccharide-binding protein and β-1, 3-glucan-binding protein, which mobilize phagocytosis and the prophenoloxidase activating system that leads to melanization.

Bacillus subtilis has an apparent probiotic effect against growth of *V. harveyi* in shrimp, with documented 90% reduction in mortality. Shrimp fed cultures of this organism grow larger and are more likely to survive to harvest.

Efficacious fish vaccines are available for *V. ordalii* and *V. salmonicida*.

SUGGESTED READINGS

Abbott SL, Cheung WK, Janda JM: The genus *Aeromonas:* biochemical characteristics, and phenotypic identification schemes, *J Clin Microbiol* 41:2348-2357, 2003.

Gonzalez-Rey C, Svenson SB, Bravo L: Serotypes and anti-microbial susceptibility of *Plesiomonas shigelloides* isolates from humans, animals, and aquatic environments in different countries, *Comp Immunol Microbiol Infect Dis* 27:129-139, 2004.

Plumb JA: Health maintenance and principal microbial diseases of cultured fishes, Ames, Iowa, 1999, Iowa State University Press.

Chapter 21

The Genera *Moraxella* and *Neisseria*

Members of the genera *Moraxella* and *Neisseria* are found on the skin, mucous membranes, and conjunctivae of mammals. The majority of these organisms are harmless commensals, but some are significant pathogens. Species-level classification in the genera *Moraxella* and *Neisseria* is evolving and to a great extent incomprehensible.

THE GENUS *MORAXELLA*

The genus *Moraxella* belongs to the family Moraxellaceae within the class γ-Proteobacteria. Organisms previously classified as *Branhamella* species are now in the genus *Moraxella*. Moraxellae are nonmotile, fastidious, and aerobic; some strains may grow, although poorly, under anaerobic conditions. Optimal growth temperatures are from 33° to 35° C. Most are short, plump, gram-negative coccobacilli, with a tendency toward pleomorphism: some species are more coccoid, whereas others are more bacillary. Species from animals include *Moraxella boevrei*, *Moraxella bovis*, *Moraxella canis*, *Moraxella caprae*, *Moraxella caviae*, *Moraxella cuniculi*, and *Moraxella ovis*, but disease as a result of species other than *M. bovis* or *M. ovis* is rare (Table 21-1). *Moraxella (Branhamella) catarrhalis* is the most important human pathogen in the genus, causing lower respiratory infection in adults with chronic lung disease, and otitis media, sinusitis, and conjunctivitis in children.

TABLE 21-1 Species of *Moraxella* and *Neisseria* with Veterinary Significance

Species	Habitat	Significance
M. boevrei	Upper respiratory tract: healthy goats	Commensal
M. bovis	Eye, nasal cavity: cattle	Pinkeye
M. canis	Upper respiratory tract: healthy dogs, cats	Dog bite infections
M. caprae	Nasal cavity, eyes: healthy goats	Commensal
M. caviae	Upper respiratory tract: guinea pigs	Commensal
M. cuniculi	Oral cavity: healthy rabbits	Commensal
	Upper respiratory tract: marine mammals	
M. ovis	Eyes: small ruminants	Pinkeye
N. animalis	Oropharynx: guinea pig	Commensal
N. canis	Oropharynx: dogs, cats	Dog bite infections
N. dentiae	Dental plaque: cattle	Commensal
N. denitrificans	Upper respiratory tract: guinea pig	Commensal
N. iguanae	Oral cavity: iguanid lizards	Rare cutaneous abscesses, septicemia
N. macacae	Oropharynx: rhesus monkeys	Commensal
N. weaveri	Oropharynx: dogs	Dog bite infections

MORAXELLA BOVIS

Moraxella bovis is the primary etiologic agent of infectious bovine keratoconjunctivitis (IBK), or pinkeye, an economically important and highly contagious disease of cattle. Surveys have concluded that IBK is the second most common disease of cattle, and that nearly half of herds are affected. Economic losses have been estimated at $200 million annually, attributable to decreased rate of growth and milk production, treatment costs, increased labor, disfigurement of the eyes of purebred cattle, and decreases in marketability and dollar value of feeder calves. IBK is painful, and affected cattle often become temporarily blind.

IBK occurs worldwide, and asymptomatic carrier animals introduce the infection into herds. Bacteria may be transmitted animal to animal by direct contact with ocular or nasal exudates or contaminated fomites, and by cows licking their newborn calves. However, intra- and even interherd transmission is mediated mainly by flies (Figures 21-1 and 21-2). The face fly *(Musca autumnalis)* is the most important species involved in transmission. Most outbreaks occur in grazing cattle in the summer and early autumn, with infection rates decreasing significantly after the first frost.

It is not uncommon for herd morbidity rates to exceed 80%. Cattle ages 2 years or greater are apparently more resistant to infection than are calves. There is a species predisposition, with *Bos taurus* breeds being more susceptible than *Bos indicus* breeds. In addition, Hereford cattle, and other varieties without pigmented ocular tissues, are more prone to develop disease.

Pinkeye is a multifactorial disease. The importance of face flies has been noted, but ultraviolet light is also an important contributing factor. Nuclear fragmentation and corneal epithelial detachment associated with exposure to solar radiation enhance colonization of the cornea by *M. bovis*. Other contributing factors are dust, wind, tall grasses, and increased environmental levels of ammonia, all of which are ocular irritants. Concurrent ocular infections with mycoplasmas, chlamydiae, and viral agents or nematode infestation may exacerbate the disease. In addition, a relationship exists between vaccination with a modified live infectious bovine rhinotracheitis vaccine and subsequent development of IBK.

Severity of clinical manifestations of IBK varies widely. Initial clinical signs are lacrimation, blepharospasm, photophobia, and chemosis, which sometimes resolve spontaneously. However, the disease may progress to severe keratitis with corneal ulceration and abscessation (Figure 21-3). Occasionally, panophthalmitis and blindness may result. One or both eyes may be affected, and there are no systemic effects. A nonhemolytic variant of *M. bovis*, called "*M. equi*," is associated with conjunctivitis in horses.

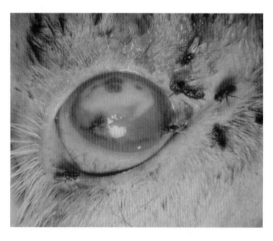

FIGURE 21-1 Face flies clustered around a bovine eye affected by infectious bovine keratoconjunctivitis. (Courtesy US Department of Agriculture, Ames, Iowa, National Animal Disease Center.)

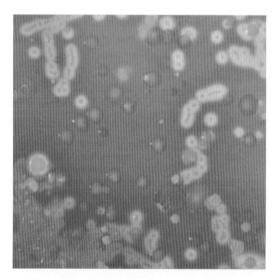

FIGURE 21-2 Hemolytic colonies of *Moraxella bovis* among bacterial contaminants on a plate inoculated by flies feeding on cattle with infectious bovine keratoconjunctivitis. (Courtesy US Department of Agriculture, Ames, Iowa, National Animal Disease Center.)

Moraxella bovis virulence factors include two functionally distinct types of pili by which the bacterium associates with corneal epithelium (Figure 21-4). The Q pilus is responsible for attachment, whereas the I pilus allows for local persistence and maintenance of an established infection. Nonpiliated strains do not cause clinical disease. Seven antigenically distinct pilus types have been identified. Virulence varies as to the infecting strain, and serotypes 3 and 4 are most often associated with pinkeye outbreaks in the United States.

After ocular colonization, the bacterium replicates and produces a cytotoxin. *Moraxella bovis* cytotoxin (cytolysin/hemolysin) is a pore-forming protein of the RTX family of toxins and is believed to promote formation of corneal ulcers through lysis of corneal epithelial cells and host neutrophils. Leakage of degradative enzymes from neutrophils into the corneal stroma ultimately results in corneal liquefaction and ulceration.

Diagnosis may be based on clinical signs and isolation of the organism from conjunctival swabs or lacrimal secretions of affected cattle. *Moraxella bovis* is extremely fragile and has limited viability outside the host, so samples should be examined promptly in the laboratory. To optimize results, clinical materials should be plated to bovine blood agar within 2 hours of collection.

In Gram-stained smears, *M. bovis* cells appear as plump coccobacilli, predominantly in pairs, that have a tendency to resist decolorization and retain crystal violet (Figure 21-5). They are nonmotile and strongly oxidase and usually catalase positive. Colonies on blood agar plates are flat to convex, friable, gray-white, and usually surrounded by a wide zone of β-hemolysis (Figure 21-6). Freshly isolated strains may corrode the agar surface.

Identification of moraxellae to the species level by cultural and conventional biochemical techniques in clinical laboratories has proven to be difficult. *Moraxella* spp. are asaccharolytic, and gelatin liquefaction, nitrate reduction, and hemolysis are the main traits used for differentiation (Table 21-2). *Moraxella bovis* does not grow on MacConkey agar, and characteristically produces a dark blue upper layer, a lighter blue middle layer, and a white bottom layer after 7 days' incubation in litmus milk.

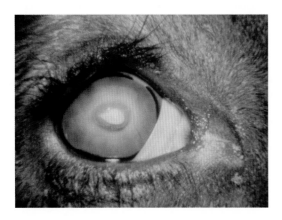

FIGURE 21-3 Corneal lesion typical of infectious bovine keratoconjunctivitis. (Courtesy US Department of Agriculture, Ames, Iowa, National Animal Disease Center.)

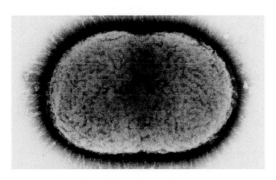

FIGURE 21-4 *Moraxella bovis* pili. (Courtesy Karen W. Post.)

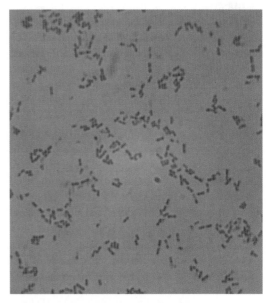

FIGURE 21-5 Gram-stained smear of pure culture of *Moraxella bovis,* revealing gram-negative coccobacilli in pairs. (Courtesy Karen W. Post.)

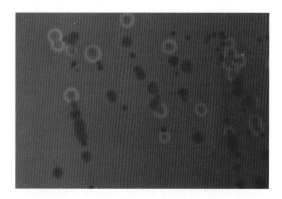

FIGURE 21-6 Small, circular, shiny, friable colonies of *Moraxella bovis* surrounded by zones of β-hemolysis. Cultivated on blood agar, 48-hour incubation. Nonhemolytic colonies are contaminants from an infected eye. (Courtesy US Department of Agriculture, Ames, Iowa, National Animal Disease Center.)

A fluorescent antibody test facilitates demonstration of the organism in lacrimal secretions. An enzyme immunoassay, which detects lacrimal or serum immunoglobulin G (IgG), is useful in determining the serogroup responsible for an outbreak, but these tests are not widely available.

Because pinkeye can be insidious, prevention rather than treatment is the best plan of attack. The key to prevention is eliminating the factors that contribute to disease development and spread. Controlling face flies, proper pasture management, proper nutrition, and provision of adequate shade are important. Use of insecticide-impregnated ear tags, sprays, back rubbers, dust bags, and systemic pour-on insecticides will help control cow-to-cow spread of pinkeye. Periodic mowing of tall grasses and noxious weeds in pastures decreases disease incidence because it limits the chance of ocular contact with coarse plant seedheads. Vitamin supplements should be used because inadequate levels of vitamin A can exacerbate pinkeye.

Treatment of pinkeye is based on the use of antimicrobials, prevention of further ocular irritation, and isolation of affected cattle. The only agent approved for the treatment of IBK is oxytetracycline. Two injections of long-acting oxytetracycline given 72 hours apart have proven effective in decreasing healing time. Mass in-feed treatment with oxytetracycline may be beneficial in an outbreak. Corticosteroids are often administered to reduce ocular inflammation and pain. The use of third-eyelid flaps, eyepatches, and tarsorrhaphy can reduce irritation associated with environmental factors.

Several commercial vaccines are available, but vaccination has met with mixed results. Lacrimal secretory immunoglobulin A (IgA) is required for resistance to infection, and current whole cell monovalent and multivalent parenteral bacterins do not increase ocular IgA levels. Furthermore, these vaccines do not protect against infection with heterologous serotypes.

MORAXELLA (BRANHAMELLA) OVIS

Moraxella ovis is the most frequently isolated aerobic organism among the normal conjunctival flora of small ruminants, and is the organism most commonly associated with infectious keratoconjunctivitis in sheep and goats. *Moraxella ovis*

TABLE **21-2** *Moraxella* Species of Veterinary Significance

Characteristic	Moraxella Species						
	M. boevrei	*M. bovis*	*M. canis**	*M. caprae*	*M. caviae*	*M. cuniculi*	*M. ovis*
Morphology	SR	R	C	R	C	C	C
Oxidase	Pos	Pos	Pos	Pos	Pos	Pos	Pos
Catalase	Pos	(Pos)	Pos	Pos	Pos	Pos	Pos
β-Hemolysis	Pos	Pos†	Pos	Pos	Wk	Neg	(Pos)
Growth on MacConkey agar	Neg	Neg	Neg	Neg	Neg	Neg	Neg
Nitrate reduction	Pos	(Neg)	Pos	Pos	Pos	Neg	Pos
Gelatinase	Pos	Pos	Neg	Neg	Neg	Neg	Neg
DNase	Neg	Neg	(Pos)	Neg	(Neg)	Neg	(Neg)
Litmus milk	Pep	Three layers	NC	NC	NC	NC	NC

M. canis produces a brownish pigment on Mueller-Hinton agar.
†*M. equi* strains that belong to the species *M. bovis* are nonhemolytic.
C, Coccus; *NC,* no change; *Neg,* negative; *(Neg),* most negative; *Pep,* peptonization; *Pos,* positive; *(Pos),* most positive; *R,* rod, *SR,* short rod; *Wk,* weak reaction.

has also been recovered from numerous outbreaks of pinkeye in cattle. Clinical signs in cattle are similar to those observed with *M. bovis* infection. Little is known about the pathogenesis of *M. ovis*–associated ocular disease, but the organism produces pili and a heat-labile protein exotoxin with both cytotoxic and hemolytic activities in vitro. Diagnosis is through culture of affected eyes. Methods for prevention, control, and treatment are similar to those used in *M. bovis* infection of cattle.

THE GENUS *NEISSERIA*

The genus *Neisseria* is a member of the family Neisseriaceae, which is classified in the β-subgroup of the Proteobacteria. Members of the genus are coccal or rod shaped and frequently occur in pairs or short chains. Some species have a distinctive diplococcal morphology. *Neisseria* spp. are commensals on the mucous membranes of mammals and some lower species. These organisms are aerobic, nonmotile, and grow optimally at 35° to 37° C. Growth is stimulated by humidity and CO_2. All species are oxidase positive and most are catalase positive. Neisseriae produce acid from carbohydrates oxidatively, which enables them to be differentiated from moraxellae. Frank pathogens of humans are *Neisseria gonorrheae*, the agent of gonorrhea, and *Neisseria meningitidis*, an agent of acute bacterial meningitis. Species of veterinary significance appear in Table 21-1.

SUGGESTED READINGS

Pettersson B, Kodjo A, Ronaghi M, et al: Phylogeny of the family Moraxellaceae by 16S rDNA sequence analysis, with special emphasis on differentiation of *Moraxella* species, *Int J Syst Bacteriol* 48:75-89, 1998.

Rogers DG, Cheville NF, Pugh GW: Pathogenesis of corneal lesions caused by *Moraxella bovis* in gnotobiotic calves, *Vet Pathol* 24:287-295, 1987.

Chapter 22

The Genus *Actinobacillus*

Disease associated with members of the genus *Actinobacillus* (family Pasteurellaceae) was first reported in 1902, in the form of bovine subcutaneous abscesses from which gram-negative rods were consistently recovered. The overwhelming majority of the species or specieslike taxa included in the genus are commensals, or pathogens, of animals (Table 22-1).

Actinobacilli are gram negative and pleomorphic, with mostly bacillary and occasional coccal elements with a "Morse code" appearance (dots and dashes) on Gram stain (Figure 22-1). Organisms are variably hemolytic on blood agar, nonmotile, usually oxidase positive, catalase variable, and nitrate-reductase positive. They are facultatively anaerobic, but added CO_2 is required

TABLE **22-1**   Relationship Between Species of *Actinobacillus* and Preferred Host

Species	Disease(s)	Host(s)
A. actinomycetemcomitans	Periodontitis	Man
A. arthritidis	Arthritis, septicemia	Horse
A. capsulatus	Arthritis, septicemia	Rabbit
A. delphinicola	Uncertain significance	Sea mammals
A. equuli ssp. equuli	"Joint ill," septicemia	Horse
	abortion, metritis, septicemia	Pig
A. equuli ssp. haemolyticus	Various disease conditions	Horse
A. genomospecies 1	Stomatitis	Horse
A. genomospecies 2	Septicemia	Horse
A. hominis	Respiratory disease	Man
A. indolicus	Uncertain significance	Pig
A. lignieresii	Pyogranulomatous lesions ("wooden tongue")	Ruminants
A. minor	Uncertain significance	Pig
A. muris	Uncertain significance	Rodents
A. pleuropneumoniae	Fibrinous pleuropneumonia	Pig
A. porcinus	Uncertain pathogenic significance	Pig
A. rossii	Abortion, metritis	Pig
A. scotia	Uncertain significance	Sea mammals
A. seminis	Epididymitis, orchitis	Sheep
A. succinogenes	Uncertain significance	Cattle
A. suis	Septicemia	Pig
A. ureae	Respiratory disease	Man

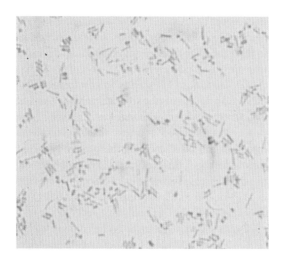

FIGURE 22-1 Typical Gram stain of *Actinobacillus* sp., denoting "Morse code" appearance. (Courtesy J. Glenn Songer.)

for growth. Carbohydrates are fermented without the production of gas. Most species grow on triple-sugar iron agar slants, yielding a typical orange cast to the medium, and most grow on MacConkey agar as tiny lactose-fermenting colonies. Colonies may be very sticky or waxy, especially on primary culture plates.

DISEASES AND EPIDEMIOLOGY

Except for *Actinobacillus pleuropneumoniae,* diseases attributed to these bacteria occur sporadically. The upper respiratory tract and oral cavity are the natural habitats of most actinobacilli. Because *Actinobacillus* spp. are incapable of long-term survival in the environment, carrier animals are important in disease transmission.

Actinobacillus lignieresii is a commensal of the ruminant oropharynx and is recovered from rumen contents. Actinobacillosis or "wooden tongue" in ruminants results in the formation of hard tumorous masses in the tongue (Figure 22-2). Affected animals suffer from dysphagia, with resulting weight loss. Soft tissue infections primarily of the head and neck have been described in cattle and sheep; these lesions contain odorless pus. The disease is often confused with actinomycosis, but true actinomycosis is found in bone, whereas actinobacillosis affects soft tissues. *Actinobacillus lignieresii* has, on occasion, been isolated from pneumonic sheep lungs, tongue lesions of dogs, swollen lymph nodes of rats, and mastitic bovine mammary glands. Young animals appear to be more susceptible to infection, based on experimental inoculation studies. Trauma is an important predisposing factor because the organism gains entrance into the underlying soft tissues through penetration of the mucosal or epithelial barriers. Infections are most often sporadic, but consumption of dry, stemmy haylage has been associated with "outbreaks" of wooden tongue in cattle.

Actinobacillus pleuropneumoniae colonizes the tonsils and upper respiratory tract of apparently healthy pigs, where it is considered an obligate parasite. No other natural hosts have been described.

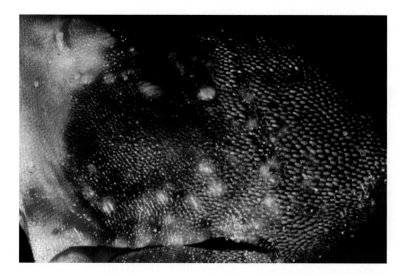

FIGURE 22-2 Gross lesions of "wooden tongue." (Courtesy Raymond E. Reed.)

Transmission is through direct contact or aerosol exposure to infected pigs. The organism is the causative agent of porcine pleuropneumonia, a highly infectious disease that causes sizable economic losses to the swine industry and has worldwide distribution. At present, 15 different serotypes and 2 biotypes have been described. The presence and prevalence of serotypes vary among countries, with serotypes 1, 5, and 7 most commonly isolated in North America, and serotypes 2 and 9 predominant in Europe. All serotypes are capable of producing disease, but they are of varying virulence. Outbreaks are usually associated with intensive pig production in which there is high-stocking density, poor ventilation, and low immunity. Animals younger than 6 months are most frequently affected. They experience a wide spectrum of signs, ranging from sudden death to chronic pneumonia, depending on the serotype of the infecting strain, the infectious dose, and the immune status of the host. Acute disease is characterized by a hemorrhagic necrotizing pneumonia of the caudodorsal aspect of the caudal lung lobe and fibrinous pleuritis with high morbidity and mortality (Figure 22-3). Coughing and expiratory dyspnea ("thumping") are common. Pregnant sows may abort. Hemorrhagic froth may be discharged from the nose or mouth immediately before death. Morbidity and mortality rates range from 30% to 50%. Concurrent infection with porcine reproductive and respiratory syndrome virus (PRRS) and *Mycoplasma hyopneumoniae* may exacerbate the illness. Acute disease becomes less common as herd immunity increases. Survivors grow poorly because of inhibition of normal respiratory function resulting from lung scarring

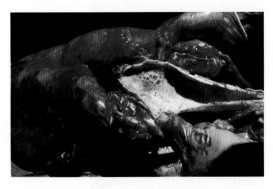

FIGURE 22-3 Gross lesions of porcine pleuropneumonia. (Courtesy J. Glenn Songer.)

with pleural adhesions. These chronically infected animals continue to harbor *A. pleuropneumoniae* in their tonsillar crypts and are the main means of transmission between herds.

Actinobacillus suis resides in the tonsils, nostrils, and vaginas of apparently healthy pigs. The prevalence of herd infections is unknown, but subclinical infection is most likely widespread. Infection can take place via the aerosol route, by various forms of close contact, or through breaks in the skin. Disease is sporadic, and is more common in high-health status or "start-up" herds following episodes of stress. In suckling or recently weaned pigs, mortality within affected litters may exceed 50%. Reports of *A. suis*–associated disease have increased in recent years and appear to parallel the shift to high-health production systems and three-site rearing facilities.

Actinobacillus suis has been isolated only from pigs. It functions as an opportunistic pathogen, and three syndromes are recognized. In pigs 2 to 30 days old, infection is characterized by an acute septicemia. Affected animals are febrile and anorectic and exhibit respiratory distress. Neurologic disturbances and arthritis can also be seen, but most piglets are simply found dead. Gross lesions include petechial and ecchymotic hemorrhages in multiple organs that include spleen, lung, kidney, heart, liver, skin, and gastrointestinal tract. Serofibrinous exudates are commonly present in the thoracic and abdominal cavities. Histologic lesions are indicative of bacteremia, and consist of foci of necrosis in multiple organs. Grow-finish animals typically experience septicemia with lung lesions that are virtually indistinguishable from *A. pleuropneumoniae* pneumonia. The course of disease in adult animals can include meningitis, abortion, metritis, and red rhomboid skin lesions that are reminiscent of those associated with erysipelas.

Actinobacillus equuli has recently been divided into ssp. *equuli* and *haemolyticus*. *Actinobacillus equuli* ssp. *equuli* resides on the mucous membranes of normal horses and pigs, whereas *A. equuli* ssp. *haemolyticus* has been recovered only from horses, where it is a component of oral and alimentary microflora. The former is associated with septicemia of neonatal foals, often referred to as "sleepy foal disease." Purulent arthritis ("joint ill") and nephritis are manifestations of chronic infection. Nearly one third of equine neonatal mortality may be associated with this organism.

The mare serves as the source of infection, via the oral, umbilical, or respiratory route either in utero, during parturition, or shortly after birth. Colostrum deprivation, stress, or parasitism may predispose to illness. Verminous aneurysms of the mesenteric artery are often culture positive for *A. equuli* ssp. *equuli,* and investigators believe the migrating larvae of *Strongylus vulgaris* carry the agent from the intestinal lumen into the circulatory system. Others have speculated that transplacental invasion by the larvae of *S. vulgaris* may result in infection in utero. *Actinobacillus equuli* ssp. *equuli* is also an opportunistic pathogen of pigs, resulting in septicemia and other infections.

Actinobacillus equuli ssp. *haemolyticus* is strictly an equine pathogen, associated with sporadic cases of endocarditis, meningitis, metritis, abortion, and respiratory and wound infections.

Human infections with actinobacilli have been limited to periodontal disease caused by *Actinobacillus actinomycetemcomitans,* sporadic infections of the respiratory tract, blood, or cerebrospinal fluid caused by *Actinobacillus hominis* and *Actinobacillus ureae,* and upper respiratory or bite wound infections with *A. equuli* or *A. suis* in people who have had contact with horses or pigs.

PATHOGENESIS

Direct inoculation of *A. lignieresii* into the submucosal tissue following abrasion by sharp objects or coarse feedstuffs initially results in deep, nonhealing ulcers of the tongue, soft palate, pharynx, or buccal mucosa. Lesions typically form several days after the traumatic insult, with leukocytosis followed by a granulomatous reaction. Purulent foci containing club-shaped clusters of *A. lignieresii* microcolonies form within the center of the lesion and enlarge into tumorous masses as they become surrounded by layers of connective tissue. The organism may disseminate via the regional lymphatics to internal organs such as the lung.

The pathogenesis of porcine pleuropneumonia is complex. *Actinobacillus pleuropneumoniae* infection begins with inhalation of the organism and subsequent colonization of the lower respiratory tract, where the bacterium adheres to the cilia of the terminal bronchioli and epithelial cells of the alveoli. Adhesion leads to production and localization of a high concentration of toxins.

Early in the course of disease there is a marked infiltration of neutrophils, followed later by macrophage infiltration. The associated inflammatory response to the toxins rapidly induces focal necrotizing vasculitis, leading to localized thrombosis, edema, ischemic necrosis, and fibrinous pleuritis. Pulmonary hemorrhage follows continued breakdown of the blood-lung barrier.

The pathogenicity of *A. suis* is not well understood, but infection likely disseminates from the tonsils or nostrils to other parts of the body, especially the lung. Bacterial emboli are apparently trapped within the walls of blood vessels, forming microcolonies that eventually cause vascular necrosis and hemorrhage.

Relatively little is known about the pathogenesis of equine actinobacillosis. The organism disseminates by the blood to many organs in infected foals, and these septic emboli lead to microabscess formation in affected tissue. Bacterial colonies are evident histologically and most frequently observed in the glomeruli and intertubular capillaries, where there is intense suppuration. Polyarthritis results from an increase in synovial fluid, followed by congestion and swelling of the joint capsule and leukocytosis.

Virulence factors associated with actinobacilli include polysaccharide capsule, pore-forming exotoxins (RTX toxins), lipopolysaccharide, iron acquisition mechanisms, urease production, secreted proteases, and possibly fimbriae. Capsules protect the bacteria from phagocytosis by host immune cells and lysis by complement. RTX toxins, named for their repetitive sequences, are widespread within the Pasteurellaceae. These host-cell–specific toxins act on immune cells, either by inducing production of inflammatory mediators or exerting cytotoxic effects that result in inflammation or cell death by apoptosis or necrosis. Four types of RTX toxins identified in *A. pleuropneumoniae* (ApxI, ApxII, ApxIII, and ApxIVA) play a predominant role in pathogenicity. RTX toxins have also been discovered in *A. suis, A. actinomycetemcomitans,* and *A. lignieresii.* In *A. equuli* ssp. *haemolyticus* the hemolysin is the Aqx protein, a member of the RTX toxin family.

The lipopolysaccharide moiety plays a major role in adhesion of *A. pleuropneumoniae* to porcine respiratory epithelial cells, which facilitates colonization. In addition, lipopolysaccharide binds porcine hemoglobin and facilitates iron uptake. Iron acquisition is essential to bacterial metabolism and is limited in the host. Actinobacilli acquire iron by means of a siderophore-independent receptor-mediated mechanism.

Urease-negative mutants of *A. pleuropneumoniae* do not establish infection when inoculated into pigs, suggesting a role for urease activity in pathogenesis. Urease activity has been considered a mechanism by which actinobacilli obtain ammonia, a preferred source of nitrogen. Urease activity may also enable *A. pleuropneumoniae* to survive within macrophages.

Proteases secreted by *A. pleuropneumoniae* degrade IgA and hemoglobin. Degradation of IgA may facilitate mucosal spread of the organism.

Type 4 fimbrial genes have been identified in *A. pleuropneumoniae,* but the role of fimbriae in adhesion is not yet clear.

DIAGNOSIS

Direct examination of Gram-stained smears of pus from tongue lesions may reveal club-shaped forms ("sulfur granules") that contain central masses of pleomorphic gram-negative rods. However, bacteriologic culture of actinobacilli from infected tissues is the most reliable method of diagnosis. All taxa except *A. equuli* ssp. *equuli* are associated with specific animal hosts, so identification of isolates is aided by knowledge of the species of origin. Species differentiation by classical biochemical methods may prove challenging. For example, the swine respiratory tract is heavily colonized by NAD-dependent species *(Actinobacillus*

indolicus, Actinobacillus minor, Actinobacillus porcinus) that have no apparent role as pathogens. It is critical that these species be distinguished from *A. pleuropneumoniae* (Table 22-2). One of the most dependable means of recognizing *A. pleuropneumoniae* is its positive CAMP test.

Differentiation of actinobacilli can be based on hemolytic properties, their ability to grow on MacConkey agar and hydrolyze esculin, their dependency on NAD, and their ability to produce oxidase, catalase, urease, and acid in various carbohydrate substrates (Table 22-3). When phenotypic characterization fails to identify an organism, analysis of the sequence of 16S rDNA may be necessary.

Serotyping of *A. pleuropneumoniae* isolates may be valuable to swine producers because inactivated vaccines usually protect against homologous serotypes only. Serotype specificity is predominantly a result of structural differences in capsular polysaccharides. Cross-reaction between serotypes often occurs when traditional serologic assays are used for typing. Because *apx* genes are associated with specific serotypes, isolates can be typed based on the presence of these four genes. A multiplex polymerase chain reaction (PCR)–based method has largely replaced older assays. NAD-dependent strains (serotypes 1-12) are biotype I, and NAD-independent strains (serotypes 13 and 14) are biotype II.

Several serologic tests are available for antemortem diagnosis of *A. pleuropneumoniae* infections.

TABLE **22-2**   Differentiation of *Actinobacillus pleuropneumoniae* from Similar Organisms

	A. pleuro-pneumoniae Biotype I	A. pleuro-pneumoniae Biotype II	A. minor	Haemophilus parasuis	A. porcinus	A. indolicus	Haemophilus Taxon C
V factor	(Pos)	Neg	Pos	Pos	Pos	Pos	Pos
Urease	(Pos)	Pos	Pos	Neg	Neg	Neg	Neg
Indole	Neg	Neg	Neg	Neg	Neg	Pos	Neg
CAMP	Pos	Pos	Neg	Neg	Neg	Neg	Neg
β-Hemolysis	(Pos)	Pos	Neg	Neg	Neg	Neg	Neg
Catalase	Pos	Pos	Neg	Pos	Neg	Pos	Pos
Ferments arabinose	Neg	Neg	Neg	Neg	(Neg)	Neg	Pos
Ferments mannitol	Pos	Pos	Neg	Neg	Var	Neg	Neg
Ferments raffinose	Neg	Neg	Pos	Neg	Var	Pos	Pos
Ferments lactose	Neg	Neg	Pos	Neg	Var	Neg	Neg

Neg, Negative; *(Neg),* most negative; *Pos,* positive; *(Pos),* most positive; *Var,* variable.

TABLE 22-3 Differentiation of *Actinobacillus* Species of Veterinary Significance

Species	Catalase	Urease	Esculin hydrolysis	MacConkey*	β-hemolysis	Acid from					
						L-arabinose	Inositol	D-mannitol	Salicin	D-sorbitol	Trehalose
A. arthritidis	Pos	Pos	Neg	Neg	Neg	Var	Neg	Pos	Neg	Pos	Neg
A. capsulatus	Pos	Pos	Pos slow	Pos	Neg	Neg	Neg	Pos	Pos	Pos	Pos
A. delphinicola	Neg	Neg	ND	Neg	Weak pos	ND	Neg	Neg	Neg	ND	Neg
A. equuli ssp. equuli	Pos	Pos	Neg	Var	Neg	Var	Neg	Pos	Neg	Neg	Pos
A. equuli ssp. haemolyticus	Pos	Pos	(Neg)	Var	Pos	(Neg)	Neg	(Neg)	(Pos)	(Neg)	Pos
A. lignieresii	(Pos)	Pos	Neg	Var	Neg	(Neg)	Neg	Pos	Neg	(Neg)	Neg
Genomospecies 1†	(Pos)	Pos	Neg	Var	Neg	(Neg)	Neg	Pos	Neg	(Neg)	Neg
A. muris	Pos	Pos	Pos (slow)	Neg	Neg	Neg	Weak var	Pos	Pos	Neg	Pos
A. pleuropneumoniae‡	Var	Pos	Var	Neg	Pos	Neg	Neg	Pos	Neg	Neg	Neg
A. pleuropneumoniae biotype 2	Var	Pos	Neg	Pos	Pos	Pos	Neg	Pos	Neg	Neg	Neg
A. rossii	Pos	Pos	Neg	(Pos)	Var	Pos	Pos	Pos	Neg	Pos	Neg
A. scoitae	Neg	Pos	ND	Neg	Weak pos	Neg	Neg	Neg	Neg	Neg	Neg
A. seminis	Pos	Neg	Var	Neg	Neg	Var slow	Var	Var slow	Neg	Neg	Neg
A. suis	Pos	Pos	Pos	Pos	Pos	(Pos)	Neg	Neg	Pos	Neg	Pos
Genomospecies 2	Pos	Pos	Neg	Var	Neg	Var	Neg	Pos	Neg	Neg	Neg

*Growth on MacConkey agar.
†Unable to distinguish biochemically.
‡Must differentiate *A. pleuropneumoniae* from other V-factor–dependent species that are normal respiratory flora.
Neg, Negative; *(Neg)*, most negative, *ND*, not determined; *Pos*, positive; *(Pos)*, most positive; *Var*, variable.

Complement fixation offers low sensitivity, in that infected animals generally produce only low titers of complement-fixing antibodies. Enzyme immunoassay-based methods are better tools for monitoring antibody response. Apx toxins are good antigens, so immune responses to them have been used as the basis for serodiagnosis. A hemolysin neutralization test detects antibodies against ApxI, but cannot differentiate infections by causative serotype.

PREVENTION AND CONTROL

Actinobacilli are susceptible to most commonly prescribed antibiotics, including ampicillin, penicillin, macrolides, oxytetracycline, tiamulin, and ceftiofur. Systemic or local treatment with antimicrobials has proven effective in resolving lesions. Circumscribed lesions may be treated by surgical excision. Prevention of ruminant actinobacillosis includes preventing ingestion of coarse feedstuffs.

Prevention and control of porcine pleuropneumonia is best achieved through medication, vaccination, and management programs. Antimicrobial therapy is most effective for acute disease outbreaks; however, prevention can be accomplished by using continuous or pulse medication in feed or water. Several commercial vaccines reduce clinical disease and improve performance, but they cannot totally eliminate the organism. Whole-cell autogenous bacterins may reduce mortality after infection with the homologous serotype, but do not seem to confer protection against heterologous serotypes. Current research has focused on the development of a live vaccine.

Reduction of acute disease outbreaks can be achieved through improvement in management and housing. Increasing ventilation and decreasing stocking density are important factors for consideration. Farms that are disease-free should maintain measures to quarantine herd additions and develop serologic monitoring programs. Detection of asymptomatic carrier animals is essential for disease control. Other management strategies include all-in/all-out production systems and segregated early weaning programs. Because most carrier animals do not show measurable antibodies in serum, detection of the agent through tonsillar or nasal cultures or PCR assays is required for identification. Carriers should be culled.

Autogenous bacterins have not been extensively evaluated for the prevention and control of field outbreaks of *A. suis*. However, anecdotal evidence suggests their efficacy. The organism is susceptible to most antibiotics, but treatment often is initiated too late because of the unpredictability of outbreaks.

No commercial vaccines are available for prevention or control of *A. equuli* ssp. *equuli* infection. Antimicrobial therapy may be successful if initiated early in the course of disease. Good husbandry practices should be followed in the foaling barn. Foals from mares that have had a history of producing affected foals should be closely monitored and given antimicrobials prophylactically.

SUGGESTED READINGS

Bosse JT, Janson H, Sheehan BJ, et al: *Actinobacillus pleuropneumoniae*: pathobiology and pathogenesis of infection, *Microbes Infect* 4:225-235, 2002.

Christensen H, Bisgaard M, Olsen JE: Reclassification of equine isolates previously classified as *Actinobacillus equuli*, variants of *A. equuli*, *Actinobacillus suis* or Bisgaard taxon 11 and proposal of *A. equuli* subsp. *equuli* subsp. nov. and *A. equuli* subsp. *haemolyticus* subsp. nov., *Int J Syst Evol Microbiol* 52:1569-1576, 2002.

Rycroft AN, Garside LH: *Actinobacillus* species and their role in animal disease, *Vet J* 159:18-36, 2000.

Schaller A, Kuhnert P, de la Puente-Redondo VA, et al: Apx toxins in Pasteurellaceae from animals, *Vet Microbiol* 74:365-376, 2000.

Chapter 23

The Genera *Mannheimia* and *Pasteurella*

*M*annheimia and *Pasteurella* are members of the class α-Proteobacteria, order Pasteurellales, family Pasteurellaceae, that contain small, facultatively anaerobic, non-motile, gram-negative rods or coccobacilli that do not form endospores. Glucose is fermented without gas production, the oxidase reaction is normally positive, and nitrate is usually reduced to nitrite. These organisms are found as mucosal commensals of the oropharynx and gastrointestinal tract of healthy mammals, birds, and reptiles. They survive poorly outside the host.

THE GENUS *MANNHEIMIA*

The new genus *Mannheimia* was established in 1999 to include trehalose-negative members of the *Pasteurella haemolytica* complex. All strains in the genus ferment mannitol, and failure to ferment D-mannose is a key by which *Mannheimia* spp. are differentiated from members of the genus *Pasteurella*.

The five current species in the genus *Mannheimia* are *Mannheimia haemolytica, Mannheimia granulomatis, Mannheimia glucosida, Mannheimia ruminalis,* and *Mannheimia varigena* (Table 23-1).

Mannheimia haemolytica was historically classified into 17 serotypes based on indirect hemagglutination of capsular surface antigens. The organism was further divided into two biotypes A and T, based on the ability to ferment the sugars L-arabinose or trehalose, respectively. T biotype strains (serotypes 3, 4, 10, and 15) have recently been reclassified as a separate species, *Pasteurella trehalosi.* Serotype A11 is now *M. glucosida,* and the A biotype strains A1, A2, A5-A9, A12-A14, A16, and A17 remain as *M. haemolytica.*

DISEASE AND EPIDEMIOLOGY

Mannheimia haemolytica is one of the most important pathogens of domestic cattle. It is the primary bacterial agent responsible for bovine

TABLE **23-1** Hosts and Significance of *Mannheimia* Species

Species	Host(s)	Significance
M. haemolytica	Cattle	Pneumonia
	Sheep	Pneumonia, septicemia, mastitis
M. granulomatis	Cattle	Panniculitis (lechiguana)
	Deer and hares	Bronchopneumonia, conjunctivitis
M. glucosida	Sheep	Normal respiratory flora
M. ruminalis	Cattle, sheep	Normal ruminal flora
M. varigena	Pigs	Septicemia, enteritis, pneumonia
	Cattle	Septicemia, pneumonia, mastitis

pneumonic pasteurellosis, also known as "shipping fever," because of its frequent occurrence in transported animals. It is a major cause of morbidity and mortality, accounting for approximately 30% of the total cattle deaths globally. A recent study estimated the annual economic loss to the U.S. beef cattle industry at $640 million.

Historically, serotype A1 has been the predominant strain associated with pneumonic pasteurellosis. Results of a recent U.S. survey reaffirmed that fact, indicating that serotype A1 accounted for approximately 60% of the total isolates recovered from pneumonic bovine lungs, whereas serotype 6 was isolated from 26% and serotype 2 from 7%. The remaining 7% was composed of serotype 9, 11, or untypable strains.

Bovine respiratory disease is multifactorial, involving environmental factors and concurrent infections with viruses (infectious bovine rhinotracheitis, bovine viral diarrhea, parainfluenza 3, or bovine respiratory syncytial) and other bacterial agents (mycoplasmas, *Pasteurella multocida,* or *Histophilus somni*).

Mannheimia haemolytica is usually an innocuous inhabitant of the nasal cavity and tonsillar crypts. However, when calves are stressed by overcrowding, exhaustion, starvation, dehydration, or cold temperatures, they become more susceptible to illness. Organisms shed from the nasal cavity serve as a source of infection for other animals. Infections are spread by inhalation of bacteria-containing droplets, by direct nose-to-nose contact, or by ingestion of feed contaminated with nasal discharges from infected cattle. The two most important factors in determining if an exposed animal will develop pneumonia are the challenge dose of *M. haemolytica* and the immune status of the host.

Clinical signs of shipping fever, including depression, anorexia, fever, nasal discharge, and a soft, moist cough, become apparent 6 to 10 days after a stressful episode. When lung consolidation becomes extensive, dyspnea and open-mouth breathing often develop. Mortality is high because of bronchial obstruction with fibrinous exudates. Survivors have irreversible lung damage and a high relapse rate and remain lifelong chronic poor-doers.

Mannheimia haemolytica may also cause septicemia in young lambs, acute or chronic pneumonia in sheep, and an uncommon but severe mastitis in ewes.

Experimental and epidemiologic evidence supports a role for *M. granulomatis,* interacting with *Dermatobia hominis,* in the etiology of lechiguana in Brazilian cattle. The disease is characterized by large, hard, subcutaneous swellings that progress rapidly and cause the death of untreated animals after a 3- to 11-month clinical course. Microscopic lesions consist of focal proliferation of fibrous tissue, and infiltration with plasma cells, eosinophils, lymphocytes, and occasionally neutrophils. The primary lesion is an eosinophilic lymphangitis, which results in eosinophilic abscesses, with occasional rosettes containing bacteria in their centers.

Mannheimia varigena strains have been isolated from sporadic cases of bovine mastitis, calf pneumonia, and septicemia, as well as from the oral cavity and gastrointestinal tract of healthy animals. Bovine mastitis is thought to be trauma associated, perhaps from overvigorous suckling of calves or from poor milking equipment. Disease may be severe, with high fever, marked udder edema, and agalactia. Fibrosis and atrophy of affected quarters or entire udders may result in culling of an animal from the milking herd. If calves are allowed to suckle infected cows, pneumonia or septicemia may result. *Mannheimia varigena* is apparently a normal resident of the upper respiratory tract of healthy pigs, but has also been isolated from pigs with pneumonia or enteritis.

PATHOGENESIS

Study of pathogenesis of *Mannheimia* spp. infections has mainly addressed disease caused by *M. haemolytica.* Field evidence suggests that viral and mycoplasmal agents predispose the animal to pneumonic pasteurellosis by impairing normal host defenses and that synergy between these agents and *M. haemolytica* is usually responsible for natural outbreaks of bovine respiratory disease. When animals are stressed, rapid, selective proliferation of serotype A1 occurs in the nasopharynx. Organisms reaching the lungs infect alveolar epithelium, and invasion of the lower respiratory tract is associated with rapid deterioration of lung architecture and function. Within hours of infection, the bronchi, bronchioles, and alveoli are infiltrated by neutrophils, fibrin, blood, and seroproteinaceous fluid. Pulmonary damage is a direct result of action of bacterial products, as well as leukocyte- and platelet-mediated injury, the end result of which is acute fibrinous pleuropneumonia.

The primary virulence factors are leukotoxin and lipopolysaccharide (LPS). Leukotoxin, a

TABLE **23-2**   Virulence Factors of *Mannheimia haemolytica*

Virulence Factor	Activity
Leukotoxin	Pore-forming cytolysin, lethal for leukocytes and platelets; impairment of pulmonary macrophage function
Lipopolysaccharide	Stimulates production of proinflammatory cytokines, lipid mediators, procoagulant substances, oxygen radicals, proteases that damage lung parenchyma
Capsular polysaccharide	Adherence to lower respiratory mucosa, inhibits phagocytosis, mediates resistance to complement-mediated lysis, neutrophil chemoattractant
Fimbriae	Adherence
Siderophore	Iron acquisition
O-sialoglycoprotein endopeptidase	Cleaves glycoproteins, inactivates macrophages and other leukocytes
Neuraminidase	Reduces viscosity of respiratory mucus, impairs mucociliary blanket, allows bacterial penetration to respiratory epithelium

pore-forming cytotoxin of the RTX family, induces lysis of ruminant leukocytes and platelets, but not those from other species. It impairs pulmonary macrophage function and bacterial clearance and damages lung parenchyma through the release of proteolytic enzymes from lysed leukocytes. Decreased antigen-presenting capacity of macrophages aids in lung colonization, directly impairing induced pulmonary defenses.

Pulmonary exposure to LPS induces hemorrhage, edema, hypoxemia, and acute inflammation, and is an important contributor to maintenance and extension of lesions caused by *M. haemolytica* pulmonary infections. Macrophage activation by LPS (and leukotoxin) induces release of proinflammatory cytokines. There is apparent synergy between leukotoxin and LPS in diminution of alveolar macrophage function and increased inflammatory cytokine expression.

Other virulence determinants of *M. haemolytica* include capsular polysaccharide, iron-regulated proteins, enzymes, and fimbriae (Table 23-2). Antibodies against a carbohydrate surface component of *M. haemolytica* may also protect against *M. haemolytica* infection, suggesting a role in virulence for this yet-to-be characterized factor.

DIAGNOSIS

Diagnosis is based on bacterial isolation from clinical specimens. *Mannheimia* spp. grow readily on blood agar or glucose agar plates supplemented with serum. Colonial morphology is similar for all species; colonies are smooth, grayish, variably β-hemolytic, and 1 to 2 mm in diameter after 24 hours' incubation (Figure 23-1). Species are differentiated on the basis of phenotype (Table 23-3).

PREVENTION AND CONTROL

Treatment, prevention, and control of bovine pneumonic pasteurellosis involve management, vaccination, and supportive therapy. Stress and crowding should be avoided. "Preconditioning" calves before shipping, which includes vaccination against common viral respiratory pathogens at least 3 weeks before shipping and not commingling animals from different sources, has been advocated. Early disease recognition, isolation of clinically ill animals, and prompt antimicrobial therapy should be instituted.

A commercial vaccine containing leukotoxoid and surface antigens protects against pneumonic pasteurellosis. Commercial bacterins are, in general, inefficacious and may actually exacerbate disease. Vaccination with bacterins induces formation of opsonizing antibodies that facilitate phagocytosis, leading to increased phagocytic cell lysis and

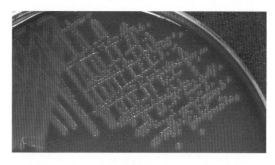

FIGURE **23-1**   *Mannheimia haemolytica* colonies on blood agar. (Courtesy Karen W. Post.)

TABLE **23-3** Differential Characteristics of the *Mannheimia* Species

Test	M. haemolytica	M. granulomatis	M. glucosidae	M. ruminalis	M. varigena
β-Hemolysis (bovine blood)	(Pos)	Neg	Pos	neg	(Pos)
Ornithine decarboxylase	Neg	Neg	Pos	Neg	(Pos)*
α-Fucosidase	Pos	Neg	Var	Neg	Pos
Fermentation of:					
L-arabinose	Neg	Neg	Var	Neg	Pos
D-sorbitol	Pos	Pos	Pos	Var	Neg
D-xylose	Pos	Var	Pos	Var	Pos
Maltose	Pos	Var	Pos	Var	Pos
Dextrin	Pos	Var	Pos	Var	Neg

*Strains from swine are negative.
Neg, Negative; *Pos,* positive; *(Pos),* most positive; *Var,* variable.

subsequent severe pulmonary inflammation. Antiinflammatory agents may be useful, and antimicrobials (macrolides, penicillins, cephalosporins, or florfenicol) are usually administered to prevent further bacterial multiplication and secondary infection. Plasmid-mediated resistance in some strains may be a significant problem.

THE GENUS *PASTEURELLA*

The genus *Pasteurella* contains veterinary pathogens (Table 23-4) that are small nonmotile

gram-negative, coccobacillary to rod–shaped or bipolar-staining cells that appear singly or in pairs. They are nutritionally fastidious and require blood or serum for growth. Several species are NAD dependent, and growth is enhanced in an environment with increased CO_2 concentration.

DISEASES AND EPIDEMIOLOGY

Pasteurella multocida is among the most fascinating bacterial pathogens, particularly in its broad host preference. The specific epithet literally

TABLE **23-4** Hosts and Significance of *Pasteurella* Species

Species	Host(s)	Significance
P. aerogenes	Swine	Normal gastrointestinal (GI) flora, rare abortion
P. avium	Chicken	Normal respiratory flora
P. bettyae	Human	Pneumonia, bacteremia
P. caballi	Horse	Respiratory, uterine infection
P. canis	Dog	Normal oropharyngeal flora, puppy septicemia
	Human	Bite wound infection
P. dagmatis	Dog, cat	Normal oropharyngeal, GI flora
	Human	Bite wound infection
P. gallinarum	Chicken, turkey	Mild fowl cholera, salpingitis
P. langaa	Chicken	Normal respiratory flora
P. lymphangitidis	Bovidae	Lymphangitis
P. mairii	Swine	Rare abortion, septicemia
P. multocida	Ruminants, swine, lab animals	Pneumonia
	Chicken, turkey	Fowl cholera
	Swine	Atrophic rhinitis
	Dog, cat	Oral flora; abscesses, bite wound infections
	Cattle	Hemorrhagic septicemia, mastitis
	Human	Bite wound infections
P. pneumotropica	Lab animals	Pneumonia
P. skyensis	Farmed Atlantic salmon	Septicemia
P. stomatis	Various mammals	Normal respiratory flora
P. testudinis	Reptiles, especially desert tortoise	Normal GI flora; pneumonia and abscesses
P. trehalosi	Sheep	Septicemia, pneumonia
P. volantium	Chicken	Normal respiratory flora

means "killer of many," and it is in fact associated with a wide range of diseases in animals. These include major diseases such as hemorrhagic septicemia in cattle and bison, bovine and porcine pneumonia (often as a secondary invader), fowl cholera, atrophic rhinitis, and rabbit pasteurellosis. The organism is zoonotic, and human infections are derived largely from animal bites. Hemorrhagic septicemia is an uncommon disease in the West, and fowl cholera is controlled with vaccines and antibiotics. However, in developing countries, pasteurellosis remains a widespread problem with serious economic consequences.

Many *P. multocida* strains express a polysaccharide capsule on their surface. Five serogroups (A, B, D, E, and F) are distinguished by indirect hemagglutination of capsular antigens, and diseases are often associated with specific capsular types. Type A strains cause fowl cholera, rabbit snuffles, and bovine pneumonia. Hemorrhagic septicemia strains belong to serogroup B or E, and swine atrophic rhinitis strains to serogroup D. Type F strains have been recovered primarily from turkeys, but their role in disease is unclear. *Pasteurella multocida* is also typed by agar gel precipitation of somatic or O antigens. At least 16 somatic types are designated numerically.

Subspeciation of *P. multocida* may be informative in epidemiologic studies. *Pasteurella multocida* ssp. *multocida* is associated with diseases in domestic animals, whereas *P. multocida* ssp. *gallicida* has been isolated exclusively from birds and may occasionally cause fowl cholera. Isolates from dogs, cats, man, and some birds have been designated *P. multocida* ssp. *septica*.

HEMORRHAGIC SEPTICEMIA

Hemorrhagic septicemia is an acute, highly fatal disease of cattle, water buffaloes, and American bison, and is caused by *P. multocida* serotypes B:2 and E:2. Buffalos appear to be the most susceptible animals, and cases occur sporadically in goats, sheep, swine, deer, camels, and elephants. The disease causes significant economic loss in tropical and subtropical regions of Asia and Africa, but is foreign to the United States; the last U.S. case was reported in bison in 1965. Disease outbreaks are usually preceded by episodes of stress, such as drastic changes in weather, poor nutrition, and overcrowding. Morbidity and mortality rates vary from 50% to 100%. About 50% of healthy animals in herds that have experienced disease harbor

the organism on their tonsils or nasopharyngeal mucosae, as compared with a 3% to 5% carrier rate in disease-free herds.

Spread occurs directly or indirectly to susceptible animals from contact with saliva or nasal discharges from normal carriers or clinically ill animals. The disease is characterized by acute septicemia, and clinical signs include high fever, profuse salivation, depression, dyspnea, submucosal petechiation, and occasional dysentery. There may also be subcutaneous edema around the throat, dewlap, brisket, or perineum. Death ensues within 24 hours, and gross lesions include generalized petechiation (especially on serous surfaces), pulmonary edema, enteritis, and lymphadenopathy.

BOVINE AND PORCINE PNEUMONIA

Pasteurella multocida serogroup A:3 is isolated frequently from beef cattle with severe fibrinous broncho- and pleuropneumonia, as part of the bovine respiratory disease complex. Illness is seen most frequently in young recently weaned animals. The organism is generally regarded as an opportunistic pathogen of low relative virulence that invades secondary to viral or bacterial pneumonias.

Pneumonic pasteurellosis of swine, which occurs in the final stage of the porcine respiratory disease complex, is one of the most economically significant diseases in swine production systems throughout the world. *Pasteurella multocida* is extremely difficult to eradicate and is found commonly even in high-health herds. The implementation of segregated early weaning programs has not resulted in complete eradication of the organism. Both type A and type D toxigenic strains have been recovered from the pneumonic lungs of affected pigs, but the role of toxigenicity in swine pneumonia has not been elucidated.

FOWL CHOLERA

Fowl cholera is a disease of historical significance. Louis Pasteur conducted his classic experiments on bacterial virulence attenuation in an attempt to produce immunity to *P. multocida* infection in poultry. The disease is highly contagious and affects a wide range of domesticated and wild birds in most countries. It usually manifests as septicemia with high morbidity and mortality (up to 70%), but may also occur in a chronic form. Fowl cholera is most prevalent in late summer, fall, and winter. Turkeys, domestic ducks, and geese are more susceptible to disease than chickens. Mature chickens are more susceptible than birds less than 16 weeks of age, and the mortality rate in these birds is 1% to 20%. Disease often results in reduced egg production and localized infections. Chronically infected birds are major reservoirs of infection. Fomites such as contaminated crates, feeders, or waterers may introduce fowl cholera to new birds placed into a house. Excretions from infected birds may spread the disease within a flock, either directly or indirectly. Signs of acute disease in turkeys are usually apparent for only a few hours before death and include fever, diarrhea, mucoid oral discharge, ruffled feathers, and tachypnea. Chronic fowl cholera may result from infection with a strain of low virulence or may be a sequel to acute disease. Localized infections are the hallmark of this form. Swollen wattles, joints, or footpads, and conjunctivitis, torticollis, rales, or dyspnea may be present.

ATROPHIC RHINITIS

Atrophic rhinitis is an upper respiratory disease occurring primarily in piglets 1 to 8 weeks of age, and is usually characterized by mild signs and lesions. The sequel to this early disease may be rapidly progressive atrophy of the nasal and ethmoid turbinates, with severe nasal deviation and decreased weight gain.

The more severe form of atrophic rhinitis occurs in swine-rearing countries throughout the world. Slaughter checks in the United States have revealed that nearly one quarter of the animals have some degree of turbinate involvement. Infection with *Bordetella bronchiseptica* may predispose pigs to atrophic rhinitis, but only *P. multocida* toxigenic capsular type D strains cause the severe, progressive form of the disease. Other risk factors for disease development include increased farrowing density, high levels of environmental ammonia or dust, and the presence of weaned pigs in farrowing buildings.

RABBIT PASTEURELLOSIS

Pasteurellosis, often called "snuffles," is the most important bacterial disease of rabbits, and is most often caused by *P. multocida*. The disease is a major concern for commercial rabbitries and research facilities, causing economic loss and compromising research efforts. Half of conventionally raised rabbits may have upper respiratory tract colonization by *P. multocida,* and many are asymptomatic.

Neonates become colonized during parturition or through nursing infected does. Environmental factors such as temperature fluctuations, increased ammonia levels, poor sanitation, gestation, and old age may initiate clinical disease. Pasteurellosis in rabbits also manifests as otitis media or interna, pneumonia, abscesses, conjunctivitis, mastitis, metritis, abscessation in nearly any site, and septicemia. Signs exhibited depend on the site infection and may include oculonasal discharge, snuffling, dyspnea, cyanosis, torticollis, vaginal discharge, subcutaneous swelling, and sudden death.

OTHER *PASTEURELLA* SPECIES

Pasteurella pneumotropica is an opportunistic pathogen of rodents. The bacterium exists in latency on respiratory or gastrointestinal mucosae and is disseminated by aerosol or fecal shedding, or by intimate contact. Any factor that lowers host resistance, such as stress or concurrent infection with viral or mycoplasmal agents, may precipitate secondary infection with *P. pneumotropica*. Dyspnea, weight loss, cutaneous abscesses, mastitis, conjunctivitis, abortion, cystitis, infertility, and vaginitis are clinical signs.

Pasteurella trehalosi is a cause of septicemia and pneumonia, particularly of feeder lambs. This economically significant disease occurs in Europe, Iceland, America, and probably other sheep-rearing countries. Disease is characterized by a sudden onset of fever, anorexia, respiratory distress, and sudden death. Animals may recover completely or become chronically affected, with reduced lung capacity and weight gain efficiency.

All breeds and sexes are equally affected. Recently weaned or transported lambs 2 to 12 months of age have the highest incidence of disease. Most outbreaks occur from late summer to early fall, or shortly after an episode of inclement weather. Infection by viruses or other bacteria increases susceptibility of lambs to infection with *P. trehalosi*. Transmission is by direct or indirect contact.

PATHOGENESIS

Mechanisms of pathogenesis and virulence determinants for most species other than *P. multocida* are still incompletely understood. The genus is complex and diverse with respect to host predilection and antigenic variation.

Pasteurella multocida strains associated with fowl cholera usually enter avian tissues through the mucous membranes of the pharynx, upper respiratory passages, conjunctivae, or rarely through cutaneous wounds. In atrophic rhinitis, toxigenic *P. multocida* strains of serogroup D attach to the membranes overlying nasal turbinates. As the organism multiplies, it produces a dermonecrotic toxin that destroys osteoblasts and causes osteoclastic lysis, resulting in turbinate destruction.

Virulence factors of *Pasteurella* spp. include capsule, endotoxin, exotoxin, adhesins, hemagglutinins, and proteases. Strains with the hyaluronic acid capsule are more resistant to phagocytosis and intracellular killing by macrophages. Endotoxin or lipopolysaccharide is pyrogenic. Strains of serogroups A, B, and D have type 4 fimbriae, which are associated with adhesion to host epithelial cell surfaces. Swine strains possess hemagglutinins and fimbriae.

Pasteurella multocida expresses a siderophore called multocidin, which scavenges iron from host iron-binding glycoproteins. *Pasteurella trehalosi* produces collagenase, which may destroy collagen in lung parenchyma, allowing for deeper penetration of the bacterium and further pulmonary inflammation.

DIAGNOSIS

Diagnosis of pasteurellosis is based on isolation of the causative organism from affected tissues.

FIGURE 23-2 Gram-stained smear of *Pasteurella multocida*. (Courtesy Public Health Image Library, PHIL #3621, Centers for Disease Control and Prevention, Atlanta, 1971, R. Weaver.)

The routine isolation medium is blood agar, although V factor–dependent *Pasteurella* spp. grow better on chocolate agar. Plates should be incubated under 3% to 5% CO_2 at 37° C for 24 to 48 hours. Isolates are gram negative with variable morphology (Figure 23-2) and colonial characteristics (Table 23-5).

Pasteurella spp. are phenotypically similar to *Actinobacillus* and *Mannheimia* spp. No single test can distinguish pasteurellae from actinobacilli. Fermentation of D-mannose differentiates *Pasteurella* from *Mannheimia* spp. (Tables 23-6

TABLE **23-5** Colonial Characteristics of Selected *Pasteurella* Species

Pasteurella Species	Colonial Morphology on Blood Agar
P. aerogenes	Circular, smooth, entire, convex, translucent, 0.5-1 mm diameter
P. caballi	Round, nonhemolytic, slightly raised, smooth, shiny, grayish yellow, 1-1.5 mm diameter
P. gallinarum	Nonhemolytic, iridescent, circular, smooth, entire, convex, ≤1.5 mm diameter
P. lymphangitidis	Round, grayish, semitransparent, ~2.5 mm diameter after 48 hr incubation; may cause greenish discoloration of red cells
P. mairii	Round, grayish, semitransparent, ~3 mm diameter after 48 hr; may cause greenish discoloration of red cells
P. multocida	May be mucoid and smooth (see Figure 23-3) or more dry, somewhat rough; smooth colonies may be iridescent; distinctive odor; some strains cause greenish discoloration on blood agar
P. pneumotropica	Smooth, gray, translucent, butyrous, nonhemolytic, ≤2 mm diameter after 48 hr; may have odor like P. *multocida*
P. skyensis	Circular, entire, convex, smooth, gray, 0.5 mm diameter, nonhemolytic to weakly β-hemolytic after 48 hr at 22° C; no growth above 32° C or on medium without 1.5% salt
P. testudinis	Whitish, mucoid colonies ≤1 mm diameter after 24 hr; β-hemolytic on sheep blood agar
P. trehalosi	Round, grayish, semitransparent, ≤2.5 mm diameter after 48 hr incubation; pronounced zones of β-hemolysis (often double-zoned); occasional strains may produce greening of red cells

TABLE 23-6　Differential Characteristics of *Pasteurella* Species

	Catalase	Oxidase	Nitrate Reductase	ONPG	ODC	Indole	Urease	β-Hemolysis	Growth on MacConkey	Glucose with Gas	Fermentation of:			
											Lactose	Maltose	Mannose	Sucrose
P. aerogenes	Pos	D	Pos	D	D	Neg	Pos	Neg	Pos	Pos	Pos	Neg	D	Pos
P. anatis	Pos	Wk pos	Pos	Pos	Neg	Neg	Neg	Neg	Wk pos	Neg	Pos	Neg	Pos	Pos
*P. avium**	Wk pos	Pos	Pos	Neg	Neg	Neg	Neg	Neg	Neg	Neg	Neg	Neg	Neg	Neg
P. caballi	Neg	Pos	Pos	Pos	Pos	Neg	Neg	Neg	Neg	Pos	Pos	Pos	Pos	Pos
P. canis	Pos	Pos	Pos	Neg	Pos	Wk pos	Neg	Neg	Neg	Neg	Neg	Neg	Neg	Pos
P. dagmatis	Pos	Pos	Pos	Neg	Neg	Pos	Pos	Neg	Neg	Wk pos	Neg	Pos	Neg	Pos
P. gallinarum	Pos	Pos	Pos	Neg	Neg	Neg	Neg	Neg	Neg	Neg	Neg	Pos	Neg	Pos
P. langaa	Neg	Wk pos	Pos	Pos	Neg	Neg	Neg	Neg	Neg	Neg	Pos	Neg	Pos	Pos
P. lymphan-gitidis	Pos	Neg	Neg	Neg	Neg	Neg	Pos	Neg	D	Neg	Neg	D	Pos	D
P. mairii	Pos	Pos	Pos	D	Pos	Neg	Pos	D	D	Neg	Neg	D	Pos	Pos
P. multocida	Pos	Pos	Pos	Neg	D	Pos	Neg	Neg	Neg	Neg	Neg	Neg	Pos	Pos
P. pneumo-tropica	Pos	Pos	Pos	Pos	Pos	Pos	Pos	Neg	D	D	D	D	Neg	Pos
P. skyensis	Neg	Wk pos	Neg	Neg	Pos	Pos	Neg	D	ND	Pos	Pos	Pos	Pos	Neg
P. stomatis	Pos	Pos	Pos	Neg	Neg	Wk pos	Neg	Neg	Neg	Neg	Neg	Neg	Neg	Pos
P. testudinis	Pos	Pos	Pos	Neg	Neg	Pos	Neg	Pos	D	Neg	Neg	Pos	D	Pos
P. trehalosi	Neg	Pos	Pos	Neg	Neg	Neg	Neg	Pos	Pos	Neg	Neg	Pos	Pos	Pos
*P. volantium**	Pos	Pos	Pos	Pos	D	Neg	Neg	Neg	Neg	Neg	Wk pos	Neg	Pos	Pos
Species A	Pos	Pos	Pos	Pos	D	Neg	Neg	Neg	Neg	Neg	Neg	D	Pos	Pos
Species B	Pos	Pos	Pos	Pos	Pos	Pos	Neg	Neg	D	Neg	Neg	Pos	Neg	Pos

P. avium and *P. volantium* require NAD for growth.

D, 21%–79% of strains are positive; *indole*, test performed in SIM medium; *ND*, not determined; *Neg*, negative; *ODC*, ornithine dihydrolase; *ONPG*, hydrolysis of ortho–nitrophenyl-p-galactopyranoside; *Pos*, positive; *urease*, Christensen's medium; *Wk*, weak.

TABLE 23-7 Differentiation of Subspecies of *Pasteurella multocida*

	P. multocida		
	ssp. *multocida*	ssp. *septica*	ssp. *gallicida*
D-sorbitol fermentation	Positive	Negative	Positive
Trehalose fermentation	Positive	Positive	Negative

and 23-7). *Pasteurella* spp. ferment mannose, whereas *Mannheimia* spp. do not. An essential part of the identification process is the knowledge of the animal from which the isolate was recovered because many species have unique host predilections (e.g., *Pasteurella testudinis* or *Pasteurella caballi*).

Serologic tests for diagnosis of fowl cholera (plate agglutination or agar gel diffusion precipitation tests) have limited value in chronic disease and no value in acute forms of the disease.

PREVENTION AND CONTROL

Safe and effective vaccines for *P. multocida* in cattle are not available. Vaccines currently available are killed bacterins or live attenuated products, and the efficacy of most of these has not been critically evaluated. Vaccination with killed bacterins is practiced in areas where hemorrhagic septicemia is endemic. Vaccination may reduce disease incidence, but duration of immunity is short lived and disease outbreaks still occur.

Practices for prevention and control of bovine pneumonia are the same as those for *M. haemolytica*. Prevention of porcine pneumonic pasteurellosis is best achieved through management, including modification of the environment or decreasing the spread of the organism. Increasing ventilation, decreasing levels of ammonia and dust, and maintaining stable temperatures in swine units are recommended, as are all-in/all-out production flow, maintaining closed herds, reducing stocking density, and minimal commingling of pigs from mixed sources. Control by using antimicrobials and vaccination has been variably successful. Efficacy of antimicrobial therapy varies greatly and depends on strain susceptibility and route of administration of the antimicrobial; swine isolates are usually susceptible to cephalosporins and tetracyclines. Killed bacterins for disease prevention in pigs are marketed, but are of questionable efficacy. Prevention and control of other diseases in the porcine respiratory

disease complex (*Actinobacillus pleuropneumoniae*, porcine respiratory and reproductive syndrome virus, swine influenza virus, and *Mycoplasma hyopneumoniae*) is an important means to control *P. multocida* infections.

Management practices necessary for the prevention and control of atrophic rhinitis are virtually identical for those of pneumonic pasteurellosis and are also covered in Chapter 18.

Methods for prevention of fowl cholera include elimination of the reservoirs of infection and implementation of sound husbandry practices, with an emphasis on sanitation. Primary sources of infection are sick birds or chronically infected, asymptomatic carrier birds, which should be identified and culled from the flock. Replacement stock should originate from farms known to be free from fowl cholera, and new additions should be isolated for a period before introduction into existing flocks. Additional preventive measures are refraining from raising different species of birds on the same premises and eliminating access to poultry areas by farm dogs and cats, rodents, and wild birds. In the face of an outbreak, the entire flock should be placed

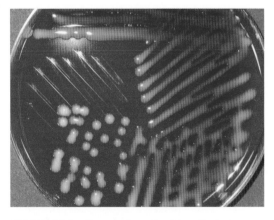

FIGURE 23-3 *Pasteurella multocida* cultivated on blood agar. (Courtesy Karen W. Post.)

under quarantine and ultimately disposed of when economically feasible. In areas where fowl cholera is most prevalent, vaccination with commercial bacterins or live vaccines should be considered. Antimicrobial chemotherapy has been used both for control and treatment of fowl cholera, with potentiated-sulfa drugs and tetracyclines administered most frequently.

Prevention of pasteurellosis in rodent or rabbit colonies requires placement of disease-free animals into clean barrier-sustained facilities. New additions should be placed under quarantine before placement into the existing colony. Control by treatment with antimicrobials such as chloramphenicol or tetracyclines is relatively easy but will not eliminate the organism from a colony.

SUGGESTED READINGS

Ackermann MR, Brogden KA: Response of the ruminant respiratory tract to *Mannheimia (Pasteurella) haemolytica, Microbes Infect* 2:1079-1088, 2000.

Angen O, Mutters R, Caugant DA, et al: Taxonomic relationships of the *(Pasteurella) haemolytica* complex as evaluated by DNA-DNA hybridizations and 16S rRNA sequencing with proposal of *Mannheimia haemolytica* gen. nov., comb. nov., *Mannheimia granulomatis* comb. nov., *Mannheimia glucosida* sp. nov., *Mannheimia ruminalis* sp. nov. and *Mannheimia varigena* sp. nov., *Int J Syst Bacteriol* 49:67-86, 1999.

Bisgaard M, Mutters R: Re-investigations of selected bovine and ovine strains previously classified as *Pasteurella haemolytica* and description of some new taxa within the *Pasteurella haemolytica* complex, *Acta Path Microbiol Immunol Scand* 94:185-193, 1986.

DiGiacomo RF, Garlinghouse LE, Van Hoosier GL: Natural history of infection with *Pasteurella multocida* in rabbits, *J Am Vet Med Assoc* 183:1172-1175, 1983.

Lo, RYC: Genetic analysis of virulence factors of *Mannheimia (Pasteurella) haemolytica* A1, *Vet Microbiol* 83:21-35, 2001.

Ribiero GA, Carter GR, Frederiksen W, et al: *Pasteurella haemolytica*–like bacterium from a progressive granuloma of cattle in Brazil, *J Clin Microbiol* 27:1401-1402, 1989.

Chapter 24

The Genera *Haemophilus, Histophilus,* and *Taylorella*

THE GENUS *HAEMOPHILUS*

Haemophilus spp. are assigned to the family Pasteurellaceae and are common commensal organisms of the mucous membranes of animals and humans. They are highly susceptible to desiccation and, in consequence, cannot survive for long periods in the environment. Most species are opportunists in stressed or compromised hosts, but some, such as *Haemophilus parasuis* in swine, cause more serious disease. Most animals and birds harbor at least one species-specific strain (Table 24-1). Human disease caused by species other than *Haemophilus influenzae* has, with some exceptions, been considered unusual.

All members of the genus *Haemophilus* are small, pleomorphic, facultatively anaerobic, nonmotile, gram-negative rods to coccobacilli that may form filaments during periods of environmental stress. The genus name is in reference to the fact that these organisms require factors X (hemin) and/or V (NAD) in blood for growth. Species designated with the prefix "*para*" require only V factor. Optimal growth is obtained in an atmosphere of 5% to 10% CO_2. The most uniformly satisfactory medium for propagation of *Haemophilus* species is chocolate agar because it provides both X and V factors. On blood agar, *Haemophilus* colonies cluster around a *Staphylococcus* streak line in a phenomenon called satellitism. Phenotypic characteristics allow differentiation of *Haemophilus* spp. (Table 24-2).

HAEMOPHILUS PARAGALLINARUM

Haemophilus paragallinarum is the agent of infectious coryza, an upper respiratory disease of laying and growing chickens worldwide. Disease is exacerbated by concurrent mycoplasmal or viral infections and, in those situations, mortality may be high. A characteristic swelling of the infraorbital region, oculonasal discharge, swollen wattles, diarrhea, and inappetence are common clinical signs (Figure 24-1). Losses result from decreased feed consumption, which impacts egg and meat yield.

TABLE **24-1** *Haemophilus* Species of Veterinary Significance

Organism	Host(s)	Disease condition(s)
H. felis	Cat	Rhinitis, conjunctivitis
H. influenzaemurium	Rodents	Respiratory, ocular disease
H. haemoglobinophilus	Dog	Normal preputial flora; rare vaginitis, cystitis, balanoposthitis
H. paracuniculus	Rabbit	From animals with mucoid enteritis; virulence unknown
H. paragallinarum	Chicken	Infectious coryza
H. parasuis	Pig	Glässer's disease, meningitis, myositis, pneumonia, septicemia

TABLE **24-2**   Differential Characteristics of *Haemophilus* Species

Species	Oxidase	Catalase	X-factor Require-ment	V-factor Require-ment	Indole Produc-tion	ODC	Urease Produc-tion	CO_2 Require-ment
H. felis	Neg	Pos	Neg	Pos	Neg	Neg	Neg	Pos
H. influenzaemurium	Neg	Pos	Pos	Neg	Neg	Neg	Neg	Neg
H. hemoglobinophilus	Pos	Pos	Pos	Neg	Pos	Neg	Neg	Neg
H. paracuniculus	Pos	Pos	Neg	Pos	Pos	Pos	Pos	Pos
H. paragallinarum	Neg	Neg	Neg	Pos	Neg	Neg	Neg	Pos
H. parasuis	Var	Pos	Neg	Pos	Neg	Neg	Neg	Neg

Neg, Negative; *Pos,* positive; *Var,* variable.

Unusual clinical presentations in developing countries include arthritis and septicemia. Lesions observed at necropsy are associated with catarrhal inflammation of the respiratory tract, and include sinusitis with congestion, edema, and sloughing. Disease transmission is via the respiratory route or through contact with contaminated drinking water. Susceptible birds exposed to the agent usually develop clinical signs within 3 days. Birds that recover from acute illness may be a source of infection for young chicks that become susceptible 4 weeks after hatching. Serogroups A, B, and C of *H. paragallinarum* are currently recognized, with four serovars in groups A and C. Infectious coryza has been infrequently diagnosed in pheasants, guinea fowl, quail, and companion birds. Ducks, turkeys, and pigeons are refractory to experimental infection.

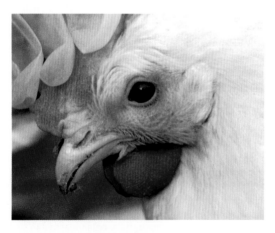

FIGURE **24-1**   Chicken infected with *Haemophilus paragallinarum.* Note swollen infraorbital region and visible purplish discoloration of the skin. (Courtesy H.M. Opitz.)

There is a paucity of information on the pathogenesis of infectious coryza. Adherence to and colonization of the nasal mucosa is apparently the initial step in pathogenesis. Potential virulence attributes of *H. paragallinarum* include a polysaccharide capsule, which may mediate attachment of the organism to cilia of the nasal mucosa. The hyaluronic acid component of the capsule and the lipopolysaccharide in the cell wall may contribute to pathogenesis, but these interactions with the host have not been clearly defined. The principal lesion is acute catarrhal inflammation of the upper respiratory tract, primarily the nasal cavity and paranasal sinus. Mast cell infiltration into the lamina propria of the mucous membrane of the nasal cavity follows. Mast cells may be responsible for the clinical signs of infectious coryza, through the activation of inflammatory mediators.

Diagnosis of infectious coryza is based on the characteristic clinical signs (facial swelling), recovery of the bacterium from clinical materials, and results of serologic testing. Although fastidious, *H. paragallinarum* is easily recovered from the sinuses of affected birds in the acute stage of infection, by bacteriologic culture on chocolate agar. The strain characterized originally apparently required both X and V factors, but the current representatives of *H. paragallinarum* require only V factor, and V-factor independent strains have been recovered from chickens in South Africa. Differentiation of the pathogenic *H. paragallinarum* from *Haemophilus*-like commensals of the avian upper respiratory tract can be based on phenotypic differences (Table 24-3). Several serologic assays allow detection of antibodies to *H. paragallinarum,* and the test of choice appears to be hemagglutination inhibition, which detects both vaccinal titers and those resulting from infection.

TABLE **24-3**   Characteristics Useful in the Differentiation of *Haemophilus paragallinarum* from Avian *Haemophilus*-like Organisms

Test	H. paragallinarum	Pasteurella avium	Pasteurella volantium	Pasteurella sp. taxon A
Catalase	Neg	Pos	Pos	Pos
Growth in ambient air	Neg	Pos	Pos	Pos
V-factor dependent	Var	Var	Var	Var
β-galactosidase	Pos	Neg	Pos	Var
ACID FROM:				
Arabinose	Neg	Neg	Neg	Pos
Galactose	Neg	Pos	Pos	Pos
Maltose	Pos	Neg	Pos	Var
Mannitol	Pos	Neg	Pos	Var

Neg, Negative; *Pos,* positive; *Var,* variable.

A polymerase chain reaction (PCR) test allows rapid diagnosis of coryza but has limited availability.

A killed vaccine containing serovars A and C has been available for many years for prevention of infectious coryza. A commercial trivalent vaccine containing serotypes A, B, and C has been developed, but outbreaks of coryza have been reported in vaccinated flocks in several countries, suggesting that there may be new serotypes. Macrolides, sulfonamides, or tetracyclines are administered in feed or water in the face of outbreaks, as a control method. These agents are bacteriostatic, so the carrier state is not eliminated and relapses after therapy are not uncommon. Management of disease should include use of coryza-free replacement birds and an all-in/all-out flow of birds. Often it is necessary to depopulate a flock for disease elimination.

HAEMOPHILUS PARASUIS

In 1910, Glässer described a disease of pigs associated with infection by a gram-negative bacillus and characterized by polyserositis, polysynovitis, and meningitis. Today the organism is ubiquitous in the nasal cavity, tonsil, and trachea of healthy pigs, and can occasionally be isolated from healthy lungs. However, disease caused by *H. parasuis* has become increasingly significant in swine-producing countries throughout the world, despite changes in production methods. Segregated early weaning (SEW) programs that have been advocated to reduce pathogens are ineffective in controlling *H. parasuis* colonization because the bacterium is transferred from the sow to her piglets before 10 days of age. Morbidity and mortality can be especially high in

conventional herds infected with porcine reproductive and respiratory syndrome (PRRS) virus, and in naïve swine populations, such as those that are specific pathogen free (SPF) or raised by SEW. Survivors grow poorly and add to production losses.

More than 15 serotypes of *H. parasuis* have been described, based on heat-stable antigens extracted from bacterial cultures and detected either in an agar gel precipitation test or an enzyme immunoassay. Up to 25% of isolates remain untypable. Some data suggest that serotypes 1, 5, and 12 through 14 may be more virulent than others. In North America, serotypes 2, 4, 5, 12, 13, and 14 account for approximately 75% of isolates recovered from clinically ill animals.

Haemophilus parasuis is a primary agent in nursery mortality. Disease severity, as well as the age of the affected animals, depends on the health status of the herd and the virulence of the infecting strain. In some herds, disease can occur within a week of weaning, and this reflects a deficiency in maternal immunity. Animals are affected at 4 to 6 weeks postweaning in the majority of herds. Glässer's disease is characterized by a high fever (107° C), swollen joints, respiratory distress, and central nervous system (CNS) signs. Severe lesions observed at necropsy include fibrinous exudates in the pleura, pericardium, synovia, meninges, brain, and peritoneal cavity (Figures 24-2 and 24-3). Acute pneumonia without polyserositis has been reported in older animals in endemically infected, stable herds. Acute septicemia or arthritis may occur in adult populations, especially sow herds.

Other disease manifestations include acute fasciitis and myositis in primary SPF sows, in the absence of lesions of septicemia, pneumonia, or polyserositis.

The pathogenesis of Glässer's disease is not well defined. The organism initially colonizes nasal mucosa, and then breaches the mucosal barrier, gains access to the bloodstream, and replicates at serosal sites to produce systemic infection and fibrinopurulent inflammation. Destruction of alveolar macrophages by PRRS virus may be a factor in the development of systemic infection. Endotoxin induces disseminated intravascular coagulation, resulting in the formation of microthrombi in the liver, lungs, and kidney. Some strains of *H. parasuis* are apparently more virulent than others, but virulence markers remain to be identified, and there is no absolute correlation between serotype and pathogenicity. A Na⁺ pump is hypothesized to allow the organism to grow in the face of superoxide radicals produced during the host immune response to infection, and a putative modulator of the heat shock response may prevent bacterial cell damage.

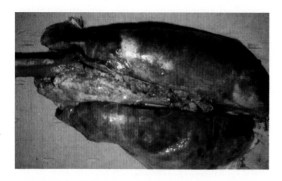

FIGURE 24-2 Respiratory lesions of Glässer's disease in a finishing pig. (Courtesy Raymond E. Reed.)

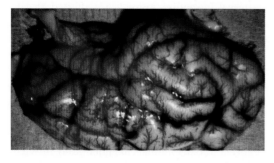

FIGURE 24-3 Brain lesions associated with Glässer's disease in a finishing pig. (Courtesy Raymond E. Reed.)

Neuraminidase may aid in scavenging nutrients, unmasking receptors, and interfering with immunity by effects on secretory antibody half-life.

Virulence can also differ among strains recovered from distinct systemic sites. Upper respiratory isolates are genetically heterogeneous, generally of low virulence, and are predominantly serotype 3. Pneumonic lung strains are highly genetically diverse and somewhat more virulent, whereas systemic isolates are closely related and of higher virulence. Some systemic isolates have a tropism for the brain.

Diagnosis of *H. parasuis*–related diseases is usually based upon clinical signs, gross lesions, bacterial isolation from affected tissues, serological testing, immunohistochemistry, and PCR assays. Recovery of *H. parasuis* may be difficult in field cases because the organism can die very quickly in the carcass; cultures may be negative even in the presence of lesions. Dilution plating or selective culture can improve recovery rates from contaminated specimens. Optimal specimens for culture are aseptically collected fluids from serosal surfaces, joints, or meninges. Once isolated, *H. parasuis* must be carefully distinguished from NAD-dependent members of the family Pasteurellaceae that are commensal respiratory flora in swine (*Actinobacillus porcinus*, *Actinobacillus indolicus*, *Actinobacillus minor*, and *Haemophilus* sp. Taxon C), and must also be distinguished from *Actinobacillus pleuropneumoniae* (Table 24-4). *Haemophilus parasuis* is distinct from *A. pleuropneumoniae* in its lack of hemolysis, urease, and CAMP factor production; its production of catalase; and its pattern of sugar fermentation. Serologic testing with an enzyme immunoassay, based on evaluation of paired samples, is available for diagnosis of herd disease. Immunohistochemistry allows detection of nonviable organisms in affected tissues; however, some polyclonal antibodies used for diagnosis of *H. parasuis* infection may cross-react with *A. pleuropneumoniae*. PCR assays can detect as few as 100 colony-forming units (CFUs) per ml in samples from lesions.

Prevention and control should be based on serotypic characterization of the prevalent strain isolated from systemic sites and selection of commercial vaccines accordingly. In contrast with cross-immunity that appears in response to natural infection, immunity after vaccination seems to be dependent on the serovar of the strain. Therefore commercial vaccines vary in efficacy,

TABLE **24-4** Differentiation of *Haemophilus parasuis* from Similar Organisms

	Actino-bacillus pleuro-pneumoniae	Actino-bacillus pleurop-neumoniae 2	Actino-bacillus minor	H. parasuis	Actino-bacillus porcinus	Actino-bacillus indolicus	Haemo-philus taxon C
V-factor requirement	(Pos)	Neg	Pos	Pos	Pos	Pos	Pos
Urease production	(Pos)	Pos	Pos	Neg	Neg	Neg	Neg
Indole production	Neg	Neg	Neg	Neg	Neg	Pos	Neg
CAMP	Pos	Pos	(Neg)	Neg	Neg	Neg	Neg
β-Hemolysis	(Pos)	Pos	(Neg)	Neg	Neg	Neg	Neg
Catalase production	(Neg)	(Neg)	(Neg)	Pos	Neg	Pos	Pos
ACID FROM:							
L-Arabinose	Neg	Neg	Neg	Neg	(Neg)	Neg	Pos
Mannitol	Pos	Pos	Neg	Neg	(Pos)	Neg	Neg
Raffinose	Neg	Neg	Pos	Neg	(Pos)	(Pos)	Pos
Lactose	Neg	Neg	Pos	Neg	(Pos)	(Neg)	Neg

Neg, Negative; *(Neg),* most negative; *Pos,* positive; *(Pos),* most positive.

in part due to the lack of cross-protection between serovars. Autogenous vaccines are another option, and they should contain at least one representative from each prevalent serotype in a production system.

Vaccination schedule is an important consideration in control of *H. parasuis* infections, and should be based upon the epidemiology of the disease in a given herd. When disease occurs shortly after weaning, piglets should be vaccinated twice, once at processing and again at weaning. Vaccination may be delayed until weaning and 2 weeks postweaning if disease occurs predominantly 4 to 6 weeks into the nursery phase of rearing. Control of *H. parasuis* in herds concurrently infected with PRRS virus may depend on stabilization of viral circulation. Herd profiling by enzyme immunoassay screening may be helpful in identifying naïve animals.

Traditional use of antimicrobials to control severe outbreaks does not offer consistent responses, partly because of the sudden onset of disease. Also, some strains of the organism are resistant to penicillin and tetracycline. Results of in vitro studies suggest that ceftiofur, pleuromutilin, and macrolide antimicrobials are efficacious.

An alternative method for reduction of mortality in herds is controlled exposure, in which 3- to 5-day-old piglets are colonized by way of a low dose of the prevalent virulent serotypes of *H. parasuis*

involved in herd mortality. Exposed piglets do not develop clinical disease postexposure because of the presence of maternal antibodies.

THE GENUS *HISTOPHILUS*

The genus *Histophilus* has recently been reorganized after phylogenetic analysis of 16S rDNA and *rpoB* sequences confirmed that phenotypically similar bacteria with the status of *species incertae sedis, Haemophilus somnus, Histophilus ovis,* and *Haemophilus agni,* comprise a novel genus within the family Pasteurellaceae. Further analyses have demonstrated that these organisms should be regarded as *Histophilus somni.*

Histophilus somni is a gram-negative, nonmotile, pleomorphic rod that is catalase negative and usually oxidase positive. Growth is capnophilic and independent of X or V factors. Organisms are also alkaline phosphatase and nitrate reductase positive, and ferment glucose. They fail to grow on Simmons' citrate agar, fail to produce urease, arginine dihydrolase, or ornithine decarboxylase, and are Voges-Proskauer negative.

Thromboembolic meningoencephalitis (TEME), or "thrombo," a CNS disease of feedlot cattle caused by a gram-negative rod, was first reported in 1956. The name *Haemophilus somnus* was proposed in 1969, even though the organism did not require X or V factors for its growth. Similar bacteria, isolated from various disease conditions in sheep, had been named *H. ovis* and *H. agni.*

Histophilus somni is the sole species of the reorganized genus. The organism generally has yellowish pigmentation and usually produces indole, although a few strains previously designated *H. agni* may be indole negative. Carbon dioxide (5%-10%) and thiamine monophosphate are growth requirements. Hemolysis is variable, but most isolates are α-hemolytic when cultivated on bovine blood agar. Pinpoint colonies form after 24 hours' incubation and grow to 1 to 1.5 mm in diameter in 48 hours.

Histophilus somni colonizes mucosal surfaces of ruminants, but it may also be the causative agent of multisystemic diseases, including bronchopneumonia, TEME, necrotic laryngitis, myocarditis, arthritis, otitis, conjunctivitis, myelitis, mastitis, myositis, abortion, and reproductive tract disorders. The organism spreads through direct contact with infected animals. Because of its association with a variety of disease conditions, the syndrome has been referred to as the *H. somnus* complex. Economic losses are high and disease is found worldwide.

Bronchopneumonia in lightweight calves is the most common disease manifestation, and outbreaks typically occur within 2 weeks of arrival in a feedlot. Clinical signs are nonspecific and resemble those associated with any of the other agents of bovine respiratory disease. Morbidity and mortality rates are highest among young, naïve calves. In some cases, sudden death can occur from bronchiolitis obliterans. Stress from weaning, weather, and shipping appears to be an important predisposing factor to illness. Pneumonia in adult cattle is rare and usually associated with the introduction of new herd additions.

CNS infection with *H. somni* usually follows an episode of pneumonia by 1 to 2 weeks and may result in blindness, depression, ataxia, convulsions, and coma. Onset to death can be less than 12 hours. This condition has been referred to as the "sleeper syndrome." Grossly, the affected portions of the brain contain multiple, reddish brown foci of necrosis (Figure 24-4). Brain and meninges are inflamed, and thrombi in vessels are composed of leukocytes, fibrin, and bacteria, giving rise to the name, thromboembolic meningoencephalitis. These lesions are considered pathognomonic for *H. somni* infection.

Necrotic laryngitis in feeder calves is associated with the "honker syndrome," so named because affected animals have a characteristic deep,

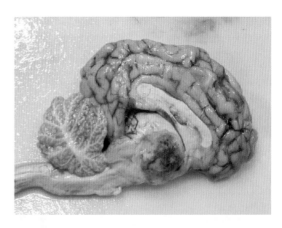

FIGURE 24-4 Bovine brain with gross lesions of thromboembolic meningoencephalitis. (Courtesy Peter Moisan.)

nonproductive cough that is exacerbated by dusty conditions. Sick calves may become unthrifty, but continue to eat and drink.

Myocarditis is a frequently diagnosed form of *H. somni* infection and a common sequel to bronchopneumonia. Pen riders in feedlots describe animals suddenly falling over and dying. Chronic myocarditis results in signs of heart failure, including dyspnea, pulmonary edema, and hydrothorax.

Arthritis in calves also follows pneumonia by 7 to 10 days, and fetlocks and tarsi are frequently affected. Joints become hot and swollen with serofibrinous fluid that is a thinner consistency than normal joint fluid.

Otitis is associated with chronic pneumonia and is caused by the ascension of *H. somni* in the eustachian tube. Animals may exhibit facial paralysis, nystagmus, and ear drooping. Brainstem involvement at the level of the seventh and eighth cranial nerves may result in vestibular signs.

Conjunctivitis may occur independently of pneumonia, but more commonly follows an acute episode. Large numbers of animals may be involved.

Myelitis occurs in weaned calves when organisms embolize to the brainstem and spinal cord. Animals may exhibit hindlimb or quadrilateral paresis, usually concurrently with TEME.

Histophilus somni causes inflammatory disease of the genital tract in association with vulvitis, vaginitis, endometritis, and, rarely, orchitis. Isolation of *H. somni* from semen and prepuce of apparently healthy bulls suggests possible venereal transmission. The organism has also been recovered from the bladder and urine, so urinary contamination of the environment may disseminate the infection in a herd.

Histophilus somni lacks a capsule, a clearly defined exotoxin, and fimbriae or other surface structures that would explain its virulence. Infection often results in septicemia, and lesions are characterized by multifocal vasculitis, thrombosis, and infarction, with a large influx of neutrophils. The organism adheres to endothelial cells in vitro and induces cytotoxic changes. *Histophilus somni* lipooligosaccharide induces apoptosis of bovine endothelial cells in vitro, leading to vasculitis in vivo. Bacterial induction of apoptosis appears to be important in evasion of destruction by host neutrophils. Lodging of organisms in smaller vessels and production of fibrin thrombi are likely involved in pathogenesis of neurologic signs, myocarditis, and arthritis. Experimental data indicate that *H. somni* is embryocidal, suggesting a role in early embryonic death. Retrograde infection of the pregnant uterus from the lower genital tract may account for endometritis. Abortion appears to result from necrotic placentitis and formation of fibrinoid thrombi in the vessels of fetal brain, lungs, and glomeruli.

Intracellular survival and replication may be an important virulence factor in the dissemination of infection within the host. *Histophilus somni* multiplies in bovine neutrophils and mononuclear phagocytes, such as alveolar macrophages and blood monocytes. The organism resides in discrete intracellular vacuoles, and phagosome-lysosome fusion apparently does not occur.

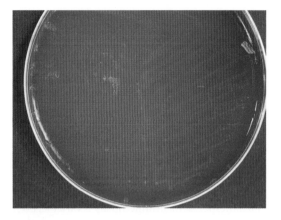

FIGURE 24-5 *Histophilus somni* on bovine blood agar, showing characteristic α-hemolysis. (Courtesy Karen W. Post.)

Lipooligosaccharide phase variation may further facilitate evasion of the host immune response.

Laboratory diagnosis is based primarily on bacterial cultivation and identification. However, isolation of the organism from the reproductive tract does not provide adequate evidence of infection because *H. somni* may be a normal resident. Traditional phenotypic methods of identification (Figure 24-5 and Table 24-5) have been used extensively, but generally lack the discriminatory power of molecular or immunologic assays such as in situ hybridization and immunohistochemical methods. PCR has been suggested as a diagnostic adjunct to cultivation of *H. somni*. Serologic methods, such as microscopic agglutination, complement fixation, or the more sensitive and specific enzyme immunoassays, have been used

TABLE **24-5** Phenotypic Characteristics That Allow Separation of the Genus *Histophilus* from Similar Genera

Test	Histophilus	Haemophilus	Actinobacillus	Pasteurella	Mannheimia
β-Hemolysis (bovine blood)	Neg	Neg	Var	Var	Var
Yellow pigmentation	Pos	Neg	Neg	Neg	Neg
X- or V-factor dependence	Neg	Pos	Var	Neg	Neg
Capnophilia	Pos	Neg	Neg	Neg	Neg
Catalase	Neg	Neg	Pos	(Pos)	Pos
Indole	(Pos)	Var	(Neg)	Var	(Neg)
Urease	Neg	Var	(Pos)	Var	Neg
FERMENTATION:					
Maltose	Neg	Pos	Pos	Var	Var
Sucrose	Neg	Neg	Pos	Pos	Pos

Neg, Negative; *(Neg),* most negative; *Pos,* positive; *(Pos),* most positive; *Var,* variable.

for antemortem diagnosis. Cattle with respiratory or systemic infections will exhibit at least a fourfold increase in titer within 14 to 21 days of exposure.

Satisfactory prevention and control of diseases attributed to *H. somni* is perhaps best achieved by preinfection immunization. Whole-cell killed vaccines do not adequately protect against systemic infection, offering only slight reductions in morbidity and mortality.

Control requires early and accurate identification of carrier animals. Serologic surveillance of calves and early antimicrobial therapy are advocated. Response to antimicrobials is variable, even though the organism is susceptible to many agents. Individuals with TEME, septicemia, and pneumonia frequently die before antimicrobial therapy is initiated. Once a diagnosis has been obtained, prophylactic mass medication of penmates is usually instituted with ceftiofur, spectinomycin, enrofloxacin, or florfenicol.

THE GENUS *TAYLORELLA*

The gram-negative coccobacillus *Taylorella equigenitalis* is the etiologic agent of contagious equine metritis (CEM), an important equine venereal disease. CEM was first reported in 1977 in Thoroughbred mares in the United Kingdom, where it was initially described as *Haemophilus equigenitalis* because of its fastidious growth requirements. Within 2 years the disease had spread to Ireland, France, Australia, Belgium, the United States, and Germany. 16S rDNA sequencing revealed a phylogenetic position in the β-subclass of the Proteobacteria, and resulted in the transfer of *H. equigenitalis* into the new genus *Taylorella*. *Taylorella equigenitalis* is most closely related to *Pelistega europaea*, a novel bacterium associated with pigeon respiratory disease, and more distantly related to both *Alcaligenes xylosoxidans* and *Bordetella bronchiseptica*.

A second species, *Taylorella asinigenitalis*, was isolated from the urethral fossa of donkeys in Kentucky and California. It grows more slowly than *T. equigenitalis*, reacts weakly in an indirect fluorescent antibody test with *T. equigenitalis*–specific antibody, and is substantially different in DNA-DNA hybridization assays. *Taylorella asinigenitalis* does not appear capable of producing disease in mares or jacks.

Stallions do not develop clinical signs of disease, but harbor the bacterium in the prepuce and urethral fossa for extended periods.

Taylorella equigenitalis introduced during coitus replicates in the uterus and causes severe endometrial inflammation, from which mares usually recover. The influx of neutrophils, mononuclear phagocytes, and plasma cells is the basis for the copious mucopurulent vaginal discharge that is characteristic of CEM. Temporary infertility is common, and early embryonic death or abortion is not uncommon. About 25% of infected mares become longtime carriers. Foals born to infected mares may become infected, either in utero or during parturition.

Diagnosis has been based on culture of the bacterium from its sites of predilection in the reproductive tracts of mares and stallions. Cervix, clitoral fossa, and clitoral sinuses of mares are often culture positive, as are the urethra, urethral diverticulum and fossa, and prepuce in stallions. Swabs from these sites should be transported in Amie's medium with charcoal, and should reach the laboratory in a refrigerated state within 48 hours of collection. Other specimens for culture include vaginal and uterine discharges, placentae, and fetal tissues. Although *T. equigenitalis* is not dependent on X or V factors, growth is enhanced in the presence of hemin. Primary isolation media include Eugon chocolate agar with and without streptomycin, and CEM Timoney, a selective medium supplemented with equine blood,

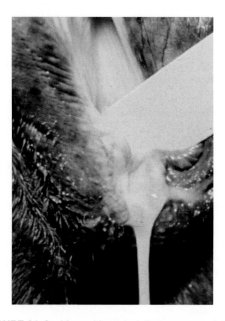

FIGURE 24-6 Mare with vaginal discharge associated with contagious equine metritis. (Courtesy J. Glenn Songer.)

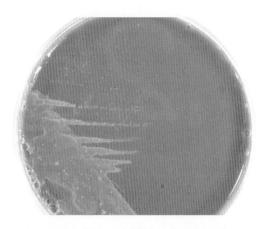

FIGURE 24-7 Colonies of *Taylorella equigenitalis* on chocolate agar. (Courtesy Karen W. Post.)

trimethoprim, clindamycin, and amphotericin B. Plates are incubated at 37° C in 5% to 10% CO_2 and examined daily for up to 1 week (Figure 24-6).

Colonies are approximately 1 mm in diameter, entire, convex, opaque, grayish, and butryous in consistency after growth on Eugon chocolate agar for 48 hours (Figure 24-7). Staining reveals gram-negative pleomorphic coccobacilli. The organism is oxidase and catalase positive, does not reduce nitrate, does not produce indole, produces alkaline phosphatase, does not hydrolyze urea or esculin, and is asaccharolytic. It does not grow on MacConkey agar, on Eugon chocolate agar plates incubated in ambient air, or anaerobically at 37° C. Slide agglutination or commercial latex agglutination tests, using high-titered antiserum to *T. equigenitalis,* can be performed on suspect isolates to confirm their identity.

Serologic tests, such as enzyme immunoassay and complement fixation, have been used to diagnose disease in mares, which, unlike stallions, develop antibodies demonstrable during the early convalescent phase of infection. PCR assays allow rapid detection of *T. equigenitalis* in clinical specimens. A multiplex PCR assay distinguishes *T. equigenitalis* and *T. asinigenitalis.*

Because of the highly contagious and costly nature of CEM, prevention and control measures have been instituted in every country heavily involved in the equine breeding industry. All horses and donkeys imported to or exported from the United States are tested for *T. equigenitalis,* primarily by bacterial culture. Breeding farm management measures include quarantine of new herd additions, early detection and treatment of infected individuals, and sound hygienic practices. Treatment protocols are available for elimination of the carrier state. One method involves the daily washing of the external genitalia of the stallion with 2% chlorhexidene followed by topical application of nitrofurazone ointment. Daily uterine infusions of penicillin have been used to eradicate the infection from mares.

SUGGESTED READINGS

Angen O, Ahrens P, Kuhnert P, et al: Proposal of *Histophilus somni* gen. nov., sp. nov. for the three species in *certae sedis* 'Haemophilus somnus,' 'Haemophilus agni' and 'Histophilus ovis,' *Int J Syst Evol Microbiol* 53:1449-1456, 2003.

Beeman KB: *Haemophilus somnus* of cattle: an overview, *Compend Cont Ed Pract Vet* 7:S259-S264, 1985.

Blackall PJ: Infectious coryza: overview of disease and new diagnostic options, *Clin Microbiol Rev* 12: 627-632, 1999.

Rapp-Gabrielson VJ: *Haemophilus parasuis.* In Straw B, Mengeling W, eds: *Diseases of Swine,* ed 8, Ames, Iowa, 1999, Iowa State University Press.

Chapter 25

The Genus *Brucella*

Brucellosis was first described by British physician David Bruce, who in 1886 isolated a bacterium from the spleens of patients with a fatal disease known as Malta or Mediterranean fever. He named the agent *Micrococcus melitensis*. L.F. Benhard Bang, a Danish veterinarian, recovered what we now know as *Brucella abortus* from a bovine fetus in 1895. Recognition of brucellosis as a zoonosis in the early twentieth century contributed to establishment of requirements for pasteurization of milk.

Brucella spp. are gram-negative, strictly aerobic, nonmotile, coccobacilli or small rods. They are facultative intracellular parasites that are taxonomically categorized in the class α-Proteobacteria, order Rhizobiales, family Brucellaceae. They produce oxidase, catalase, nitrate reductase, and urease (except *Brucella ovis*); fail to produce indole; are nonhemolytic; do not liquefy gelatin; and have negative methyl red and Voges-Proskauer tests. Most (again except *B. ovis*); utilize glucose as an energy source. *Brucella* spp. have been classified as potential agents of bioterrorism because they may be spread by aerosol and there are no human vaccines.

According to the strict phylogenetic definition of a species, taxonomists have proposed that the genus comprise a single species, *Brucella melitensis*. However, historical precedent has led to retention of the six classical "species," *B. abortus*, *B. melitensis*, *Brucella suis*, *B. ovis*, *Brucella canis*, and *Brucella neotomae*. Each "species" has a preferred host that serves as a main reservoir for infection (Table 25-1). These have been further divided into biovars based on agglutination by monospecific antisera prepared against A and M lipopolysaccharide antigens, and other phenotypic properties.

DISEASES AND EPIDEMIOLOGY

Members of the genus *Brucella* are the agents of brucellosis, a worldwide zoonotic illness. The disease is highly endemic in Mediterranean countries, Africa, the Middle East, India, central Asia, and Central and South America. It has virtually been eliminated from the United States and Canada as a result of extensive eradication programs. The host range includes humans, ruminants, swine, cervids, lagomorphs, rodents, canids, and marine mammals. Cats appear to be resistant to infection because there have been no reports of naturally occurring disease. Brucellosis remains a reportable disease in both the United States and Canada. Infection occurs through inhalation or ingestion of organisms.

Since brucellae are intracellular pathogens of animal hosts, they are not known to pursue an independent lifestyle. Animals are the reservoirs and can be the source of infection. Organisms reside inside cells of the reticuloendothelial system and reproductive tract and cause lifelong, chronic infections. They are the leading cause of abortion and sterility in domestic animals. High numbers of bacteria are shed in urine, milk, vaginal discharges, semen, and the products of birth.

TABLE 25-1   Species of *Brucella,* Hosts, and Diseases

Primary Host	Principal Species	Disease(s)	Biovars	Other Species Isolated
Cattle	*B. abortus*	Abortion, orchitis, epididymitis	7	*B. melitensis* *B. suis*
Goats	*B. melitensis*	Abortion, mastitis, lameness, orchitis	3	*B. abortus*
Sheep	*B. ovis*	Ram epididymitis, orchitis, infertility, nephritis.	1	*B. abortus*
		Sporadic abortion, vaginitis.		*B. melitensis*
Pigs	*B. suis*	Abortion, arthritis, infertility, orchitis,	5	*B. abortus*
Hares, caribou, reindeer, rodents		discospondylitis, abscesses		*B. melitensis*
Dogs	*B. canis*	Abortion, discospondylitis, epididymitis, infertility, uveitis, dermatitis, meningitis, glomerulonephritis, osteomyelitis	1	*B. abortus* *B. melitensis* *B. suis*
Wood rats	*B. neotomae*	Nonpathogenic	1	None
Marine mammals	*B. cetaceae* *B. pinnipediae*	Abortion, epididymitis, discospondylitis, abscesses, meningitis	?	None

Under appropriate conditions, *Brucella* can survive outside the host in the environment for extended periods. They may remain viable in carcasses and tissues for up to 6 months at approximately 0° C. They survive up to 125 days in dust or soil, and for as long as 1 year in feces. Brucellae are susceptible to many disinfectants, including 1% sodium hypochlorite, phenolics, 70% ethanol, iodophors, glutaraldehyde, and formaldehyde. The presence of organic matter or use in low temperatures may greatly reduce the efficacy of the disinfectant. The organisms are physically inactivated by moist heat (121° C, ≥15 minutes) and by dry heat (160°-170° C, ≥1 hour).

Brucella abortus is the etiologic agent of bovine brucellosis (Bang's disease), and is found in most cattle-producing areas of the world. The organism preferentially infects bovidae, but is sometimes transmitted to other animals, including cervids, camels, dogs, horses, sheep, goats, and pigs. American bison and elk in the Yellowstone area are one remaining reservoir of *B. abortus* in the United States.

In cattle, brucellosis is primarily a disease of the cow. Bulls can be infected but they do not readily transmit the organism venereally. *Brucella abortus* localizes in the testicles, resulting in unilateral orchitis, epididymitis, and inflammation of the accessory reproductive organs, with decreased libido and impaired fertility. In the cow there is a predilection for udder, endometrium, and associated lymph nodes. Clinical signs in infected cows include abortion during or after the fifth month of gestation, birth of weak calves, or retained placenta. Although infected cows typically abort only once, the placenta becomes colonized by brucellae during each pregnancy. These subsequent offspring may be born weak or apparently healthy. Because of in utero infection or ingestion of contaminated milk in the neonatal period, apparently healthy heifer calves may become carriers and pose a significant risk to herd and human health. *Brucella abortus* is shed in large numbers in the afterbirth, placental fluids, aborted fetus, and vaginal discharge. Cattle become infected when they ingest contaminated forage or lick calves or aborted fetuses.

Horses may be naturally infected with *B. abortus,* and the organism has a tendency to localize in joints, bursae, or tendon sheaths. It has been recovered from lesions of fistulous withers, poll evil, and hygroma. The current opinion is that horses are relatively refractory to infection with *Brucella* and present a minimal hazard to other animals. Sporadic infections with *B. abortus* have been reported in dogs ingesting reproductive material from infected cows. Abortion, epididymitis, and joint lesions occur in affected animals. There is also circumstantial evidence that dog-to-cattle transmission occurs under field conditions.

Brucella melitensis most commonly infects sheep and goats. The organism is regarded as the most virulent of the *Brucella* species and accounts for most cases of human brucellosis.

It has occasionally been isolated from camels and alpacas. Disease is endemic in the Middle East, the Iberian Peninsula, China, the former Soviet Union, parts of Africa, and Latin America. The epidemiology and pathogenesis are similar to that of *B. abortus*. The main risk factors are contact with contaminated genital discharges and ingestion of raw milk. Sexual transmission is more frequent than in bovine brucellosis. Breed susceptibility is variable in sheep, but goat breeds are highly susceptible. Some animals may spontaneously recover from infection, but the majority remain chronic carriers. Clinical signs include abortion, mastitis, lameness, and orchitis.

Brucella ovis has long been recognized as a pathogen of sheep and displays a high degree of host specificity. Ovine brucellosis is of great economic significance in most sheep-rearing countries. Although it occasionally is associated with abortion, it primarily affects rams. Infectious epididymitis, orchitis, and infertility are common disease manifestations. Persistent nephritis can develop in rams and is the most serious complication of infection. Ewes are often transiently infected, with vaginitis, stillbirths, or birth of weak lambs. Ovine brucellosis is most commonly spread directly from ram to ram by sexual contact, or indirectly, from sexual contact with ewes that have been inseminated by infected rams.

The host range of *B. suis* is variable. Swine are primary hosts for biovars 1, 2, and 3, and hares are important natural reservoirs of biovar 2. Disease in reindeer and caribou is associated with biovar 4, whereas biovar 5 is maintained by certain species of rodents in the Caucasus region of Eurasia. All biovars of *B. suis* can cause serious infections in man.

Swine brucellosis affects pigs of all ages and breeds. Males and females are equally susceptible to infection. In piglets, *B. suis* may produce a self-limiting infection that remains confined to the lymph nodes. However, most animals develop bacteremia that results in localization of the agent in the bones, joints, reproductive tract, and the organs of the reticuloendothelial system. The formation of abscesses or miliary lesions is a characteristic of infection. Swine brucellosis may cause no overt clinical signs, but in most instances, abortion, infertility, orchitis, lameness, or posterior paralysis is observed. Abortions occur between the fourth and twelfth weeks of gestation. Aborted placentae are usually edematous, hemorrhagic, and covered with yellowish brown exudates. Pregnancies proceeding to term may result in birth of weak, stillborn, or mummified piglets, or piglets may be completely normal.

Brucella canis is isolated from dogs in kennels, although natural disease has also been described in foxes and coyotes. Infection usually results from ingestion or inhalation of organisms aerosolized from aborted fetuses, vaginal discharges, milk, semen, or urine. Dogs become infected after 4 to 6 months of cohabitation with an infected individual. Only the uterine epithelial cells of the gravid bitch are colonized. This may result in early embryonic death or abortion. If pups are carried until term, both live and stillborns may be whelped in the same litter. Rarely do live infected pups survive. Nonpregnant bitches show no overt clinical signs of illness, but may shed organisms in salivary, nasal, or vaginal secretions. In the male, brucellosis manifests as infertility, with epididymitis, rather than orchitis, as the prominent feature. Spermatogenesis is severely reduced. The prostate remains persistently infected, explaining the presence of high numbers of brucellae shed in urine, but clinical signs of prostatitis are not evident. *Brucella canis* also infects other sites, causing anterior uveitis, osteomyelitis, discospondylitis, meningitis, pyogranulomatous dermatitis, and glomerulonephritis.

The desert wood rat *(Neotoma lepida)*, which is native to the American West, is the natural host for *B. neotomae*. This organism has been isolated from rodents on few occasions, and apparently not in association with pathogenic processes. No verified cases of natural infection have been in other species, including humans.

Isolation of brucellae from marine mammals, in particular dolphins, porpoises, seals, and European otters, was first reported in 1994. Presumptive diagnosis in these cases was by demonstration of serum anti-*Brucella* antibodies, and additional hosts identified by this method include whales and walruses. Most isolations have been from animals without lesions, but a wide range of associated pathology has also been found, including placentitis and possible abortion, epididymitis, meningitis, subcutaneous abscessation, and discospondylitis. Proposed new species are *B. cetaceae*, for dolphin and porpoise isolates, and *B. pinnipediae*, for seal strains.

Brucellosis in humans is known as undulant fever because of fluctuations in body temperature that are characteristic of the disease. It is an occupational disease of veterinarians, abattoir workers, laboratorians, and farmers. All brucellae are potentially pathogenic for humans, but *B. abortus, B. melitensis, B. canis,* and *B. suis* are responsible for most clinical disease. Ruminants are the primary reservoirs for human infection and the most common mode of transmission is consumption of unpasteurized dairy products. Other routes of infection are contamination of abraded or unbroken skin, inhalation of infectious aerosols, and contamination of conjunctiva or other mucous membranes. The infectious dose by the inhalation route has been estimated at 10 to 100 organisms. The incubation period is variable, ranging from 5 days to 2 months. Human brucellosis is a systemic illness with an acute or insidious onset. Symptoms include intermittent fever, chills, sweating, headache, arthralgia, and weakness. Subclinical infections are frequent. Localized suppurative infections may also develop. The case fatality rate in untreated cases is less than 5%, and the relapse rate is high. Person-to-person transmission is very rare because humans tend to be dead-end hosts.

PATHOGENESIS

Most information on pathogenesis has been based on our understanding of *B. abortus,* and disease caused by most species is much the same. Brucellae are shed near the time of abortion or parturition, as well as in milk from chronic infection of supramammary lymph nodes and from other body sites. Susceptible animals ingest bacteria that invade the oral mucosa and gain entry to regional lymph nodes either in a free state or within phagocytes. The organism localizes and proliferates in the lymph nodes during an incubation period that ranges from 2 weeks to 7 months. After a subsequent bacteremic period, *Brucella* spp. localize in cells of the reticuloendothelial system (spleen, liver, supramammary lymph nodes, or bone marrow), mammary glands, and reproductive organs. During midgestation, *B. abortus* proliferates in and around placental cotyledons, in large part due to the growth-stimulatory effects of erythritol, which is present in high concentrations in cotyledons and fetal fluids of ruminants. Necrotic placentitis results and abortion is attributed to fetal anoxia and endotoxemia.

Unlike most other pathogenic bacteria, no classical virulence factors, such as exotoxins, cytolysins, fimbriae, capsules, or apoptosis inducers have been described for the brucellae. The true virulence of *Brucella* spp. appears to be in their ability to invade and survive within host cells. They use mechanisms that avoid or inhibit the fusion of the initial phagosome with the lysosome. Inhibition of tumor necrosis factor-α (TNF-α) production may be another virulence mechanism because TNF-α is involved in intracellular killing. Some species of *Brucella* secrete a heat- and protease-sensitive factor that is important for survival inside human macrophages and contributes to the chronic nature of the disease.

DIAGNOSIS

Laboratory diagnosis is based on direct examination of clinical specimens using modified acid-fast stains, bacterial culture, and serology. Although *Brucella* species are not acid fast, they resist decolorization with mild acids, a property that provides the basis for differential staining methods such as the modified Koster's stain. Brucellae stain red by this method. Direct examination of tissues with a fluorescent antibody preparation can be useful when applied to clinical specimens that are heavily contaminated.

The most valuable specimens for bacterial culture are aborted fetal tissues (especially lung, spleen, and stomach contents), placentae, lymph nodes, postparturient uterus, vaginal discharge, semen, urine, and bone marrow. Blood culture is the single best diagnostic test for canine brucellosis. Brucellae are fastidious and some species have specific growth requirements, including amino acids, nicotinamide, thiamine, and magnesium ions. Growth may be further enhanced by addition of blood or serum to plated agar medium and incubation in an environment of 8% to 10% CO_2. Tryptose or trypticase soy agar containing 5% serum is recommended for a nonselective medium. Addition of antibiotics (cycloheximide, bacitracin, and polymyxin B) or dyes (crystal violet) to tryptose or trypticase serum agar has proven effective in suppressing overgrowth of bacterial contaminants. Plates are incubated up to 14 days at 37° C before being discarded as negative.

Brucella colonies generally become visible after cultures have been incubated for 3 to 5 days. They are usually small (0.5-1 mm in diameter), round with entire margins, translucent, and have a pale, honey color (Figure 25-1). Older colonies are larger (2-4 mm diameter) and more brown.

Microscopically, cells are 0.5 to 0.7 μm wide by 0.6 to 1.5 μm long, and are arranged singly or occasionally in short chains (Figure 25-2).

Brucella spp. and their biovars have traditionally been distinguished in the clinical laboratory based on host specificity, sensitivity to the dyes thionin and basic fuchsin, requirement for CO_2, production of hydrogen sulfide, rate of urease activity, agglutination in monospecific rabbit antisera, and phage typing (Table 25-2). All smooth strains of *Brucella* spp. possess major surface antigens A and M in varying amounts on their polysaccharide chains. Rough strains of brucellae (*B. ovis* and *B. canis*) do not agglutinate in A or M antisera, but will agglutinate in R antiserum.

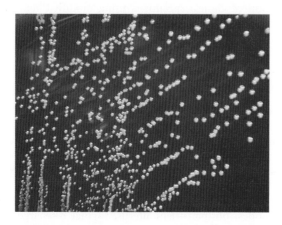

FIGURE 25-1 Smooth, pinpoint, entire, translucent, nonhemolytic colonies of *Brucella melitensis*. (Courtesy Public Health Image Library, PHIL #1902, Centers for Disease Control and Prevention, Atlanta, 2002, Larry Stauffer, Oregon State Public Health Laboratory.)

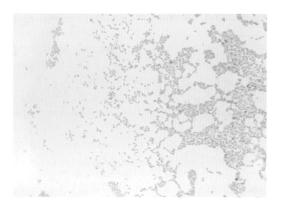

FIGURE 25-2 *Brucella melitensis* (Gram stain). (Courtesy Public Health Image Library, PHIL #1937, Centers for Disease Control and Prevention, Atlanta, date unknown.)

Bacteriophages are often used to identify and type isolates. The most common is the Tbilisi phage. The phage is used at the so-called routine test dilution (RTD), which correlates to 10^4 to 10^5 plaque-forming units per ml.

Brucellosis has remained one of the most common laboratory-acquired infections. Biosafety level 2 practices should be followed for all activities involving clinical specimens, whereas biosafety level 3 practices, containment, and facilities are recommended for all manipulation of bacterial cultures. Protective clothing should include a laboratory coat and gloves when directly handling clinical materials such as infected body fluids (urine, blood, vaginal discharge, or semen), contaminated tissues, aborted fetuses, and placentae. Gloves and a gown (tight wrists and tie in back) should be worn for all work with live bacterial cultures in a biosafety cabinet. Primary laboratory hazards include exposure to aerosols, direct skin contact with bacterial isolates, and accidental inoculation.

No other bacterial disease has a greater variety of serodiagnostic tests than those available for detection of *B. abortus* infection in cattle. These detect different immunoglobulin classes. The usual serologic screening test for *B. abortus* antibodies is the buffered acidified plate antigen (BAPA) test. Although this test is economical, interpretation of results is prone to subjectivity, with variation between individual technicians and laboratories. Rivanol, complement fixation, rapid agglutination presumptive, and particle concentration fluorescence immunoassay (PCFIA) tests are official supplemental tests. The latter two have recently been adopted in order to standardize testing (Table 25-3). Serologic cross-reactions may occur in cattle exposed to *Yersinia*, *Francisella*, and *Escherichia coli* O157:H7.

Serologic tests are used for diagnosis in other animal species. The intradermal test for delayed hypersensitivity is used as a herd- or flock-screening test for diagnosis of *B. melitensis* infection. A tube agglutination test is useful for detection of antibodies to *B. canis*, but agar gel immunodiffusion remains the gold standard to confirm a serologic diagnosis. Enzyme immunoassays are routinely used to screen sheep flocks for exposure to *B. ovis*. Although no single test is reliable in the serologic diagnosis of swine brucellosis, the buffered plate test is still the most effective and practical means for testing large numbers of animals.

TABLE **25-2** Phenotypic Identification of *Brucella* Species and Biovars

Brucella Species	Biovar	CO₂ Required	H₂S Produced*	Urease <5 Minutes	Urease >5 Minutes	Growth with Thionin†	Growth with Fuchsin†	Agglutination in Monospecific Antisera: A	M	R	Lysis by Phage RTD‡	RTD × 10⁴
B. abortus	1	(Pos)	Pos	Neg	Pos	Neg	Pos	Pos	Neg	Neg	Pos	Pos
	2	(Pos)	Pos	Neg	Pos	Neg	Neg	Pos	Neg	Neg	Pos	Pos
	3	(Pos)	Pos	Neg	Pos	Pos	Pos	Pos	Neg	Neg	Pos	Pos
	4	(Pos)	Pos	Neg	Pos	Neg	Pos	Neg	Pos	Neg	Pos	Pos
	5	Neg	Neg	Neg	Pos	Pos	Pos	Neg	Pos	Neg	Pos	Pos
	6	Neg	(Neg)	Neg	Pos	Pos	Pos	Pos	Neg	Neg	Pos	Pos
	7	(Neg)	Pos	Neg	Pos	Pos	Pos	Neg	Pos	Neg	Pos	Pos
B. canis		Neg	Neg	Pos		Pos	Neg	Neg	Neg	Pos	Neg	Neg
B. melitensis	1	Neg	Neg	Var	Pos	Pos	Pos	Neg	Pos	Neg	Neg	Neg
	2	Neg	Neg	Var	Pos	Pos	Pos	Pos	Neg	Neg	Neg	Neg
	3	Neg	Neg	Var	Pos	Pos	Pos	Pos	Pos	Neg	Neg	Neg
B. neotomae		Neg	Pos	Neg	Neg	Neg	Neg	Pos	Neg	Neg	Neg	Pos
B. ovis		Pos	Neg	Neg	Neg	Pos	(Pos)	Neg	Neg	Pos	Neg	Neg
B. suis	1	Neg	Pos	Pos		Pos	Neg	Pos	Neg	Neg	Neg	Pos
	2	Neg	Neg	Pos		Pos	Neg	Pos	Neg	Neg	Neg	Pos
	3	Neg	Neg	Pos		Pos	Pos	Pos	Neg	Neg	Neg	Pos
	4	Neg	Neg	Pos		Pos	(Neg)	Pos	Pos	Neg	Neg	Pos
	5	Neg	Neg	Pos		Pos	Neg	Neg	Pos	Neg	Neg	Pos
B. pinnipediae		Pos	Neg	ND		Pos	Pos	Pos	(Neg)	Neg	(Neg)	(Pos)
B. cetaceae		Neg	Neg	ND		Pos	Pos	Pos	Var	Neg	(Neg)	Var

*H₂S produced in heart infusion agar.

†1/50,000 w/v.

‡Routine test dilution for Tbilisi phage.

ND, Not determined; *Neg*, negative; *(Neg)*, most negative; *Pos*, positive; *(Pos)*, most positive; *RTD*, routine test dilution; *Var*, variable.

TABLE **25-3**   Serologic Tests for Diagnosis of Bovine Brucellosis

Test	Predominant Antibody Class(es) Detected	Test Principle
BAPA	IgM, IgG	Agglutination (quantitative)
Card	IgG	Agglutination (qualitative)
Rivanol	IgG	Tube or plate agglutination test (quantitative); rivanol destroys IgM
Complement fixation	IgG	Complement fixation, erythrocyte lysis as indicator (quantitative)
Milk ring	IgG	Agglutination; detects milk antibody
RAP	IgG	Rapid automated presumptive test; microscopic agglutination
PCFIA	IgG	Antigen on submicron polystyrene particles in microtiter plates binds to its specific antibody; reacts with fluorescein-labeled affinity-purified antibovine IgG; solid phase separated by filtration; total particle-bound fluorescence determined by front-surface fluorimetry

BAPA, Buffered acidified plate antigen; *IgG,* immunoglobulin G; *IgM,* immunoglobulin M; *PCFIA,* particle concentration fluorescence immunoassay; *RAP,* rapid agglutination presumptive.

Numerous polymerase chain reaction (PCR) assays have been developed for identification of *Brucella* to improve diagnostic capabilities. These can discriminate among the classical species and biovars, but are not widely available.

PREVENTION AND CONTROL

Testing and elimination of infected animals is the only proven method to control brucellosis in animals. Efforts to eradicate *B. abortus* in the United States began in 1934, with the inception of the State-Federal Brucellosis Eradication Program. Primary surveillance was through the market cattle testing program and milk ring testing. Serologic testing is still performed at all livestock markets and slaughterhouses, using the card agglutination test. Milk from commercial dairy herds is screened periodically by the milk ring test for antibodies to brucellae. These methods have been combined with herd quarantine and repeated testing of suspect herds to facilitate disease eradication in most states.

The use of vaccines has been a major factor in the success of the brucellosis eradication program in cattle in the United States. Strain 19 was officially approved for vaccine use in 1939. Whole herd vaccination included the use of a reduced dose of Strain 19 in adult cows, in addition to its administration to heifers 4 to 12 months of age. Adult vaccination increased herd resistance and decreased the degree of bacterial shedding during parturition or abortion. Its use resulted in false-positive serologic tests, in that tests were unable to discriminate between vaccinal and natural antibodies. In 1996, the U.S. Department of Agriculture (USDA) approved use of a new brucellosis vaccine that, like the Strain 19 vaccine, is based upon a live, avirulent strain, in this case designated RB-51. Unlike Strain-19, antibodies stimulated by the RB-51 vaccine are not detected by standard brucellosis serologic tests. Thus, under ideal circumstances, false positives due to brucellosis-vaccinated cattle have been alleviated. The RB-51 vaccine is administered only by state and federal brucellosis program personnel and USDA-accredited veterinarians. The vaccination age of heifers is 4 to 10 months of age, and permanent identification, in the form of a USDA brucellosis eartag and ear tattoo, is required for all vaccinated cattle. The only other commercially available vaccine is for *B. melitensis.* REV1 is a live, attenuated strain of *B. melitensis,* which is used in many countries to immunize goats and sheep. The strain is very stable, of low virulence, and imparts a high level of protection.

Brucella spp. are susceptible in vitro to a wide range of antimicrobial agents, including tetracyclines, streptomycin, rifampin, fluoroquinolones, and aminoglycosides. Treatment of infected animals is not advocated. No therapeutic regimen is 100% effective. Unsuccessfully treated animals remain a source of infection for other animals and pose a significant zoonotic threat to their owners. Transmission is much less likely in neutered animals, but brucellae can still persist in tissues of these animals.

The standard therapy for uncomplicated human infections consists of a combination of doxycycline and rifampin for 6 weeks. For disease complications such as endocarditis or meningoencephalitis, triple therapy with rifampin, a tetracycline, and an aminoglycoside has been recommended.

SUGGESTED READINGS

Ficht TA: Intracellular survival of *Brucella:* defining the link with persistence, *Vet Microbiol* 92:213-223, 2003.

Jahans KL, Foster G, Broughton ES: The characterization of *Brucella* strains isolated from marine mammals, *Vet Microbiol* 57:373-382, 1997.

Johnson CA, Walker RD: Clinical signs and diagnosis of *Brucella canis* infection, *Compend Contin Educ Pract Vet* 14:763-773, 1992.

Ko J, Splitter GA: Molecular host-pathogen interaction in brucellosis: current understanding and future approaches to vaccine development for mice and humans, *Clin Microbiol Rev* 16:65-78, 2003.

Chapter 26

The Genus *Francisella*

*F*rancisella tularensis was isolated in 1912, during studies of a plaguelike disease in rodents in Tulare County, California, from which the specific name is derived. This organism spent many decades in the genus *Pasteurella,* but was reclassified in 1947 into a new genus named for Edward Francis, a U.S. Public Health Service physician who first cultivated the organism and described its transmission and the clinical syndromes resulting from infection. Tularemia (rabbit fever, hare fever, deerfly fever, lemming fever, or Ohara's disease) remains an important zoonosis, as well as a primary pathogen of wild and domestic animals. The high infectivity of *F. tularensis,* its ready dissemination by aerosol, its ability to cause severe respiratory disease, and its documented weaponization by various biological warfare programs worldwide have led to its classification as a Category A select agent. Before and during World War II, Japanese research units studied weaponization of *F. tularensis,* as did the United States from the war's end until biological weapons programs were dismantled in 1969.

Francisella tularensis is found in association with many hosts, ranging from mammals to birds to arthropods, and in the environment. It is broadly distributed in the Northern Hemisphere, including extensive occurrence throughout North America.

DISEASE

Francisella tularensis is a small pleomorphic, facultatively intracellular, Gram-negative coccobacillus, belonging to the class γ-Proteobacteria, order Thiotrichales, and family Francisellaceae. It is fastidious, usually requires cysteine for growth, and utilizes glucose as a carbon source, but is otherwise biochemically inert.

The organism is divided into four subspecies. *Francisella tularensis* ssp. *tularensis* (formerly Jellison type A) ferments glycerol, is highly virulent (particularly for laboratory rabbits), is found solely in North America, and is perhaps the most important in the context of disease. *Francisella tularensis* ssp. *holarctica* (formerly Jellison type B) is less virulent, but still an important cause of tularemia, and is found predominantly in Asia and Europe and only occasionally in North America. *Francisella tularensis* ssp. *mediaasiatica* has not been isolated from diseased humans and is found in Central Asia. *Francisella tularensis* ssp. *novicida* was previously *F. novicida* and is of low virulence for humans, with cases reported in the United States and Canada. Strains of *F. tularensis* ssp. *tularensis* cause the most severe disease in humans and rabbits, although all members of the species are highly mouse virulent. *Francisella philomiragia* is often found in water and causes disease only in the immunosuppressed.

Based on both 16S rDNA sequence comparisons and DNA–DNA hybridizations, *F. tularensis* has no close relatives, although the family Francisellaceae is relatively closely related to *Piscirickettsia salmonis* and ciliate and tick endosymbionts. The most closely related human pathogens (which are nonetheless distant) are

TABLE 26-1 Clinical Syndromes Associated with *Francisella tularensis* Infection

Syndrome	Description
Ulceroglandular	Mucosal or other epithelial ulcer, extension to lymph nodes
Glandular	Lymph node infection without apparent local ulceration
Oropharyngeal	Localized to oropharynx; necrotizing lesions of pharynx and upper digestive tract, gastrointestinal symptoms
Oculoglandular	Localized to eye; conjunctivitis, regional lymphadenopathy
Primary pneumonic	Lung infection following inhalation
Typhoidal	Fever, abdominal pain, prostration; no skin involvement, no lymphadenopathy; primary intestinal infection? dissemination from mesenteric lymph nodes?
All forms	Secondary pleuropneumonic involvement, meningitis, sepsis

Coxiella burnetii and *Legionella* spp., both of which have lifestyle similarities with *F. tularensis.*

Tularemia can take multiple clinical forms, depending on the portal of entry (Table 26-1). On the whole, it is plaguelike, and the infectious dose of highly virulent strains is astonishingly low, at only 10 to 50 colony-forming units. Most human cases result from arthropod bites (usually mosquitoes and ticks) previously fed on infected animals. If bacterial replication in skin at the point of entry causes formation of a distinct ulcer (Figure 26-1), the ensuing disease is called ulceroglandular tularemia. Organisms are transported from the ulcer to regional lymph nodes, where subsequent lesions resemble the buboes encountered in plague. Flulike signs appear after an incubation period of 3 to 5 days, with malaise, chills and fever, headache, sore throat, and myalgia; early misdiagnosis is common as a result of symptom nonspecificity. The organism may disseminate from the lymph node lesions to other sites throughout the body, including the lungs, in which case secondary pneumomic tularemia can result. Glandular tularemia is similar, but without an obvious route of entry. Glandular and ulceroglandular tularemia are the most common forms of the disease in humans. Hunters, trappers, and others in contact with infected animals or with arthropod vectors are the highest-risk groups, and infection is rarely fatal. Infection with low-virulence strains probably goes frequently undiagnosed.

Primary pneumonic tularemia is rare, but is the most severe of all the forms of the disease. It follows inhalation of *F. tularensis* and is a much more serious form of the disease. The case fatality rate in untreated respiratory infection with *F. tularensis* ssp. *tularensis* is as high as 60%. Hilar lymph node enlargement, dry cough, pleural effusion, and retrosternal pain are common symptoms, although radiography may reveal interstitial infiltrates with minimal pulmonary symptoms.

Francisella tularensis infects more than 100 species of wild and domestic mammals, 25 species of birds, and even fish, amphibians, and reptiles. Lagomorphs and rodents are important reservoir hosts because they often develop fulminant disease when infected and are hosts for Ixodid ticks (genera *Dermacentor, Ixodes,* and *Amblyomma*), which are both reservoirs and vectors of disease. *Francisella tularensis* may be able to pass transovarially in ticks. Other biting or blood-sucking arthropods, including mosquitoes, may also be porters of infection. The role of arthropods in transmission of tularemia, and in particular the specific relationship between bacterium and arthropod, is poorly understood. Transmission of *F. tularensis* to predator species is simplified by the lethargy and sluggishness induced by the disease in its terminal phase.

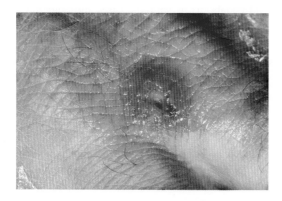

FIGURE 26-1 Ulcer caused by *Francisella tularensis* on the hand. (Courtesy Public Health Image Library, PHIL #2037, Centers for Disease Control and Prevention, Atlanta, 1963, P. Brachman.)

Clinical disease in livestock is rare. Natural infection has occurred in captive nonhuman primates, including squirrel monkeys, black and red tamarins, talapoins, and a lowland gorilla, all with depression, anorexia, vomiting, diarrhea, lymphadenopathy, and petechial hemorrhage.

Dogs may be reservoirs for *F. tularensis* or maintenance hosts for tick vectors, but clinical illness is more common in cats. The infectious dose for cats is quite high in comparison with that for humans, but manifestations of tularemia in cats range from subclinical to mild lymphadenopathy with fever to fulminant, ultimately fatal disease. Signs can include anorexia, dehydration, listlessness, lingual or oral ulceration, lymphadenopathy, hepatomegaly, icterus, and pneumonia.

Gross lesions in cats include small multifocal necrotic foci throughout mandibular, cervical, mesenteric, and hilar lymph nodes, as well as liver, spleen, and lungs. Necrosis of cortical lymph node follicles and splenic white pulp is conspicuous. Submucosal lymphoid follicles in intestines are likewise affected, with ulceration of Peyer's patches. Microscopic lesions manifest as focal or diffuse caseous necrosis surrounded by neutrophils, macrophages, and lymphocytes, in numbers varying with the stage of disease. Neither gross nor microscopic lesions are pathognomonic.

Natural infection in dogs is often associated with ingestion of wild rabbits, and is characterized by acute onset of anorexia, fever, lymphadenopathy, and necrotizing tonsillitis. Patients recover with supportive therapy. Experimental infections produce similar signs, and include fever, mucopurulent discharge from nose and eyes, and regional lymphadenopathy. Common seroconversion in dogs suggests that infection is equally common, and that illness is inapparent or mild.

Ovine tularemia can cause considerable morbidity and mortality, particularly in sheep in poor body condition, with poor nutritional status, and with heavy tick infestations. Affected sheep are pyrexic and anorexic, and have regional lymphadenopathy and diarrhea. Seroconversions suggest infection in cattle, but no definite clinical syndrome has been described. Infected mares and foals are febrile, dyspneic, depressed, tick infested, and lack coordination.

EPIDEMIOLOGY

Although fastidious in the laboratory and incapable of forming spores, *F. tularensis* survives for months in soil, mud, water, and on animal hides and carcasses. Organisms remain viable for more than 6 months in dry straw litter; more than 4 months in carcasses and organs, dust, grain, and bedbugs; nearly 3 months in tapwater and in mud or water stored at 7° C; and 1 month in rabbit meat. Transmission can occur by inoculation of skin, conjunctivae, oropharyngeal mucosa with infected blood, tissue, or arthropods; rarely by bites of infected animals; ingestion of contaminated food or water; inhalation of contaminated dust; and, as noted, bites of infected arthropods. The agent is thought to penetrate unbroken skin.

Predation by domestic carnivores is a significant risk factor for tularemia, as is ingestion of blood-sucking arthropods during grooming. The tick vectors most likely to transmit tularemia in the United States are the American dog tick (*Dermacentor variabilis*), the Lone Star tick (*Amblyomma americanum*), and the Rocky Mountain wood tick (*Dermacentor andersoni*). Deerflies and mosquitoes transmit the organism mechanically. Increased incidence in reservoir species is correlated with epidemics in humans and domestic animals.

Francisella tularensis replicates in amebae in a process that resembles *Francisella* spp. infection of macrophages. Replication is slow, and 25% to 40% of the amebae are killed, but the organism is found within amebal cysts. Thus these organisms may be important environmental reservoirs and the bacterium-ameba association could explain the ability of *F. tularensis* to survive in water.

Annual incidence in humans has declined from more than 2000 cases in 1939 to an average of about 125 cases. Most occur in Arkansas, Missouri, and Oklahoma as sporadic cases and epidemics. The most significant risk factors for humans in the United States are arthropod bites and direct contact with infected tissues. The peak number of cases in the United States and elsewhere occurs in late spring and summer, when arthropod bites are more likely to occur. There has also been a winter incidence peak in association with rabbit hunting. Direct contact with infected cats is also a means of transmission, usually by cat bite or scratch. Cats with subclinical illness can transmit, and many cases of feline tularemia are diagnosed retrospectively, after a primary diagnosis in human contacts. Dogs may transmit the bacterium mechanically, by mouth or by shaking contaminated water out of a coat. Human disease has followed shearing of dogs and sheep. Outbreaks of human disease have occurred following contact with muskrats, beavers, lagomorphs, squirrels, and pheasants, and epizootics occur in many of these species. Laboratory-acquired cases are not uncommon, and this is related to the ease of aerosolization. Person-to-person transmission of *F. tularensis* has not been documented.

Early in World War II, nearly 70,000 cases of tularemia occurred in the region surrounding Rostov-on-Don in the former Soviet Union. Similar, though less dramatic, experience during the recent conflicts in Bosnia and Kosovo suggests that tularemia, like other zoonotic diseases, may increase significantly in association with war and other disasters that interfere with standard hygiene and sanitary conditions.

Some of the more high-profile outbreaks have taken place in the northeastern United States, including specifically Martha's Vineyard. *Francisella tularensis* was imported to Cape Cod and Martha's Vineyard with cottontail rabbits, which were introduced from Arkansas and Missouri by game clubs in the late 1930s. Occurrence of disease in humans is significantly associated with mowing lawns or cutting brush in endemic areas, and many of the resulting cases are pneumonic. In one widely publicized case, two boys mowing a lawn discovered, by virtue of flying fur, that they had mowed over a dead rabbit. The event was sufficiently entertaining to induce them to repeat it, and both developed tularemia in due course.

PATHOGENESIS

Francisella tularensis enters the host by ingestion, inhalation, or injection. As noted, the infectious dose is quite small for ulceroglandular or pneumonic tularemia; however, it can be as high as 10^8 colony-forming units by the oral route. After entry and local multiplication, the organism disseminates by invading vascular endothelium (resulting in bacteremia) or by lymphatic spread (resulting in lymphadenitis). *Francisella tularensis* is readily phagocytosed, but survives and multiplies intracellularly. Thrombosis follows effects of the organism on capillary endothelium, and focal necrosis affects liver, spleen, lymph nodes, lung, and bone marrow. Necrotic foci enlarge and coalesce to form abscesses, and the inflammation becomes granulomatous. The humoral immune response manifests as nearly simultaneous

IgG, IgM, and IgA production 2 to 3 weeks after initiation of infection, but does not alter the course of infection with virulent strains. In keeping with the facultative intracellular pathogen status of *F. tularensis*, cell-mediated immunity is the key factor in host defense.

Few, if any, classical virulence factors have been identified for *F. tularensis*. Given its routes of infection, it seems likely that *F. tularensis* produces adhesins and invasins. However, these have not been described. Capsule is probably a virulence factor, but its composition and precise role in virulence are not known. Secreted toxins are apparently not produced.

Francisella tularensis can be cultivated in cell-free media, but is an intracellular pathogen in vivo. It replicates in macrophages, and apparently at about the same rate as in cell-free media. The organism is not detected in plasma of mice at various stages of disease, but is found readily in the leukocyte fraction. An acid phosphatase potently inhibits the respiratory burst in macrophages. An eventual result of infection of macrophages by *F. tularensis* is induction of apoptosis.

Macrophages treated with compounds that block endosome acidification have reduced capacity to support growth of *F. tularensis,* perhaps because of negative effects on iron acquisition by the organism. *Francisella tularensis* manipulates antimicrobial effector mechanisms of macrophages, inhibiting the release of proinflammatory cytokines by targeting the nuclear factor-B system and mitogen-activated protein kinase pathways.

The availability of a genome sequence for *F. tularensis* has allowed microarray-based strain comparisons with the end goal of identifying genes that are unique to high-virulence isolates.

DIAGNOSIS

Clinical diagnosis can be difficult because signs are nonspecific. In cats, white cell counts are not diagnostically useful, but there may be a left shift, thrombocytopenia, toxic effects on neutrophils, elevated serum transaminase activity, and hyperbilirubinemia. In dogs, laboratory findings are typically within normal ranges, except for occasionally elevated plasma fibrinogen concentration. Antemortem diagnosis is based on clinical signs, history, culture of bone marrow and lymph node aspirates, and serology. A minimum fourfold increase in anti–*F. tularensis* antibodies, detected by tube agglutination, microagglutination, hemagglutination, or enzyme-linked immunosorbent assay (ELISA), is considered diagnostic. A single specimen with a titer greater than or equal to 1:160 strongly suggests tularemia in a cat with other compatible diagnostic findings. Antibodies may not be detected until 2 to 3 weeks after the first signs appear.

At necropsy, lesions suggestive of tularemia must be confirmed by bacteriologic culture for *F. tularensis* from blood, exudates, or lymph node lesions. Cysteine-supplemented media, such as glucose cysteine blood agar, thioglycolate broth, chocolate agar, modified Thayer-Martin medium, or buffered charcoal-yeast agar, are suitable for isolation of *F. tularensis*. Antibiotics can be incorporated into blood-glucose-cysteine agar to suppress contaminants. Plates are incubated at 35° C, and smooth gray colonies, surrounded by a characteristic green zone of discoloration on blood-based media, reach a maximum size of 2 to 3 mm in 48 to 72 hours (Figure 26-2). The risk for airborne transmission to laboratory workers is significant, and many laboratories actively avoid opportunities to cultivate it. Biosafety level 2 is recommended for handling clinical material and biosafety level 3 conditions are required for handing cultures beyond simple isolation.

The organism is rarely observed in Gram-stained smears of clinical specimens, but can be

FIGURE 26-3   *Francisella tularensis,* direct fluorescent antibody staining. (Courtesy Public Health Image Library, PHIL #1907, Centers for Disease Control and Prevention, Atlanta, 2002, Larry Stauffer, Oregon State Public Health Laboratory.)

rapidly and specifically detected by fluorescent antibody staining (Figure 26-3). Rapid diagnosis is also facilitated by a polymerase chain reaction (PCR) assay based on 16S rDNA, although its use is not yet widespread.

PREVENTION AND CONTROL

Francisella tularensis is widely distributed in nature and its life cycle is potentially complex. Preventive measures for cats focus on avoiding exposure by control of ectoparasites and limiting hunting, scavenging, and drinking from possibly contaminated water sources. Cat-to-cat transmission has not been documented, but cat-to-human transmission is not uncommon. Given the difficulties in antemortem diagnosis of feline tularemia, veterinarians in endemic areas (or treating patients that have been in endemic areas) should include tularemia in differential diagnosis of febrile illness, with or without lymphadenopathy, as a matter or course. Nearly 15% of veterinarians in endemic areas have elevated titers of anti–*F. tularensis* antibodies, as compared with about 1% of the general population in the same areas. Routine precautions in patient care and at necropsy should reduce risks of transmission. It should be obvious that medical attention should be sought promptly if signs compatible

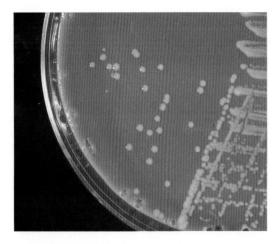

FIGURE 26-2   Colonies of *Francisella tularensis* on chocolate agar, after 48 hours' incubation at 35° C. (Courtesy Karen W. Post.)

with tularemia develop in an exposed person. Untreated human tularemia can persist for months, but is not transmitted directly from person to person.

In addition to veterinarians, laboratory workers, farmers, and hunters and trappers are at increased risk of developing tularemia. In certain areas, mowing lawns and clearing brush are also risk factors. Gloves should be worn when skinning and dressing wild game, and equipment should be disinfected and meat cooked thoroughly. Dieoffs in rodent and lagomorph populations should be reported because of possible public health consequences and even the chance that it is an indicator of a bioterrorism event.

Flies feeding on material from lesions can carry viable organisms for 2 weeks, but ticks remain infected for life. *Francisella tularensis* is susceptible to common disinfectants, including 1% sodium hypochlorite, 70% ethanol, glutaraldehyde, and formaldehyde, and is inactivated by autoclaving and dry heat ($160°$-$170°$ C for ≥ 1 hr).

Inactivated vaccines provide limited protection against *F. tularensis* infection, but live-attenuated vaccines have been used extensively (e.g., in the former Soviet Union, where up to 60 million people may have been immunized before 1960). Live vaccine strain (LVS)–based vaccines developed in the United States in the 1950s and 1960s are efficacious, but no commercially licensed project is available.

Individuals exposed to known cases of tularemia can receive prophylaxis in the form of a 2-week course of tetracyclines. The treatment of choice is streptomycin or gentamicin, although tetracyclines and chloramphenicol (especially for meningitis) may also be used. The bacteriostatic nature of the latter two makes it important to complete a full 14-day course. Fluoroquinolones may also be effective, and oral ciprofloxacin is recommended for prophylaxis or therapy after a bioterrorist event. The organism is resistant to β-lactam antimicrobials, and macrolides are not recommended for treatment.

In the absence of systematic trials to determine treatment regimens for animals with tularemia, therapeutic approaches are extrapolated from experience in human medicine. Initial treatment is usually based on clinical suspicion, and the antibiotic of choice is gentamicin, administered intravenously. Oral tetracycline and chloramphenicol are alternatives, and fluoroquinolones, such as enrofloxacin, are promising. Response to therapy usually provides conspicuous clinical improvement in 48 hours.

SUGGESTED READINGS

Belding DL, Merrill B: Tularemia in imported rabbits in Massachusetts, *N Engl J Med* 224:1085-1087, 1941.

Dennis DT, Inglesby TV, Henderson DA, et al: Tularemia as a biological weapon—medical and public health management, *J Am Med Assoc* 285:2763-2773, 2001.

Ellis J, Oyston PC, Green M, Titball RW: Tularemia, *Clin Microbiol Rev* 15:631-646, 2002.

Fortier AH, Green SJ, Polsinelli T, et al: Life and death of an intracellular pathogen: *Francisella tularensis* and the macrophage, *Immunol Ser* 60:349-361, 1994.

McCarthy VP, Murphy MD: Lawnmower tularemia, *Pediatr Infect Dis J* 9:298-300, 1990.

Sjöstedt A: Virulence determinants and protective antigens of *Francisella tularensis, Curr Opin Microbiol* 6:1-6, 2003.

Chapter 27

Infrequently Encountered Gram-Negative Rods

BARTONELLA SPECIES

Bartonella is the only genus of the family Bartonellaceae. These aerobic, slowly growing, facultatively intracellular, gram-negative organisms are placed in the α-division of the Proteobacteria based on their 16S rDNA sequences. The genus includes bacteria formerly classified in the genera *Grahamella* and *Rochalimaea;* some of the 18 species are presented in Table 27-1. All are fastidious, argyrophilic, hemotrophic, and highly adapted to a mammalian reservoir host. They cause a variety of clinical syndromes in both immunocompetent and immunocompromised humans and animals. Diseases caused by bartonellae are usually vector-borne, with transmission by arthropods (lice, fleas, ticks, biting flies, mites, chiggers). Transmission as a result of blood transfusions has also been documented.

Bartonella bacilliformis is the agent of classic human bartonellosis. This disease occurs in regions of South America and manifests as progressive anemia (Oroya fever) or as cutaneous disease (verruca peruana).

Bartonella henselae is the etiologic agent of cat-scratch fever, which is also transmitted by cat fleas. Manifestations of human and canine disease may include prolonged fever, meningitis, bacillary angiomatosis, and peliosis hepatis. Bacillary angiomatosis is a neovascular proliferative disorder that may involve skin, regional lymph nodes,

TABLE 27-1 Pathogenic *Bartonella* Species, Their Diseases, and Epidemiology

Bartonella Spp.	Disease(s)	Reservoir(s)	Arthropod Vector(s)
B. bacilliformis	Oroya fever and verruca peruana	Humans	Sandflies
B. clarridgeiae	Cat-scratch disease; canine valvular endocarditis	Domestic cats	?
B. elizabethae	Human endocarditis	Norway rat	?
B. grahamii	Human neuroretinitis	Rodents	Fleas
B. henselae	Human, canine cat-scratch fever, endocarditis, peliosis hepatis	Domestic cats; dogs?	Cat flea
B. quintana	Human trench fever	Humans	Body lice
B. vinsonii ssp. *arupensis*	Human endocarditis	Mice, voles	?
B. vinsonii ssp. *berkhoffii*	Human, canine endocarditis; canine granulomatis lymphadenitis, rhinitis, peliosis hepatis	Rodents, dogs	Ticks
B. washoensis	Human myocarditis	Ground squirrels	?

liver, spleen, brain, bones, bowel, and lungs. Peliosis hepatis–affected tissue contains numerous blood-filled partially endothelial cell-lined cystic structures. Chronically bacteremic cats are the reservoir. *Bartonella henselae* may also be an important emerging pathogen of dogs. Polyarthritis, weight loss, seizures, epistaxis, and endocarditis may result from inoculation by way of cat scratches.

Bartonella quintana causes human trench fever, which was a leading cause of morbidity among Allied troops in World War I. Lymphadenopathy and bacillary angiomatosis have also been related to this agent, which is transmitted by the human body louse.

Based on current evidence, *Bartonella vinsonii* ssp. *berkhoffii* is the species most often associated with canine disease, which manifests as endocarditis, myocarditis, and granulomatous lymphadenitis. Endocarditis, typically preceded by fever of unknown origin and intermittent leg lameness, occurs mainly in large-breed dogs, and there is a predisposition to aortic valve disease. Focal areas of myocardial inflammation can be found in dogs infected with *B. vinsonii* ssp. *berkhoffii*. This organism has also been recovered from a human endocarditis patient.

Both *Bartonella clarridgeiae* and *B. henselae* can be maintained as intravascular microflora of apparently healthy cats for years. Persistent infection in cats may also yield chronic disease manifestations. There may be an association between high antibody titers and increased risk for development of renal and urinary tract abnormalities. Chronic *Bartonella* infection may also be a cause of uveitis and myocardial inflammation.

Pathogenesis of *Bartonella*-induced disease in animals remains to be elucidated. It likely involves bacterial dissemination from regional lymph nodes and the bloodstream, or via the portal system following enteric infection, but virulence determinants have not been clearly defined. Bartonellae interact with both erythrocytes and endothelial cells. Mechanisms of deformation, invasion, and proliferation have been studied, and an extracellular protein, deformin, in *B. bacilliformis*, produces deep invaginations of the red blood cell membrane. These invaginations are likely portals of entry for invading bacteria. Polar flagella have been implicated in adhesion and erythrocyte invasion. Bundle-forming pili have been described

in *B. henselae* and *B. quintana*, and appear to play an important role in host cell attachment. *Bartonella henselae* undergoes phase variation in its outer-membrane proteins, which may facilitate immune evasion. This organism is unable to synthesize heme, but possesses a protein that is involved in heme acquisition. Induction of endothelial cell proliferation is common to many pathogenic bartonellae. Colonization and invasion of vascular endothelium is a crucial step in the establishment of proliferative lesions by *B. bacilliformis*, *B. henselae*, and *B. quintana*. Proliferation of nonlymphoid cells results in formation of new blood vessels, and this angioproliferation might be a strategy for expanding bacterial habitat in vivo.

Bartonella quintana appears to be able to inhibit apoptosis, which may enhance its intracellular survival and proliferation. Its intraerythrocytic localization is a unique strategy for bacterial persistence. Colonization of red blood cells in the absence of hemolysis preserves the bacteria for efficient vector transmission, provides protection from the host immune response, and possibly contributes to the decreased efficacy of antimicrobials in eradicating the infection.

Diagnosis of bartonellosis may be extremely difficult because the typical clinical features are not distinctive. Etiologic diagnosis is usually established by serologic testing and detection of the organisms by bacteriologic culture, polymerase chain reaction (PCR) assays, and histologically with Warthin-Starry silver staining or immunohistochemistry. Serologic testing is by an immunofluorescence assay, in which cross-reactions with *Coxiella burnetii* and chlamydiae may occur. Diagnosis relies heavily on the detection of the agent or its DNA in affected tissue.

Lymph node biopsies or aspirates, affected portions of liver or spleen, and blood are the specimens of choice. Efficiency of blood culture is increased by lysis of erythrocytes. Blood collected in EDTA is held at $-70°$ C for 24 hours before inoculation onto plated isolation media. Colonies of *Bartonella* spp. appear in 10 days or more on solid media, and freshly prepared heart infusion agar with 5% to 10% horse or rabbit blood supports better growth than chocolate or sheep blood agar. Primary culture plates should be sealed against dehydration after 24 hours' incubation and incubated for up to 6 weeks before being discarded as negative. Growth is optimal at $37°$ C in 5% to 7% CO_2 for all species except *B. bacilliformis*,

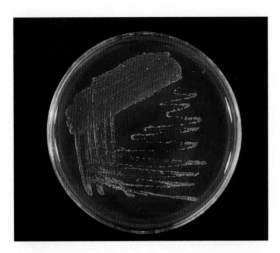

FIGURE 27-1 *Bartonella* sp. on blood agar. (Courtesy Edward Breitschwerdt.)

which has an optimal growth temperature of 25° to 28° C and grows best without supplemental CO_2.

Bartonella colonies usually exhibit two morphotypes (Figure 27-1). One is irregular, whitish, raised, rough, and dry, and may be cauliflower-like in appearance. The other type is small, tan, circular, moist, entire, and adherent to the agar. Gram stains of the colonies reveal tiny, slightly curved, faintly staining, gram-negative bacilli. Most *Bartonella* spp. are oxidase, catalase, urease, and nitrate reductase negative, and carbohydrates are not utilized. Genus and species identification is best accomplished by molecular methods.

Bartonellae are highly susceptible in vitro to some β-lactams, aminoglycosides, macrolides, and tetracyclines, but less so to penicillin and clindamycin. Considerable variation occurs in susceptibility to fluoroquinolones. Azithromycin is probably the drug of choice for treatment of canine bartonellosis. Evidence suggests that *Bartonella* spp. may be transmitted by fleas and ticks to cats and dogs, so use of insecticides and acaricides may be important in prevention and control.

CDC GROUP EF-4A

A group of gram-negative, nonmotile, coccoid to short, facultatively anaerobic bacilli has been assigned by the Centers for Disease Control and Prevention (CDC) to a group designated eugonic fermenter (EF)-4A. These organisms share phenotypic features with Pasteurellaceae, but are members of the emended family Neisseriaceae. Group EF-4A bacteria are part of the normal flora of the oral and nasal cavity of cats, dogs, and rodents. However, they have been recovered from bite wounds and scratches in man and animals and are associated with acute pneumonia of domestic cats and dogs and captive felids. Pulmonary disease is rather distinctive, in that lesions are multifocal, granulomatous, and involve all lung lobes. There are also rare extrapulmonary infections such as purulent peritonitis, hepatic abscessation, retrobulbar abscesses, otitis, and sinusitis.

Diagnosis is by culture of affected tissues. After 48 hours of aerobic incubation on blood agar plates, colonies are 1 mm in diameter, non-hemolytic, convex, round, opaque, and nonpigmented to yellowish with a distinctive popcornlike odor. Isolates are catalase and oxidase positive, and growth is sometimes seen on MacConkey agar. Triple-sugar iron (TSI) agar (butt and slant) have an initial weak acid reaction. Other distinguishing features include nitrate reductase, gelatinase, and arginine dihydrolase activities, acid production from glucose, and inability to produce urease or indole (Table 27-2).

TABLE 27-2 Selected Biochemical Reactions of *Chromobacterium violaceum,* EF-4A, and *Streptobacillus moniliformis*

Reaction	C. violaceum	EF-4A	S. moniliformis
Catalase	Pos	Pos	Neg
Oxidase	Var	Pos	Neg
Growth on MacConkey agar	Pos	Var	Neg
TSI butt, acid	Pos	Var	Var
Arginine dihydrolase	Pos	Var	Pos
Nitrate to nitrite	Pos	Pos (gas)	Neg
Gelatinase	Var	Var	Neg

Neg, Negative; *Pos,* positive; *TSI,* triple-sugar iron; *Var,* variable.

These organisms are reported to be susceptible in vitro to ampicillin, aminoglycosides, sulfa drugs, and tetracyclines. Resistance to narrow-spectrum cephalosporins, trimethoprim-sulfamethoxazole, penicillin, and erythromycin has been reported.

THE GENUS *CHROMOBACTERIUM*

Violet-pigmented bacteria, described since the late 1800s as a cause of fatal septicemias in animals and humans, have now been placed in the genus *Chromobacterium*, which is the closest neighbor to the Neisseriaceae. *Chromobacterium violaceum*, the sole species in the genus, is a motile, facultatively anaerobic, short to medium-length, gram-negative rod. Pigmentation is caused by the production of a nondiffusible pigment, violacein; nonpigmented strains are quite rare.

Chromobacterium violaceum is a saprophyte inhabiting soil and water, but is also an opportunistic pathogen of extreme virulence, especially in compromised hosts. Sporadic cases have been reported worldwide, primarily from tropical and subtropical regions. Infections in swine, dogs, buffaloes, Barbary sheep, nonhuman primates, and a panda have resulted in necrotizing pleuro-pneumonia, septicemia, and skin, pulmonary, splenic, or hepatic abscesses. Most human infections are trauma associated, with skin as the portal of entry, but infection may also be by the oral route.

Little is known about pathogenesis. The organism has elastase activity in vitro, which may in part explain its ability to produce necrotizing lung lesions. Violacein is cytotoxic in vitro, especially for fibroblasts, which are primary components of the integument.

Diagnosis is based on bacterial isolation and identification. Colonies are 0.5 to 1.5 mm in diameter, smooth, and convex with entire edges and β-hemolysis. Growth may occur at 25° and 42° C. A faint violet tint generally develops after 24 hours' incubation on blood agar, and the color becomes deeper in subsequent days. Colonies on MacConkey agar are colorless. Most isolates produce oxidase and catalase, but are negative for Voges-Proskauer reaction and do not hydrolyze esculin. There is an acid reaction on TSI slants, but H$_2$S is not produced. Arginine dihydrolase is produced. Oxidase-positive nonpigmented strains can be differentiated from *Aeromonas* or *Vibrio* spp. by the ability of the former to grow in nutrient broth without salt and to ferment glucose,

mannitol, and maltose, and by their lack of lysine and ornithine decarboxylase activities. Oxidase-negative strains can be mistaken for enteric bacilli (see Table 27-2).

Chromobacterium violaceum is susceptible to fluoroquinolones and tetracyclines, variably susceptible to aminoglycosides, but commonly resistant to β-lactam antibiotics.

THE GENUS *GALLIBACTERIUM*

Hemolytic organisms resembling *Pasteurella* species were first reported in the 1950s, in association with peritonitis and salpingitis in laying hens. These organisms are prevalent in the upper respiratory and lower genital tracts of healthy poultry, ducks, geese, pheasants, pigeons, and psittacine birds. Isolates have been recovered from a variety of pathologic conditions, in addition to salpingitis and peritonitis, septicemia, hepatitis, pericarditis, airsacculitis, and enteritis have been described. The genus *Gallibacterium*, in the family Pasteurellaceae, has recently been established to contain bacteria formerly classified within the avian *[Pasteurella haemolytica]-'Actinobacillus salpingitidis'-Pasteurella anatis* complex. *Gallibacterium* spp. have rarely been isolated from mammals (cattle and pigs).

The genus is composed of gram-negative, facultatively anaerobic to microaerophilic non-motile, rod-shaped to pleomorphic bacteria that are catalase and oxidase positive. Nitrate is reduced to nitrite and acid is produced (without gas) from glucose, glycerol, xylose, mannitol, galactose, sucrose, and raffinose. ONPG tests are positive, and growth on MacConkey agar varies from species to species. Other phenotypic traits are lack of symbionic growth and growth on Simmons' citrate agar, failure to produce urease, arginine dihydrolase, ornithine decarboxylase, lysine decarboxylase, and indole, and negative Voges-Proskauer test. Differentiation from other Pasteurellaceae is through differences in catalase production, V-factor dependency, hemolysis, carbohydrate fermentation patterns, and results of urease, indole, and ONPG tests (Tables 27-3 and 27-4).

The only species is *Gallibacterium anatis,* which is divided into biovars *haemolytica* and *anatis*. These have been isolated from chickens, ducks, geese, cattle, parakeets, psittacine birds, turkeys, partridges, pigs, and guinea fowl. Two genomo-species have been recovered from chickens and pigeons in association with pathologic lesions.

TABLE 27-3 Differentiation of *Gallibacterium* from Closely Related Organisms

	Gallibacterium	Pasteurella gallinarum	Pasteurella volantium	Pasteurella langaaensis	Pasteurella avium
Catalase	Pos	Pos	Pos	Neg	Weak pos
β-Hemolysis	Var	Neg	Neg	Neg	Neg
ONPG	Pos	Neg	Pos	Pos	Neg
V-factor required	Neg	Neg	Pos	Neg	Pos
D-mannitol	Pos	Neg	Pos	Neg	Neg
D-sorbitol	Neg	(Neg)	Var	Neg	Neg
Maltose	Var	Pos	Weak pos	Pos	Neg
Raffinose	Pos	Pos	Neg	Neg	Neg
D-xylose	Pos	Neg	Var	Neg	(Pos)

Neg, Negative; *(Neg)*, most negative; *Pos*, positive; *(Pos)*, most positive; *Var*, variable.

TABLE 27-4 Phenotypic Characteristics of Members of the Genus *Gallibacterium*

	Gallibacterium Species			
	anatis BIOVAR anatis	anatis BIOVAR haemolytica	Genomospecies 1	Genomospecies 2
β-Hemolysis	Neg	Pos	Pos	Pos
	Acid Production from:			
L-arabinose	Neg	Neg	Var	Var
Dextrin	Neg	Var	Pos	Pos
L-fucose	Neg	Pos	Pos	Var
Maltose	Neg	Var	Pos	Pos
D-sorbitol	Var	Var	Neg	Neg
Trehalose	Pos	Var	Pos	Var

Neg, Negative; *Pos*, positive; *Var*, variable.

Biovars of *G. anatis* have the role of opportunists, and virulence varies strain to strain.

Diagnosis is based on bacteriologic culture. *Gallibacterium* colonies on bovine blood agar are initially gray, nontransparent, smooth, shiny, circular, and raised, with entire margins and butyrous consistency. After 24 to 48 hours, colonies are 1 to 2 mm in diameter and eventually become translucent at the periphery. Biovar *anatis* is not β-hemolytic (see Table 27-4).

THE GENUS *LEGIONELLA*

The genus *Legionella* and the family Legionellaceae were established in 1979 to accommodate a previously unrecognized gram-negative bacterium that was isolated from patients in an epidemic of acute respiratory disease at an American Legion convention in 1976. The original species, *Legionella pneumophila*, has been joined by many others, and the genus now comprises 48 species. They are ubiquitous in freshwater environments and are intracellular parasites of amebae, ciliated protozoa, and slime molds. More than half of these species have been implicated in human disease, but *L. pneumophila* is the organism most often responsible for illness.

The organisms gain entry to and colonize man-made water supplies and, as a consequence, have been isolated from the water systems of large buildings. Most outbreaks of legionellosis have been traced to air conditioners, whirlpool spas, and evaporative condensers. Temperature is a critical determinant for proliferation of legionellae. Colonization of hot water tanks is most likely if the temperature is greater than 40° C, although *L. pneumophila* can multiply at 25° to 42° C.

Legionellosis in humans presents as severe pneumonia progressing to multisystemic disease, or Pontiac fever, which is a mild, flulike illness.

Animals appear to be relatively refractory to *L. pneumophila* infection. Attempts to infect horses, cattle, pigs, dogs, goats, sheep, rabbits, and several wild animal species have been unsuccessful. Horses have the highest prevalence of antibodies in response to experimental exposure, exhibiting a marked increase in agglutinating antibodies as early as 4 days postinoculation, with titers persisting for up to 4 months. Prevalence of antibodies to *L. pneumophila* in the equine population may exceed 30%. The organism was recovered from lungs and liver of a calf with dyspnea, diarrhea, fever, anorexia, and ultimately fatal pneumonia. Bilateral pneumonia involved the cranial lobes, with fibrinous pleurisy. Microscopic examination of lung tissue revealed acute necrotic and fibrinous pneumonia. *Legionella pneumophila* was isolated from water heater sediment on the farm, and contaminated water used to dilute milk may have been aspirated by the affected animal.

Respiratory disease occurs when a susceptible host inhales aerosols or aspirates water contaminated with the bacterium. Growth in monocytes and macrophages is the primary basis for pathogenesis. Bacteria are phagocytosed, and reside intracellularly in a phagosome, which does not fuse with lysosomes. *Legionella pneumophila* induces apoptosis in macrophages and alveolar epithelial cells and causes necrosis by the action of a pore-forming molecule in infected phagocytes. Virulence factors include cytotoxins, phospholipases, lipopolysaccharides, iron acquisition compounds, and metalloproteases.

Diagnosis by bacteriologic culture is the most specific diagnostic procedure. *Legionella pneumophila* is difficult to isolate and identify, and culture requires the use of both selective and nonselective media. Charcoal yeast extract agar is the basal medium used most frequently, and hemoglobin and L-cysteine are essential requirements. Media can be prepared with indicator dyes (bromothymol blue or bromocresol purple) and selective antimicrobials, such as anisomycin, polymyxin B, vancomycin, and cefamandole. Plates are incubated at 35° to 37° C in a non-CO_2 environment up to 7 days. Early colonies have a ground glass appearance with iridescent edges that are speckled green, blue, pink, or purple. Mature colonies form in 72 to 96 hours and are 3 to 4 mm in diameter, entire, and convex. In stained smears, *L. pneumophila* is thin, faintly staining, and gram-negative. The usual basis of identification includes culture characteristics, Gram-stain morphology, negative oxidase test, requirement for L-cysteine, demonstration of nonfermentative metabolism, and serotyping by slide agglutination or direct fluorescent antibody tests.

Erythromycin has been the drug of choice for treatment of legionellosis. The newer, currently recommended antimicrobials are azithromcyin and levofloxacin.

ORNITHOBACTERIUM RHINOTRACHEALE

Ornithobacterium rhinotracheale (ORT) is a unique gram-negative rod that was first characterized in the early 1990s in association with respiratory disease, increased mortality, and growth retardation in poultry. ORT has since been isolated from diseased ducks, pheasants, quail, chukar, geese, ostriches, pigeons, guinea fowl, partridges, and rooks. The phylogenetic position of this organism is in the rRNA superfamily V within the "flavobacter" subgroup of the "Flavobacter-Bacteroides" phylum. Phenotypically similar bacteria include *Riemerella anatipestifer* and *Capnocytophaga* species.

ORT has been isolated from turkeys and chickens throughout the world. Infections are most often associated with respiratory disease, but decreased egg production and arthritis have been reported. ORT may be transmitted horizontally by the aerosol route, or possibly by the egg, either transovarially or through cloacal contamination. Respiratory disease may be acute and is highly contagious, especially in turkeys. Affected birds exhibit nasal discharge and coughing, sometimes with bloody expectorations. There may be extreme variability in the severity of clinical signs, disease duration, and mortality of ORT outbreaks. Poor ventilation, increased stocking density, high ammonia levels, and concurrent diseases appear to be directly related to disease severity. Mortality may be as high as 10%.

Seven serotypes of ORT, designated A through G, have been distinguished by agar gel precipitation. Serotype A is probably predominant.

ORT attaches to ciliated epithelium on the respiratory side of the air sacs. Congestion, edema, and macrophage infiltration progress to airsacculitis. The lungs then become infiltrated and necrotic. Gross lesions include severe necrotizing fibrinopurulent pneumonia, airsacculitis, hepatomegaly, and suppurative pericarditis.

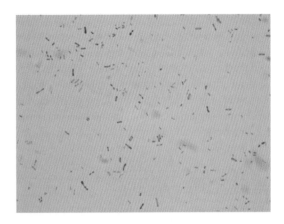

FIGURE 27-2 Gram stain of *Ornithobacterium rhinotracheale* depicting extreme pleomorphism. (Courtesy Karen W. Post.)

To date, no specific virulence factors have been identified. Origin or serotype has no apparent effect on virulence. ORT may be a primary pathogen in turkeys.

Diagnosis is by bacteriologic culture of affected lungs or air sacs. Rapid and accurate identification can be frustrating because the organism grows slowly, producing only pinpoint-sized colonies on blood agar plates after 24 hours' incubation. Optimal growth occurs when plates have been incubated more than 48 hours in an atmosphere of 5% to 7% CO_2 at 37° C. Colonies are gray to grayish white, opaque, convex, and circular, with a diameter of 1 to 3 mm. Gram-stain morphology is unique, with gram-negative, nonsporulating rods exhibiting extreme pleomorphism, with a tendency toward clubbing (Figure 27-2). Phenotypic traits useful for presumptive identification include production of oxidase, lack of catalase production and motility,

slow production of acid from glucose, production of β-galactosidase, inability to reduce nitrate to nitrite, and lack of growth on MacConkey agar (Table 27-5). Immunohistochemical methods have been employed to detect the organism in tissue, and both PCR and enzyme immunoassays have been described.

Use of autogenous, inactivated, oil-adjuvant vaccines has proven efficacious in reduction of airsacculitis and pneumonia. The antimicrobial susceptibility of ORT varies considerably by infecting strain, but the organism is uniformly resistant to aminoglycosides. The most consistent therapeutic control measure has been administration of chlortetracycline in feed at a dose of 500 mg/L or amoxicillin at 250 mg/L in water.

RIEMERELLA ANATIPESTIFER

Riemerella anatipestifer, previously classified as *Pfeifferella, Moraxella,* or *Pasteurella anatipestifer,* is an important pathogen of ducks, causing infectious serositis, new duck disease, duck septicemia, or anatipestifer septicemia. This gram-negative bacillus belongs to the family Flavobacteriaceae in rRNA superfamily V, and is most closely related to the genera *Bergeyella* and *Chryseobacterium*. To date, 21 serotypes have been recognized, and serotypes 1, 2, 3, 5, and 15 are most prevalent in severe outbreaks of infectious serositis.

Infectious serositis occurs worldwide and is responsible for major economic losses in the duck industry, associated with high mortality, decreased growth, poor feed conversion, and increased condemnations. Other avian species such as geese and turkeys may be affected. The disease occurs as an acute or chronic septicemia characterized by airsacculitis, fibrinous pericarditis, perihepatitis, caseous salpingitis, and meningitis.

TABLE 27-5 Selected Phenotypic Properties of *Ornithobacterium rhinotracheale* and *Riemerella anatipestifer*

	O. rhinotracheale	R. anatipestifer
Catalase	Neg	Pos
Oxidase	Pos	Pos
Growth on MacConkey agar	Neg	Neg
Acid from glucose	Slow pos	Neg
Nitrate reduction	Neg	Neg
Gelatinase	Neg	Pos
Arginine dihydrolase	Neg	Pos

Neg, Negative; *Pos,* positive.

The organism has been recovered from wild birds, and rarely from pigs.

The mechanism by which infection becomes established in a flock is unknown because routes of natural infection have not been definitively established. *Riemerella anatipestifer* may be a normal component of the pharyngeal flora of healthy ducks. Skin punctures, particularly of the feet, are a possible route of infection. Disease in turkeys may be transmitted by arthropod vectors. The bacterium is rarely a primary disease agent; predisposing factors include adverse environmental conditions and concomitant bacterial or viral infection. Disease severity varies with the infecting strain.

Virulence factors have not been identified. Potential virulence determinants include the product of gene *vapD1*, which has homology to virulence-associated proteins of other bacteria and a CAMP cohemolysin. The latter may be an iron-scavenging mechanism.

Diagnosis is by bacteriologic culture. *Riemerella anatipestifer* strains are usually identified by their morphologic, biochemical, and serologic characteristics. The bacterium grows well on blood agar, and forms colonies that are 1 to 2 mm in diameter, convex, entire, butyrous, and transparent after 24 hours' incubation at 37° C in an environment enriched with CO_2 (Figure 27-3). Gram staining reveals non–spore-forming bacilli, occurring singly or in pairs with occasional filamentous forms and ranging from 0.2 to 0.4 μm wide to 1 to 5 μm long. Biochemical identification is based on its ability to produce oxidase and catalase,

hydrolyze gelatin, arginine, and hippurate, and its inability to ferment carbohydrates in conventional media or grow on MacConkey agar (see Table 27-5).

Bacterins and live vaccines confer protection against homologous serotypes but offer no cross-protection against heterologous serotype exposure. This limits the usefulness of immunization as a means of disease prevention and control. Antimicrobials may be used to control disease in the face of an outbreak. Ceftiofur and penicillin have demonstrated in vitro activity against *R. anatipestifer,* but the organism has high minimal inhibitory concentrations (MICs) to many agents, including aminoglycosides, aminocyclitols, tetracyclines, and trimethoprim.

STREPTOBACILLUS MONILIFORMIS

The genus *Streptobacillus,* a member of the family Fusobacteriaceae, consists of a single species, *Streptobacillus moniliformis,* which is a normal inhabitant of the naso- and oropharynx of rodents and possibly cats. The organism is a facultatively anaerobic, nonmotile gram-negative rod.

Streptobacillus moniliformis causes septicemia, arthritis, otitis media, hepatitis and abortion in laboratory and wild rodents. The bacterium infects turkeys, usually following rat bites, resulting in polyarthritis and synovitis. Nonhuman primate disease has occurred in a rhesus macaque (valvular endocarditis) and a titi monkey (septic arthritis). The organism has also been recovered from a guinea pig with cervical abscesses and pneumonia, and from a koala with pleuritis.

Disease in humans is called rat-bite fever, and is associated with bites by rodents or cats that prey on rodents. Human illness resulting from ingestion of contaminated foodstuffs or water is called Haverhill fever. Flulike illness and then a rash follow a 2- to 10-day incubation period. Septicemia, polyarthritis, meningitis, endocarditis, cutaneous abscesses, pneumonia, and amnionitis may be complications of infection. Most cases are in children younger than 12 years old.

Diagnosis is by bacteriologic culture. Gram stains reveal extremely pleomorphic bacilli with tapered to pointed ends that appear as long wavy chains or filaments. Single rods may have a central swelling or chains of rods may have swellings that give the appearance of a "string of beads." Diff-Quik staining is useful for demonstration of the

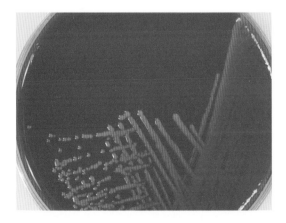

FIGURE 27-3 Colonial morphology of *Riemerella anatipestifer* on blood agar. (Courtesy Karen Post.)

organism in clinical materials. Round, convex, grayish, smooth, glistening, butyrous colonies develop after 3 days' incubation on blood agar in 5% to 10% CO_2. Occasional L-phase colonial variants have a fried-egg appearance on agar. Liquid media are useful for initial isolation, and *S. moniliformis* grows as grayish "puffballs" with 2 to 6 days' incubation. The organism is catalase and oxidase negative and produces a weak acid reaction in the butt portion of a TSI tube. Glucose is fermented without gas production. Acid is produced from maltose, salicin, and inulin but not from lactose, sorbitol, trehalose, mannitol, or sucrose. Hydrogen sulfide and arginine dihydrolase are produced, but gelatinase, urease, indole, and nitrate reductase are not (see Table 27-2).

Antibodies to *S. moniliformis* in laboratory mice and rats can be demonstrated by enzyme immunoassay, and the organism can be detected by PCR in tissues of affected animals.

Streptobacillus moniliformis is susceptible to a variety of antimicrobials. Penicillin and doxycycline are recommended for treatment.

SUGGESTED READINGS

Breitschwerdt EB, Kordick DL: *Bartonella* infection in animals: carriership, reservoir potential, pathogenicity, and zoonotic potential for human infection, *Clin Microbiol Rev* 13:428-438, 2000.

Christensen H, Bisgaard M, Bojesen AM, et al: Genetic relationships among avian isolates classified as *Pasteurella haemolytica, Actinobacillus salpingitidis* or *Pasteurella anatis* gen. nov., comb. nov. and description of additional genomospecies within *Gallibacterium* gen. nov., *Int J Syst Evol Microbiol* 53:275-287, 2003.

Drolet R, Kenefick KB, Hakomaki MR, Ward GE: Isolation of group eugonic fermenter-4 bacteria from a cat, *J Am Vet Med Assoc* 189:311-312, 1986.

Fabbi M, Pastoris M, Scanziani E, et al: Epidemiological and environmental investigations of *Legionella pneumophila* infection in cattle and case report of fatal pneumonia in a calf, *J Clin Microbiol* 36:1942-1947, 1998.

Fields BS, Benson RF, Besser RE: *Legionella* and legionnaires' disease: 25 years of investigation, *Clin Microbiol Rev* 15:506-526, 2002.

van Empel PC, Hafez HM: *Ornithobacterium rhinotracheale*: a review, *Avian Pathol* 28:217-227, 1999.

Wullenweber M: *Streptobacillus moniliformis*: a zoonotic pathogen. Taxonomic considerations, host species, diagnosis, therapy, geographical distribution, *Lab Anim* 29:1-15, 1995.

Chapter 28

The Genera *Campylobacter, Helicobacter,* and *Arcobacter*

CAMPYLOBACTER

Members of the genus *Campylobacter* are gram-negative, slender, spiral to curved rods (Figures 28-1 and 28-2). Many were formerly in the genus *Vibrio,* leading to continuing references to the diseases they cause as vibriosis. *Campylobacter* spp. are motile, with a characteristic darting or corkscrew motion, best seen by darkfield or phase contrast microscopy. They are microaerophilic and require 3% to 5% CO_2 and 3% to 15% O_2 for growth.

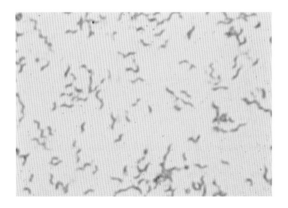

FIGURE 28-1 Gram-stained cells of *Campylobacter fetus* ssp. *fetus.* (Courtesy J. Glenn Songer.)

They are distinguished from true *Vibrio* species by their lack of oxidation and fermentation of carbohydrates. All are oxidase positive, some produce catalase, and most reduce nitrate. Urease negativity is common, and this trait is useful in distinguishing them from many members of the genus *Helicobacter.*

Campylobacter spp. frequently live as commensals in the intestinal tracts of mammals and birds. *Campylobacter jejuni,* the leading cause of bacterial food-borne illness, and *Campylobacter coli,* which contributes a minor share of cases, colonize food animals without producing illness. Non-*jejuni* and non-*coli* species have a role in animal disease. Animal-derived foods, especially those from poultry, are the major source of *Campylobacter* spp. for infection of humans. Species encountered in veterinary medicine are presented in Table 28-1.

Diseases, Epidemiology, And Pathogenesis

Campylobacter fetus. Subspecies of *C. fetus* have been recognized causes of ovine and bovine abortion for decades and, before the mid-1970s, were the major organisms of interest in the genus. Sheep infected with *Campylobacter fetus* ssp. *fetus,* by ingestion of the organism in contaminated food or water, develop bacteremia. Infection is sporadic, but in at least some cases, deposition of *C. fetus*

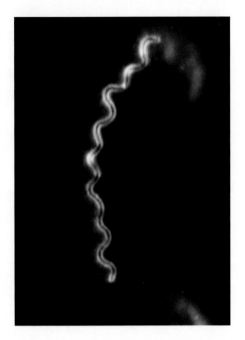

FIGURE 28-2 *Campylobacter* sp. viewed by darkfield microscopy. Note the chaining of individual organisms, which are often mistaken for spirochetes. (Courtesy J. Glenn Songer.)

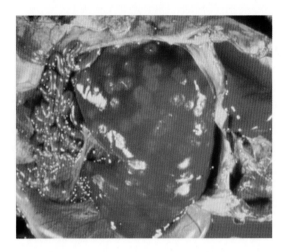

FIGURE 28-3 Ovine abortion resulting from *Campylobacter fetus* ssp. *fetus*. (Courtesy J. Glenn Songer.)

ssp. *fetus* in placenta initiates an inflammatory process that is followed by abortion, usually in the third trimester (Figure 28-3). Infection by *Campylobacter fetus* ssp. *venerealis,* known as bovine venereal campylobacteriosis, is transmitted from bulls to cows in the normal process of breeding or by way of artificial insemination. The organism can typically be recovered from the glans penis and distal urethra of infected bulls, and deposition in the female reproductive tract results in ascending colonization that extends to the fallopian tubes. The syndrome usually manifests as infertility, and abortion occurs in less than 10% of infected cows.

Serum resistance probably plays a major role in virulence of *C. fetus*, and high-molecular-weight proteins composing the S (surface)-layer are the

TABLE 28-1 *Campylobacter* Species Encountered in Veterinary Medicine

Species	Comments
C. coli*	Porcine, poultry normal intestinal flora; rare mild porcine diarrhea
C. fetus ssp. fetus*	Ovine abortion; sporadic bovine abortion; ruminant normal intestinal flora
C. fetus ssp. venerealis	Venereally transmitted bovine abortion and infertility
C. helveticus	Feces of normal and diarrheic dogs and cats
C. hyointestinalis ssp. hyointestinalis	Porcine normal intestinal flora; once thought to cause porcine proliferative enteropathy
C. hyointestinalis ssp. lawsonii	Stomachs of pigs; unknown virulence
C. jejuni ssp. jejuni*	Diarrhea in young dogs, cats, pigs, calves, lambs, ferrets, mink; sporadic ruminant abortion; "avian vibrionic hepatitis" in chickens and ratites; normal intestinal flora in most birds, ruminants, dogs, cats, rabbits, primates
C. lari	Feces of healthy gulls, other birds, dogs
C. mucosalis	Porcine normal oral, intestinal flora
C. sputorum ssp. bubulus	Normal genital flora in cattle and sheep of both sexes; differentiate from C. fetus
C. sputorum ssp. fecalis	Sheep feces, bovine semen and vagina; questionable virulence
C. upsaliensis*	Feces of healthy and diarrheic dogs and from healthy cats

*Zoonotic agent.

key components in this resistance. The S-layer is not effectively opsonized by complement component C3b, so neutrophil phagocytosis is limited. A 135-kD protein mediates resistance to phagocytosis by preventing binding of O-specific antibody. Mutants lacking the S-layer are serum sensitive and have reduced virulence in mice, suggesting that the S-layer masks *Campylobacter* lipopolysaccharide (LPS), perhaps in a bacterial strategy to decrease immunogenicity. S-layer proteins of *C. fetus* ssp. *venerealis* may be subject to antigenic shifts over time in experimentally infected heifers, and genetic analysis suggests that the basis for this phenomenon is in genomic rearrangements. The *sapA* promoter is on an invertible DNA fragment, which allows expression of two oppositely oriented S-layer gene cassettes, and recombination of 5′ conserved regions of multiple *sapA* homologs also contributes to antigenic variation. The S-layer is not required for adherence to epithelial cells in vitro.

Campylobacter jejuni and Campylobacter coli. Campylobacter jejuni and *C. coli* occur in large numbers (as many as 10^7 colony-forming units [CFUs] per g) as commensals in the intestinal tract of companion and food animals. Humans are infected by consumption of undercooked meats, especially poultry, contaminated by either *C. jejuni* (95%) or *C. coli* (5%); an incubation period of 24 to 72 hours is followed by severe diarrhea, with blood and leukocytes in feces, fever, vomiting, and abdominal pain. Illness is usually self-limiting.

Prevalence of campylobacters in companion animals varies inversely with age. Nonetheless, dogs and cats may be involved in transmission of campylobacteriosis to humans. Healthy dogs harbor *C. jejuni,* but there is a strong correlation between the occurrence of diarrhea and recovery of *C. jejuni* from these animals. The organism is found in clinically normal cats. Symptoms of campylobacteriosis are mild in food animals, consisting of soft to watery feces with mucus and flecks of blood.

Extraintestinal infections with *C. jejuni* have been reported in sheep, goats, cattle, and pigs. The organism can cause abortion in sheep and goats, with symptoms similar to those of *C. fetus* abortions, and mastitis in cattle. *Campylobacter jejuni* is frequently isolated from milk contaminated by feces or via mastitic infections, and is a major source of infection in countries where raw milk is consumed. *Campylobacter jejuni* and *C. coli* infections have been associated with abortion in sheep and pigs, but infections in these species are usually more benign.

Pathogenesis of *C. jejuni* infections is initiated when the organism penetrates the intestinal mucus layer and invades enterocytes. This adherence facilitates resistance to elimination by peristalsis, and is mediated by constitutively expressed proteins. Attachment factors include a fibronectin binding protein (CadF), a lipoprotein (JlpA), and possibly flagellin, pilus proteins, and LPS. Binding is followed by invasion, the extent of which is highly strain dependent; environmental isolates are much less invasive than clinical isolates, and isolates from noninflammatory diarrheal disease are less invasive than those from colitis patients. Internalization of *C. jejuni* is by directed endocytosis, and requires fully functional bacterial metabolism. Cia proteins play an important but undefined role in pathogenesis. They are synthesized on bacterium-cell contact, and reach the cytoplasm via a type III secretion system. Intracellular membrane-bound *C. jejuni* initially decreases in numbers, but then undergoes exponential growth over a 72-hour period. It gains access to deeper tissues by transcytosis, and can be found in granulocytes, parenchymal cells, and mononuclear cells in the lamina propria and submucosa. Experimental disease in newborn piglets mimics human campylobacteriosis. Macrophages and neutrophils appear in the lamina propria and submucosa within three days of infection, and many contain internalized *C. jejuni.* In vitro, uptake is strain and host dependent, and is facilitated by antibodies.

Survival of *C. jejuni* in macrophages may contribute to disease severity, duration of symptoms, and rate of relapse. *Campylobacter* superoxide dismutase (from *sod*B) might be expected to facilitate intracellular survival of *C. jejuni,* but survival of a *sod*B mutant was no different than that of the parent strain. In contrast, a catalase (*kat*A) mutant was susceptible to intracellular killing, whereas the parent strain remained viable through 72 hours of intracellular residence.

Campylobacter upsaliensis, Campylobacter hyointestinalis, and Campylobacter mucosalis. The high carriage rate of *C. upsaliensis* among domestic animals makes it difficult to associate this organism with disease. Two thirds of cats carry *C. upsaliensis,* and it is the most common species in canine stools. *Campylobacter upsaliensis* has been isolated from human patients with gastroenteritis, and accounts for 20% of *Campylobacter* isolates among Australian and South African pediatric patients with diarrhea.

Campylobacter upsaliensis binds to epithelial cells in vitro, a process perhaps mediated by its interaction with small intestinal mucin. A cytolethal distending toxin (CDT) has been demonstrated in epithelial cells, which undergo apoptosis after exposure.

Campylobacter hyointestinalis has been isolated from hamsters, cattle, and monkeys *(Macaca nemestrina)*. Genetic similarities suggest that a strain causing diarrhea and vomiting in a human was of porcine origin. The organism has been isolated from pigs with enteritis, but little is known about pathogenesis of these infections. Many porcine-derived isolates produce a cytotoxin, perhaps similar to CDT of *C. upsaliensis*.

Campylobacter hyointestinalis and *C. mucosalis* are found in most pigs with proliferative enteritis. Large numbers of *C. mucosalis* are isolated from cases of porcine intestinal adenomatosis.

Diagnosis

Diagnosis of venereal campylobacteriosis is relatively straightforward, but requires bacteriologic culture. Vaginal or preputial washings should be cultured immediately or held in an appropriate transport medium (such as Clark's) or thioglycollate broth. Fetal and placental tissues should be preserved at 4° C. Columbia blood agar is sufficient for isolation if specimens are collected aseptically, and plates should be incubated under microaerophilic conditions at 37° C. Contaminated vaginal or preputial washes should be inoculated directly onto selective medium. They may also be filtered (0.65 or 0.45 μm pore diameter) before inoculation onto blood agar. Incubation should be continued through 5 days before discarding plates. *Campylobacter fetus* is distinguished from *C. jejuni* by optimal growth at 37° C and susceptibility to cephalothin. It can also be identified by means of a polymerase chain reaction (PCR) assay using primers to the 16S rDNA.

Specimens to be examined for *C. jejuni* can be transported in Cary-Blair or Campy-thio media maintained at 4° C until processing. Plates of Columbia blood agar (for specimens collected aseptically or filtered) and selective agar should be inoculated and incubated under microaerophilic conditions, but at 42° C. *Campylobacter upsaliensis* can be isolated by these same methods. *Campylobacter hyointestinalis* is differentiated from other *Campylobacter* spp. by differences in the pulsed field gel electrophoresis pattern and the sequence of the 16S rRNA gene. It is an H_2S producer when cultivated in an H_2-containing atmosphere. *Campylobacter mucosalis* requires hydrogen for growth in vitro.

Colonial morphologies for common pathogens in the genus *Campylobacter* are presented in Table 28-2. Biochemical properties are important in speciation within the genus (Table 28-3).

TABLE 28-2 Colonial Morphology of *Campylobacter* Species from Domestic Animals

Species	Colonial morphology
C. coli	Round, raised, convex, smooth, glistening, white to tan; nonhemolytic; 1-2 mm diameter; on moist agar, low, flat, gray colonies spread in direction of streak
C. fetus ssp. *fetus*	Smooth, ~1 mm diameter, colorless to cream
C. fetus ssp. *venerealis*	Rough, 1-2 mm diameter, round, granular, opaque, white, cream or tan, low, flat, gray to tan, translucent, irregular edge, may spread along line of streak All nonhemolytic
C. hyointestinalis	2 mm diameter after 48 hr; circular, convex, slightly mucoid, yellowish cast
C. jejuni ssp. *jejuni*	Low, flat, grayish, finely granular, translucent, irregular margin round, raised, convex, smooth, glistening, 1-2 mm diameter, translucent at edge with darker, dirty brown to tannish, opaque center, entire margin Both nonhemolytic
C. mucosalis	1.5 mm diameter, circular, raised, flat, dirty yellow; may swarm on moist agar
C. sputorum ssp. *bubulus*	Similar to *mucosalis* but without yellow pigment
C. sputorum ssp. *fecalis*	Pinpoint to 3.5 mm diameter, shiny, smooth, convex, round, entire edges
C. upsaliensis	Pinpoint after 48 hr incubation; nonhemolytic, swarm on moist agar

TABLE 28-3 Phenotypic Characteristics of Members of the Genus *Campylobacter*

Characteristic	coli	C. fetus ssp. fetus	C. fetus ssp. venerealis	C. hyointestinalis	C. jejuni ssp. jejuni	C. sputorum ssp. bubulus	C. sputorum ssp. fecalis	C. mucosalis	C. hyoilei	C. hyointestinalis*	C. upsaliensis
Oxidase	Pos	Pos	Pos	Pos	Pos	Pos	Pos	Pos	Pos	Pos	Pos
Catalase	Pos	Pos	Pos	Pos	Pos	Neg	Pos	Neg	Pos	Pos	Pos
Urease	Neg	Neg	Neg	Neg	Neg	Neg	Neg	Neg	Neg	Neg	Neg
Nitrate reductase	Pos	Pos	Pos	Pos	Pos	Pos	Pos	Pos	Pos	Pos	Pos
H$_2$S from TSI	Neg	Neg	Pos	Neg	Neg	Pos	Pos	Pos	Pos	Neg	Neg
H$_2$S from Pb acetate strip	Pos	Var	Var	Neg	Pos	Pos	Pos	Pos	Pos	Neg	Neg
Growth 25° C	Neg	Pos	Pos	Weak pos	Neg	Var	Neg	Neg	Unk	Weak pos	Neg
Growth 42° C	Pos	(Neg)	(Neg)	Pos	Pos	Neg	Pos	Pos	Pos	Pos	Pos
Growth in 1% glycine	Pos	Pos	Neg	Pos	Pos	Pos	Pos	Neg	Pos	Pos	Pos
Growth in 3.5% NaCl	Neg	Neg	Neg	Neg	Neg	Pos	Pos	Neg	Neg	Neg	Neg
Hippurate hydrolysis	Neg	Neg	Neg	Neg	(Pos)	Neg	Neg	Neg	Neg	Neg	Neg
Nalidixic acid sensitivity	S	R	R	R	(S)	Var	R	Var	S	R	S
Cephalothin sensitivity	R	S	S	S	R	S	S	S	R	S	S
Indoxylacetate production	Pos	Neg	Neg	Neg	Pos	Neg	Neg	Neg	Unk	Neg	Pos

*Differentiate ssp. *hyointestinalis* from ssp. *lawsonii* by growth of the former in 1.5% bile.
Neg, Negative; *(Neg)*, most negative; *Pos*, positive; *R*, resistant; *S*, sensitive; *(S)*, most sensitive; *TSI*, triple-sugar iron; *Unk*, unknown; *Var*, variable.

Control And Prevention

Infection by campylobacters transmitted by the fecal-oral route can be controlled by heightened attention to sanitation. Proper food handling from slaughter to consumption can be expected to reduce the incidence of human infections by *C. jejuni*.

Most campylobacters are susceptible to antimicrobial agents, but this form of therapy is not often practical. Penicillin and streptomycin are sometime used in outbreaks of bovine venereal campylobacteriosis, and tetracyclines may be useful in preventing ovine abortions. Bacterins are of some use in cattle, but immunity is usually short lived. There is apparently a sound scientific basis for the widely held belief that vaccination can eliminate the carrier state in bulls. Semen is treated with penicillin and streptomycin, and use of artificial insemination can eliminate *C. fetus* ssp. *venerealis*. Elimination of *C. fetus* ssp. *fetus* from a herd is extraordinarily difficult.

HELICOBACTER

Helicobacter spp. infections have been widely documented in mammals and birds, largely as part of the frenzy generated by the description of *H. pylori*–induced gastric disease in humans. They may be zoonotic, and cause gastritis, gastric cancer, hepatitis, hepatic cancer, and gastroenteritis (Table 28-4).

Helicobacter species are helical, curved or straight, unbranched gram-negative rods. They have darting motility and may appear coccoid when in stationary phase. They are microaerophilic, they neither ferment nor oxidize carbohydrates, and they grow optimally at 37° C. Hydrogen is required for growth of some species and stimulates growth of others (Table 28-5).

Disease, Pathogenesis, And Epidemiology

Helicobacter hepaticus and Helicobacter bilis. *Helicobacter hepaticus* is a clearly documented mouse pathogen, and infections by this organism and *H. bilis* are common in rodent colonies and commercial breeding facilities. Initial lesions of *H. hepaticus* infection include focal hepatic necrosis or subacute, nonsuppurative hepatic inflammation. Lesions progress to involve more lobes of the liver and become chronic, with bile duct hyperplasia. Lesions become preneoplastic foci and, eventually, hepatocellular tumors. *Helicobacter bilis* colonizes liver, gallbladder, and intestine. It can be isolated readily from bile and has been associated with multifocal, but not hyperplastic, hepatitis (see Table 28-4).

Helicobacter pylori. *Helicobacter pylori* infections cause chronic inflammation of the stomach

TABLE 28-4 *Helicobacter* Species Associated with Animals

Species	Host	Colonization Site	Disease
H. acinonyx	Cheetah	Stomach	Gastritis
H. bilis	Mouse	Bile duct, liver, intestine	Hepatitis
H. bizzozeronii	Dog	Stomach	None
H. canis	Dog	Intestine	Gastroenteritis
H. cholecystus	Hamster	Gallbladder, pancreas	Cholangiofibrosis and pancreatitis
H. cinaedi	Human, hamster	Intestine	None; hamster normal flora
H. felis	Cat, dog	Stomach	Gastritis
H. fennelliae	Human, dog	Intestine	None
*H. heilmanni**	Human, other mammals	Stomach	Unknown
H. hepaticus	Mouse, rat	Liver, intestine	Hepatitis
H. muridarum	Mouse, rat	Stomach, intestine	Gastritis
H. mustelae	Ferret	Stomach	Gastritis
H. nemestrinae	Macaque	Stomach	Gastritis
H. pamentensis	Wild birds, pig	Intestine	None
H. pullorum	Poultry, human	Intestine	Gastroenteritis, hepatitis
H. pylori	Monkey, cat, human	Stomach	Primate gastritis
H. rappini†	Mouse, rat, dog, sheep	Intestine	Ovine abortion
H. trogontum	Rat	Colon	Unknown

*Not cultured in vitro.
†Formerly *Flexispira rappini*.

TABLE 28-5 Phenotypic Characteristics of Members of the Genus *Helicobacter*

Species	Catalase	Oxidase	Alkaline Phosphatase	Indoxyl Acetate	Growth at 42° C	Growth in 1% glycine	Nitrate Reductase	Urease	Nalidixic Acid*	Cephalothin*
H. acinonyx	Pos	Pos	Pos	Neg	Neg	Neg	Neg	Pos	R	S
H. bilis	Pos	Pos		Neg	Pos	Pos	Pos	Pos	R	R
H. bizzoz	Pos	Pos	Pos	Pos	Pos	Neg	Pos	Pos	R	S
H. canis	Neg	Pos	Pos	Pos	Pos		Neg	Neg	S	I
H. cholecystitis	Pos	Pos	Pos	Neg	Pos	Pos	Pos	Neg	I	R
H. cinaedi	Pos	Pos	Neg	Neg	Neg	Pos	Pos	Neg	S	I
H. felis	Pos	Pos	Pos	Neg	Pos	Neg	Pos	Pos	R	S
H. fennelliae	Pos	Pos	Pos	Pos	Neg	Pos	Neg	Neg	S	S
H. hepaticus	Pos	Pos		Pos	Neg	Pos	Pos	Pos	R	R
H. muridarum	Pos	Pos	Pos	Pos	Neg	Neg	Neg	Pos	R	R
H. mustelae	Pos	Pos	Pos	Pos	Pos	Neg	Pos	Pos	S	S
H. nemestrinae	Pos	Pos	Pos	Neg	Pos	Neg	Neg	Neg	R	S
H. pamentensis	Pos	Pos	Pos	Neg	Pos	Pos	Pos	Neg	S	S
H. pullorum	Pos	Pos	Neg	Neg	Pos		Pos	Neg	S	S
H. pylori	Pos	Pos	Pos	Neg	Neg	Neg	Neg	Pos	R	S
H. rappini	Pos	Pos	Neg		Pos	Neg	Neg	Pos	R	R
H. trogontum	Pos	Pos	Neg		Pos	Neg	Neg	Pos	R	R

*Susceptibility to 30 μg disk.

I, Intermediate; *Neg,* negative; *Pos,* positive; *R,* resistant; *S,* sensitive.

in humans, leading to chronic atrophic gastritis, intestinal metaplasia, and gastric cancer. It maintains residence by attaching to gastric epithelial cells, and attachment is accomplished through expression of an antigen-binding adhesin, phospholipase A, flagellins, and urease. Damage to gastric epithelium is associated with delivery of virulence proteins via a type IV secretion system. VacA cytotoxin is an autotransporter that ensures the availability of urea for utilization by *H. pylori*. VacA is also implicated in mitochondrial targeting and cytochrome C release during induced apoptosis, and may induce inflammation via mediation of release of tissue-damaging cytokines from mast cells. CagA proteins, which induce changes in the tyrosine phosphorylation state of host cell proteins, are also delivered by the type IV secretion machinery of *H. pylori*. These intracellular changes cause abnormal growth of gastric epithelial cells and promote the development of gastric cancer.

Gastric ulcers in food animals (especially in swine) have been linked to the presence of *Helicobacter* spp., but the exact role of the bacterium in lesion development is unclear.

Diagnosis

Gastric or intestinal mucosa or liver is refrigerated in sterile saline or Stuart's transport medium. Feces from live animals can also be collected. Tissue homogenates are plated on Columbia sheep blood agar, brucella blood agar with trimethoprim-vancomycin-polymyxin B (TVP), or Skirrow's medium. Fecal specimens are plated directly onto brucella blood agar with TVP and/or Campy-Skirrow. Plates are incubated in an atmosphere suitable for *Campylobacter* spp., at 37° C for up to 7 days. Colonies are 1 to 2 mm in diameter, and are flat, gray to grayish white, nonhemolytic, and translucent, with a flat, irregular morphology. On moist agar plates, colonies may appear as a thin, spreading film.

ARCOBACTER

Arcobacter spp. have campylobacter-like morphology, but are aerotolerant and grow at 30° C. This genus comprises the former aerotolerant *Campylobacter* sp. *cryaerophila* and *nitrofigilis* (a strictly environmental species), and two recently described species, *skirrowii* and *butzleri*. They are small gram-negative curved to spiral shaped, non–spore-forming rods (Table 28-6). Their possible importance as pathogens is only just being explored.

Diseases, Pathogenesis, And Epidemiology

Arcobacter cryaerophilus (*Campylobacter cryaerophila*, *Campylobacter*-type Neill strain) is associated with late-term abortion in swine, cattle, horses, sheep, and dogs. It has also been isolated from mastitic bovine milk and ovine feces. *Arcobacter cryaerophilus* is isolated from mild mastitis in newly freshened dairy cows, and acute mastitis has been reproduced experimentally. This organism is aerotolerant, and was first isolated from aborted fetuses in semisolid leptospiral media. It can also be isolated from normal bovine and porcine fetuses. Organisms are initially microaerophilic but grow in air after subculture. Growth is optimal at 30° C.

Arcobacter butzleri causes diarrheal disease in humans and other primates, but has also been isolated from the diarrheic feces of horses, cattle,

TABLE 28-6 Phenotypic Characteristics of *Arcobacter* Species

	Species			
	A. butzleri	*A. cryaerophilus*	*A. nitrofigilis*	*A. skirrowii*
Catalase	Pos	Pos	Pos	Pos
Nitrate reductase	Pos	Neg	Pos	Pos
DNase	Pos	Pos	Pos	Pos
Growth on MacConkey agar	Pos	Neg	Var	Neg
Growth at 42° C	Pos	Neg	Neg	Neg
H$_2$S from cysteine	Pos	Neg	Var	Neg
1% Glycine growth	Pos	Neg	Neg	Pos
3.5% NaCl growth	Neg	Neg	Var	Pos
Nalidixic acid susceptibility	Pos	Pos	Pos	Pos
Cephalothin susceptibility	Neg	Neg	Var	Pos

Neg, Negative; *Pos*, positive; *Var*, variable.

and swine. Isolates have been obtained from cases of abortion in swine and cattle and from an ostrich yolk sac. Diarrhea in humans is often accompanied by acute abdominal cramps, and may be persistent. Both *A. butzleri* and *A. cryaerophilus* may be zoonotic agents.

Arcobacter skirrowii has been isolated from diarrheic humans, from abortions in swine and cattle, and from cases of diarrhea in lambs and calves. It is often found in bovine preputial washings and must be differentiated from *C. fetus* ssp. *venerealis.*

Diagnosis

Vaginal discharges and fetal stomach contents, as well as supernatant fluids from mascerated tissues, are inoculated into semisolid leptospiral medium and incubated at 25° C; growth may occur as early as 48 hours or as late as 5 weeks. Samples are checked periodically by darkfield or phase-contrast microscopy, for motile organisms with *Campylobacter*-like morphology. Growth occurring as turbidity just below the surface of the medium is subcultured onto Columbia blood agar and incubated microaerophilically for 48 to 72 hours at 30° C. Microaerophilic conditions are required for optimal growth, but these organisms can grow in ambient air. All species produce white, gray, yellow, or colorless colonies that are translucent to wet, and may swarm.

Catalase activity of arcobacters is variable, with most *A. butzleri* strains being negative or weakly positive and other species being positive. Other generic traits include oxidase positivity, indoxyl acetate positivity (useful for differentiation from *C. fetus* subspecies), nitrate reduction (most strains), and failure to produce indole or hydrolyze gelatin or hippurate. Given the difficulties in establishing an identity by traditional biochemical means, many veterinary diagnostic laboratories report "*Arcobacter* spp. isolated" on the basis of (1) initial isolation in leptospiral semisolid medium, (2) characteristic Gram-stain morphology, (3) darting motility, (4) growth in ambient air at room temperature and at 37° C, (5) little or no growth at 42° C, and (6) ability to grow on *Yersinia* selective medium (CIN agar).

SUGGESTED READINGS

Babakhani FK, Bradley GA, Joens LA: Newborn piglet model for campylobacteriosis, *Infect Immun* 61: 3466-3475, 1993.

Blaser MJ, Pei Z: Pathogenesis of *Campylobacter fetus* infections: critical role of high-molecular-weight S-layer proteins in virulence, *J Infect Dis* 167:372-377, 1993.

Day WA Jr, Sajecki JL, Pitts TM, Joens LA: Role of catalase in *Campylobacter jejuni* intracellular survival, *Infect Immun* 68:6337-6345, 2000.

Eaton KA, Dewhirst FE, Radin MJ, et al: *Helicobacter acinonyx* sp. nov., isolated from cheetahs with gastritis, *Int J Syst Bacteriol* 43:99-106, 1993.

Konkel ME, Joens LA: Adhesion to and invasion of Hep-2 cells by *Campylobacter* spp., *Infect Immun* 57: 2984-2990, 1989.

Lee A, Krakowka S, Fox JG, et al: Role of *Helicobacter felis* in chronic canine gastritis, *Vet Pathol* 29:487-494, 1992.

Supajatura V, Ushio H, Wada A, et al: Cutting edge: VacA, a vacuolating cytotoxin of *Helicobacter pylori*, directly activates mast cells for migration and production of proinflammatory cytokines, *J Immunol* 168:2603-2607, 2002.

Ward JM, Fox JG, Anver MR, et al: Chronic active hepatitis and associated liver tumors in mice caused by a persistent bacterial infection with a novel *Helicobacter* species, *J Natl Cancer Inst* 86:1222-1225, 1994.

Chapter 29

The Genus *Brachyspira*

The family Spirochaetaceae contains pathogens in the genera *Treponema* and *Borrelia* (see Chapter 32), and *Brachyspira*. Many species of *Brachyspira* were formerly in the genus *Serpulina,* which now contains only the nonpathogenic species *Serpulina intermedia* and *Serpulina murdochii*. It is apparently inevitable that both of these will move to the genus *Brachyspira,* leaving the genus *Serpulina* without legitimate members. They will be referred to here as members of the genus *Brachyspira*.

Spirochetes in general are slender, flexible, and helically coiled. Their three basic elements are an outer sheath, axial filaments or fibrils, and the cell wall and cell membrane comprising the protoplasmic cylinder. The axial filaments insert at either end of the protoplasmic cylinder, overlapping in the center and enabling the corkscrewlike motility, along a helical path, which is characteristic of spirochetes. Spirochetes are gram negative, but stain poorly.

Brachyspira species of veterinary significance are *Brachyspira hyodysenteriae, Brachyspira pilosicoli, Brachyspira aalborgi, Brachyspira intermedia,* and *Brachyspira alvinipulli* (Table 29-1). *Brachyspira innocens* is a commensal. *Brachyspira* spp. are oxygen-tolerant anaerobes.

BRACHYSPIRA HYODYSENTERIAE

Disease and Epidemiology

Swine dysentery is a severe mucohemorrhagic diarrheal disease characterized by extensive inflammation and epithelial necrosis of the large intestine (Figure 29-1). Pigs of any age may be affected, although disease is uncommon in neonates and is seen primarily in grower/finisher pigs. Bloody diarrhea can be fatal if not treated, or may become chronic, with dehydration and emaciation and pseudomembrane formation in the cecum, colon, and rectum. Less acute disease

TABLE 29-1   *Brachyspira* Species of Veterinary Importance

Brachyspira Species	Role in Animal Disease
B. hyodysenteriae	Swine dysentery
B. pilosicoli	Colonic spirochetosis in pigs, chickens, humans
B. aalborgi	Colonic spirochetosis in humans, nonhuman primates, opossums
B. alvinipulli	Colonic spirochetosis in poultry
B. intermedia	Colonic spirochetosis in poultry
B. innocens	Nonpathogen; colonizes pigs, dogs, chickens
B. murdochii	Nonpathogen; colonizes dogs, chickens

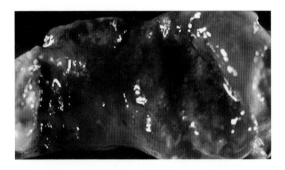

FIGURE 29-1 Mucohemorrhagic colonic lesion typical of swine dysentery. (Courtesy J. Glenn Songer.)

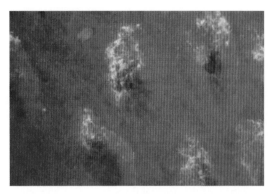

FIGURE 29-2 *Brachyspira hyodysenteriae* in colonic crypts (fluorescent antibody stain). (Courtesy Lynn A. Joens.)

manifests as weight loss and mild diarrhea. Economic losses result mainly from growth retardation, medication costs, and mortality.

The causative agent of swine dysentery, now known as *B. hyodysenteriae* (formerly *Treponema hyodysenteriae, Serpula hyodysenteriae,* and *Serpulina hyodysenteriae*) was identified and characterized in the early 1970s. Nine serotypes of *B. hyodysenteriae* are based on differences in lipopolysaccharide (LPS) antigens.

Infection with *B. hyodysenteriae* is by the fecal-oral route. Reservoir hosts for *B. hyodysenteriae* include pigs and wild rodents, but farm dogs can also spread the infection by way of coprophagia and subsequent excretion. Recovered, asymptomatic pigs can excrete *B. hyodysenteriae* in feces for 3 months or more. Environmental survival of *B. hyodysenteriae* is usually short lived (24-48 hours).

Swine dysentery is a relatively common disease in some major pig-producing countries, but is now relatively uncommon in the United States. When a naive herd is first exposed, disease may appear in only a few pigs, but as environmental accumulations of the organism are increasingly refreshed from diseased and asymptomatic carrier pigs, larger numbers of pigs are affected. The characteristics of an outbreak are influenced by the types of contact with infectious material allowed by the particular management system and housing type. Endemic swine dysentery can manifest a spectrum of severity ranging from mild and transient to severe and occasionally fatal. Disease can be inapparent because of specific medication schemes.

Pathogenesis

Brachyspira hyodysenteriae has two bundles of 7 to 13 periplasmic flagella, which make the organism highly motile in mucus and facilitate colonization

of colonic crypts (Figure 29-2) and other mucus-covered enterocytes. Flagella are composed of three antigenically related core polypeptides and two sheath polypeptides. Flagellar mutants are avirulent in swine, suggesting that motility is an important virulence factor.

Neither specific nor nonspecific adherence to enterocytes has been demonstrated in vivo. *Brachyspira hyodysenteriae* and *B. innocens* adhere equally well in vitro to cultured intestinal and epithelial cells. Thus a role for adhesion in virulence of *B. hyodysenteriae* remains unproven.

Brachyspira hyodysenteriae is found in epithelial cells in pigs with swine dysentery, but dogma has been that invasion is not an obligate part of pathogenesis. Furthermore, invasion of colonic enterocytes in vitro has not been demonstrated. The organism may invade goblet cells and disseminate to enteroabsorptive cells. Tight junctions between colonic enterocytes may be weakened in response to *B. hyodysenteriae* infection.

The pathology observed in acute cases of swine dysentery suggests involvement of one or more cytotoxins, possibly in the form of the widely observed β-hemolysin. Lesions similar to those in natural cases develop in intestinal loops exposed to purified hemolysin. Three distinct hemolysin genes, *tlyA, tlyB,* and *tlyC,* have been cloned and sequenced. Each gene is present as a single-copy chromosomal locus. Recombinant proteins are hemolytic and cytotoxic, but by an unknown mechanism; *tlyA*-minus mutants display decreased hemolysis in vitro and are attenuated in mice and in pigs. LPS, however, is of uncertain importance in pathogenesis, in that biological activity of LPS from *B. hyodysenteriae* differs little from that of *B. innocens*.

Protease may also contribute to virulence of *B. hyodysenteriae*. Damage to and detachment of epithelial cell monolayers are partially abrogated by serine protease inhibitors, although only a minority of strains produce demonstrable protease activity.

Dysentery cannot be produced in gnotobiotic pigs with pure cultures of *B. hyodysenteriae*, and the organism may require interaction with members of the normal flora (e.g., *Fusobacterium necrophorum, Bacteroides vulgatus,* and *B. fragilis*).

Diagnosis

Diagnosis of swine dysentery is based, in the first instance, on compatible clinical signs. However, signs may be similar in other types of enteritis (e.g., salmonellosis, colonic spirochetosis, and proliferative enteropathy), so demonstration of *B. hyodysenteriae* in lesions is the basis for a presumptive diagnosis of swine dysentery.

Mucosal scrapings from affected large intestine, rectal swabs, or feces should be subjected to direct examination and bacteriologic culture. Wet mounts can be examined by darkfield or phase contrast microscopy, and fixed smears should be Gram stained (using carbol fuchsin as the counterstain) and examined by brightfield microscopy. Staining with dilute carbol fuchsin, Victoria blue 4-R, or silver impregnation is also useful; the last is commonly used to demonstrate organisms in tissue. Fluorescent antibody techniques have been described. Demonstration of three to five spirochetes per high-power field is significant (Figure 29-3).

Brachyspira hyodysenteriae (and other members of the genus) grow slowly and are nutritionally fastidious. Specimens are plated onto selective blood agar (containing colistin, vancomycin, and spectinomycin, or spectinomycin alone). Plates incubated at 42° C in an anaerobic environment containing hydrogen and carbon dioxide are examined at 48-hour intervals for up to 10 days. Key features in identification of *B. hyodysenteriae* are colonial morphology, degree of β-hemolysis, production of indole, and hippurate hydrolysis. *Brachyspira hyodysenteriae* produces small, translucent colonies with a zone of clear hemolysis after approximately 48 hours' incubation. Incorporation of 1% sodium RNA into media enhances growth, but also accentuates the difference in hemolysis

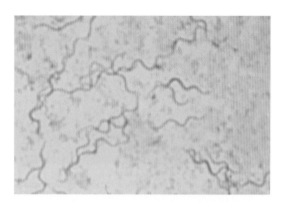

FIGURE 29-3   *Brachyspira hyodysenteriae* (Victoria blue 4R-stained smear from colon). (Courtesy D.L. Harris.)

between *B. hyodysenteriae* and *B. innocens,* the latter being weakly β-hemolytic. *Brachyspira hyodysenteriae* is indole positive and hippurate negative (Table 29-2).

Isolation of the organism from affected untreated animals is straightforward, but detection of individual asymptomatic carrier animals is often unsuccessful. Diagnosis is sometimes facilitated by use of nucleic acid-based assays. Polymerase chain reaction (PCR) may be able to detect as few as 10 cells per gram of feces, but the practical limit is probably closer to 10^3 to 10^4 cells per gram of feces. This relative lack of sensitivity limits the utility of PCR for detection of carrier animals with subclinical infections.

Colonization by *B. hyodysenteriae* elicits a strong immunologic response. Antibody titers may be maintained at low levels, even in animals long recovered from swine dysentery. Many methods for detection of circulating antibodies against *B. hyodysenteriae* have been developed. Tests based on whole-cell antigens are prone to false positives as a result of cross-reactivity among shared antigens. Lipopolysaccharide antigen–based assays are more specific, but decreased sensitivity may be an issue because of serotype variation. Specific assays include indirect fluorescent antibody tests, hemagglutination, microscopic agglutination, complement fixation, and enzyme immunoassays. Serology is best applied to herds rather than to individual pigs. A 30-kD outer-membrane lipoprotein (BmpB) is *B. hyodysenteriae*–specific and is immunoreactive in natural and experimental infections. This antigen may form the basis for more useful serologic tests,

TABLE 29-2 Characteristic Features of Members of the Genus *Brachyspira*

Brachyspira Species	B-Hemolysis	Indole	Hippurate Hydrolysis	Colony Morphology
hyodysenteriae	Strong	Pos	Neg	Thin film, sometimes with "ground
pilosicoli	Weak	Neg	Pos	glass" appearance; β-hemolysis
aalborgi	Weak	Neg	Neg	appears before surface growth;
alvinipulli	Weak	Neg	Pos	visible colonial surface growth in
intermedia	Weak	Pos	Neg	2-4 days; discrete colonies
innocens	Weak	Neg	Neg	become confluent with age
murdochii	Weak	Neg	Neg	

Neg, Negative; *Pos*, positive.

but at present no specific serologic assays are commercially available.

Prevention and Control

It was at one time common practice to treat swine dysentery with arsanilic acid. Producers were advised to treat until pigs developed signs of arsenic poisoning. In the 1970s, producers frequently resorted to off-label use of imidazole compounds (ipronidazole, dimetridazole) that were strictly prohibited from use in food animals. A more useful approach today is treatment or prophylaxis with lincomycin, tylosin, erythromycin, bacitracin, carbadox, gentamicin, tiamulin, virginiamycin, or spiramycin in feed or water. Antimicrobial susceptibility testing is not routinely practiced, but may nonetheless be useful because of apparent development of resistance.

Immunity is predominantly humoral, and hyperimmune serum is protective. Bacterins protect against infection, at least to some degree.

INTESTINAL OR COLONIC SPIROCHETOSES: *BRACHYSPIRA PILOSICOLI, BRACHYSPIRA AALBORGI, BRACHYSPIRA INTERMEDIA,* AND *BRACHYSPIRA ALVINIPULLI*

Diseases and Epidemiology

Brachyspira pilosicoli is likely the primary etiologic agent of intestinal spirochetosis in humans and domestic and wild animals. *Brachyspira aalborgi, B. intermedia,* and *B. alvinipulli* also cause such infections, all of which are characterized by attachment of spirochetes to the epithelial surface of the colon, cecum, and rectum. North American opossums are infected with spirochetes

resembling *B. aalborgi.* Colonic spirochetosis may be a more accurate description of *B. pilosicoli* infection because colonization and lesion development is restricted to the colon (Figure 29-4). The closely related *B. aalborgi* causes colonic spirochetosis in humans, nonhuman primates, and opossums.

Brachyspira pilosicoli from animals is similar in many respects to isolates from humans. Disease has been produced experimentally in pigs, chicks, and mice by inoculation with *B. pilosicoli* isolated from humans, monkeys, pigs, dogs, and birds. Genetically similar strains of *B. pilosicoli* have been obtained from humans and dogs in the same community. In sum, it seems likely that *B. pilosicoli* is zoonotic.

DISEASE IN NONHUMAN PRIMATES

Most monkeys with intestinal spirochetosis have no clinical signs or gross lesions. The extent of spirochetal surface colonization varies among

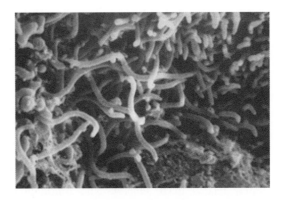

FIGURE 29-4 Spirochetal colonization of colonic epithelium. (Courtesy D.L. Harris.)

infected macaques, but often extends from the cecum to the rectum. End-on attachment of spirochetes is commonly demonstrated in wild-caught, colony-housed primates.

Histologic lesions comprise focal to diffuse brush border thickening extending into crypts in the cecum, colon, and rectum. End-on attachment of spirochetes to the brush border surface of colonic enterocytes resembles a picket fence and results in displacement or effacement of microvilli and rarefaction of terminal-web microfilaments. Spirochetes are also found in basolateral spaces, in membrane-bound vesicles or free in enterocyte cytoplasm, in subepithelial connective tissue of lamina propria, and in macrophages. Inflammation is usually minimal, although some monkeys have inflammatory cell infiltrates suggestive of ulcerative colitis.

Rates of infection by various species remains to be thoroughly defined, but most are probably caused by *B. aalborgi* or *B. pilosicoli*.

DISEASE IN OPOSSUMS

Opossums may represent a reservoir of infection for other species. Information is not complete, but spirochetes apparently disrupt the brush border of cecal enterocytes, after the manner of colonic spirochetosis in humans and nonhuman primates. Growth characteristics of spirochetes recovered from opossums are consistent with *B. aalborgi,* but sequence analysis of 16S and 23S rDNA suggests that they share characteristics with *B. aalborgi* and *B. pilosicoli.*

DISEASE IN DOGS

Symptomatic dogs are usually less than 1 year old and have a history of chronic mucoid diarrhea and wasting. End-on attachment of spirochetes along enterocyte brush borders causes microvillous effacement in the cecum and colon, and spirochetes are often found attached to underlying stromal connective tissue in erosions at the extrusion area between crypts. Invasiveness is suggested by the occurrence of spirochetes in basolateral spaces and free in the cytoplasm of enterocytes. Older dogs may be asymptomatic carriers.

Genetic characterization indicates that spirochetes found in dogs with intestinal spirochetosis are *B. pilosicoli*. Those from healthy dogs are more closely related to *B. innocens* and *Brachyspira murdochii,* and have been provisionally named *Brachyspira canis.*

DISEASE IN PIGS

Porcine colonic spirochetosis (CS) was identified more than 20 years ago in the United Kingdom, and is now recognized as a cause of reduced performance in intensively raised swine worldwide. Disease is characterized by rapid onset of loose stools and a clinical course of 7 to 10 days. Persistent infection causes reduced feed efficiency and extended time to market, varying with the severity and the extent of colonic involvement.

Cecum and spiral colon of affected pigs may be gas filled and contain loose to watery feces. Mesocolonic edema is common, and fibrinonecrotic exudate over coalescing mucosal erosions is sometimes present. Spirochetal colonization can be demonstrated by microscopic examination of hematoxylin and eosin- or silver-stained sections of cecum and spiral colon, although a more definitive approach involves immunohistochemistry (based on antiflagellar antibodies) or in situ hybridization. Attached spirochetes may take on the appearance of a false brush border or of spirochetal rosettes (spirochetes attached to membrane fragments in the colonic lumen).

As the infection progresses, attenuation of cecal and colonic epithelia is accompanied by multifocal erosion. Spirochetes attach to exposed extracellular matrix and submucosal capillary walls in erosions, and are seen inside macrophages. Hyperplasia of crypt epithelium, elongation of crypt columns, and depletion of goblet cells accompany repair. When infection persists, spirochetes can be demonstrated in mucus-filled, dilated colonic glands. Concurrent infection with other bacteria increases the severity of clinical cases. Clinical recovery from experimentally induced CS can occur, but may require up to 7 weeks after challenge

Binding of spirochetes to epithelial cells is not always demonstrated, suggesting that it is transitory or perhaps patchy. However, persistence of the organism in crypts and invasion of lamina propria may be important components of pathogenesis. Dissemination to extraintestinal sites (lymph nodes and pericardial sac) suggests the existence of invasive properties.

Diet influences the clinical presentation of infections caused by *B. pilosicoli*. A highly digestible diet, in which relatively little fermentable carbohydrate enters the cecum and spiral colon, may result in elevated colonic pH and reduced volatile fatty acid production, both of which are unfavorable for spirochetal colonization. Poorly digestible diets heighten clinical signs and colitis in *B. pilosicoli* infections.

DISEASE IN DOMESTIC, WILD, ZOO, AND GAME BIRDS

Avian intestinal spirochetosis has emerged as a problem in commercial layer and meat breeder chickens. It was first reported in the mid-1980s in the Netherlands and is now known to occur in the United States, Europe, United Kingdom, Australia, and elsewhere. Initial diagnosis of the condition was likely delayed by lack of suitable diagnostic methods; avian intestinal spirochetes stain poorly in histologic sections, and specialized media and techniques are required for isolation. Furthermore, they do not all induce characteristic histologic lesions. Surveys have revealed a two- to fivefold higher colonization rate in symptomatic flocks of broiler breeder and layer flocks than in flocks without disease, and age is a risk factor for colonization.

Avian intestinal spirochetes have the expected gram-negative cell wall structure. Axial flagella are most commonly arranged in an 8:16:8 or 5:10:5 pattern. All species are oxygen-tolerant anaerobes, and they can be cultivated under much the same conditions as *B. hyodysenteriae.* Incubation at 42° C inhibits growth of some contaminants while allowing spirochetes to grow. Discrete colonies are not formed, and evidence of growth is found in a thin hazelike film that forms on the agar surface after 3 or more days' incubation. Some strains are hemolytic.

Three members of the genus *Brachyspira* have been associated with intestinal spirochetosis in fowl (see Table 29-1). In Europe and Australia, *B. intermedia* and *B. pilosicoli* predominate, whereas in the United States, most cases involve *B. pilosicoli* or *B. alvinipulli.* The nonpathogens *B. innocens* and *B. murdochii,* as well as the proposed species *B. pulli,* may also be found. In addition to domestic poultry, zoo and game birds may be infected with *B. pilosicoli* and *B. intermedia,* and infection of captive rheas with *B. hyodysenteriae* has been reported.

Disease associated with *B. intermedia* is characterized by growth retardation, increased fecal moisture content, chronic diarrhea, and delayed or reduced egg production, and chicks experimentally inoculated with *B. intermedia* or *B. pilosicoli* (but not with *B. innocens*) develop diarrhea. Increased fecal lipids is a commonly observed phenomenon,

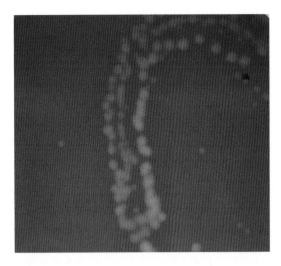

FIGURE 29-5 Mechanical carriage of colonic spirochetes (illustrated here by *Brachyspira hyodysenteriae*) by house flies. (Courtesy J. Glenn Songer.)

but its genesis is unknown. Fecal staining of eggs and the problems associated with wet litter (problems in cage cleaning, odor control, and flies) (Figure 29-5) are additional economic issues.

The most consistent finding upon microscopic examination of affected tissues is segmental, basophilic thickening of the cecal enterocyte brush border. This comprises a layer of spirochetes arrayed end-on along enterocyte membranes. Multifocal necrosis and spirochetal invasion of lamina propria are common. The likelihood of cecal wall inflammation increases with age.

Avian intestinal spirochetosis occurs rarely, if at all, in broiler flocks, although retarded growth is common in experimentally inoculated chicks. Inoculation of broiler breeding hens, however, causes persistent infection comparable to that seen in layer hens. Furthermore, chicks hatched from eggs produced by these birds have reduced growth rates, poor feed conversion, and poor feed digestion, although they are not colonized by spirochetes. There is also a tendency toward an increased number of weak chicks. Thus intestinal spirochetosis can affect broiler performance through effects on the breeding flock.

Treatment of avian intestinal spirochetosis has been with lincospectin (which produced slimy diarrhea of 2 to 3 weeks' duration and absence of spirochetes for 3 months) and tiamulin (which reduced the level of infection by two thirds for 3 months posttreatment).

Pathogenesis

Pathogenesis of intestinal spirochetosis has been best studied in *B. pilosicoli*. It is probably initiated by chemotaxis of spirochetes toward mucin. Spirochetal motility in viscous environments and mucin glycoproteins could be important nutrients. Thus motility and attraction to mucin could facilitate attachment by placing the spirochete in proximity to enterocytes. End-on attachment of spirochetes to the enterocyte apical membrane forms parallel arrays by way of interaction of a specific spirochete adhesin with a host-cell receptor. Attachment is accompanied by formation of plasma membrane caplike structures that resemble (at least superficially) the result of interaction of *Helicobacter pylori* with gastric epithelial cells. Pathophysiology of the diarrhea is based on massive spirochetal attachment and disruption of absorption, as well as reduction in the number of crypts and interference with absorption of specific amino sugars.

Damage in *B. pilosicoli* infection is in the extrusion zone between crypts. Penetration of the epithelium occurs primarily between enterocytes, by paracytosis. Attachment at intercellular junctions may allow a *B. pilosicoli* serine protease to affect integrity of tight junctions and facilitate penetration; invasion of epithelial cells in vitro is minimal. The organism spreads extracellularly in connective tissue beneath the lamina propria. It is phagocytosed by macrophages, but may also enter submucosal blood capillaries, consistent with frequent isolation from lymph nodes of affected pigs.

Bracyhspira pilosicoli persists in crypt luminae and in cecal and colonic goblet cells. Infiltration of lamina propria by macrophages and lymphocytes in chronic disease is reminiscent of the pattern seen in chronic leptospiral interstitial nephritis. A humoral immune response occurs several weeks after challenge.

Diagnosis

Gross lesions are likely to be absent in intestinal spirochetoses, and initial diagnosis is often based on microbiologic findings. Spirochetes may be observed in wet mount preparations of feces or cecal droppings, but this is not a sensitive method, especially in avian disease. Sensitivity of bacteriologic culture depends heavily on the condition of the sample. It may not be possible to isolate spirochetes from birds given antimicrobial therapy, even if organisms are observed microscopically.

Media inoculation, incubation, and examination of cultures should be done under conditions described for isolation of *B. hyodysenteriae*.

Identification to species is difficult. Biochemical profiling and carbohydrate fermentation can be useful (see Table 29-2). However, the most definitive methods of identification have been multilocus enzyme electrophoresis or PCR assays for 16S or 23S rDNA.

Prevention and Control

Attention to biosecurity may limit opportunities for introduction of spirochetes on contaminated machinery, boots, and clothing. Elevated standards for hygiene in housing areas will often allow a producer to break a transmission cycle. Measures that minimize contact with infected feces should be instituted.

Antimicrobial susceptibility testing of chicken isolates of *B. pilosicoli* and *B. alvinipulli* reveals susceptibility to lincomycin, carbadox, and tiamulin; compounds used for the treatment of *B. hyodysenteriae* infections are likely to be useful in treating intestinal spirochetosis in pigs and chickens. Infections may recur, especially in birds that are heavily infected when treatment is initiated.

SUGGESTED READINGS

Atyeo EF, Oxherry SL, Combs BG, Hampson DJ: Development and evaluation of polymerase chain reaction tests as an aid to the diagnosis of swine dysentery and intestinal spirochaetosis, *Lett Appl Microbiol* 26:126-130, 1998.

Boyne M, Jensen TK, Moller K, et al: Specific detection of the genus *Serpulina*, *S. hyodysenteriae* and *S. pilosicoli* in porcine intestines by fluorescent rRNA in situ hybridization, *Mol Cell Probes* 12:323-330, 1998.

Buckles EL, Eaton KA, Swayne DE: Cases of spirochete-associated necrotizing typhlitis in captive common rheas *(Rhea americana)*, *Avian Dis* 41:144-148, 1997.

Duhamel GE, Elder RO, Muniappa N, et al: Colonic spirochetal infections of nonhuman primates associated with *Brachyspira aalborgi*, *Serpulina pilosicoli*, and unclassified flagellated bacteria, *Clin Infect Dis* 25(Suppl 2):186-188, 1997.

Duhamel GE, Muniappa N, Gardner I, et al: Porcine colonic spirochetosis: a diarrheal disease associated with a newly recognized species of intestinal spirochaetes, *Pig J* 35:101-110, 1995.

Duhamel GE, Muniappa N, Mathiesen MR, et al: Certain canine weakly hemolytic intestinal spirochetes are phenotypically and genotypically related to spirochetes associated with human and porcine intestinal spirochetosis, *J Clin Microbiol* 33:2212-2215, 1995.

Fellström C, Pettersson B, Thomson J, et al: Identification of *Serpulina* species associated with porcine colitis by biochemical analysis and PCR, *J Clin Microbiol* 35:462-467, 1997.

Kinyon JM, Harris DL, Glock RD: Enteropathogenicity of various isolates of *Treponema hyodysenteriae, Infect Immun* 15:638-646, 1997.

Lymbery AJ, Hampson DJ, Hopkins RM, et al: Multilocus enzyme electrophoresis for identification and typing of *Treponema hyodysenteriae* and related spirochaetes, *Vet Microbiol* 22:89-99, 1990.

Songer JG, Glock RD, Schwartz KJ, Harris DL: Isolation of *Treponema hyodysenteriae* from sources other than swine, *J Am Vet Med Assoc* 172:464-466, 1978.

Taylor DJ, Simmons JR, Laird HM: Production of diarrhoea and dysentery in pigs by feeding pure cultures of a spirochaete differing from *Treponema hyodysenteriae, Vet Rec* 106:326-332, 1980.

Trott DJ, McLaren AJ, Hampson DJ: Pathogenicity of human and porcine intestinal spirochetes in one-day-old specific-pathogen-free chicks: an animal model of intestinal spirochetosis, *Infect Immun* 63:3705-3710, 1995.

Chapter 30

The Genus *Lawsonia*

Lawsonia intracellularis is the etiologic agent of an intestinal hyperplastic disease called proliferative enteropathy. It is an obligate intracellular pathogen, and has not been cultivated on artificial media. Disease in pigs was described more than 70 years ago and was reproduced with homogenates of intestine from affected pigs nearly 30 years ago. In the past decade, the organism was isolated from hamsters and pigs and cultivated in vitro in pure culture and used to infect pigs.

Lawsonia intracellularis is gram negative, curved, and without fimbriae or spores. A single polar flagellum is responsible for the darting motility of extracellular organisms. Cultivation in vitro requires dividing eukaryotic cells and an atmosphere of 82% nitrogen, 9% carbon dioxide, and 9% oxygen. The organism is more than 90% similar to *Desulfovibrio desulfuricans* and approximately 92% similar to *Bilophila wadsworthia* in 16S rDNA sequence, but a distinct physiologic and biochemical profile justified establishment of a new genus and species. Isolates from several animal species have more than 98% 16S rDNA sequence similarity to pig isolates, and phenotypic analysis has demonstrated only minor differences among isolates.

DISEASE AND PATHOGENESIS

Proliferative enteropathy (proliferative enteritis, porcine intestinal adenomatosis, proliferative hemorrhagic enteropathy, ileitis, wet-tail disease, and intestinal adenomatous hyperplasia) is best described in pigs and hamsters. The same disease process occurs sporadically in cats, dogs, ferrets, foxes, and horses.

A major form of the disease in pigs is acute hemorrhagic diarrhea (proliferative hemorrhagic enteropathy; Figure 30-1) in older animals, including breeding stock, characterized by marked hemorrhage from thickened, proliferated mucosa, in the absence of visible bleeding points. Disease can also take the form of chronic mild diarrhea and reduced performance in growing pigs (porcine intestinal adenomatosis), with marked reductions in rate of gain, lasting 4 to 6 weeks. A portion of these animals may develop necrotic ileitis, with deep coagulative necrosis of the adenomatous ileum and permanent stunting

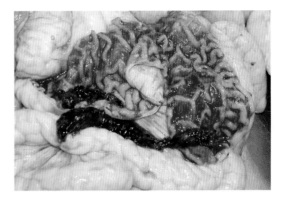

FIGURE 30-1   Gross lesions of the hemorrhagic form of proliferative ileitis. (Courtesy Peter Moisan.)

and unthriftiness. Lesions in hamsters are comparable with those in the chronic porcine disease, although later stages are characterized by pyogranulomatous inflammation.

Oral inoculation of conventional pigs with pure cultures of *L. intracellularis* leads to rapid association with and endocytic internalization by enterocytes. Vacuolar escape and cytoplasmic multiplication occurs through day 6 postinfection. Mitosis continues, and organisms are found in cytoplasmic protrusions of daughter cells. Bacteria are eventually released from enterocytes at villous apices, and infection spreads throughout the ileum, distal jejunum, cecum, and colon. The organism is detected only in intestine, lymph node, and tonsil, the last of which has no apparent role in pathogenesis.

Macroscopic lesions occur almost coincidentally in time with microscopic lesions. Microcolonies of *L. intracellularis* are found in apical cytoplasm of crypt epithelial cells during the first week postinfection, but enterocyte hyperplasia is not in evidence until nearly 1 week later and can continue for more than 6 weeks. Gross lesions are usually found in terminal ileum, but also in jejunum, cecum, and proximal colon. In the acute form, intestinal tissue is thickened and turgid, with a corrugated serosal surface and lumenal blood clots. Chronically affected intestines have irregular, patchy, subserosal edema, mainly at the mesenteric insertion. Ileal mucosa is thickened, with deep folds and patches of pseudomembrane. Surviving animals may have hypertrophic and thickened muscularis mucosa. Microscopic lesions consist of adenomatous proliferation of crypt enterocytes (Figure 30-2), in association with morphologically compatible organisms (Figure 30-3). Crypts are elongated and enlarged, and immature epithelial cells are highly mitotic. Goblet cells are reduced in numbers or absent in affected areas; inflammatory cell infiltration is minimal. Intestines of acutely affected pigs are congested, and blood is found in the intestinal lumen. Infected enterocytes usually have short irregular microvilli. Resolution of lesions is closely related to disappearance of intracellular organisms. Inflammation is a factor only in later-stage lesions and is not characteristic of the primary lesion. Following initiation of mucosal hyperplasia in hamsters, there is progressive replacement of mature villous columnar absorptive cells by undifferentiated crypt-type cells.

Specific humoral and cell-mediated immune responses are detected 2 weeks after exposure, and levels peak near the end of the third week. There is a mild infiltration of cytotoxic T cells, macrophages, and B-lymphocytes (major histocompatibility complex [MHC] class II) at the beginning of the cell-mediated immune response to *L. intracellularis*. Interferon-γ may limit intracellular infection and secretory IgA has been demonstrated in the apical cytoplasm of proliferating enterocytes. Convalescent pigs have a degree of immunity to reinoculation.

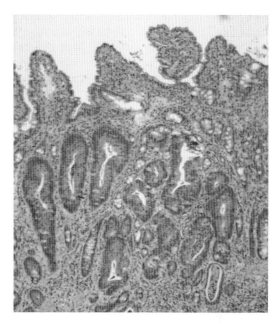

FIGURE 30-2 Proliferative lesions in the non-hemorhagic form of *Lawsonia intracellularis* infection. (Courtesy Lynn A. Joens.)

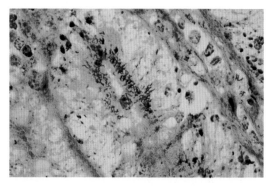

FIGURE 30-3 Silver-stained *Lawsonia intracellularis* in proliferative lesions. (Courtesy Lynn A. Joens.)

Virulence of *L. intracellularis* is not well characterized. The infection process requires the presence of normal intestinal flora, in that germ-free pigs are not susceptible to infection by pure cultures. Enterocyte attachment and entry occur from the apical surface. Neither adhesins nor receptors have been described, but invasion apparently does not require bacterial viability; eukaryotic cells internalize formalin-fixed organisms. Invasion is reduced, but not eliminated, by effects of cytochalasin D on the enterocytoskeleton.

Lawsonia intracellularis escapes from the endocytic vacuole and lives free in cytoplasm. Phagosomal or endosomal escape is facilitated by lytic toxins in some organisms, and a protein hemolysin has been associated with attachment and invasion by *L. intracellularis*, both in vitro and in vivo. Cellular proliferation characteristic of proliferative enteropathy has not been reproduced in vitro, and its mechanism of induction is unknown. Proliferating enterocytes have poor MHC class II expression, perhaps providing an immunologically safe environment for *L. intracellularis*. Enterocyte proliferation is apparently not a result of reduced apoptosis. Cell division may be required for bacterial multiplication, in that cell growth inhibitors also inhibit multiplication of *L. intracellularis.*

Partial genomic sequencing of *L. intracellularis* has identified putative flagellar biosynthesis genes, as well as Yop (*Yersinia* outer protein) and LvrV gene homologs, suggesting that *L. intracellularis* has a type III secretion system.

EPIDEMIOLOGY

Proliferative enteropathy has been described in a broad range of hosts, including pigs, nonhuman primates, hamsters, rabbits, rats, guinea pigs, foals, sheep, white-tailed deer, ferrets, arctic foxes, dogs, and birds. There are no reports of proliferative enteropathy in human beings. The source of infection for these animal species has not been determined, but the habitat of *L. intracellularis* may be limited to the glandular ileal epithelium of infected animals. Species-to-species transmission occurs, and pig isolates infect hamsters, mice, and horses.

Little is known about the carrier state, including the time during which animals shed the organism following the clinical disease. Fecal matter from infected pigs is a source of infection, and pig-to-pig contact is an important route of transmission. Mechanical vectors (such as boots) and biologic vectors (such as mice, birds, and insects) may carry the infection from one group of pigs to another.

Isolation of *L. intracellularis* is difficult, so there is a paucity of information about environmental survival. Pigs become colonized after oral inoculation with feces (from culture-positive animals) stored for as long as 2 weeks at temperatures approximately 15° C. Pure cultures are susceptible to quaternary ammonium disinfectants, but 1% povidone-iodine is less effective. The organism is resistant to 1% potassium peroxymonosulfate or a 0.33% phenolic mixture.

DIAGNOSIS

Laboratory diagnosis has usually been based on herd history, clinical signs, gross and microscopic lesions, and detection of morphologically compatible intracellular bacteria. The last is accomplished by silver staining, immunofluorescence assays, immunoperoxidase stains, and by hybridization with DNA probes. An enzyme-linked immunosorbent assay (ELISA) is used on a herd basis and a polymerase chain reaction (PCR) assay facilitates detection of individual infected pigs.

CONTROL AND TREATMENT

Control begins with preventing introduction of infection by carriers, and there is some support for a strategy in which replacement stock is acquired only from ELISA-negative herds. Infection can be controlled by a variety of antibiotics in feed, including carbadox, spectinomycin, and tylosin. A commercial vaccine, based on a live attenuated strain of *L. intracellularis,* is widely used and is considered to be quite effective.

SUGGESTED READINGS

Guedes RMC, Gebhart CJ: Onset and duration of fecal shedding, cell-mediated and humoral immune responses in pigs after challenge with a pathogenic isolate or attenuated vaccine strain of *Lawsonia intracellularis, Vet Microbiol* 91:135-145, 2003.

Joens LA, Nibbelink S, Glock RD: Induction of gross and microscopic lesions of porcine proliferative enteritis by *Lawsonia intracellularis, Am J Vet Res* 58:1125-1131, 1997.

Jones GF, Davies PR, Rose R, et al: Comparison of techniques for diagnosis of proliferative enteritis of swine, *Am J Vet Res* 54:1980-1985, 1993.

Lawson GH, McOrist S, Jasni S, Mackie RA: Intracellular bacteria of porcine proliferative enteropathy: cultivation and maintenance in vitro, *J Clin Microbiol* 31: 1136-1142, 1993.

Lomax LG, Glock RD: Naturally occurring porcine proliferative enteritis: pathologic and bacteriologic findings, *Am J Vet Res* 43:1608-1621, 1982.

McOrist S, Gebhart CJ, Boid R, Barns SM: Characterization of *Lawsonia intracellularis* gen. nov., sp. nov., the obligately intracelullar bacterium of porcine proliferative enteropathy, *Int J Syst Bacteriol* 45:820-882, 1995.

McOrist S, Jasni S, Mackie RA, et al: Reproduction of porcine proliferative enteropathy with pure cultures of ileal symbiont intracellularis, *Infect Immun* 61: 4286-4292, 1993.

McOrist S, Lawson GH, Rowland AC, MacIntyre N: Early lesions of proliferative enteritis in pigs and hamsters, *Vet Pathol* 26:260-264, 1989.

Rowland AC, Lawson GH, Maxwell A: Intestinal adenomatosis in the pig: occurrence of a bacterium in affected cells, *Nature* 243:417, 1973.

Chapter 31

The Genus *Leptospira*

eptospirosis is encountered commonly by those dealing with animal infectious disease. Its occurrence as a zoonotic infection of humans is strongly influenced by connections to animal production, tropical climates, at-risk occupations, and behavior; it is counted by some as an emerging infectious disease of humans and by others as the most widespread zoonosis. The highest incidence of leptospirosis in the United States is in Hawaii. Interest in human leptospirosis has increased in recent times as a result of several large and well-publicized flood-associated case clusters in Central and South America. This might, as some have suggested, result from increased leptospiral virulence, but it is perhaps more likely to be caused by altered interaction among humans, reservoir species, and the environment.

Manifestations of human disease vary from nearly subclinical flulike illness to fulminant and fatal pulmonary hemorrhage and hepatic and renal failure. Icteric leptospirosis with renal failure was reported in the nineteenth century, and although much of the credit for this has been given to Adolf Weil, the description of the syndrome predates his work. Leptospirosis was recognized as an occupational disease in ancient China, and akiyami (autumn fever) is a part of modern Japanese medicine. Early in the twentieth century, physicians studying yellow fever in New Orleans found spirochetes in tissues of jaundiced patients and briefly advocated an etiologic role for them. The link between spirochetes and what we now know as leptospirosis was established

later, when Japanese and German workers detected spirochetes and specific antibodies in the blood of miners and soldiers with infectious jaundice.

Leptospirosis is strongly environmentally associated, and transmission depends on direct or indirect interactions between humans and mammalian (usually rodent) reservoir hosts. *Leptospira interrogans* serovar *icterohaemorrhagiae* may have reached western Europe in the 1700s, coincident with extension of the range of *Rattus norvegicus* from Eurasia; the role of rats in epidemiology of the disease was discovered early in the twentieth century.

Epidemiologic patterns of leptospirosis fall roughly into three categories. Few serovars are involved in human disease in temperate climates, and infection is inevitably associated with direct contact with infected farm animals. In wet tropical areas, many more serovars infect humans, domestic animals, and large numbers of reservoir species; human exposure is often caused by widespread environmental contamination. Also, rodent-borne leptospirosis occurs in the urban environment, especially with infrastructure disruption by natural or man-made disasters. Human leptospirosis has not been a reportable disease in the United States for nearly 10 years, but urban disease in humans is not uncommon and is frequently misdiagnosed.

Until recently, the genus *Leptospira* was divided into species *interrogans* (the name deriving from the question mark shape of the organism and comprising pathogenic strains) and *biflexa* (encompassing saprophytic, mainly environmental,

244

TABLE 31-1 Genomospecies of the Genus *Leptospira*

Genomospecies of the Genus *Leptospira*
L. alexanderi
L. biflexa
L. borgpetersenii
L. fainei
L. inadai
L. interrogans
L. kirschneri
L. meyeri
L. noguchii
L. parva
L. santarosai
L. weilii
L. wolbachii

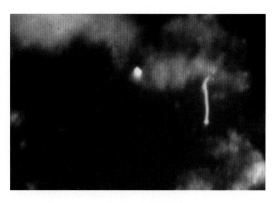

FIGURE 31-1 Fluorescent antibody stain of *Leptospira interrogans* in kidney. (Courtesy William A. Ellis.)

strains). Growth at 13° C, 8-azaguanine resistance, and failure to form spherical cells in 1 M NaCl distinguished *L. biflexa* from *L. interrogans*. Both species were divided into numerous serovars (>60 in *L. biflexa* and >200 in *L. interrogans*), and related serovars are placed in serogroups. Many serovars appear to have a certain species as a natural host, but animals and humans can be infected with a wide variety of serovars. The serovars causing disease in animals vary among countries and sometimes among regions in the same country. Most infections in domestic animals are caused by only a few serovars.

Genetic typing of leptospirae has yielded 13 genomospecies (Table 31-1), and this is likely the future of leptospiral taxonomy. However, there is little correlation between serologic type and genomospecies; it is not uncommon for serogroups and even serovars to be represented in multiple genomospecies. Furthermore, methods for genomospeciation are not widely available, and it seems likely that the antigen-based approach to classification will be the standard for some time to come.

DISEASES, EPIDEMIOLOGY, AND PATHOGENESIS

A few key concepts form the foundation for understanding leptospirosis and its pathogenesis. First, leptospires often colonize proximal convoluted kidney tubules and may be excreted in urine for extended periods by reservoir hosts without clinical signs (Figure 31-1). The carrier state may be as short as a few days or may extend throughout the life of the animal. This is considered a major means of host-to-host transmission. Indirect exposure depends on environmental moisture, neutral soil pH, and a sufficiently mild climate to favor survival of leptospires. Streams and ponds contaminated by the urine of wild rodents or domestic and wild animals can be a source of infection for domestic animals and humans, as can urine aerosols in milking parlors (especially those of the herringbone configuration). The organism can also be isolated from milk of infected cows, and this probably serves as a means of transmission to humans and calves (Figure 31-2).

Second, localization in tissues from which the organism cannot be readily shed is common in infection of at least some hosts with specific serovars. In some urban areas more than 90% of Norway rats have serovar *icterohaemorrhagiae* localized in brain, and horses not infrequently experience localization in the eye.

Third, many serovars of leptospirae can be roughly categorized as host adapted or nonadapted. Infections by the former tend to be relatively mild and sporadic, with venereal transmission and lifelong colonization of the genitourinary tract; serovars *hardjo* in cattle and *bratislava* and *tarassovi* in swine are examples. Nonadapted strains, however, are more likely to produce catastrophic infections, with abortion storms in pregnant animals and, not infrequently, death of adult hosts. The carrier state is generally brief. Serovar *pomona* is nonadapted for swine and cattle, as is serovar *canicola* for dogs. Serovars of serogroups Icterohaemorrhagiae and Ballum are adapted to rats, the latter adapted to mice. The relationship between hosts and adapted strains gives rise to a

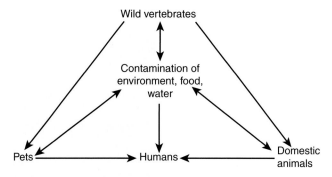

FIGURE 31-2 Transmission and maintenance of *Leptospira interrogans*. (Courtesy Ashley E. Harmon.)

minor but long-lasting serologic response, whereas nonadapted strains provoke high antibody titers. It should be obvious that a serovar may be adapted to one species and not others. It seems reasonable to speculate that most, if not all, species have host-adapted strains, including perhaps humans.

Fourth, certain steps seems to be common to *Leptospira*-induced disease, although all need not occur in every case and in some infections can lead only to very mild clinical signs. Exposure by mucosal or conjunctival routes, or through broken skin, is followed by invasion and eventual development of leptospiremia. Organisms proliferate in parenchymatous organs, including liver, kidneys, spleen, and meninges. Venereal transmission may result only in colonization of reproductive organs. The period of leptospiremia may be shorter (with host-adapted strains) or longer (with nonadapted strains), but in either case gives rise to circulating antibodies that mediate clearance of leptospirae by complement-mediated bacteriolysis. Damage to the maternal-fetal interface or active invasion beyond the placenta may cause fetal death and abortion, or birth of weak offspring. Fetuses infected in the third trimester (and perhaps earlier) may be born with specific antibodies. Organisms are cleared by the effects of antibodies and complement, or if antimicrobial therapy is applied, but may localize for days to years in kidney, reproductive tract, brain, or other tissues.

Fifth, mechanisms of pathogenesis are largely unknown, although the recently demonstrated ability to genetic transform leptospirae should facilitate detailed analysis of leptospiral virulence genes. Leptospiral endotoxin is of low potency, compared with that of many other gram-negative bacteria. Lipopolysaccharide (LPS) mediates adherence of neutrophils to endothelial cells and platelets, suggesting a role in development of thrombocytopenia. LPS is immunogenic and responsible for serovar specificity. In acute leptospirosis, damage to vascular endothelium is common, with resulting hemorrhage and disseminated intravascular coagulation (DIC). The last may be mediated, at least in part, by endotoxin, but sphingomyelinase hemolysins produced by many serovars may be responsible for this vascular damage and for specific clinical signs such as hemoglobinuria. Hemolysis by organisms of serovar *lai* is not related to sphingomyelinase activity, but is apparently due to a pore-forming protein. Protein and glycoprotein cytotoxins have been described.

Leptospiral attachment to epithelial cells can be enhanced by antibody. Virulent strains can bind to fibronectin. On the negative side (for the leptospirae), antibodies and complement are opsonizing; the outer envelope may be antiphagocytic. Leptospires induce apoptosis in vivo and in vitro.

Some symptoms may be immune mediated. Immune complexes may be associated with central nervous system (CNS) inflammation, although this apparently does not occur in the kidney. Autoantibodies, including IgG anticardiolipin antibodies, are detected in acute human illness. Antileptospiral antibodies cross-reacting with equine ocular tissues are apparently involved in pathogenesis of recurrent uveitis because retinal damage relates to the presence of B lymphocytes in the retina.

Finally, there is sufficient leptospiral promiscuity in host selection that it is difficult to say with certainty that a given serovar *cannot* infect a specific host. Certain strains are more commonly associated than others with disease in a given species, but even that varies with geographic region. Thus it is probably best for veterinary practitioners and diagnosticians to become familiar with the serovars infecting animals in the specific locale in which they practice (Table 31-2).

Disease in Cattle

Cattle are commonly infected by serovars *hardjo* and *pomona,* although infections by serovars *grippotyphosa, icterohaemorrhagiae,* and *canicola* are not uncommon. Serovar *hardjo* is apparently adapted to the bovine host, and produces sporadic abortions and infertility, often without other clinical signs. Fetal expulsion is delayed by several days after fetal death as a result of serovar *hardjo* infection. Colonization of the female upper reproductive tract is as common as that of kidneys. Thus the organism is available locally for interaction with embryos. Localization in the seminal vesicle is also quite common, and bulls and cows likely pass the infection back and forth at breeding. A common misconception is that transmission cannot occur under dry conditions. Given venereal transmission and the potential for exposure at congregation sites (such as water sources), *hardjo* and other serovars are quite efficiently transmitted in arid environments. Cows may experience mild to moderate mastitis during the acute phase of disease.

Infection by nonadapted strains often produces more dramatic signs. Infected animals are usually febrile, can be anemic and icteric, are often hemoglobinuric, and may be diarrheic. Abortion is common, with immediate expulsion of the dead fetus. Depending on the nature of the exposure,

the number of animals in a group, and management of remaining animals after initial cases, abortions may occur because storms affect as much as 90% of pregnant females in a herd. With early recognition it is sometimes possible to interrupt the progress of an outbreak by administration of antimicrobials such as streptomycin, but in most cases they have no positive effect.

Disease in Pigs

Porcine leptospirosis is often caused by serovar *pomona* or serovar *bratislava.* Serovars *canicola, grippotyphosa,* and *icterohaemorrhagiae* may also be involved. Disease caused by serovar *pomona* is similar to infections by this serovar in cattle; signs are acute, with abortion in pregnant females. Affected animals often experience fever, icterus, anemia, metritis, and meningoencephalitis, and growing pigs may be generally unthrifty. Sources of infection include carrier pigs, cattle, and wildlife (such as skunks, raccoons, opossums, and deer). Serovar *bratislava* is apparently pig adapted, and causes a clinical picture similar to that associated with serovar *hardjo* infection in cattle. Subclinical disease is the common presentation in adult animals, and lifelong shedding is apparently common. This serovar is extraordinarily difficult to culture from affected animals, and most indications of infection have been obtained as serologic observations.

Disease in Horses

Horses are most commonly affected by serovars *pomona, kennewicki,* and *bratislava.* The first two of these produce acute disease, with fever, icterus, and abortion. Serovar *bratislava* causes

TABLE 31-2 Examples of *Leptospira* Serovars Associated with Disease in Specific Hosts

Serovar	Hosts and Associated Disease
L. kennewicki	Equine abortion, repeat breeding (United States, Northern Ireland, England)
L. bratislava	Equine abortion, repeat breeding (United States, Northern Ireland, England)
	Porcine abortion, infertility (worldwide)
L. pomona	Porcine, bovine, equine abortion
	Skunks
L. canicola	Canine renal, systemic disease
	Porcine systemic disease, abortion
L. icterohaemorrhagiae	Canine septicemia
	Bovine, porcine abortion
	Classic association with rats
L. hardjo	Bovine abortion, infertility
L. grippotyphosa	Canine renal, systemic disease
	Wildlife infections, especially raccoons, skunks

mild and sporadic infection of adults but may be associated with late-term abortions. Most serovars can cause recurrent iridocyclitis (moon blindness or periodic ophthalmia) as a sequel to active infection.

Disease in Companion Animals

Primary routes of infection are direct contact (oral or conjunctival), venereal and placental transfer, bite wounds, and ingestion of infected or contaminated meats. Dogs that have direct or indirect contact with wild rats are often infected, and indirect transmission may occur by way of contaminated food and water. Incidence is perhaps highest when ambient temperatures are 50° to 60° C, and organisms may become concentrated in stagnant or sluggish water. Canine carriers may shed indefinitely, and neutral to slightly basic urinary pH favors both shedding and subsequent survival of spirochetes.

Leptospiremia is detectable after an incubation period of 3 to 8 days, with clinical signs appearing shortly thereafter; these figures vary widely with size and breed of the dog, inoculum size, infecting serovar, and immune status of the host. Peracute disease is characterized by high fever, myalgia, and bloody vomition. Vascular damage by leptospirae and their toxins leads to DIC, with associated melena, epistaxis, petechial hemorrhage, and hematochezia. Renal localization occurs in most infected animals and leptospiruria is evident by about 2 weeks postinfection. Microcolonies of leptospirae can be seen in proximal convoluted tubules, where they are largely protected from opsonization. Acute nephritis in this stage may progress to chronic interstitial nephritis and renal failure. Hepatic lesions comprise centrilobular necrosis and subcellular damage, and clinical manifestations include icterus, but liver failure is uncommon, except in peracute cases. Dogs may experience mild meningitis or encephalitis, immune-mediated uveitis, and abortion. Acute disease may also be accompanied by coughing, dyspnea, and conjunctivitis.

Given that rather grim picture, it is somewhat of a relief to acknowledge that most cases are chronic or subclinical. Coincident occurrence in dogs of apparently idiopathic fevers and anterior uveitis suggests a diagnosis of leptospirosis and should prompt serologic investigation. As noted, recovery depends on the humoral immune response, and immunity is serovar specific.

Serologic evidence indicates that a variety of leptospiral serovars can infect cats, but disease appears to be uncommon in this animal.

DIAGNOSIS

Diagnosis is based on bacteriologic culture, serology, detection of gross and microscopic lesions, and detection of leptospirae by fluorescent antibody testing on body fluids or impression smears or darkfield examination of body fluids.

Leptospiral Culture and Typing of Isolates

Effective culture for leptospirae is labor intensive, and is not widely practiced. Organisms are rarely cultivated on solid media. In acute leptospirosis, the organism can often be recovered from the kidney, reproductive tract, liver, brain, lung, and body fluids (thoracic, cerebrospinal, urine, and blood). However, leptospiremia is often of short duration (or does not occur at all) in infections by host-adapted strains. Accordingly, bacteriologic diagnosis in these cases often results only from examination of tissues where the infection is focused (such as aborted fetal tissues, placenta, uterus, and oviduct). If delays to processing are anticipated, 20 ml of urine can be mixed with 1.5 ml of 10% formalin for examination by darkfield microscopy. Liquid specimens or mascerated tissues are serially diluted in tubes of semisolid leptospiral culture medium, which contains 1% bovine serum albumin and long chain fatty acids (Tweens). A few drops of blood can be inoculated directly into semisolid medium. Tubes incubated aerobically at 30° C are examined weekly for growth, which may manifest as slight, subsurface turbidity. Detection of growth requires examination of wet mounts by darkfield microscopy for organisms with the appropriate morphology and motility. Contamination is common, and early examination and transfer of such cultures (~24 hr postinoculation) is often indicated. Media can be made at least semiselective by addition of 5-fluorouracil and other antimicrobials (such as cefoperazone, vancomycin, fungizone, and novobiocin), and leptospirae in heavily contaminated cultures can sometimes be recovered by filtration (pore diameters 220-800 nm).

Leptospires are indistinguishable by biochemical testing, and classification is based on agglutination in serovar-specific antisera. Difficulties in serologic identification of leptospirae have led to development of molecular methods for identification and subtyping. Restriction endonuclease assays (REA) have been useful, demonstrating distinct genotypes (hardjoprajitno and multiple subtypes of hardjobovis) among bovine isolates. North American serovar *balcanica* isolates have REA patterns identical to those of genotype hardjobovis isolates. Examination of serovar *pomona* revealed a similar pattern; North American isolates are subtype kennewicki, whereas those from Europe are serovar *pomona* or serovar *mozdok*. Application of restriction fragment length polymorphisms (RFLP) and pulsed field gel electrophoresis (PFGE) to isolates of a single REA type has revealed multiple clones within geographic areas, suggesting possible epidemiologic significance. However, differences are not consistently demonstrated by REA between serovars *copenhageni* and *icterohaemorrhagiae,* and isolates of these two serovars cannot be distinguished by PFGE. In general, PFGE analysis has revealed that leptospiral genomes are remarkably conserved over time and across geographic distributions.

Molecular methods, including dot-blotting and in situ hybridization, have been used as alternatives or adjuncts to culture procedures. Polymerase chain reaction (PCR) assays, most of which target 16S or 23S rRNA genes or repetitive elements, are used in many veterinary diagnostic laboratories. Some appear to be more sensitive than culture, whereas others are subject to false negatives. Determination of the offending serovar is usually not possible.

Diagnosis by Serology

Examination of paired sera by microscopic agglutination test (MAT) is probably still the best approach to serologic diagnosis of leptospirosis. The preferred format uses live leptospiral antigens. Use of formalinized antigens surmounts the difficulties of maintaining multiple serovars at equivalent cultural densities, but titers are lower and cross-reactions more common. The desired collection interval depends on the stage of the infection, but can range from approximately 5 days (in acute disease) to as long as 14 days (if the first is collected early in the course). A single elevated titer detected in association with an acute febrile illness suggests acute infection. The relative insensitivity of the MAT is well documented, especially on samples collected early in the acute phase.

Inclusion of multiple leptospiral serovars as antigens in the MAT allow, in many cases, identification of the infecting serogroup or serovar. However, interpretation of test results is often complicated by cross-reactions between serogroup antigens. Highest titers may even be to a serogroup unrelated to the infecting strain. Serologic diagnosis may also be complicated by the anamnestic response arising from previous infection with a member of a different serogroup.

There are no firm rules for interpretation of antileptospiral titers in domestic animals, but some generalizations can be drawn. A fourfold rise in titer is generally considered to confirm infection, especially in nonvaccinated animals. The MAT detects IgM approximately 7 to 9 days after the onset of clinical disease. Leptospirosis in maintenance hosts is characterized by a low serologic response of long duration, whereas incidental hosts develop severe disease and high MAT titers.

It may be possible to differentiate animals with active infection from vaccinates or animals with past infection by comparison of IgG and IgM titers. IgM is predominant in active cases, whereas IgG is the primary isotype in the others.

MAT titers greater than 1:12,800 to serovar *pomona* are common in cows and sows at the time of abortion. The serologic response of cattle to serovar *hardjo* may be minimal, with only approximately 50% of infected animals developing titers greater than 1:100 and very few having titers greater than 1:1600. Titers greater than 1:400 in nonvaccinated animals are usually considered positive. Aborting cows will often have reached or passed their maximum titer at the time of fetal expulsion.

The serologic response to serovar *bratislava* is often poor, and some infected animals will not have detectable titers, whereas others may have titers 1:800 to 1:1600. Antibody titers following specific vaccination are often higher than those in natural infection and may persist for approximately 3 months. Herd titers averaging more than 1:100 in nonvaccinated animals may indicate endemic infection. As with serovar *hardjo* in cattle, fetal death is followed by expulsion in 1 to 3 weeks, so the MAT titer in paired serum samples may remain static or drop. In general, it is useful to sample approximately 10% of a potentially affected herd, or a minimum of 10 normal and diseased animals. Titers greater than 1:800 in most samples from a nonvaccinated herd are a significant finding, as is conversion from negative to positive in most samples.

Alternative screening tests for antileptospiral antibodies include complement fixation (which has been widely used but not standardized) and enzyme-linked immunosorbent assay (ELISA). The latter is more applicable to diagnosis of human infections in which broadly reactive assays are desirable, than to veterinary diagnosis, in which serovar-specific diagnosis is more important. Macroscopic slide agglutination is still widely used, but this assay is more prone to false positives and false negatives than the MAT.

CONTROL AND PREVENTION

Immunity to leptospirosis is largely humoral, and is passively transferred by antibodies alone. Sodium dodecyl sulfate (SDS) extracts of whole cells are immunogenic, but protection is only against homologous or closely related serovars. Several leptospiral outer-membrane proteins (OMPs) are conserved, suggesting the possibility of subunit vaccines.

Both IgG and IgM are produced in response to vaccination with commercial bacterins, although the latter falls below the detection limits of the MAT within a few weeks. Duration of immunity may be as long as 6 to 12 months, and is often of little impact in eliminating the carrier state.

Penicillin and streptomycin may be useful for treating acute leptospirosis or for prophylaxis in contacts within a group of animals. Doxycycline is often used in humans and dogs, especially during leptospiruria in the latter. During canine leptospiremia, antibiotics of choice are penicillin G, ampicillin, or amoxicillin, with dosages adjusted for degree of renal insufficiency. Antimicrobials may be of little use if renal damage is extensive.

Supportive care should be tailored to individual cases, with attention to the extent of liver and kidney dysfunction and the presence of DIC.

Dogs in renal failure should receive intravenous fluids with potassium, and those that are oliguric are given a diuretic. Transfusion and low-dose heparin may be useful in cases in which DIC is an issue.

Prevention strategies should focus on elimination of carrier animals and environmental contamination. Suspected carriers should be eliminated or, especially in the case of carrier dogs, treated with doxycycline. Control of rodents is important, as is environmental cleaning and decontamination.

SUGGESTED READINGS

Blackmore DK, Schollum LM: Risks of contracting leptospirosis on the dairy farm, *N Z Med J* 95:649-652, 1982.

Bolin CA, Koellner P: Human-to-human transmission of *Leptospira interrogans* by milk, *J Infect Dis* 158:246-247, 1988.

Bolin CA, Zuerner RL: Correlation between DNA restriction fragment length polymorphisms in *Leptospira interrogans* serovar *pomona* type kennewicki and host animal source, *J Clin Microbiol* 34:424-425, 1996.

Brenner DJ, Kaufmann AF, Sulzer KR, et al: Further determination of DNA relatedness between serogroups and serovars in the family Leptospiraceae with a proposal for *Leptospira alexanderi* sp. nov. and four new *Leptospira* genomospecies, *Int J Syst Bacteriol* 49:839-858, 1999.

Brown CA, Roberts AW, Miller MA, et al: *Leptospira interrogans* serovar *grippotyphosa* infection in dogs, *J Am Vet Med Assoc* 209:1265-1267, 1996.

Hathaway SC, Little TWA, Stevens AE: Isolation of *Leptospira interrogans* serovar *hardjo* from aborted bovine fetuses in England, *Vet Rec* 111:58, 1982.

Zuerner RL, Alt D, Bolin CA: IS1533-based PCR assay for identification of *Leptospira interrogans* sensu lato, *J Clin Microbiol* 33:3284-3289, 1995.

Zuerner RL, Bolin CA: Differentiation of *Leptospira interrogans* isolates by IS1500 hybridization and PCR assays, *J Clin Microbiol* 35:2612-2617, 1997.

Chapter **32**

The Genera *Treponema* and *Borrelia*

THE GENUS *TREPONEMA*

Treponema spp. are motile, helical rods with tight, regular to irregular spirals (Figure 32-1). Many species are normal flora in the oral cavities, genital tract, or rumen of animals.

Treponema pallidum ssp. *pallidum* is well known as the cause of human syphilis, and *Treponema pallidum* ssp. *carateum* and *Treponema pallidum* ssp. *pertenue* cause the related diseases, pinta and yaws, respectively. Although it is not an animal pathogen per se, *T. pallidum* ssp. *pallidum* is included in this chapter because of its overwhelming importance as a human pathogen. The endemic treponematoses affect at least 2.5 million persons worldwide.

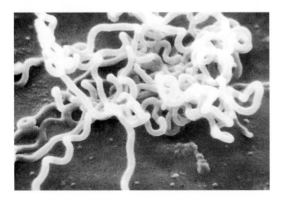

FIGURE 32-1 Electron photomicrograph of *Treponema pallidum* on cottontail rabbit epithelial cells. (Courtesy Public Health Image Library, PHIL #1971, Centers for Disease Control and Prevention, Atlanta, 1980, David Cox.)

Species pathogenic for domestic animals include *T. paraluis-cuniculi* (associated with venereal disease in rabbits ["rabbit syphilis"]) and *T. brennaborense* (which causes interdigital dermatitis in cattle ["hairy foot warts"]). Many of the pathogenic treponemes have not been cultivated in vitro, and genome sequencing suggests that *T. pallidum* ssp. *pallidum* has been subject to reductive evolution through centuries of association with human hosts.

Treponema pallidum and Human Syphilis

There is substantial controversy over the origin and spread of venereal syphilis, and current thought (a term fraught with danger in this case) is that non-venereal treponemal disease has existed worldwide since the emergence of the genus *Homo* and that the first epidemic outbreak of venereal syphilis in Europe occurred in the late fifteenth and the early sixteenth centuries. Examination of bone lesions has long been a common means to study historical aspects of syphilis and other treponematoses. Molecular methods that allow identification of *T. pallidum* ssp. *pallidum* in paleo-pathologic material may make it possible to clarify issues relating to the origin and spread of syphilis.

DISEASE AND PATHOGENESIS

The incidence of human syphilis is increasing, as is often the case with diseases having such a strong sociologic component. Primary syphilis is evidenced by the development of a circumscribed

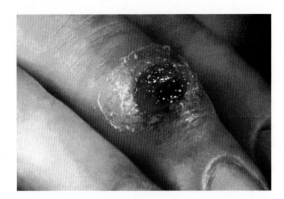

FIGURE 32-2 Extragenital syphilitic chancre on the right middle finger. (Courtesy Public Health Image Library, PHIL #4146, Centers for Disease Control and Prevention, Atlanta, date unknown.)

lesion, called a *chancre,* at the inoculation site (Figure 32-2). It is initially maculopapular, but eventually develops an inflamed, necrotic, moist center. Exudate from the chancre teems with spirochetes, and this is the most infectious stage of the disease for person-to-person transmission. The chancre may be in a location that is not readily visible and may thus go unnoticed. Treatment at this stage results in a nearly 100% cure rate, but the lesion disappears without treatment in 10 to 14 days.

This return to seeming normalcy is deceptive. Spirochetes move, from their primary location on mucous membranes, to the bloodstream, which in due time leads to the development of secondary syphilis. Fever and rash are characteristic of this stage of the disease, and *T. pallidum* is found in the erythematous skin lesions. These clinical signs occur in most, but not all, infected people, and treatment is generally effective at this stage. However, the secondary symptoms will also resolve spontaneously, and a surprising number of cases go untreated.

Treponemes remaining after the secondary stage invade cardiac muscle, the musculoskeletal system, and the central nervous system (CNS) in tertiary syphilis. The antibody response remains strong, and this stage is relatively noninfectious. Symptoms of the tertiary stage develop slowly; cardiac damage and CNS symptoms are common, and an enormous portion of healthcare dollars in the United States are devoted to providing care for the syphilitic insane.

A major concern is transplacental transmission during latent infections, resulting in congenital syphilis at a rate approaching 1000 U.S. cases annually. The infection manifests in malformed teeth and long bones, cardiac lesions, and CNS effects leading to learning disabilities and mental retardation.

Elucidation of virulence mechanisms of *T. pallidum* has been limited by failure of all attempts to cultivate it in vitro. Furthermore, there is no suitable in vivo model of human disease. *Treponema pallidum* can be maintained by serial passage in rabbit testicles, a process in which laboratory technicians have approximately the same risk of occupational exposure to the organism as street-based sex workers. However, symptoms (in the rabbits) are limited to rather severe orchitis in steroid nontreated animals, and no visible symptoms at all if steroidal antiinflammatory drugs are used. Chancres resembling those in human syphilis are produced by intradermal inoculation of rabbit skin, and these resolve much as would be expected in humans. However, the infection does not become systemic. Information gleaned from study of natural cases and limited work with in vivo–grown organisms has revealed that *T. pallidum* adheres to and invades cell monolayers (Figure 32-3).

Treponema pallidum has a surprising lack of outer-membrane proteins, and the treponemal equivalent of porin activity (to allow diffusion of nutrients through the outer membrane) remains undiscovered. There is likely some sort of active transport mechanism, because *T. pallidum* is

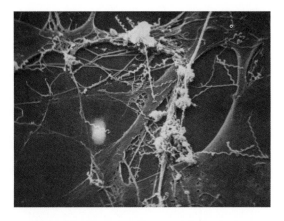

FIGURE 32-3 Electron photomicrograph of *Treponema pallidum* on cottontail rabbit epithelial cells. (Courtesy Public Health Image Library, PHIL #1975, Centers for Disease Control and Prevention, Atlanta, 1980, David Cox.)

susceptible to β-lactam antibiotics, and these are not thought to diffuse through membranes.

Treponema pallidum may protect itself from the immune response by cloaking with host proteins such as α_2-macroglobulin, albumin, and class I major histocompatibility complex (MHC) proteins. This strategy is obviously not completely successful because individuals with syphilis do produce antibodies against the organism. Fibronectin may mediate treponemal attachment to host cells, and in processing a treponemal antigen–fibronectin complex, the immune system may produce antibodies against fibronectin itself, with subsequent immune-mediated damage to cardio-pulmonary, musculoskeletal, and central nervous systems in tertiary syphilis.

Indirect effects of *T. pallidum* may cause local tissue damage. Binding of the organism to cultured endothelial cells stimulates expression of intercellular adhesion molecule 1 (ICAM-1), which in turn binds to integrins on the surface of neutrophils and enables their emigration into surrounding tissue. Endothelial cells are also stimulated to produce cytokines, and treponemal lipoproteins activate tumor necrosis factor-α (TNF-α) and interleukin-1 (IL-1) production by macrophages. Both may contribute to the inflammation, which plays such a prominent role in pathogenesis of primary and secondary syphilis.

DIAGNOSIS

The Wassermann test, and other tests based on anticardiolipin (rather than antitreponemal) antibodies are useful, but prone to false positives. A variety of specific tests now available are based on bacterial immobilization by antibodies, fluorescent antibody assay, and other detection systems.

Treponema brennaborense and Hairy Footwart

Disease and Etiology. Bovine papillomatous digital dermatitis (PDD; digital dermatitis, hairy footwart) was first described nearly 30 years ago in Italy and shortly thereafter in the United States. It is now widely distributed in North America, affecting cattle in more than 40% of U.S. dairy herds. There is at least one report of papillomatous pastern dermatitis, of apparent spirochetal etiology, in a horse.

The incubation period of PDD is about 3 weeks. Its clinical presentation is episodic lameness of variable severity, as a result of acute or chronic

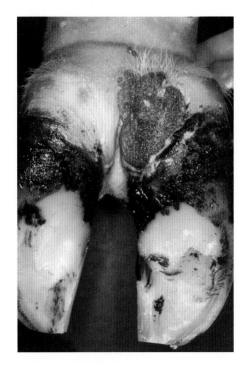

FIGURE 32-4 Gross lesions of papillomatous digital dermatitis. (Courtesy Deryck Read.)

ulceration of the skin on the bulbs of the heel or the interdigital cleft and often just above the perioplic horn of the heels. In intense cases, cows often walk on their toes and hooves are clubbed. Lesions are most commonly associated with plantar or palmar skin adjacent to the interdigital space (Figure 32-4). Both medial and lateral digits of individual limbs are involved in most animals.

Erosions can encompass the superficial layers of the epidermis, and epithelial hyperplasia and hypertrophy, hemorrhage, pain, swelling, and foul odor are hallmarks of the disease. Lesions average 4 cm in diameter, are circular to oval, and are most common on the hind feet. They have the granular, red appearance of a strawberry and are often surrounded by a ridge of hyperkeratotic skin with hypertrophied hairs. Proliferation of filiform papillae increases as lesions mature, with formation of long wartlike projections. Microscopic examination reveals epidermopoiesis and papilloma formation, with perivascular aggregation of inflammatory cells. Silver staining of sections reveals invasive spirochetes deep in lesions, invading the stratum spinosum in company with coccoid and large bacillary forms. However, spirochetes are also found, essentially alone, in deeper tissues.

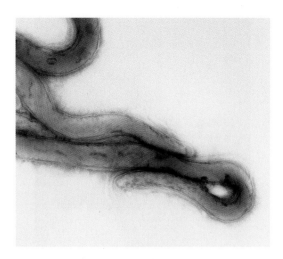

FIGURE 32-5 Electron photomicrograph of *Treponema brennaborense*, showing axial fibrils. (Courtesy Richard L. Walker.)

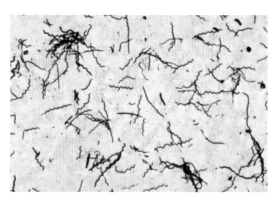

FIGURE 32-6 *Treponema brennaborense* in a stained smear from a papillomatous digital dermatitis (PDD) lesion. (Courtesy Richard L. Walker.)

A novel treponeme isolated from typical lesions was determined, based on chemotaxonomy, protein profiling, and analysis of 16S rDNA sequences, to be a new species, and was named *T. brennaborense*. It is small and highly motile, with two periplasmic flagella arranged in a 1-2-1 pattern (Figure 32-5). It has α-glucosidase and N-acetyl-β-glucosaminidase activity, and growth is inhibited by rabbit serum. Comparative 16S rDNA sequence analysis of multiple isolates revealed three phylotypes clustered with the saprophytic human oral (*Treponema denticola* and *Treponema vincentii*) or genital (*Treponema phagedenis*) treponemes. *Treponema brennaborense* is probably most closely related to *Treponema maltophilum*, from human periodontitis. Differential distribution in lesions suggests that development of deep lesions may correlate with the presence of a particular phylotype or combination of phylotypes. Immunohistochemical examination of lesion biopsies reveals that organisms from many countries are antigenically related.

Pathogenesis of *T. brennaborense* infections has not been explored.

Epidemiology

There may be breed-related differences in susceptibility, and the severity of diseases increases with parity. The risk of infection increases with stage of lactation. Highest incidence is in late spring and summer. Regions of the United States with the highest percent of affected herds are the Southwest, Northwest, and Northeast. Morbidity in affected herds may be as low as 0.5% per month, but may be more than 10% per month.

PDD is associated with wet environmental conditions, and hooves caked with mud have a higher occurrence of disease. Flooring type is also important, presumably for the same reasons. Occurrence of disease in specific herds has also been associated with failure to wash hoof-trimming equipment between cows.

Diagnosis

Diagnosis of PDD is based on observation of typical clinical signs and lesions and detection of morphologically compatible spirochetes in biopsies stained by silver impregnation or other methods (Figure 32-6).

Prevention, Control, and Therapy

PDD can persist for months if not treated, leading to significant economic losses caused by reduced milk production, infertility, culling, and treatment costs.

Parenteral antibiotics can be useful, and there are good claims for penicillin and ceftiofur. Deep scraping of the hoof surface and local application of an antibacterial aerosol is probably the most effective treatment. Topical oxytetracycline, benzathine penicillin, or formaldehyde are effective, although regardless of form of treatment, more than half are likely to have recurrent or new infections within a few weeks.

Recurrences are most often due to continuing to house animals in a contaminated environment. Disease control can often be effected by frequent scraping of floors in dairy barns and routine use

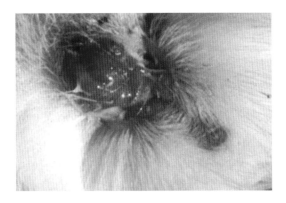

FIGURE 32-7 Rabbit syphilis (vent disease), resulting from infection by *Treponema paraluis-cuniculi*. (Courtesy Raymond E. Reed.)

of zinc sulphate (20%) or oxytetracycline (6 g/L) footbaths; these can be therapeutic in mild cases. Powerwashing of heels boosts the effectiveness of footbaths. Isolation of herd additions is also important because disease may be introduced to a herd from infected replacement stock. Field experience with a commercial vaccine is yet insufficient to assess its usefulness.

Spirochetes have also been isolated from severe cases of ovine foot disease, and 16S rDNA sequence analysis revealed that it is related to *T. vincentii*, which has been associated with human periodontal disease. Another spirochete from ovine footrot more closely resembles *T. brennaborense*.

Treponema paraluis-cuniculi causes the venereal disease rabbit syphilis (vent disease) (Figure 32-7). Lesions include vesicles and scabs on the prepuce, vagina, and perineum, and scales and crusts persist long term in females. These infections can confound experimental work on *T. pallidum* ssp. *pallidum* because of serologic cross-reactions between the organisms. *Treponema paraluis-cuniculi*

can be demonstrated by darkfield microscopy, and has not been cultivated in vitro. Penicillin therapy is effective, but affected animals remain seropositive for long periods.

THE GENUS *BORRELIA*

Borrelia species are microaerophilic to anaerobic spirochetes with loose, irregular coils, many of which have not been cultivated in vitro. They are best demonstrated in tissue sections by way of silver stains, through darkfield examination of body fluids, or by Giemsa staining of impression smears of spleen or liver or smears of body fluids.

Borrelia species are highly adapted to arthropod transmission. Relapsing fever, caused by *Borrelia recurrentis* and other *Borrelia* spp., occurs sporadically in the United States and is distributed worldwide. It is transmitted animal to animal and from animals to humans by ticks, and human to human by lice. The organism can be recovered from the blood during the recurrent febrile attacks that give the disease its name.

Animal pathogenic borreliae include *Borrelia anserina* (avian spirochetosis), *Borrelia burgdorferi* (Lyme disease), *Borrelia theileri* (tick spirochetosis of cattle), and *Borrelia coriaceae* (epizootic bovine abortion) (Table 32-1).

Borrelia burgdorferi

Lyme borreliosis is the most prevalent human tick-borne disease in the United States, Europe, and parts of Asia. Canines are the domestic animals at greatest risk of infection, although infections occur in horses, cattle, and cats.

Lyme disease was first recognized in the late 1970s in the northeastern United States. A woman in Old Lyme, Connecticut, harassed state public health authorities with her observation of a much higher than expected incidence of arthritis in area

TABLE 32-1 Non-Lyme Borrelioses in Domestic Animals

Borrelia Species	Vector	Hosts	Disease	Distribution
B. anserina	Argasid ticks; *Argas persicus*	Domestic and wild birds	Avian spirochetosis; high mortality in young birds	Worldwide
B. theileri	*Rhipicephalus* spp., *Boophilus* spp., others	Cattle; horses, sheep	Bovine borreliosis; fever, anemia; one or two relapses typical; minor clinical problem in sheep, horses	United States, South Africa, Australia, Europe
B. coriaceae	*Ornithodoros coriaceus*	Cattle	Foothills abortion, enzootic bovine abortion	Western United States

children, and this led to the description of Lyme disease. In the United States, disease is found only in endemic areas, with 90% of cases occurring in 10 northeastern states. These findings were later connected to similar observations of European physicians, dating to the early 1900s, who had been sufficiently convinced of a bacterial etiology that they were treating with antimicrobials. The causative spirochete, *B. burgdorferi*, has since been found in museum voucher specimens of mice and ticks from the early twentieth century.

Similar to other *Borrelia* spp., these spirochetes have both circular and linear plasmids, as well as linear chromosomes.

Disease and Pathogenesis

The incubation period in humans (through onset of erythema migrans) is typically 7 to 14 days, but ranges from 3 to 30 days. Some infected individuals are subclinical, or manifest only nonspecific symptoms including fever, headache, and myalgia.

The first clinical sign is erythema migrans. A rash appears in days to weeks after the bite, surrounding the site of inoculation, expanding in concentric rings, and disappearing spontaneously after several weeks. About one fifth of infected individuals do not develop this rash, so falsely negative diagnoses may result if based on this sign alone.

The second stage, which follows in weeks to months, is characterized by fever, chills, malaise, and stiffness, and, in a small proportion of patients, central nervous system (CNS) signs (facial palsy, meningitis, chronic axonal polyneuropathy, and encephalitis with cognitive disorders, sleep disturbance, fatigue, and personality changes), and cardiac damage (myocarditis and transient atrioventricular blocks) may occur. Musculoskeletal signs include migratory joint and muscle pains.

The third stage follows in months to years and involves persistent joint inflammation, fatigue, and occasionally paralysis. Fatalities are rare.

Lameness caused by acute arthritis, with increased synovial fluid, and/or myalgia is the most common sign of Lyme disease in dogs (Table 32-2). Dogs of any breed, age, or sex may be affected. The onset is often sudden, combined with lethargy, inappetence, and sometimes fever and swelling of draining lymph nodes. Painful swelling of one or more joints may be noticed, which may include carpus, elbow, shoulder, tarsus, or stifle. Synovial fluid cell counts are high (≥80,000 cells/ml, with 90% neutrophils, 1% lymphocytes and macrophages, and the remainder synovial lining cells). Fibrin and neutrophils accumulate in the joint space. Axillary and popliteal nodes near the affected limb are often swollen and edematous.

A less acute form of disease manifests as intermittent, nonspecific lameness or reluctance to move, some lethargy, and decreased appetite. Experimentally infected dogs develop lameness, of 3 to 4 days' duration, 2 to 5 months after tick exposure. Lameness is recurrent at 2- to 4-week intervals, and although clinical signs disappear after two or three relapses, mild polyarthritis and spirochetal joint infection persists for at least a year.

Lyme disease in dogs may also manifest as CNS infection, with cervical pain, severe depression, anorexia, seizures, behavioral changes, and fever, all of which are responsive to antimicrobial therapy. In rare instances cardiac arrhythmias or heart block, and a fatal renal disease have been reported, with Lyme-specific immune complexes and complement deposition in glomeruli.

Clinical pathology is generally unremarkable. Experimentally infected dogs have normal white blood cell counts, hematocrits, and serum enzyme panels. Creatine kinase levels may be slightly elevated during acute lameness.

Arthritis, encephalitis, uveitis, and laminitis have been recognized in infected horses and cows. Recovery of *B. burgdorferi* from the liver of a passerine bird is of unknown significance.

TABLE 32-2 Phases of Canine Lyme Borreliosis

Phase	Signs	Length of Phase
Incubation	None	2-5 months
Acute	Fever, swollen joints and lymph nodes, polyarthritis, lameness	1-3 weeks
Subclinical	None	Up to 3 years
Chronic	Lameness, polyarthritis, cardiac and central nervous system symptoms, acute renal failure	Indefinite; possibly fatal

Methods for cultivation of *B. burgdorferi* are even now sufficiently difficult that research on this organism is not for the faint of heart. Its generation time is 10 to 12 hours under optimal conditions. Nonetheless, substantial progress toward understanding pathogenesis has been made during the past three decades.

In the primary stage of Lyme disease, bacteria multiply in skin, but quickly enter circulation. Circulating organisms are killed by phagocytes, complement-mediated bacteriolysis, and complement-independent antibody effects. Lack of lipopolysaccharide (LPS) presumably limits formation of a functional membrane-attack complex in the absence of an antibody response to specific proteins. A primary target of this response is the outer surface proteins, or Osps. Animals immunized with OspA or OspB are protected against infection. However, the humoral response in humans or other animals infected with *B. burgdorferi* develops slowly. Antibody titers to Osps rise slowly, and antibodies formed early (for example, against flagella) are not bactericidal because they are not available at the surface. Bactericidal antibodies reach maximal levels only after 3 to 5 weeks. Reasons for delayed immune recognition and antibody formation are not known. Blebbing (shedding of outer membrane vesicles containing Osps) may bind some proportion of the antibodies that do form, away from the bacterial surface, making them unavailable for opsonization.

Borrelia burgdorferi causes bacteremia in rodents, but there is fairly strong sentiment on the part of some researchers that the dissemination of *B. burgdorferi* from the site of inoculation in dogs is by active migration rather than spirochetemia. Target organs other than joints are lymph nodes, muscle, pericardium, peritoneum, and meninges, and incubation period is probably a function of speed of migration.

Despite the ability to delay the humoral response, most spirochetes are eventually cleared (in experimental infections in rodents) from circulation. Survivors localize inside host cells. Crossing of endothelium is accomplished by disruption of tight junctions, or by transcytosis (with or without intracellular replication). Nonmotile mutants cannot cross endothelia, nor can mutants lacking OspB. In the latter case, ID_{50}s for severe combined immunodeficient (SCID) mice are increased by two logs, and inflammation

of tibiotarsal joints is pronounced in wildtype infections but absent in mice inoculated intradermally with the mutant. Thus OspB may play a role in invasiveness. Invasion of cells is also a key factor in other aspects of pathogenesis that affect cardiac muscle and the CNS. Transplacental transmission has been reported in humans.

Inflammation is likely the root cause of the symptoms of Lyme disease. Colonization of synovial cells activates IL-8 production, which is potently chemotactic for neutrophils. This may be mediated by an LPS analog or by outer-membrane lipoproteins (which stimulate TNF-α and IL-1 production by macrophages). Fibrin deposition and fluid accumulation accompany neutrophils, and the cellular response shifts to lymphocytes and plasma cells as the infection progresses. Immune complexes have not been demonstrated in affected joints.

Field strains become permanently avirulent when passaged in vitro. Cataloging of these lost attributes has been one basis for elucidation of virulence. Infections by wildtype and mutant strains can be modeled in rabbits (for skin lesions similar to those in humans), SCID mice (for arthritis and to determine attributes involved in invasiveness, on the one hand, or immune system evasion, on the other). Attachment and invasion can be modeled in cultured cells.

Chronic disease may be autoimmune mediated; antiflagellar antibodies bind to cardiac and CNS antigens and, combined with the expected T-cell response, serve as the basis for the antiself reaction. Heat shock proteins, as well as Osps, may also be involved.

Epidemiology

Encroachment of humans into the habitat of an expanding white-tailed deer population allowed Lyme disease to emerge as a human condition. *Borrelia burgdorferi* is spread from deer or mice to humans by the bite of adults or nymphs of soft ticks of the genus *Ixodes*, primarily *Ixodes scapularis (dammini)* (Figure 32-8), but also *Ixodes pacificus, Ixodes ricinus,* and others. It has also been isolated from *Dermacentor variabilis*. As part of a 2-year life cycle, adult female ticks produce approximately 2000 eggs in the spring, which hatch as uninfected larvae. Those feeding on initial, infected hosts (e.g., the white-footed mouse [*Peromyscus leucopus*] in the northeastern United States) emerge from dormancy the following spring as infected nymphs (Figure 32-9) and quest for new hosts. Those not infected as larvae may become infected by feeding on infected hosts. Nymphs mature into adults in late autumn, and mate after attaching to deer or other mammalian hosts. The female feeds to repletion and drops off, remaining on the ground until spring, when the cycle is complete.

The infection rate in nymphs is 10% to 25%, compared with as many as 60% of adult ticks. An important part of the epidemiology is spirochete migration in the tick during feeding; *B. burgdorferi* migrates, over a 24- to 48-hour period, from the midgut to the salivary glands. Thus short-term tick exposure does not result in infection.

Intrauterine transmission of spirochetes has been reported in dogs. Transplacental infections,

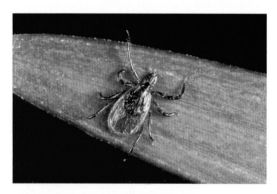

FIGURE 32-8 Female *Ixodes scapularis (dammini)*. (Courtesy Public Health Image Library, PHIL #1669, Centers for Disease Control and Prevention, Atlanta, date unknown, James Mathany.)

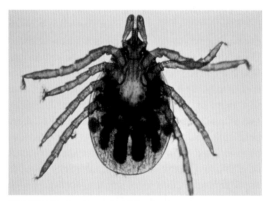

FIGURE 32-9 Nymphal tick of the genus *Ixodes*. (Courtesy Public Health Image Library, PHIL #3808, Centers for Disease Control and Prevention, Atlanta, 1975, World Health Organization.)

but not other direct human-to-human transmission, have also occurred. Dogs may be sentinels, but are apparently not reservoirs for human infection. Results of experimental studies do not support a role for infected canine urine in infection of humans.

Diagnosis

A history of tick exposure in an enzootic area, compatible clinical signs, positive serology, and response to antibiotic therapy are typical criteria for diagnosis of canine Lyme disease. Physical exam, radiography, and the nature of the animal's response to antimicrobials usually rule out other causes of lameness. Tests for antinuclear antibodies, lupus erythematosus, and rheumatoid arthritis can eliminate immune-mediated diseases from consideration. Mono- or oligoarthritis, rather than polyarthritis, is most common with Lyme disease.

A definitive and unequivocal diagnosis can be based on isolation of *B. burgdorferi* from skin biopsies near the tick bite. In humans, at least 80% of biopsies from early erythema migrans lesions are culture positive. However, culture of borreliae is extraordinarily difficult and time consuming. Modified Barbour-Stoenner-Kelly medium is inoculated and then incubated and observed for protracted periods. Attempts to isolate *B. burgdorferi* from canine blood or urine have been mainly unsuccessful. Polymerase chain reaction (PCR) has been applied to specimens of skin, blood, cerebrospinal fluid, and synovial fluid, but has not been standardized for routine use.

Thus, in canine Lyme disease, appropriate use of serologic testing is crucial. The enzyme-linked immunosorbent assay (ELISA) is most commonly used and is more reliable than the fluorescent antibody test. Current recommendations are for application of the highly sensitive ELISA, followed by Western blotting to confirm equivocal or positive results. Early application of antimicrobial therapy may limit or eliminate a diagnostically useful antibody response, but there is usually strong serologic reactivity during and after early disseminated disease. Antibodies may persist for months or years.

Western blotting increases the specificity of diagnostic serology. It differentiates between vaccinated and tick-exposed dogs, in that the former have an OspA response only (if vaccinated with OspA vaccine), or antibodies to a few *B. burgdorferi* proteins, including OspA (if vaccinated with a killed bacterin). Dogs experiencing tick phlebotomy have antibodies to many different *B. burgdorferi* proteins. IgM antibodies may persist for months, and thus their presence does not necessarily confirm early stage infection. Serology in Europe is complicated by the variety of *Borrelia* spp. that cause Lyme disease. *Borrelia garinii* and *Borrelia afzelii,* in addition to *B. burgdorferi,* produce clinical or subclinical infections.

A recently described ELISA method promises increased sensitivity and specificity in diagnosis of Lyme disease. It is based on the so-called invariable region 6, which is antigenically conserved among strains and genospecies of *B. burgdorferi sensu lato* and immunodominant in human and canine hosts. Sensitivity in humans ranges from 75% to 100%, depending on the stage and type of infection. Patients infected with *B. garinii* or *B. afzelii* produce equivalent responses.

There is a strong antibody response in dogs, beginning 4 to 5 weeks after experimental infection, and about one third are positive 3 weeks after infection. Responses remain through at least 17 months, suggesting that chronic infections are also detected by this method. The assay is also highly specific.

Furthermore, no antibodies were detected by this assay in OspA-vaccinated monkeys or dogs, or in dogs vaccinated with the bacterin. These so-called C6-based tests have been approved by the U.S. Department of Agriculture for use in canines and are available commercially.

PREVENTION, CONTROL, AND THERAPY

Lyme disease usually resolves with antimicrobial therapy, if applied early in the course of disease. Treatment of secondary or tertiary disease is often unsuccessful. Tetracyclines, such as doxycycline, or β-lactam antibiotics, such as amoxicillin, are very effective, and dogs recover clinically in 24 to 48 hours. Duration of therapy is usually 4 weeks because of slow multiplication and in vivo persistence. Experimentally infected dogs treated with high doses of amoxicillin or doxycycline remained infected after 30 days. Canine Lyme nephritis is uncommon, but it is refractory to antimicrobial therapy and therefore often fatal. Serum antibody levels decline with treatment of uncomplicated Lyme arthritis, but often rise again over subsequent months, suggesting persistent infection. Corticosteroids are useful in antiinflammatory doses, but larger doses may be immunosuppressive.

Long courses of antibiotic therapy may be required for chronic infection of humans, and convalescence is often extended and the clinical outcome uncertain.

Neither positive serologic test results nor even previous infection by *B. burgdorferi* ensures protective immunity. There is a consensus that dogs in endemic areas should be vaccinated. However, vaccination is effective only if administered to naive dogs. Vaccine consisting of killed *B. burgdorferi* appears satisfactory, but studies in hamsters have suggested that this bacterin may induce delayed adverse reactions. An OspA vaccine (used in dogs and humans) induces formation of borreliacidal antibody; *B. burgdorferi* is killed in the tick early in the 24- to 48-hour feeding period, before the spirochete migrates from the midgut of the tick to the salivary gland to the host. Persistent infection is not eliminated by either vaccine.

Tick control is an important part of preventing Lyme disease. Use of acaricides or repellents is helpful, as is daily grooming. A genocidal approach to deer populations has little useful impact on tick populations because of the large number of alternate hosts.

Borrelia theileri

Borrelia theileri, the agent of bovine borreliosis, was described in the early twentieth century, but its relationship to relapsing fever spirochetes or *B. burgdorferi* and Lyme-associated organisms is only partially understood. This organism, along with the so-called *Amblyomma* agent are part of a natural group distinct from the relapsing fever spirochetes and more distantly related to the Lyme agents. The disease in cattle is characterized by a conspicuous spirochetemia, possibly strengthening the hypothesized relationship of *B. theileri* to the relapsing fever spirochetes. The spirochete referred to as the *Amblyomma* agent has been detected in Lone Star ticks (*Amblyomma americanum*) (Figure 32-10), and interest in them has increased because of their association with a human syndrome (of unknown etiology) known as southern tick-associated rash infection or Masters' disease. The degree of sequence similarity between the *Amblyomma* agent and *B. theileri* strongly suggests that they are the same species.

Borrelia anserina

Borrelia anserina causes avian spirochetosis in domestic and wild birds. It is not common in the

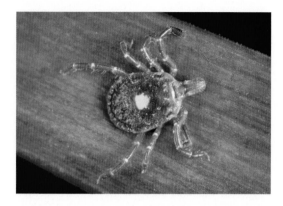

FIGURE 32-10 Female Lone Star tick *(Amblyoma americanum),* vector of bovine borreliosis. (Courtesy Public Health Image Library, PHIL #4407, Centers for Disease Control and Prevention, Atlanta, 2003, James Mathany.)

United States, but is of considerable economic consequence in many countries. The infection is characterized by acute septicemia, with fever, diarrhea, lassitude, and emaciation. The principal vector is *Argas persicus,* although other arthropods may also be involved.

Affected birds are usually anemic, and the spleen may be enlarged and mottled. Some affected birds die, but many recover after a clinical course of about 2 weeks and have lifelong immunity.

Diagnosis is based on demonstration of *B. anserina,* in smears of blood, spleen, or liver, stained with carbol fuchsin, Giemsa, or fluorescein-labeled specific antibodies, or examined directly by darkfield microscopy. The organism can also be cultivated in chick embryos.

Penicillin, streptomycin, kanamycin, tylosin, and tetracyclines are effective in treatment, and a crude bacterin from chicken embryo–derived cultures may be used for prevention. Tick control is important in controlling avian spirochetosis.

Borrelia coriaceae

Borrelia coriaceae was first recognized in 1985, isolated from and named after its tick vector, *Ornithodoros coriaceus.* This spirochete is passed transstadially and occasionally via eggs. There is circumstantial evidence that *B. coriaceae* causes epizootic bovine abortion (congenital spirochetosis) in range cattle in the western United States, but this etiologic link has not been confirmed. The spirochete is found in fetal blood. Epizootic bovine abortion–affected fetuses, with evidence of spirochetemia, were aborted by cows on which wild-caught ticks from endemic areas were allowed to feed. Clinically inapparent spirochetosis has been documented in fetuses in clinically normal cattle at slaughter. Clinical disease may result only as a result of repeated infection.

SUGGESTED READINGS

Berger BW, Johnson RC, Kodner C, Coleman L: Cultivation of *Borrelia burgdorferi* from erythema migrans lesions and perilesional skin, *J Clin Microbiol* 30:359-361, 1992.

Bujak DI, Weinstein A, Dornbush RL: Clinical and neurocognitive features of the post Lyme syndrome, *J Rheumatol* 23:1392-1397, 1996.

Dressler F, Whelan JA, Reinhart BN, Steere AC: Western blotting in the serodiagnosis of Lyme disease, *J Infect Dis* 167:392-400, 1993.

Johnson BJ, Robbins KE, Bailey RE: Serodiagnosis of Lyme disease: accuracy of a two-step approach using a flagella-based ELISA and immunoblotting, *J Infect Dis* 174:346-353, 1996.

Nowakowski J, Schwartz I, Nadelman RB: Culture-confirmed infection and reinfection with *Borrelia burgdorferi, Ann Intern Med* 127:130-132, 1997.

Osebold JW, Spezialetti R, Jennings MB, et al: Congenital spirochetosis in calves: association with epizootic bovine abortion, *J Am Vet Med Assoc* 188:371-376, 1986.

Anaerobic Bacteria

Anaerobic Gram-Positive Rods and Cocci

Chapter 33

The Genus *Clostridium*

Clostridia are large, sporulating, gram-positive, oxygen-tolerant to strictly anaerobic rods. *Clostridium piliforme* is the exception, in that it is gram negative. The source of clostridia can be exogenous (most commonly the soil) or endogenous (often from the intestinal tract). Most pathogenic clostridia produce one or more toxins, and direct or indirect evidence links many of these with pathogenesis (Table 33-1). Myonecrosis often follows mechanical injury, with clostridial spores germinating in damaged, ischemic muscle. Toxemia can also ensue when spores are deposited in wounds, or when spore-containing tissues are damaged. Disruption of normal flora by antibiotic therapy or sudden dietary changes may precede enteric infection, which is frequently accompanied by intestinal lesions; in some types of enterotoxemias, intestinal lesions are minimal. Disease can also result from ingestion of preformed clostridial toxins. Death is a frequent endpoint, and is often acute or peracute. Vaccination with bacterin-toxoids or toxoids is an effective prophylactic measure for many clostridial diseases.

Animal pathogenic clostridia can be conveniently categorized as neurotoxic, enteric, and histotoxic (see Table 33-1). Some (e.g., *Clostridium perfringens*) are heterogeneous and thus rather cosmopolitan in terms of hosts and systems affected, whereas others (e.g., *Clostridium colinum*) cause a single, well-defined syndrome.

NEUROTOXIC CLOSTRIDIA
Diseases and Epidemiology

Tetanus usually results from inoculation of a traumatic wound with spores of *Clostridium tetani*. Minor penetrating wounds or abrasions, surgical incisions, docking, castration or eartag wounds, injection sites, and postpartum lesions in the reproductive tract may be portals of entry. The wound may be trivial, even unnoticed, but the reduced oxygen and Eh resulting from necrosis are usually required. The typical source of *C. tetani* is soil, and both vegetative cells and spores are detected in the digestive tracts of animals. Disease occurs frequently in horses, less often in other herbivores, and infrequently in pigs and carnivores. Cattle may develop tetanus following growth of *C. tetani* in the rumen.

After germination in the wound, *C. tetani* produces a neurotoxin that causes the majority of the

TABLE 33-1 Animal Pathogenic Clostridia

Pathotype	Species	Disease
Neurotoxic	C. botulinum	Botulism
	C. tetani	Tetanus
Histotoxic	C. perfringens	Myonecrosis, gas gangrene
	C. septicum	Malignant edema, braxy
	C. chauvoei	Blackleg
	C. novyi	Myonecrosis, infectious necrotic hepatitis (black disease), bacillary hemoglobinuria (redwater)
	C. sordellii	Myonecrosis, enteritis
Enteric	C. perfringens	Enteritis, enterotoxemia
	C. difficile	Diarrhea, antibiotic-associated diarrhea, pseudomembranous colitis, colitis X
	C. colinum	Quail disease
	C. spiroforme	ι-Enterotoxemia
	C. piliforme	Tyzzer's disease

symptoms of tetanus. The incubation period ranges from 24 hours to 2 weeks, varying with the toxogenicity of the infecting strain, the rate at which toxin is transferred to target tissues, and host sensitivity. Ascending tetanus follows retrograde, intraaxonal transport of toxin along the peripheral motor nerves to the central nervous system (CNS). Toxin crosses the synapse and binds to presynaptic axonal terminals, causing motoneuron hyperactivity, with sustained spasms in the innervated muscles. Other muscle groups are affected when toxin travels within the spinal cord. Descending tetanus results from vascular dissemination of toxin, and clinical effects often begin in sites distant from the infection.

Muscular tremor and increased stimulus response appear early in the course of the disease, and are followed by impaired muscle function in the head and neck. Difficulty in chewing and swallowing is sometimes exacerbated by trismus. In horses with tetanus, nostrils may be flared, the third eyelid retracted, and the ears stiffly erect. Permanent rigidity follows the tetanic spasms, and muscles of the back and tail become rigid, with orthotonus. Mechanical respiratory failure and death occur in a few days to 2 weeks.

Botulism is typically an intoxication with one of several serologically distinct neurotoxins that cause neuroparalysis by blocking acetylcholine release from cholinergic nerve endings. Spores of *Clostridium botulinum* are found in soil and sediment, and on plants growing in contaminated soil. The primary form of botulism in humans has shifted from intoxication to toxicoinfection, primarily in the form of infant botulism ("floppy baby syndrome"). Toxicoinfectious botulism can arise from a variety of foods, but one of the most common is honey. Botulinum spores are a microbiologic bonus for bees collecting pollen and nectar, and even the low concentration of spores (approximately 0.25 spore/g) can lead to initiation of disease in infants. Toxicoinfectious botulism also occurs in users of illicit injected drugs, particularly so-called black tar heroin, especially when injection is intramuscular ("muscle popping") rather than intravenous.

Clostridium botulinum producing toxin serotypes A and B are found in soil, and types C, D, E, F, and G are common in wet environments. Spores germinate in animal carcasses or rotting vegetation and produce enough toxin to cause disease outbreaks in ruminants, horses, mink, and fowl; other carnivores, swine, and fish are occasionally affected. The most common types are C and D, although this varies geographically and among animal species. Loin disease and lamziekte (cattle), limberneck and western duck sickness (waterfowl), and spinal typhus and shaker foal syndrome (horses) are distinctive names applied worldwide to the various clinical syndromes.

Phosphorus-deficient animals may develop pica and ingest botulinum toxin with the bones of animals. The common name lamziekte (lame sickness) is applied because lameness often accompanies phosphorus deficiency. Poultry litter can also be a source of toxin. The lethal dose of toxin orally is larger than that by other routes, probably because of degradation by rumen bacteria. Equine botulism is also most commonly associated with adulterated feed, but shaker foal syndrome follows toxin production in the gut of the affected animal.

Outbreaks of type C botulism in waterfowl may originate with, and be sustained by, toxin in tissues of dead invertebrates. Invertebrate larvae ingest toxin from vertebrate carcasses and are consumed by fowl. Sporadic outbreaks of type E botulism in wild birds may be associated with consumption of toxin-bearing fish. Dabbling ducks are commonly affected, as are shorebirds. Mortality in migratory populations can exceed 50,000 birds in a single season.

Type C botulism is the most common form in domestic poultry, and multiplication of *C. botulinum* in the gut may be responsible for some outbreaks. Botulism in farmed mink is also caused most often by type C.

Type D botulism occurs in cattle, and a 1990 outbreak on the Darling Downs in Queensland, Australia, killed nearly 20% of a herd of 30,000 cattle. Spent poultry litter, fed as a source of non-protein nitrogen, was contaminated with dead birds. In this outbreak, deaths continued after contaminated feed had been removed from the ration, suggesting toxicoinfectious botulism due to multiplication of the organism in the rumen.

The gene for botulinum toxin resides on a bacteriophage in some strains of *C. botulinum,* and the finding of *Clostridium baratii* and *Clostridium butyricum* toxins, which are serologically and pharmacologically similar to botulinum toxin, suggests gene transfer via this mobile element.

Clinically, botulism is characterized by anorexia, incoordination, ataxia, and flaccid paralysis. Paralysis of the tongue and pharynx leads to difficulty in swallowing, and death eventually results from respiratory paralysis. Horses experience tremors, and paralysis of facial muscles is common in cattle. In waterfowl, loss of ability to fly and a drooping head ("limberneck") are common. Chickens often have diarrhea.

Pathogenesis of tetanus and botulism. Neurotoxins of *C. tetani* and *C. botulinum* inhibit neurotransmitter release at CNS and peripheral synapses, respectively. Tetanus toxin bound to the presynaptic membrane of the neuromuscular junction is internalized and transported retro-axonally to the spinal cord. The result is spastic paralysis through toxin action on spinal inhibitory interneurons. The neurotoxins produced by *C. botulinum* are the most potent toxins known. They induce flaccid paralysis through intoxication of the neuromuscular junction.

These neurotoxins are zinc metalloproteinases that enter the cytoplasm and cleave specific protein components of the neuroexocytosis apparatus. They are composed of two disulfide-linked polypeptide chains, the larger of which is responsible for neurospecific binding and cell penetration. Upon reduction, the smaller chain is released into the cytoplasm, where its zinc-endopeptidase activity is expressed.

Tetanus neurotoxin and botulinum neurotoxins serotypes B, D, F, and G cleave VAMP/synaptobrevin, a membrane protein of the synaptic vesicles (Figures 33-1 and 33-2). Cleavage is at different, single sites for each toxin. Botulinum A and E neurotoxins cleave synaptosomal-associated protein–25 (SNAP-25), a component of the presynaptic membrane, at two different carboxyl-terminal peptide bonds. Serotype C specifically cleaves syntaxin, another protein of the nerve plasmalemma. These three proteins are conserved from yeast to humans and are essential in a variety of docking and fusion events in every cell. The end result of toxin action on target cells is blockage of acetylcholine release, and muscle paralysis.

The target specificity of these toxins is based on interaction with the cleavage site and with a noncontiguous segment containing a structural motif common to VAMP, SNAP-25, and syntaxin. VAMP contains two copies of a nine-residue motif, also present in SNAP-25 and syntaxin. Antibodies against this motif cross-react among the three proteins, and inhibit the proteolytic activity of the neurotoxins.

Two additional *C. botulinum* toxins, designated C_2 and C_3, are not neurotoxic. They are also binary toxins, but have ADP–ribosylating activity, similar to ι-toxins of *C. perfringens* and *Clostridium spiroforme.* In addition, they are much less toxic (mouse lethal dose values >45 ng) than botulinum toxin (minimum lethal dose [MLD] <0.01 ng).

HISTOTOXIC CLOSTRIDIA
Diseases, Epidemiology, and Pathogenesis

Histotoxic clostridia are common pathogens of humans and domestic animals, and a limited group causes most of the infections (Table 33-2). The hallmark is enthusiastic toxinogenesis, but common themes are acquisition of the infecting organism from soil or an endogenous source (such as the intestinal tract), entry to tissue

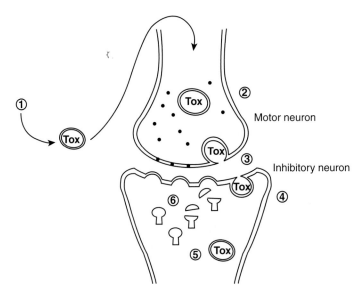

FIGURE 33-1 Tetanus neurotoxin inhibits neurotransmitter release at central nervous system (CNS) synapses. Tetanus toxin bound to the presynaptic membrane of the neuromuscular junction is internalized and transported retroaxonally to the spinal cord. Tetanus toxin (Tox) produced at a distant site *(1)* moves retrograde along peripheral nerve fibers to motoneurons *(2)*. Toxin exocytosed by the motor neuron *(3)* is endocytosed by the inhibitory neuron *(4)*. Release of the smaller chain of tetanus toxin to the cytoplasm *(5)* is followed by cleavage of VAMP/synapto-brevin, a membrane protein of the synaptic vesicles *(6)*, with spastic paralysis as the clinical result. (Courtesy Ashley E. Harmon.)

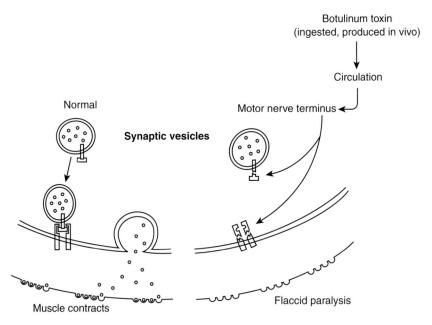

FIGURE 33-2 Botulinum neurotoxins serotypes B, D, F, and G cleave VAMP/synaptobrevin, a membrane protein of the synaptic vesicles, while those of serotypes A and E cleave synaptosomal-associated protein–25 (SNAP-25), a component of the presynaptic membrane; serotype C toxin specifically cleaves syntaxin in the nerve plas-malemma. The end result is inhibition of docking and fusion events, blockage of acetylcholine release, and muscle paralysis. (Courtesy Ashley E. Harmon.)

TABLE 33-2 Clostridia as Agents of Myonecrosis

Organism	Major Toxin(s)	Disease(s)	Species Affected
C. perfringens type A	α, θ	Gas gangrene, myonecrosis	All warm blooded
C. septicum	α	Abomasitis (sheep) Malignant edema (cattle, sheep)	Humans; sheep, cattle
C. chauvoei	α, β	Blackleg	Sheep, cattle
C. novyi types A and B	α, β	Wound infections ("bighead"), infectious necrotic hepatitis	Humans; sheep, goats
C. novyi type D (*C. haemolyticum*)	β	Bacillary hemoglobinuria	Cattle
C. sordellii	Hemolytic, lethal	Myonecrosis	Humans; sheep, cattle

following trauma, local multiplication and toxin production, occurrence of extensive local (and often systemic) tissue damage, and rapid death of the host. In animals, control by vaccination has decreased the incidence, and perhaps also the visibility, of some clostridial diseases, but renewed interest in mechanisms of pathogenesis, and to some degree the continuing interest in prevention of battlefield clostridial infections or intoxications, has yielded new information, particularly about modes of toxin action.

Clostridium septicum. *Clostridium septicum* is commonly found in soil, and has been isolated from the feces of domestic animals and humans. It is frequently a postmortem invader from the gut, particularly in ruminants. The organism has been isolated from snails that play a role in the life cycle of liver flukes, as well as from flukes recovered from sheep experimentally infected with the parasites. Further, there is evidence that *C. septicum* can enter animals from the environment in one of the life stages of the fluke.

The organism causes malignant edema in humans, with infections often associated with traumatic wounds, occult bowel carcinomas, diabetes mellitus, liver cirrhosis, and peripheral vascular disease. Nontraumatic clostridial myonecrosis is an uncommon but often fatal condition that requires immediate medical and surgical therapy. Clinical features include rapidly evolving acute illness with pain, tachycardia, and bulla formation, followed by hypotension and acute renal failure; palpation and radiography reveal gas in soft tissues. Hemorrhage, edema, and necrosis develop rapidly as the infection spreads along muscular fascial planes. Early lesions are initially painful and warm, with pitting edema, but with time, the tissue becomes crepitant and cold. Death follows,

often in less than 24 hours. The source of the organism is gastrointestinal in more than 50% of patients and the mortality rate varies from 33% to 58%, depending on method of management.

In addition to its role in myonecrosis, *C. septicum* may also cause enteric infections. In lambs or older sheep the organism penetrates the abomasal lining and produces a disease known as braxy or bradsot, which is characterized by hemorrhagic, necrotic abomasitis and fatal bacteremia. Braxy causes heavy mortality in sheep in Great Britain, Ireland, Norway, Iceland, and the Faroe Island archipelago, and has been reported in Europe, Australia, the United States, and elsewhere. A similar disease syndrome occurs in calves.

Clostridium septicum infection can manifest as gangrenous dermatitis in chickens. Iatrogenic infections are more common in horses than in other species.

Malignant edema in domestic animals (Figure 33-3) usually follows direct contamination of a traumatic wound. Genital infections can be associated with mismanaged attempts at delivery, and umbilical infections are not infrequent

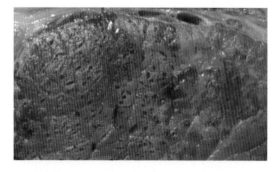

FIGURE 33-3 *Clostridium septicum*–associated necrotic myositis (malignant edema). (Courtesy Raymond E. Reed.)

in lambs. Hemorrhage, edema, and necrosis spread rapidly along fascial planes from the point of infection. As in human infections, the developing lesion is initially painful, warm, and it pits on pressure, but gradually becomes crepitant and cold, with loss of feeling. Death follows a period of fever, anorexia, and depression, often in less than 24 hours.

The pathogenetic mechanism by which *C. septicum* invades the abomasal lining (leading to development of braxy) is not known, but ingestion of cold or frozen feed is frequently an associated factor in both sheep and dairy calves; impaired mucosal function may allow entry of the organism, followed by local multiplication and dissemination throughout the body, producing local lesions and toxemia. Abomasal and proximal small intestinal walls are edematous, hemorrhagic, and sometimes necrotic.

Toxic or potentially toxic products of *C. septicum* include α-toxin (oxygen-stable hemolysin), β-toxin (DNase, leukocidin), γ-toxin (hyaluronidase), δ-toxin (oxygen-labile hemolysin), neuraminidase, chitinase, and sialidase. Recent work has demonstrated the pivotal role of α-toxin in pathogenesis of malignant edema and related infections. The effect of the purified toxin mimics some of the features of the animal and human diseases caused by *C. septicum*. α-Toxin is secreted as a 46 kD protoxin, which is activated by proteolytic cleavage and release of a 45 amino-acid fragment from the COOH terminus. The deduced primary sequence of α-toxin has 72% similarity (over a 387-residue region) with the primary structure of the *Aeromonas hydrophila* toxin aerolysin. There is good evidence that the propeptide is a chaperone, which stabilizes α-toxin monomers and escorts them to the membrane, where protease activation and oligomerization are followed by pore formation in the plasma membrane and colloidal-osmotic lysis. In vitro activation can be by trypsin cleavage, but furin and other eukaryotic proteases are involved in activation of toxin on the cell surface in vivo. α-Toxin likely binds to glycosylphosphatidylinositol-anchored protein receptors. Activated toxin forms 230 kD aggregates in erythrocyte membranes, causing release of potassium ions and hemoglobin.

A role for potential virulence attributes other than α-toxin has not been proven, but they may, in combination, increase capillary permeability and contribute to myonecrosis and systemic toxicity.

Clostridium novyi. *Clostridium novyi* type C is nontoxigenic (and therefore avirulent), but types A and B, as well as D (also called *Clostridium haemolyticum*), cause disease in humans and domestic animals. Differential production of α- and β-toxins determines toxin phenotype. However, *C. novyi* types B, C, and D may be one independent species arising from a single phylogenetic origin. 16S rDNA sequences of type B and D strains are identical, and are nearly identical to sequences from types C and A.

Strains of type A cause gas gangrene in humans and wound infections in animals. The hallmark lesion is edema, and "bighead" of young rams is illustrative; rapidly spreading edema of the head, neck, and cranial thorax follows bacterial invasion of subcutaneous tissues damaged by fighting. *Clostridium novyi* type A has been recently recognized with alarming frequency as a cause of septicemia in drug addicts who inject themselves intramuscularly.

Infectious necrotic hepatitis ("black disease") of sheep and cattle results from *C. novyi* type B infection. Dormant spores germinate in liver tissue, often damaged by fluke migration, and systemic effects with acute or peracute death follow dissemination of α-toxin. Its cardio-, neuro-, histo-, and hepatotoxic effects apparently produce edema, serosal effusion, and focal hepatic necrosis. The name "black disease" derives from the characteristic darkening of the underside of the skin as a result of venous congestion.

Clostridium novyi type D (*C. haemolyticum*) causes bacillary hemoglobinuria of cattle and other ruminants. Strains of type D resemble those of type B, except that type D strains produce no α-toxin and much more β-toxin.

Bacillary hemoglobinuria is most common in well-nourished animals more than 1 year of age. Deposition of type D spores or vegetative cells in the digestive tract and liver follows ingestion. Immature flukes migrate through the liver, causing hepatic necrosis and hypoxia, and inducing germination of spores in Kupffer cells. β-Toxin causes hepatic necrosis, and dissemination through the bloodstream leads to intravascular hemolysis and hemorrhage. Fever, pale mucous membranes, anorexia, abdominal pain, and hemoglobinuria (from which the common name "redwater" is derived) are typical clinical signs; when hemoglobinuria appears, 40% to 50% of red cells have been lysed, and death ultimately results from anoxia. Serosal effusions and a large circumscribed liver infarct are pathognomonic, and gram-positive rods are abundant in the sinusoids. Thus the pathogenesis of bacillary hemoglobinuria is similar to that of black disease of sheep, except that the primary toxin is β- rather than α-toxin. A typical case fatality rate is 90% to 95%.

Type B may be involved in an emerging problem with sudden death in sows (Figure 33-4), which is associated with multiplication of the organism in the liver at or about the time of parturition. This disease has not been reproduced by experimental inoculation of sows.

Clostridium novyi α-toxin causes rounding of cultured cells by effects on the cytoskeleton. It belongs to the family of large clostridial cytotoxins that modify small GTP-binding proteins. The substrate range includes N-acetylglucosamine and the active site is near the NH_2-terminus. Full enzyme activity of the intact toxin resides on an approximately 550 amino-acid fragment, and mutation of aspartic acid residues within this fragment dramatically reduces enzyme activity. α-Toxin specifically modifies the Rho subfamily proteins Rho, Rac, Cdc42, and RhoG, by N-acetylglucosaminylation of a threonine molecule at position 37.

Little is known about pathogenesis of type D infections, but β-toxin probably plays a major role. It is a phospholipase C with lethal, necrotizing, and hemolytic activities. The phage that mediates α-toxin production in type B can transduce type D to α-toxin production.

Clostridium chauvoei. Blackleg is a necrotizing emphysematous myositis caused by *Clostridium chauvoei*. The organism inhabits primarily the intestines of cattle and sheep, although persistence in soil may be important, based on observed year-to-year occurrence of the disease on the same pastures. *Clostridium chauvoei* and *C. septicum* are closely related, based on sequence analysis of 16S rRNA genes.

Blackleg (Figure 33-5) occurs most commonly in well-fed cattle less than 3 years of age. Lesions usually occur in hindlimb muscle mass, but may be seen only in myocardium, or possibly the diaphragm or tongue. In sheep the disease more frequently presents as a wound infection resembling malignant edema (*C. septicum* infection) or gas gangrene (*C. perfringens* infection). Clinical signs include high fever, anorexia, depression, and lameness. Many lesions are internal, but superficial ones may be crepitant on palpation. Sudden death, without observed clinical signs, is common.

The periphery of lesions is typically edematous and hemorrhagic, with myonecrosis, whereas the central areas of the lesions are often dry and emphysematous. Bacterial production of butyric acid lends a rancid-butter odor to the lesions. Microscopically, evidence of leukocytic infiltration is negligible, but degenerative changes occur in muscle fibers, and edema, emphysema, and hemorrhage are common.

Ingestion is the most probable route of exposure in cattle, and various tissues, especially

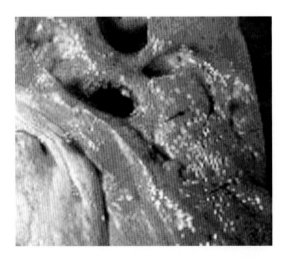

FIGURE 33-4 "Aerochocolate" liver from a sow with *Clostridium novyi* type B infection. (Courtesy Raymond E. Reed.)

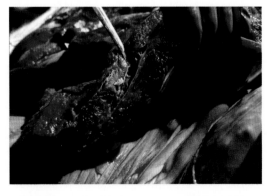

FIGURE 33-5 Bovine blackleg. (Courtesy Raymond E. Reed.)

skeletal muscle, are seeded with spores. Outbreaks may be due to spread of infection or a common source of local muscle anoxia, such as overexercise induced by encounters with phlebotomous insects. Damage to the muscle provides conditions favoring germination of dormant spores, with subsequent multiplication and toxin production. Acute indigestion may also initiate these events.

The roles of α-toxin, which is necrotizing, hemolytic, and lethal, and β-toxin, a DNase, remain undefined. Hyaluronidase (γ-toxin), oxygen-labile hemolysin (δ-toxin), and neuraminidase are of uncertain importance. Phase variation in motility and flagellation occurs, and flagellar expression is associated with virulence. *fliC* has been cloned and characterized, but immunization with recombinant flagellin protein does not protect mice against challenge.

Clostridium sordellii. *Clostridium sordellii* is a common inhabitant of soil and of the intestine of domestic animals. Isolates have been obtained from myositis, liver disease, and sudden death in cattle, sheep, and horses. Edema of subcutaneous tissues and fascial planes, with subendocardial hemorrhage, is a common lesion, with terminal septicemia in experimentally infected cattle. *Clostridium sordellii* is sometimes found in the intestines of cattle experiencing "sudden death syndrome," and bovine enteritis has been produced experimentally with the organism.

The organism has rarely been encountered in human clinical specimens, but a recent series of cases of fatal postoperative infection has raised its visibility. The potential for lethality requires that it be given serious attention when found. It is a rare cause of postpartum endometritis and, even more rarely, of spontaneous endometritis. Onset is typically sudden, with flulike symptoms and progressive refractory hypotension. Edema begins locally and spreads rapidly, and laboratory findings include marked leukocytosis and elevated hematocrit. Death follows rapidly in most cases.

Numerous putatively toxic substances are produced, including an edemagenic, lethal factor, two phospholipases C, an oxygen-labile hemolysin, neuraminidase, and a DNase. Most have not been characterized, but it is assumed that these toxins play a role in pathogenesis.

Two toxins, one hemolytic and one lethal, are antigenically and pathophysiologically similar to *C. difficile* toxins A and B, respectively. *Clostridium sordellii* lethal toxin (TcsL) glucosylates Ras, Rac, and Ral, differing from other large clostridial toxins in its modification of Ras.

Clostridium piliforme. The etiologic agent of Tyzzer's disease is *Clostridium piliforme* (Figure 33-6). Formerly known as *Bacillus piliformis*, recent studies of the 16S rRNA sequence have yielded a phylogenetic tree that suggests that the organism's closest relatives are *Clostridium coccoides*, *Clostridium oroticum*, *Clostridium clostridiiforme*, *Clostridium symbiosum*, and *Clostridium aminovalericum*. It has never been cultivated in cell-free medium, but has been propagated in a mouse-embryo fibroblast cell line.

Tyzzer's disease is typically characterized by severe diarrhea and high mortality. It occurs epizootically in many mammals, including rabbits, mice, rats, gerbils, guinea pigs, dogs, foals, calves, marsupials, and other laboratory, wild, and domesticated animals. The disease is apparently rare in birds, and there is one report of *C. piliforme* infection in a human with concurrent human immunodeficiency virus (HIV) infection.

Acutely affected, recently weaned rabbits manifest profuse watery diarrhea, with mortality ranging from 15% to 50%. Survivors may be chronically affected, with depression, anorexia, weight loss, and cachexia. Necrotic and hemorrhagic enteritis are observed mainly in the ileum, cecum, and colon, with marked serosal and submucosal edema, congestion, and distinct reddening of cecal tissues. Multifocal hepatic

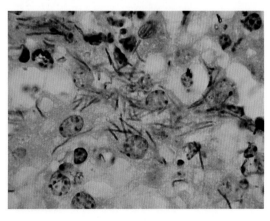

FIGURE 33-6 *Clostridium piliforme* infection in a foal. (Courtesy Karen W. Post.)

necrosis generally appears after the acute phase of the disease in rabbits. Focal myocardial necrosis may also occur. Bundles of slightly gram-negative and silver-positive rod-shaped bacilli can be seen in viable hepatocytes bordering necrotic foci, in myocytes around necrotic foci in the heart, and in enterocytes and smooth muscle cells of the muscularis mucosa of the intestine. The occurrence of antibodies to *C. piliforme* in some species suggests that subclinical infection is common.

The disease in foals usually occurs before 5 weeks of age, and in Arabian foals, combined immunodeficiency may play a role in susceptibility. Clinicopathologic abnormalities include leukopenia, hyperfibrinogenemia, metabolic acidosis, and hypoglycemia. Gross lesions include icterus, focal pale tan areas in the liver, and catarrhal enterocolitis. Focal, dark red lesions may be present in the small intestine, and the mesenteric lymph nodes may be enlarged and hyperemic. Multiple discrete and confluent foci of hepatic necrosis, hemorrhage, sinusoid congestion, infiltration of the portal triads with inflammatory cells, and bile duct hyperplasia are observed microscopically. Intestinal lesions may be mucohemorrhagic, and consist of mucosal necrosis with inflammatory cell infiltration and submucosal lymphoid hyperplasia. Hemorrhage, and necrosis of lymphoid follicles, is also present in spleen and mesenteric lymph nodes. As in the manifestation of the disease in other species, bacilli can be demonstrated in hepatocytes at the margin of liver lesions. The dams of affected foals may be carriers of the disease, and, judging by antiflagellar antibody titers, infection of horses may be quite common.

Rats with subclinical infections can transmit *C. piliforme* to naive rats. It seems likely that strains of *C. piliforme* display host specificity, and use of sentinels of one species may fail to demonstrate the presence of strains that are specific for another. Furthermore, certain strains of rats are more susceptible than others, which is a factor of major importance in colonies containing animals of multiple genotypes. Murine susceptibility varies with host strain, age, and immune status.

In dogs the infection is typically seen in the very young. Pups display widely disseminated lesions, with hepatitis, myocarditis, and enterocolitis. Disease in older dogs is less common and may be related to an immunocompromised state.

Resistance to infection in mice is correlated with antibody titers, but neutrophils and natural killer cells may play an important role in the pathogenesis of murine Tyzzer's disease. In juvenile mice, experimental depletion of either neutrophils or natural killer (NK) cells increases the severity of the disease, whereas in adults, NK cell depletion significantly increases the severity of disease in resistant (C57BL/6) but not in susceptible (DBA/2) mice. Macrophage depletion does not alter the course of infection.

Rats inoculated orally with spores of *C. piliforme* develop necrotic lesions in the intestines, liver, and heart during the first 2 weeks after inoculation, and infective spores are shed in feces. Rats that are clinically recovered can remain infected, with recrudescence of infections following steroid treatment.

Some isolates of *C. piliforme* are cross-infective (affecting more than one laboratory animal species) and others have a more limited host range. The reasons for this host specificity are not known. There are recent reports of cytotoxin production.

Clostridium perfringens. *Clostridium perfringens* causes myonecrosis and gas gangrene in humans and domestic animals. The general assumption is that most cases of human myonecrosis are caused by type A strains (Table 33-3). However, toxin typing of myonecrosis strains is rare, either by traditional in vivo neutralization tests or polymerase chain reaction (PCR) genotyping; thus occasional cases may be caused by strains of other toxin types.

Disease manifestations in humans and domestic animals are much the same. Spores germinate, vegetative cells multiply in ischemic tissues, and the infection spreads to healthy muscle, often leading to mortality. Human endomyometritis, sometimes called "pink lady syndrome," can follow cesarean delivery or bungled obstetric procedures; early recognition and aggressive management may prevent fulminant and ultimately fatal disease. *Clostridium perfringens*–associated mastitis is not uncommon in cattle and goats.

As with the other histotoxic clostridia, toxins are the major virulence factors; direct and indirect evidence implicate α- and θ-toxins in pathogenesis.

TABLE 33-3 Toxin Types of *Clostridium perfringens* and Associated Diseases

Type	α	β	ε	ι	Common Diseases
		Major Toxins Produced			
A	X				Myonecrosis, fowl necrotic enteritis, bovine and ovine enteritis, porcine necrotic enterocolitis
B	X	X	X		Ovine hemorrhagic enterotoxemia, equine and bovine hemorrhagic enteritis
C	X	X			Neonatal hemorrhagic or necrotizing enterotoxemia (ovine, porcine, bovine, caprine, equine)
D	X		X		Ovine enterotoxemia, caprine enterocolitis
E	X			X	Bovine hemorrhagic enteritis

ENTERIC AND ENTEROTOXEMIC CLOSTRIDIA

Diseases, Epidemiology, and Pathogenesis

Clostridium perfringens. *Clostridium perfringens* is broadly distributed in the environment and in the intestinal tracts of humans and domestic and wild animals. Thus infecting organisms may be from an exogenous source, but are often endogenous, through contamination of traumatic or surgical wounds or multiplication of organisms in the gut under appropriate conditions.

It is perhaps the most frequently isolated pathogenic bacterium; it is certainly the anaerobe most commonly found in human infections and is the most important cause of clostridial disease in domestic animals. The widely known typing system divides the species into five toxin types based on production of α-, β-, ε-, and ι-toxins, as determined by in vivo protection tests in guinea pigs or mice (Table 33-4; see also Table 3-3).

Truly nontoxigenic strains of *C. perfringens* (not producing any of the four major toxins) are rare.

Type A. Enteric disease in ruminants remains a diagnostic and management challenge. Lamb enterotoxemia (yellow lamb disease) occurs rarely in the northwestern United States. Affected animals exhibit depression, anemia, icterus, and hemoglobinuria, dying after a clinical course of 6 to 12 hours. Large numbers of *C. perfringens* are often found in the intestine. Type A–associated disease is much more common in beef and dairy calves, including those raised for veal (Figure 33-7). Infection may originate in contaminated colostrum, and the method of administration provides risk factors; ingestion of icy colostrum in large volumes is associated with development of disease. Bloating is common, and affected animals die quite rapidly. Gross lesions consist typically of hemorrhagic gastroenteritis. The abomasum is often grossly dilated, with thickened, emphysematous walls and folds.

TABLE 33-4 Toxins of *Clostridium perfringens*

Toxin	Activity
α	Major toxin, produced by all isolates; multifunctional phospholipase, acts on cell membrane phospholipids; hemolytic, dermonecrotic, lethal
β	Major toxin; mucosal necrosis, CNS signs, cardiac effects; homology of *cpb* with genes for *Staphylococcus aureus* α-toxin, γ-toxin, leukocidin; dermonecrotic, lethal
ε	Major toxin; synthesized as prototoxin, activated by proteolysis; induces increased permeability, facilitates uptake to circulation; affects CNS, causing encephalomalacia; necrotizing, potently lethal; placed on CDC Select Agent List
ι	Major toxin; binding, entry of Ia component (ITXa) mediated by Ib (ITXb); Ia ADP-ribosylates globular skeletal muscle, nonmuscle actin; similar in activity to spiroforme toxin, *C. botulinum* types C, D C2 toxin; dermonecrotic, lethal
θ	Perfringolysin O; cholesterol-binding toxin, pore former; oxygen labile; role in myonecrosis
Enterotoxin	Food poisoning toxin; production coregulated with sporulation; cytotoxic N-terminus, receptor binding by C-terminus; pore formation, cytoskeletal disintegration, cytolysis

ADP, Adenosine diphosphate; *CDC,* Centers for Disease Control and Prevention; *CNS,* central nervous system.

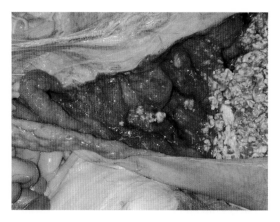

FIGURE 33-7 Hemorrhagic abomasitis in a dairy calf (*Clostridium perfringens* type A). (Courtesy J. Glenn Songer.)

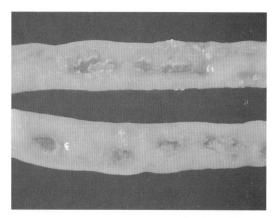

FIGURE 33-8 Chicken necrotic enteritis (*Clostridium perfringens* type A). (Courtesy J. Glenn Songer.)

Microscopic lesions include severe necrosis and hemorrhage, with microcolonies of large rod-shaped bacteria and gas bubbles observed in the mucosa and submucosa. Anaerobic culture usually results in heavy growth of *C. perfringens* from abomasum and small intestine, which are most often of genotype A.

Necrotic enteritis of domestic poultry is usually caused by *C. perfringens* type A or type C (Figure 33-8). Captive and free-living wild birds may also be affected. Soil, dust, and contaminated feed and litter are potential sources of infection, and disease can result from raising chicks on litter on premises with a history of the disease or by administration of contaminated feed; challenge with cultures of *C. perfringens* or culture supernatant fluids, under proper conditions, also produces lesions of necrotic enteritis. Mild forms of necrotic enteritis result in poor feed efficiency. In others, depression, inappetence, anorexia, and diarrhea occur, but many birds are simply found dead. Jejunal and ileal necrosis are common, and lesions in the lower intestine consist of acute catarrh without necrosis. Gram-positive bacilli are usually found on the mucosa.

Neonatal foals may develop hemorrhagic diarrhea as a result of *C. perfringens* infection, with lesions including diffuse necrosis of the villous mucosa, and hyperemia and hemorrhage of the lamina propria, submucosa, and subserosa. Intravenous inoculation of ponies with type A organisms has caused acute colic and hemorrhagic enterocolitis, although these results are of uncertain meaning in explaining the natural disease.

Type A infection in neonatal pigs is most often characterized by mild necrotizing enterocolitis and damage to the tips of the villi, affecting primarily the jejunum and ileum. A form of the disease has been reproduced by oral or intragastric inoculation of conventional and gnotobiotic colostrum-deprived pigs, in which enteropathy follows substantial adherence and multiplication of α-toxigenic *C. perfringens* in the gut. α-Toxin administered alone to neonatal piglets causes mild enteritis and villous edema, with epithelial and vascular damage.

Hemorrhagic canine gastroenteritis is sometimes associated with *C. perfringens*. Watery to mucoid diarrhea with blood is common, as is peracute death, with hemorrhagic mucosal necrosis.

Type B. Lamb dysentery typically develops after infection of neonates by the dam or from the environment. Multiplication of type B organisms in the gut results in enterotoxemia, accompanied by extensive hemorrhage and ulceration of the small intestine. Death is often sudden, but may be preceded by cessation of feeding, severe abdominal pain, bloody diarrhea, recumbency, and coma; case fatality rates approach 100%. A disease called "pine" occurs in older lambs and manifests as chronic abdominal pain without diarrhea. Type B may also be associated with hemorrhagic enteritis in goats, calves, and foals.

Type C. Newborn animals are typically most susceptible to infections by *C. perfringens* type C, perhaps because of ready colonization of the gut in the absence of established normal intestinal flora. Alteration of flora by sudden dietary changes may also be an inciting factor. Sows are thought to be a common source of the infection for newborn pigs, but numbers of *C. perfringens* in sow feces may be too low to be detected by conventional culture methods.

Morbidity rates of 30% to 50% and case fatality rates of 50% to 100% are not uncommon among 1- to 2-day-old piglets in affected herds (Figure 33-9). Neonatal pancreatic secretion deficiencies and protease inhibitors in colostrum favor the action of β-toxin. Intestinal lesions are usually extensive and severe, but death is probably due ultimately to toxemia. Peracute disease in piglets 1 to 2 days of age is characterized by diarrhea and dysentery, with blood and necrotic debris in feces. Hemorrhagic necrosis of the mucosa, submucosa, and muscularis mucosa is extensive, with gas accumulation in tissue and hemorrhagic exudate in the lumen. Piglets affected at 1 to 2 weeks of age often have a longer clinical course, experiencing yellowish nonbloody diarrhea and jejunal mucosal necrosis. The cecum and proximal colon are affected in some pigs.

Infection of neonatal calves, lambs, and goats with type C causes hemorrhagic necrotic enteritis and enterotoxemia, accompanied at times by nervous signs, including tetany and opisthotonos. Adult sheep can be affected by a form of enterotoxemia often referred to as "struck." Rapid death is common, leaving the impression that the animal has been struck by lightning. Damage to the gastrointestinal mucosa, often by poor quality feed, precedes multiplication of type C in the abomasum and small intestine. Mucosal necrosis and toxemia result, usually without dysentery or diarrhea.

Type C is also an enteric pathogen of foals, producing disease that is often indistinguishable from that caused by enterotoxigenic or nonenterotoxigenic type A strains. Depression, hemorrhagic diarrhea, dehydration, and colic accompany jejunal and ileal lesions that usually consist of acute hemorrhagic enteritis with necrosis of villi. Isolates of type C have also been obtained from dogs with peracute to acute lethal hemorrhagic enteritis.

Type D. Type D causes enterotoxemia (sudden death, "overeating") in sheep of all ages except neonates. It is common in suckling lambs 3 to 10 weeks old and in feedlot animals. Disease often follows upsets in the gut flora, which can result from sudden changes to a rich diet or continual feeding of concentrated rations. Rapid multiplication of type D and production of ε-toxin are favored by excess dietary starch in the small intestine. ε-Toxin facilitates its own absorption, resulting in toxemia with little evidence of enteritis. The effects of ε-toxin on the central nervous system (CNS) and other tissues cause sudden death, preceded in some cases by clinical signs such as opisthotonos and convulsions, with agonal struggling. Focal encephalomalacia (Figure 33-10) is likely a chronic manifestation of enterotoxemia, and affected sheep display blindness, head pressing, and anorexia. "Pulpy kidney," another common name for type D enterotoxemia, derives from a hallmark lesion that results from rapid postmortem autolysis in toxin-damaged tissue.

Enterotoxemia in suckling calves is similar to disease in sheep, but catarrhal, fibrinous, or hemorrhagic enterocolitis is a consistent lesion in goats, and the classic pulpy kidney is absent.

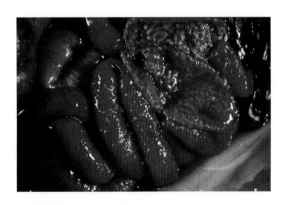

FIGURE 33-9   Porcine necrotic enteritis (*Clostridium perfringens* type C). (Courtesy D.L. Harris.)

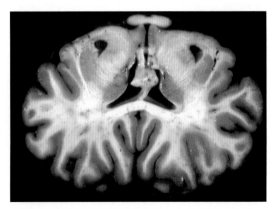

FIGURE 33-10   Encephalomalacia associated with *Clostridium perfringens* type D enterotoxemia. (Courtesy Raymond E. Reed.)

Type D is apparently a rare cause of disease in adult cattle, deer, domesticated camels, and horses.

Type E. Type E has been associated with enterotoxemia of lambs, calves, and rabbits (see Table 33-3). ɩ-Enterotoxemia in calves and lambs was reported in the late 1940s in Britain, and accounts published since that time have been of hemorrhagic necrotic enteritis of calves and of detection of type E organisms and ɩ-toxin in ovine or bovine intestines at postmortem. Strains of type E are distinguished from other toxinotypes by their production of ɩ-toxin, which is composed of two noncovalently associated components which ADP-ribosylate actin. Little is known of the pathogenesis of type E infections, although ɩ-toxin is assumed to play an important role. Suspected type E–induced disease in rabbits must be differentiated from that caused by *C. spiroforme,* which produces a toxin quite similar to ɩ-toxin.

Dogma has held that type E isolates are quite rare, especially in North America. In fact, strains of type E are quite common in certain niches, representing 3% to 5% of strains of *C. perfringens* from domestic animals with enteritis, and perhaps as many as 50% of isolates from calves with hemorrhagic enteritis. The enterotoxin gene, *cpe,* can be detected by PCR in most, if not all, type E isolates, but is silent.

Enterotoxigenic *C. perfringens.* Enterotoxigenic strains of *C. perfringens* have been detected in many species of animals, including diarrheic dogs and cats, horses, cattle, poultry, and sheep. Dogs develop hospital-acquired infections, with mild depression, anorexia, and soft to watery diarrhea, in some cases with blood and mucus. Colic and hemorrhagic gastroenteritis have been produced in ponies by inoculation with enterotoxin (CPE). Involvement of CPE in pathogenesis of colitis X has been suggested, based on observations of large numbers of enterotoxigenic *C. perfringens* in the gut of affected horses and lesions produced in experimental infections with type A.

CPE is probably also an etiologic factor in diarrheal disease of pigs. Superficial mucosal necrosis and villous atrophy are detected in animals with naturally occurring disease attributable to CPE-producing strains; spore counts in affected animals are often more than two logs higher than in nondiarrheic pigs.

Animal-to-human transmission of CPE-producing strains is suggested by epidemiologic evidence.

Pathogenesis. More than 15 exotoxins of *C. perfringens* have been described, but a definitive role in pathogenesis has been demonstrated for only a few.

α-Toxin (CPA), a multifunctional phospholipase, is produced in varying amounts by all animal isolates. Hydrolysis of cell membrane phospholipids by α-toxin causes lysis or other deleterious effects, resulting in hemolysis, necrosis, and lethality. Genes with varying degrees of homology to the CPA structural gene, *cpa,* have been found in other clostridia.

The dominant role of CPA in pathogenesis of myonecrosis was established by immunization against lethal challenge and by the demonstration that specific mutants have reduced virulence in a mouse myonecrosis model. Protective epitopes are apparently in the C-terminal third of the molecule because immunization with the genetically truncated C-terminal portion protects mice against challenge with toxin or with 10 LD_{50} of *C. perfringens.*

CPA may also be a virulence factor in enterotoxemia, in that large amounts may be found in feces of affected animals. α-Toxigenic *C. perfringens* causes enteropathy after substantial multiplication in the gut of piglets; CPA alone causes only mild enteritis and villous edema, with minimal damage to the epithelium and blood vessels and no ultrastructural changes in villi, lymphatics, or other tissues. The syndrome in lambs and calves is often consistent with a hemolytic toxin (such as CPA) acting in the circulation, causing intravascular hemolysis and capillary damage, inflammation, platelet aggregation, shock, and cardiac effects, culminating in death.

β-Toxin (CPB) is responsible for mucosal necrosis and possibly for CNS signs. Dermonecrosis can be produced in guinea pigs with as little as two ng of CPB, and the intravenous LD_{50} for mice is approximately 500 ng per kg. Intravenous administration causes increased blood pressure and decreased heart rate, with electrocardiographic disturbances suggestive of atrioventricular block. The CPB gene *(cpb)* resides on a large extrachromosomal element, and its homology with genes for *Staphylococcus aureus* α-toxin, γ-toxin, and leukocidin lend credence to suggestions that CPB may directly affect the CNS.

In pigs, CPB acts in the jejunum under conditions of decreased proteolytic activity that arise from neonatal pancreatic secretion deficiency or ingestion of protease inhibitors in colostrum. Production of experimental disease in pigs requires viable bacteria as well as toxin, and acute hemorrhagic enterotoxemia occurs in lambs inoculated with cultures of type C and soybean flour (as a protease inhibitor), but not with cell-free culture supernatant fluid. Damage to microvilli, mitochondria, and terminal capillaries precedes adhesion of *C. perfringens* to the jejunal mucosa. Widespread, progressive, mucosal necrosis follows, with cycles of bacterial invasion, multiplication, and toxin production, and epithelial cell death and desquamation. Gram-positive bacilli can be demonstrated across extensive areas of the mucosa. Intestinal lesions are extensive and severe, but death is probably a result of β-toxemia. Acute or peracute deaths are common.

ε-Prototoxin is converted to the greater than 1000-fold more toxic ε-toxin (ETX) by proteolytic cleavage, which removes 14 N-terminal amino acids. Its precise biological activity is not known, but ETX is necrotizing and lethal, and possesses approximately 3×10^6 IV minimum lethal doses per mg in mice. A small amount of ETX in the gut of normal animals is probably innocuous, but high concentrations of toxin cause increased permeability, with subsequent absorption into circulation. Foci of liquefactive necrosis, perivascular edema, and hemorrhage occur in the CNS, especially in the meninges. Vascular endothelial cells bear a receptor for ETX, and a sialoglycoprotein in synaptosomal membranes may be a high-affinity binding site. In brain tissue of animals inoculated with ETX, tight junctions in the vascular endothelium degenerate, causing swelling and rupture of perivascular astrocyte processes. Increased capillary permeability, with rapid extravasation of fluid, is followed by elevated intracerebral pressure. Focal to diffuse areas of degeneration and necrosis, as well as bilateral macroscopic foci of encephalomalacia, frequently occur. The degree of incoordination and convulsions, as well as other signs of CNS derangement, is directly related to the severity of lesions.

Hemorrhage is uncommon in type D–induced disease in sheep or cattle, although hemorrhage in the small intestine, petechial hemorrhages of the endocardium, and subendocardial hemorrhage around the mitral valve is occasionally detected. Hemorrhagic enterocolitis is common in goats. Peritoneal and pericardial effusions are typical in sheep, and hyperglycemia and glycosuria are pathognomonic.

Globular skeletal muscle and nonmuscle actin are ADP-ribosylated by the Ia component of ι-toxin (ITXa), which is targeted to sensitive cells and enters the cytoplasm in a process mediated by the Ib (ITXb) component. ITX shares activities (induction of increased vascular permeability, dermonecrosis, and lethality) with the toxin of *C. spiroforme* and with C2 toxin of *C. botulinum* types C and D.

Production of CPE is coregulated with sporulation, and toxin is released upon lysis of the vegetative cell. Proteolytic cleavage removes 24 N-terminal amino acids, activating the molecule, which then consists of a cytotoxic N-terminal domain and a C-terminal domain with receptor activity. Pore formation, altered permeability, inhibition of macromolecular synthesis, cytoskeletal disintegration, and lysis occur sequentially when susceptible cells are exposed to CPE. *cpe* has been demonstrated in strains of all toxin types, in chromosomal or extrachromosomal locations, but the gene is silent in type E strains.

In human food poisoning, organisms ingested in food sporulate in the gastrointestinal tract; there is evidence in domestic animals (especially in dogs) that the organism may go through cycles of germination, sporulation, and toxin production in the gut. In either case, toxin is released, and it acts rapidly on the jejunal and ileal mucosa. Binding to a specific receptor on cell membranes is followed by insertion into the plasma membrane and complexing with membrane proteins. The toxin does not enter the cytoplasm, but there is a rapid decrease in intracellular concentrations of ions and small molecules. Inhibition of synthesis of macromolecules and decreased energy metabolism also occur. Profuse diarrhea and associated clinical signs appear rapidly.

Enterotoxin is weakly immunogenic when exposure is through the intestinal tract, and clinical disease gives rise to serum antibodies in humans, pigs, sheep, cattle, and horses.

Clostridium difficile. Pseudomembranous colitis in humans follows overgrowth of the large intestine by *Clostridium difficile,* usually after bowel flora are perturbed by antimicrobial therapy or other circumstances. The prevalence of *C. difficile* in colonies of laboratory mice can be augmented by antibiotic treatment. Hamsters and guinea pigs develop an identical condition after antibiotic treatment, although it is most often fatal in these species. *Clostridium difficile*–induced disease also occurs in a variety of domestic and wild species, including adult horses, foals, and swine, and has been reported in ostriches, a penguin, and even a Kodiak bear. *Clostridium difficile* causes cecitis in rabbits and hares, but *C. spiroforme* is more common (Table 33-5).

The organism can multiply to large numbers in unfilled (neonates, infants, or gnotobiotes) or emptied (by antimicrobial therapy) ecological niches in the bowel. Occurrence of *C. difficile*–associated disease (CDAD) without prior antimicrobial therapy suggests that antibiotic depression of normal flora is not the only circumstance that allows establishment of *C. difficile* in the bowel. The risk of developing disease is probably influenced by dose, ability to compete for nutrients, toxigenicity, perhaps the ability to adhere to colonic epithelium, the presence in the microenvironment of organisms that positively affect multiplication, and unidentified host susceptibility factors.

Clostridium difficile has been isolated from marine sediment, soil, sand, the hospital environment, feces of nondiarrheic humans, camels, horses, donkeys, dogs and cats (up to 39% prevalence rate), domestic birds, cattle, ducks, geese, seals, snakes, the environment of household pets, the human genital tract, and, rarely, from septicemias and pyogenic infections in humans and domestic animals. In horses, the organism is

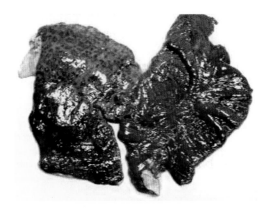

FIGURE 33-11 Equine colitis (adult) associated with *Clostridium difficile* infection. (Courtesy J. Glenn Songer.)

putatively important as a cause of both diarrhea and fatal necrotizing enterocolitis (Figure 33-11). Affected foals are usually neonates, and typically display severe hemorrhagic necrotizing enterocolitis, with colic, weakness, profuse watery diarrhea, and dehydration. Large numbers of gram-positive rods line the surface of necrotic villi. Onset of clinical signs is usually followed by death in less than 24 hours. Lesions are similar to those encountered in *C. perfringens* type C infection. The disease has been reproduced experimentally by inoculation with *C. difficile*.

The organism and its cytotoxin have been demonstrated in feces of dogs with chronic diarrhea. Pups are more commonly affected than adults, and infection with different toxigenic phenotypes in the same litter suggests transient infection with different strains. Shedding of the organism in feces of normal dogs and the possibility of false positives in toxin detection assays (enzyme immunoassays) make the significance of these findings in dogs with chronic diarrhea uncertain.

CDAD in pigs is an emerging condition, occurring typically in piglets 1 to 7 days of age and presenting with a history of scours since shortly after birth (Table 33-6). Litters from gilts and sows are affected, and decreased rates of survival to weaning are common. Gross pathology can include moderate to severe edema of the mesocolon (Figure 33-12), sometimes accompanied by hydrothorax and/or ascites. Large intestines are frequently filled with pasty to watery yellowish feces. Microscopic lesions in the colon consist of scattered foci of suppuration in the lamina propria,

TABLE 33-5 Diseases Associated with *Clostridium difficile* Infection

Species	Condition(s)
Human	Antibiotic-associated diarrhea
	Pseudomembranous colitis
	Toxic megacolon
	Septicemia
	Myonecrosis
Laboratory rodents	Typhilitis in hamsters
	Antibiotic-associated diarrhea in mice, rabbits, and guinea pigs
Horses	Hemorrhagic necrotizing enterocolitis in neonatal foals
	Nosocomial diarrhea and typhilitis in adult horses
Dogs	Chronic diarrhea
Ratites	Enterotoxemia in ostriches
Pigs	Neonatal necrotizing colitis

TABLE 33-6 Case Definition for *Clostridium difficile*–Associated Disease in Neonatal Pigs

	Features
History and clinical signs	Piglets (from gilts and sows) 1-7 days of age, often scouring from shortly after birth; loss of condition, stunting of survivors; respiratory distress, decreased survival rates common Morbidity 10%-90%, averaging 20% Case fatality rate up to 50%, averaging 20% Possible association with administration of penicillins, cephalosporins at processing
Gross pathology	Moderate to severe mesocolonic edema; hydrothorax and/or ascites occasional; pasty to watery yellowish colonic contents
Microscopic pathology	Scattered suppurative foci in colonic lamina propria; neutrophilic infiltrate in mesocolon; segmental erosion of colonic mucosal epithelium; "volcano" lesions (neutrophil and fibrin exudation into colonic lumen); large rods, sometimes with spores on mucosal surface, in lumen No remarkable lesions in small intestine
Bacteriology and toxin testing	Moderate to heavy growth of *C. difficile* Presence of toxins A and B

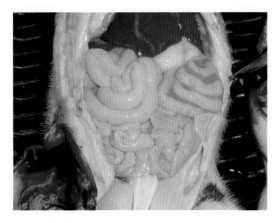

FIGURE 33-12 Mesocolonic edema in porcine *Clostridium difficile* infection. (Courtesy Sarah Probst Miller.)

with additional accumulation of neutrophils in the mesocolon. A common lesion is edema involving the colonic serosa and mesentery, and there are infiltrations of mononuclear inflammatory cells and neutrophils in the edematous areas. There may be segmental erosion of the mucosal epithelial surface of the colon. Exudation of neutrophils and fibrin from these inflamed mucosal segments into the lumen gives rise to the description of "volcano" lesions. There are usually no remarkable lesions in the small intestines of pigs with uncomplicated *C. difficile* infection. Villous blunting, congestion of mucosal vessels, atonicity, and pale contents in the small intestine suggest concurrent infection with *C. perfringens* or *Escherichia coli*. Widespread occurrence of

C. difficile–associated disease in pigs is implied by its diagnosis in laboratories throughout swine-producing areas of the United States.

Virulence attributes may include pili, capsule, and degradative enzymes, but production of toxins is essential. Toxin A (TcdA), an enterotoxin, causes fluid accumulation in the gut and is lethal when administered orally or IP to hamsters. Toxin B (TcdB), a cytotoxin, is lethal by IP and oral routes, and does not cause fluid accumulation in the bowel. Picogram amounts are toxic for culture cells (Figure 33-13). When TcdA and TcdB are produced in vivo in hamsters, the result is a severe, often fatal, hemorrhagic ileitis or cecitis with ulceration, formation of a pseudomembrane, and watery and bloody diarrhea. Immunization with both is required to protect hamsters against *C. difficile* infection.

Clostridium spiroforme. *Clostridium spiroforme* causes enterotoxemia of rabbits and other laboratory rodents. When cultivated on blood agar, this organism has a loosely coiled, spiral morphology consisting of a uniform end-to-end aggregation of semicircular cells (especially when cultivated in vivo).

Clostridium spiroforme is apparently not found normally in the rabbit bowel, but is acquired from the environment. In many cases, poor hygiene, stress, and diet have a prominent influence on development of disease. Weaning or antibiotic treatment destabilize cecal microflora, providing conditions under which diarrhea develops rapidly, and death ensues soon after. Gross lesions

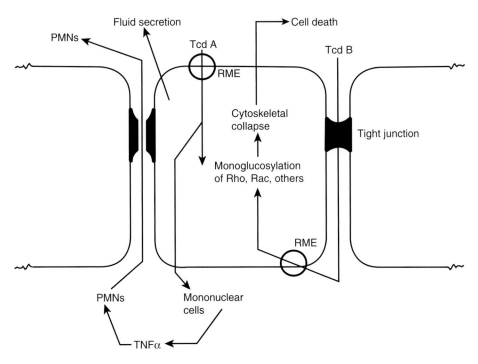

FIGURE 33-13 Toxin A (TcdA) of *Clostridium difficile* enters susceptible cells by receptor-mediated endocytosis (RME), where it monoglucosylates Rho, Rac, and other proteins, inactivating them, affecting the cytoskeleton, and leading to fluid secretion. It may also be exocytosed to the submucosa, where its interactions with mononuclear cells results in TNF-α release, recruitment of polymorphonuclear neutrophils (PMNs), and the characteristic neutrophilic colitis. Toxin B (TcdB) accesses the basolateral surface of colonic epithelial cells via tight junctions damaged by TcdA effects. It enters by RME, carries out the same monoglucosylation reaction, with cytoskeletal effects leading to cell death. (Courtesy Ashley E. Harmon.)

include an immensely dilated cecum with watery contents. Epithelial necrosis accompanies a pronounced inflammatory infiltration of the lamina propria. Affected animals have high levels of *C. spiroforme* spores in cecal contents.

Isolates of *C. spiroforme* from rabbits with enterotoxemia produce a toxin that is neutralized by antibodies against *C. perfringens* ι-toxin. It is lethal for mice and dermonecrotic for guinea pigs, and enterotoxemia can be reproduced with filtrates of cecal contents from rabbits that have died of the disease. Spiroforme toxin occurs in binary form, with two independent polypeptides expressing ADP-ribosyltransferase and binding/internalization activities, respectively. The target of the ADP-ribosylating activity is monomeric actin, which is trapped in the unpolymerized form, leading to destruction of the microfilament network.

Clostridium colinum. *Clostridium colinum* causes ulcerative enteritis of chickens, quail, and other wild and domestic fowl, including turkeys, grouse, and partridge. The condition is characterized by sudden onset and rapidly increasing mortality in a flock. It was originally known as quail disease because of its frequent enzootic occurrence in bobwhite quail *(Colinus virginianus)*, from which the causative organism derives its name. The mol% G+C of the DNA of *C. colinum* (43%) is significantly higher than that of many pathogenic clostridia.

Certain aspects of the natural history of *C. colinum* and ulcerative enteritis are relatively clear. Natural infection probably occurs orally, and the annual recurrence of infections on some premises suggests maintenance of *C. colinum* in soil. Quail with chronic disease can be carriers. Experimental infection of quail is straightforward, but chickens are much more resistant to *C. colinum* as a primary etiologic agent, with coccidiosis, aplastic anemia, stress, or infectious bursal disease often predisposing to infection.

Birds younger than 3 months of age are most commonly infected with *C. colinum,* and the disease follows a rapid and fatal clinical course. After establishing in the intestine, *C. colinum* causes duodenal hemorrhagic enteritis, cecal necrosis, and ulceration. A pseudomembrane is sometimes present, and bowel perforation can occur, followed by peritonitis. Microscopic lesions include desquamation of mucosal epithelium, edema of intestinal wall, engorgement of local blood vessels, and a prominent lymphocytic infiltration. Ulcers extend into the submucosa, and are surrounded by granulocytic infiltrations. Infection extends to liver, apparently by portal circulation, producing diffuse centrilobular or pinpoint necrosis. Splenic congestion, hemorrhage, and necrosis may also occur. Birds often die in less than 48 hours, and emaciation and pectoral muscle atrophy occur in those with a clinical course longer than 7 days. The average mortality in chickens is 10% to 30%, but may reach 100% in young quail. The course of the disease in a flock is usually about 3 weeks, with peak mortality during the second week. Filtrates of supernatant fluids are not toxic for mice, and virulence has not been further studied.

Diagnosis

Clostridial neurointoxications. Diagnosis of clostridial neurointoxications begins with observation of compatible clinical signs, but should be confirmed by toxin detection and neutralization in mice or, in the case of botulism, by an in vitro assay such as enzyme-linked immunosorbent assay (ELISA). Enzyme immunoassays have been applied to diagnosis of botulism in waterfowl, but neither kits nor reagents are commercially available.

Bacteriologic culture is also useful in confirmation of a diagnosis. *Clostridium botulinum* and *C. tetani* are particularly oxygen sensitive, so this should be taken into account when establishing culture conditions. Morphology of colonies of *C. botulinum* varies somewhat with the type of strain (A-G), but most are β-hemolytic, circular to irregular, raised to flat, translucent to opaque, and have scalloped to lobate margins. Cells are mainly straight rods with subterminal spores. *Clostridium tetani* produces colonies that may be β-hemolytic; they are flat, translucent, and gray, with matte surfaces and irregular to rhizoid margins. Swarming may be observed when *C. tetani* is cultivated on moist agar plates. Cells from cultures less than 24 hours old stain gram positive, but become gram negative with age. Spores of *C. tetani* are usually round and terminal, giving cells the characteristic "tennis racquet" appearance.

Histotoxic clostridial infections. Myonecrosis and other *C. perfringens* infections outside the gastrointestinal tract can be diagnosed by findings of gross and microscopic pathologic examinations, as well as bacteriologic culture and typing of isolates. An experienced diagnostician may be able in some cases to differentiate *C. perfringens*–induced disease from other, similar infections (such as blackleg or malignant edema), but bacteriologic culture is indicated in most instances. *Clostridium perfringens* colonies are circular, smooth, and surrounded by an inner zone of complete β-hemolysis and an outer zone of incomplete hemolysis. Cells stain gram positive to gram variable, and appear as short, plump rods with blunt ends ("boxcars"). Conjugates for fluorescent antibody tests are not available.

Diagnosis of blackleg, malignant edema, and infections by *C. novyi* and *C. sordellii* can be based on clinical signs, gross and microscopic findings at necropsy, Gram and fluorescent antibody stains of direct smears, and bacteriologic culture (Table 33-7). Colonies of *C. chauvoei* are β-hemolytic, circular, convex or raised, translucent to opaque, granular, and shiny or dull, entire to erose margins. Cells stain gram positive, although irregularly, and spores are oval and subterminal. Colonies of *C. novyi* are β-hemolytic, circular, raised to convex, translucent, gray, and shiny, with a granular surface and erose to slightly scalloped margins. Some strains grow as a film over the entire plate. Cells of *C. novyi* type D rapidly become gram negative with age, and spores are oval and subterminal. Toxin typing of *C. novyi* isolates is useful, but rarely done. *Clostridium septicum* is likely to be the etiologic agent if it predominates in specimens obtained soon after death. Colonies are circular, with rhizoid to irregular margins and are slightly raised, translucent, gray, glossy and β-hemolytic. Not unlike *C. novyi,* some strains produce a thin film over the entire agar surface. Staining may be uneven, regardless of the age of the culture. The cells are straight to curved rods, occurring singly or in pairs; they may also be pleomorphic, especially in lesions. *Clostridium sordellii* grows in circular to irregular colonies that are flat or raised and

TABLE 33-7   Use of Fluorescent Antibody Tests for Diagnosis of Histotoxic Clostridial Infections

Disease	Species	Test for *Clostridium*
Blackleg	Ruminants	*C. septicum, C. chauvoei, C. novyi, C. sordellii*
	Swine	*C. septicum, C. chauvoei*
Braxy	Sheep	*C. septicum*
Bighead		*C. novyi*
Black disease	Ruminants	*C. novyi*
Bacillary hemoglobinuria	Cattle	*C. novyi*
Malignant edema	Horses, ruminants, swine	*C. septicum*
Gangrenous dermatitis	Poultry	*C. septicum,* rarely *C. novyi, C. sordellii;* most likely etiology is *C. perfringens* (no conjugate available)

translucent to opaque; color varies from gray to chalk white and the margins are scalloped, lobate, or entire.

Clostridium piliforme has not been cultivated in cell-free media, so diagnosis of Tyzzer's disease is based on microscopic demonstration, by silver staining, of the organism within the cytoplasm and nucleus of viable cells around necrotic areas of liver or intestine.

The most useful direct and rapid differential assay for myonecrosis agents is the fluorescent antibody test (see Table 33-7). The test is performed either on smears taken directly from clinical material or on isolates for *C. chauvoei, C. novyi, C. septicum,* or *C. sordellii.*

Clostridial enteritis and enterotoxemia. Diagnosis of *C. perfringens* gastrointestinal infections requires evaluation of clinical signs and gross and microscopic lesions, bacteriologic culture of appropriate specimens, and typing of isolates. Identification is aided by the nearly invariate production of a double zone of hemolysis. About 2% of strains do not produce θ-toxin, and thus have no clear inner hemolytic zone.

Demonstration of toxins by in vivo assays is no longer a common practice. Culture supernatant fluids or eluates from gut contents (trypsin treated or untreated, neat or mixed with antiserum) are examined in mice (injected IV) for lethality or guinea pigs (injected ID) for dermonecrosis. Detection of toxins in clinical specimens does not necessarily confirm the existence of disease, and false negatives may occur because of the lability of these proteins, especially CPB. CPE can be detected by commercially available immunoassays.

PCR genotyping can be a useful complement to other diagnostic methods. Genes for the four major toxins, as well as *cpe,* can be detected in a multiplex PCR assay; the correlation between phenotype and genotype approaches 100%, suggesting that the prevalence of silent toxin genes is low. Type E isolates, all of which carry silent copies of *cpe,* are the exception.

If isolates of genotypes C, D, or E are obtained from animals with typical lesions in nonvaccinated herds, diagnosis is unequivocal. Diagnosis of genotype A infections is more complex, but if clinical signs and lesions are compatible, and if other etiologies are ruled out by concurrent microbiologic examination, a diagnosis of type A enteritis should be considered.

Clostridium difficile can usually be isolated from affected gut tissues (primarily colon and cecum), but the gold standard for diagnosis remains toxin detection. This can be accomplished by neutralization tests in Chinese hamster ovary (CHO) cells or by use of a commercial enzyme immunoassay (EIA). Excellent correlation is between clinical, pathologic, and bacteriologic diagnosis, on the one hand, and toxin detection on the other, for samples from affected piglets. No commercial supplier of EIA kits makes a claim for applicability to diagnosis of animal diseases, and, in fact, false positives are quite common in samples from dogs and ruminants. Bacteriologic culture is a useful adjunct to diagnosis. Colonies of *C. difficile* on blood agar are circular, occasionally rhizoid, flat to low convex, opaque, and whitish gray. All strains produce a pale green fluorescence under long wave ultraviolet light after 48 hours on brucella blood agar supplemented with vitamin K and hemin.

Isolates have an odor, described as that of an "elephant house" at a zoo. Cells are gram-positive rods, sometimes in chains of two to six cells. Spores are oval and subterminal.

Detection of semicircular gram-positive bacteria in feces or cecal contents of affected rabbits suggests *C. spiroforme* infection, but definitive diagnosis requires demonstration of spiroforme toxin by a lethality assay in mice or a cytotoxicity assay in Vero cells. Colonies of *C. spiroforme* are approximately 1 mm in diameter, with entire to slightly erose margins; they are convex, smooth, shiny, semiopaque and whitish or grayish. Cells stain gram positive and form tightly coiled long chains. Most strains produce round, terminal to subterminal spores that can be difficult to demonstrate.

Diagnosis of ulcerative enteritis is based on demonstration of typical lesions in the intestinal tract, liver, and spleen, and isolation of *C. colinum* from the intestine or liver. Subterminal spores may be seen in tissue, but rarely occur in vitro. Colonies of *C. colinum* are white, circular, convex, semitranslucent and nonhemolytic, and cells are individual gram-positive rods that are straight or slightly curved. *Clostridium colinum* is very similar biochemically to *C. difficile,* but ferments raffinose and does not hydrolyze gelatin.

Control and Prevention

Botulism and tetanus. Antitoxic antibodies can usually not be demonstrated in animals naturally resistant to tetanus. Acquired resistance arises from circulating antitoxin, and widespread vaccination has dramatically lessened the impact of tetanus. Passive immunity acquired by neonates from the dam protects for 2 to 3 months, after which they can be actively immunized with toxoid. Boosters are recommended at 1- to 5-year intervals.

Antibodies against botulinum toxins can be found in serum of carrion eaters, but may not be protective. Dogma states that sufficient toxin to immunize a host is more than enough to kill. Toxoids are immunogenic and have been employed for immunoprophylaxis in some species. Vaccination is usually practiced only in populations at immediate risk. Polyvalent antitoxins can be effective for therapy, depending on the amount of toxin bound to target tissues before treatment is initiated.

Neutralizing preformed toxin, eliminating toxin production, and symptomatic treatment are of paramount importance in treatment of tetanus and botulism. Antitoxin will provide immediate passive protection, but is more effective as a prophylactic than as a therapeutic. In the case of tetanus or wound botulism, surgical attention to the wound and administration of penicillin can be useful in stopping toxin production. Muscle relaxants and sedatives are useful in therapy of tetanus; artificial feeding and respiratory support may be necessary in botulism.

Infections by histotoxic and enteric/enterotoxemic clostridia. The brief clinical course of most histotoxic infections dictates prevention, rather than treatment, as a course of action. Commercial immunoprophylactic products usually consist of inactivated liquid cultures, eliciting antibody responses to bacterial surface antigens, toxic exoproducts, or both. Responses to flagella of *C. chauvoei* are apparently important in prevention of blackleg; anti-idiotypic antibodies imaging *C. chauvoei* flagella immunize mice against challenge. Toxoids containing lethal and hemolytic toxins of *C. sordellii* protect against spore challenge. Antibody responses to somatic and toxin antigens yield lifelong immunity, although differences in immunogenicity by vaccine, agent, and host species have been reported. Death losses in vaccinated feedlot cattle can be reduced by approximately 50%, with a cost: benefit ratio as high as 1:40.

Newborns of several species can be protected against *C. perfringens* enteritis and enterotoxemia by vaccinating the dam with type C or D toxoids 2 to 3 months before parturition and again 3 to 5 weeks later. Annual booster injections given 1 month before parturition will provide protection to subsequent offspring through ingestion of colostrum.

In some cases, equine hyperimmune serum is useful for passive prophylaxis in nonvaccinated animals. This is particularly true for infections by enterotoxemic *C. perfringens* (types C and D), *C. novyi,* and *C. sordellii.* Offspring delivered to nonimmunized dams can be given antitoxin or hyperimmune serum to provide passive immunity. This will last about 3 weeks, after which time the toxoid should be effective in preventing disease.

Losses caused by type D infection in lamb feedlots can be controlled by increasing dietary roughage and decreasing the ration concentrates, although this may not be economically feasible. Control of flukes is important in managing bovine and ovine health, particularly as this pertains to control of infections by *C. novyi*.

Antibiotic therapy is rarely useful. Necrotic enteritis and gangrenous dermatitis in chickens respond to therapy with penicillins, macrolides, and tetracyclines. Tyzzer's disease can be treated with oxytetracycline, but most other antibiotic regimens fail to affect the course of the disease. Latent infection in breeding colonies can sometimes be eliminated by traditional rederivation techniques and disinfection. Treatment of the chronic form of *C. perfringens* type D enterotoxemia in goats may be successful. During a herd or flock outbreak, antitoxins and oral sulfonamides should be administered to all potentially susceptible individuals. Antitoxin will provide passive immunity for up to 3 weeks, and should be administered as quickly as possible after a presumptive diagnosis, to minimize losses. Vaccines should be given, with antimicrobials, to both susceptible animals and dams.

Immunoprophylaxis is not available for some of today's most important clostridial enteritides; toxoids for prevention of infections by *C. difficile* and *C. perfringens* type A are in development. It is possible to prevent *C. perfringens* infections in swine by use of bacitracin methylene disalicylate (BMD), and tylosin may be useful in treating *C. difficile* infection in neonatal pigs. *Clostridium spiroforme* infections are usually treated with metronidazole and penicillin G. *Clostridium colinum* is susceptible to tetracyclines, chloramphenicol, clindamycin, erythromycin, penicillin G, and bacitracin.

SUGGESTED READINGS

Aktories K, Wegner A: Mechanisms of the cytopathic action of actin-ADP-ribosylating toxins, *Mol Microbiol* 6:2905-2908, 1992.

Al-Mashat RR, Taylor DJ: Production of diarrhoea and enteric lesions in calves by the oral inoculation of pure cultures of *Clostridium sordellii*, *Vet Rec* 112:141-146, 1983.

Al-Sheikhly F, Truscott RB: The interaction of *Clostridium perfringens* and its toxins in the production of necrotic enteritis of chickens, *Avian Dis* 21:256-263, 1977.

Amimoto K, Oishi E, Yasuhar H, et al: Protective effects of *Clostridium sordellii* LT and HT toxoids against challenge with spores in guinea pigs, *J Vet Med Sci* 63:879-883, 2001.

Amimoto K, Sasaki O, Isogai M, et al: The protective effect of *Clostridium novyi* type B alpha-toxoid against challenge with spores in guinea pigs, *J Vet Med Sci* 60:681-685, 1998.

Awad MM, Ellemor DM, Boyd RL, et al: Synergistic effects of alpha-toxin and perfringolysin O in *Clostridium perfringens*-mediated gas gangrene, *Infect Immun* 69:7904-7910, 2001.

Ballard J, Sokolov Y, Yuan WL, et al: Activation and mechanism of *Clostridium septicum* alpha toxin, *Mol Microbiol* 10:627-634, 1993.

Berkhoff GA: *Clostridium colinum* sp. nov., nom. rev., the causative agent of ulcerative enteritis (quail disease) in quail, chickens, and pheasants, *Int J Syst Bacteriol* 35:155-159, 1985.

Billington SJ, Wieckowski EU, Sarker MR, et al: *Clostridium perfringens* type E animal enteritis isolates with highly conserved, silent enterotoxin gene sequences, *Infect Immun* 66:4531-4536, 1998.

Borriello SP, Carman RJ: Association of iota-like toxin and *Clostridium spiroforme* with both spontaneous and antibiotic-associated diarrhea and colitis in rabbits, *J Clin Microbiol* 17:414-418, 1983.

Burke MP, Opeskin K: Nontraumatic clostridial myonecrosis, *Am J Forensic Med Pathol* 20:158-162, 1999.

Busch C, Schomig K, Hofmann F, Aktories K: Characterization of the catalytic domain of *Clostridium novyi* alpha-toxin, *Infect Immun* 68: 6378-6383, 2000.

Buxton D, Morgan KT: Studies of lesions produced in the brains of colostrum deprived lambs by *Clostridium welchii* (*C. perfringens*) type D toxin, *J Comp Pathol* 86:435-447, 1976.

Carman RJ, Perelle S, Popoff MR: Binary toxins from *Clostridium spiroforme* and *Clostridium perfringens*. In Rood JI, McClane BA, Songer JG, Titball RW, eds: *The clostridia: molecular biology and pathogenesis,* London, 1997, Academic Press.

Collins JE, Bergeland ME, Bouley D, et al: Diarrhea associated with *Clostridium perfringens* type A enterotoxin in neonatal pigs, *J Vet Diagn Invest* 1:351-353, 1989.

Ellis TM, Rowe JB, Lloyd JM: Acute abomasitis due to *Clostridium septicum* infection in experimental sheep, *Aust Vet J* 60:308-309, 1983.

Estrada-Correa AE, Taylor DJ: Porcine *Clostridium perfringens* type A spores, enterotoxin, and antibody to enterotoxin, *Vet Rec* 124:606-610, 1989.

Gibert M, Jolivet-Reynaud C, Popoff MR, Jolivet-Renaud C: Beta2 toxin, a novel toxin produced by *Clostridium perfringens*, *Gene* 203:65-73, 1997.

Gordon VM, Benz R, Fujii K, et al: *Clostridium septicum* alpha-toxin is proteolytically activated by furin, *Infect Immun* 65:4130-4134, 1997.

Hatheway CL: Toxigenic clostridia, *Clin Microbiol Rev* 3:66-98, 1990.

Hook RR, Riley LK, Franklin CL, Besch-Williford CL: Seroanalysis of Tyzzer's disease in horses: implications that multiple strains can infect Equidae, *Equine Vet J* 27:8-12, 1995.

Johannsen U, Arnold P, Köhler B, Selbitz HJ: Studies into experimental *Clostridium perfringens* type A enterotoxaemia of suckled piglets: experimental provocation of the disease by *Clostridium perfringens* type A intoxication and infection, *Monatsh für Veterinaermed* 48:129-136, 1993.

Meer RR, Songer JG: Multiplex polymerase chain reaction assay for genotyping *Clostridium perfringens*, *Am J Vet Res* 58:702-705, 1997.

Popoff MR, Boquet P: *Clostridium spiroforme* toxin is a binary toxin which ADP-ribosylates cellular actin, *Biochem Biophys Res Commun* 152:1361-1368, 1988.

Rood JI, Cole ST: Molecular genetics and pathogenesis of *Clostridium perfringens*, *Microbiol Rev* 55: 621-648, 1991.

Songer JG: Clostridial enteric diseases of domestic animals, Clin Microbiol Rev 9:216-234, 1996.

Tonello F, Morante S, Rossetto O, et al: Tetanus and botulism neurotoxins: a novel group of zinc-endopeptidases, *Adv Exp Med Biol* 389:251-260, 1996.

Chapter 34

Other Gram-Positive Anaerobes

THE GENUS *ACTINOBACULUM*

Actinobaculum suis is the current stopover on a taxonomic odyssey beginning with the genus *Corynebacterium* and moving to *Eubacterium* and *Actinomyces*. However, 16S rDNA sequence analysis demonstrated that *Corynebacterium-Eubacterium-Actinomyces* strains from cystitis in sows are a different subline within the *Actinomyces-Arcanobacterium* spp. complex and, in light of a 6% sequence divergence, became *Actinobaculum suis*.

Actinobaculum suis is a normal component of the preputial flora in boars and the vaginal flora in sows. The bacterium produces cystitis, nephritis, and metritis in sows. Boars may transmit the bacterium to sows at breeding. Piglets may be infected when they come in contact with the organism during parturition. The organism has been detected on the pen floor of pig barns and is transmitted via urine. Distribution is worldwide. In several large surveys of swine disease, cystitis/pyelonephritis caused by *A. suis* ranked as a major cause of death in the U.S. sow population.

Actinobaculum suis requires alkaline conditions for growth and replication. The healthy vaginal tract of the sow, being slightly acidic, is an unsuitable environment. During estrus, the urine pH rises in response to the rise in estrogen, enhancing the growth of *A. suis* and leading to migration into the upper urinary tract. Inadequate water supply, with resulting crystalluria, is an important predisposing factor. Sows housed in gestation stalls have a higher prevalence of infection because there is more fecal contamination of the perineum and a reduction of daily activity leading to urine stagnation.

The only clinical sign indicating initiation of cystitis is bacteriuria. In mild cases, lesions include epithelial cell hyperplasia, desquamation of superficial epithelial cells, and goblet cell metaplasia with intraepithelial cyst formation. Severe cases are characterized by necrotizing ureteritis and pyelitis (Figure 34-1), with accumulation of bacterial colonies, ascending renal infection, and uremia. Infection is frequently accompanied by hematuria and urinary pH greater than 8. The most

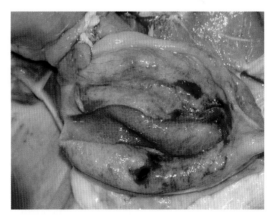

FIGURE 34-1 *Actinobaculum suis* infection in a sow. (Courtesy Peter Moisan.)

severe infections are characterized by purulent ureteritis and pyelitis/pyelonephritis, and are likely to be caused by *A. suis* in concert with other bacteria, especially *Escherichia coli*. Recent studies suggest that a toxin produced by *E. coli* may damage the ureteric valve, allowing retrograde flow of urine into the kidneys, resulting in hydronephrosis.

The known virulence attributes of *A. suis* are adhesion to transitional cells via pili and production of urease. In bladder, urease splits urea into ammonia, which damages bladder defense mechanisms and initiates the formation of urinary calculi.

Diagnosis of infection is based on isolation of the organism from urine. This is aided by using a gram-positive selective medium, such as colistin nalidixic acid agar. Small gray colonies 2 to 3 mm in diameter that have "fried-egg" morphology with shiny centers and dull edges are produced in 48 hours under anaerobic conditions. Cells are pleomorphic, gram-positive, non–spore-forming rods that occur singly or in pairs and often have a beaded appearance. Bacteria are identified using colonial morphology, growth characteristics, Gram-stain morphology, and catalase and urease reactions.

Treatment can usually be effected with injectable penicillin or ampicillin, even in cases involving hemorrhagic inflammation, if infection is restricted to the bladder. Sows with ascending infection and renal insufficiency are unlikely to recover, even with aggressive therapy. Culling chronically infected animals is usually the most cost-effective measure.

Because of the ubiquitous nature of *A. suis*, eradication of the organism from a farm is not possible. Disease may be prevented through proper husbandry. Good sanitation should be maintained. Adequate space in gestation and farrowing crates should be provided. Water consumption should be maximized through the addition of salt to the ration. The use of urinary acidifiers may significantly reduce clinical disease.

THE GENUS *EUBACTERIUM*

Eubacterium tortuosum is a newly described organism associated with hepatic and splenic granulomas in poultry. After 48 hours' incubation on blood agar, colonies are 0.5 to 4 mm in diameter, circular, entire to erose to diffuse, convex to umbonate, translucent, gray to white, and smooth to slightly rough. Colonies may have a "snowflake" morphology. Cells stain as filamentous, gram-positive, non–spore-forming rods. The role of this organism in animal disease awaits confirmation.

THE GENUS *PEPTOSTREPTOCOCCUS*

Peptostreptococcus indolicus is one of a group of organisms that cause "summer mastitis" in cows. The organism is a frequent inhabitant of teat skin, from whence it is readily available for mammary gland infection under appropriate circumstances. The high proportion of clinically healthy carriers suggests that yet-unknown factors participate with *P. indolicus* in development of clinical summer mastitis. Isolation of summer mastitis pathogens corresponds to the seasonal activity of symbovine insects, such as the headfly, *Hydrotaea irritans*.

Colonies of *P. indolicus* are circular, convex to slightly pulvinate, 0.5 to 1 mm in diameter, grayish to yellowish, and glistening, with entire margins. Some strains may be α-hemolytic. Staining reveals gram-positive rods that may occur singly or in pairs, short chains, tetrads, or clusters. The organism produces indole, alkaline phosphatase, and coagulase, and reduces nitrate.

Peptostreptococcus anaerobius is associated with periodontal disease, particularly in cats. Gram stains of clinical material or pure cultures reveal elongated cells (which are almost coccobacillary), often in chains.

THE GENUS *PROPIONIBACTERIUM*

Propionibacterium acnes is a catalase-positive, gram-positive diphtheroid that produces indole and may reduce nitrate. It is uncommonly associated with bovine mastitis, and its significance as a pathogen is uncertain. Some have claimed nonspecific immunostimulation by killed *P. acnes*, as applied to prevention of mastitis during the dry period or at freshening.

THE GENUS *FILIFACTOR*

The gram-variable rod *Filifactor villosus* (formerly *Clostridium villosum*) is normal flora of feline gingivae and is isolated frequently from cat-bite wound abscesses and feline pleural effusions.

SUGGESTED READINGS

Carr J, Walton JR: Bacterial flora of the urinary tract of pigs associated with cystitis and pyelonephritis, *Vet Rec* 132:575-577, 1993.

Lawson PA, Falsen E, Akervall E, et al: Characterization of some *Actinomyces*-like isolates from human clinical specimens: reclassification of *Actinomyces suis* (Soltys and Spratling) as *Actinobaculum suis* comb. nov. and description of *Actinobaculum schaalii* sp. nov., *Int J Syst Bacteriol* 47:899-903, 1997.

Madsen M, Hoi Sorensen G, Aalbaek B, et al: Summer mastitis in heifers: studies on the seasonal occurrence of *Actinomyces pyogenes*, *Peptostreptococcus indolicus* and Bacteroidaceae in clinically healthy cattle in Denmark, *Vet Microbiol* 30:243-255, 1992.

Anaerobic Gram-Negative Rods

Chapter 35

The Genus *Bacteroides*

Gram-negative anaerobic, non–spore-forming bacteria of veterinary importance are in the genera *Bacteroides* (the subject of this chapter) and *Fusobacterium, Prevotella, Porphyromonas,* and *Dichelobacter* (covered in subsequent chapters) (Table 35-1). Many are found in the environment in large numbers, and residence in the intestinal tract is common. The Eh in necrotic and suppurative lesions may approach −240 mV, which favors the growth of strict anaerobes. Concurrent infection with facultative organisms contributes to the lowered Eh, and these mixed infections are common. Given their common occurrence in the intestine and the environment, isolation of these organisms does not necessarily imply involvement in the genesis of an infection.

DISEASE AND EPIDEMIOLOGY

Members of the genus *Bacteroides* represent nearly 50% of isolates of anaerobic bacteria in some veterinary hospital situations. The most common conditions from which these organisms are recovered include soft-tissue abscesses, cellulitis, periodontal abscesses, lung and liver abscesses, peritonitis, pyometritis, osteomyelitis, postoperative wound infections, and mastitis. *Bacteroides* spp. have little host or tissue predilection; bile-resistant, nonpigmented members of *Bacteroides fragilis* are often encountered in the respiratory tract but less so in abscesses (Figure 35-1). *Bacteroides fragilis* has also been isolated from aborted bovine fetuses with bronchopneumonic lesions. Multiple species have been isolated from uteri of dairy cows with retained fetal membranes

TABLE 35-1 *Bacteroides* Species of Veterinary Significance

Bacteroides Species	Associated Disease
B. fragilis	Neonatal diarrhea in foals, calves, piglets, kids, lambs; bovine abortion, mastitis; feline, canine abscesses
B. ovatus, B. thetaiotaomicron, B. vulgatus	Osteomyelitis, soft tissue infections
B. asaccharolyticus	Osteomyelitis in dogs, cats, horses, cattle
B. levii	Mastitis in cows

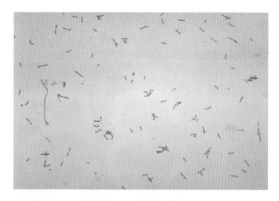

FIGURE 35-1 *Bacteroides fragilis* grown in Schaedler's broth (Gram stain). (Courtesy Public Health Image Library, PHIL #2996, Centers for Disease Control and Prevention, Atlanta, 1974, Don Stalons.)

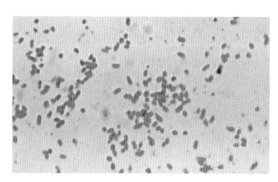

FIGURE 35-3 *Bacteroides ovatus* (thioglycollate broth, 48-hour incubation). (Courtesy Public Health Image Library, PHIL #2962, Centers for Disease Control and Prevention, Atlanta, 1972, V.R. Dowell.)

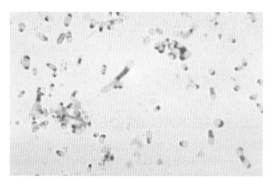

FIGURE 35-2 *Bacteroides thetaiotaomicron,* with morphology reminiscent of Greek letters (thioglycollate broth, 48-hour incubation). (Courtesy Public Health Image Library, PHIL #2956, Centers for Disease Control and Prevention, Atlanta, 1972, V.R. Dowell.)

and postparturient endometritis. *Bacteroides asaccharolyticus* has been isolated from lesions of osteomyelitis in small animals and horses, and *Bacteroides levii* is associated with bovine mastitis. Cats with empyema have been a source of *Bacteroides salivosus* (see Table 35-1). *Bacteroides thetaiotaomicron* is a member of the normal flora, but occasionally causes infections in immuno-compromised patients (Figure 35-2); *Bacteroides ovatus* and *Bacteroides vulgatus* cause osteomyelitis and soft tissue infections (Figure 35-3).

Some strains of *B. fragilis* are associated with watery nonhemorrhagic diarrhea in livestock and young children. Piglets become anorexic and dehydrated, and lesions include swelling and vacuo-lation of enterocytes, with eventual exfoliation. Attachment to and invasion of enterocytes have

not been demonstrated. Crypt hyperplasia is extensive in the colon and less so in the ileum. Experimental inoculation of rabbits with strains from pigs or humans produces watery diarrhea and dehydration, with lesions similar to those in piglets. Clinical signs and microscopic lesions suggest a mechanism based on net secretion of fluid into the small intestine and decreased absorption by the large intestine.

PATHOGENESIS

Culture supernatants of *B. fragilis* strains from diarrheic humans and other animals induce fluid secretion in ligated ileal loops in various species, and lesions in orally inoculated rabbits are similar to those in animals inoculated with pure cultures. Similar changes occur in rat, rabbit, and lamb intestinal loops exposed to purified toxin. The enterotoxic effect is apparently based on at least two zinc-dependent metalloproteases, now desig-nated BFT-1 and BFT-2, that cause cell rounding, loss of cell-to-cell contacts, and decreased transepithelial resistance. Monomeric actin is hydrolyzed, and a region of these molecules is suggestive of a membrane insertion domain. It seems likely that the toxin genes are contained in pathogenicity islands or islets, acquired by hori-zontal transfer.

DIAGNOSIS

Specimen collection and transport is a key element in diagnosis of infections by non–spore-forming anaerobes. It is important to collect proper specimens (Table 35-2) as well as transport them

TABLE 35-2 Specimens for Anaerobic Culture

Site	Specimen
Head/neck	Abscess aspirate; surgical biopsy; anaerobic swab
Lungs	Transtracheal aspirates, washes; percutaneous lung, pleural aspirates; anaerobic swabs; intact abscesses obtained at necropsy
Central nervous system	Abscess aspirate; intact brain abscesses obtained at necropsy; anaerobic swabs
Abdomen	Aspirated peritoneal fluid; abscess aspirates; anaerobic swabs; intact liver, intraabdominal abscesses obtained at necropsy
Urinary tract	Urine collected by cystocentesis; ligated bladders, intact kidneys obtained at necropsy
Female genital tract	Endometrial discharge in anaerobic transport medium; biopsies; intact uterus with ligations obtained at necropsy
Musculoskeletal system	Aspirates in anaerobic transport medium; biopsies; anaerobic swabs; joint fluid in blood culture medium (unvented); affected muscle collected at necropsy
Soft tissue	Aspirates; surgical biopsies; deep sinus tract aspirates; necrotic portions of interdigital spaces
Gastrointestinal tract	Ligated loops of small or large intestine; stools

in an appropriate commercial transport system or in laboratory-prepared Cary-Blair transport medium. An anaerobic environment is usually maintained in tissue specimens (≥ 1 in³) transported in an airtight jar. Residual air should be expelled from syringes containing aspirates, and it is often useful to seal the needle by inserting it into a rubber stopper. Specimens should be maintained at ambient temperature (rather than refrigerating or freezing) and processing should be completed within a few hours. Grossly purulent specimens should be vortexed to ensure uniform distribution of bacteria; large volumes of nonpurulent material should be centrifuged and the pellet used to inoculate media and prepare Gram stain. Bone specimens should be ground in a sterile mortar and pestle. Swabs should be plated onto solid media and then wrung out into enriched thioglycollate medium.

It is also important to examine Gram-stained direct smears of specimens. Some of these organisms will be morphologically distinctive and a suggestion of identity may be established by microscopic examination. Large gram-positive "boxcar-shaped" rods, usually without spores, suggest the presence of *Clostridium perfringens* (see Chapter 33). Gram-negative coccobacilli are often *Prevotella* spp. or *Porphyromonas* spp. (see Chapter 38). Gram-negative, slightly curved rods of above-average size, obtained from cases of ovine footrot, suggest *Dichelobacter nodosus* (see Chapter 36). Gram-negative rods that are long, filamentous, and have tapered ends, especially

from certain clinical conditions (bovine liver abscesses or footrot) may be *Fusobacterium necrophorum* (see Chapter 37). However, it is also important to compare the population seen microscopically with that isolated by bacteriologic culture. This will provide an indication of which organisms, if any, have failed to grow on culture media.

Myriad solid and liquid media are used to cultivate anaerobes, and methods of incubation are nearly as numerous. Perhaps the most common today is the anaerobe jar, in which anaerobiosis is achieved by interaction of residual oxygen with hydrogen (supplied directly as a gas or generated by a chemical reaction in a commercial generator envelope), in the presence of palladium catalyst, to produce water. Roll-tubes, in which a thin layer of agar is placed on the inner surface of a stoppered tube, are used to a small degree, and more laboratories are acquiring and using anaerobe chambers.

Differentiation among isolates is based initially on cellular and colonial morphology (Table 35-3), pigment production, fluorescence under long-wave ultraviolet light, and response to special-potency antibiotic disks (Table 35-4). It is, of course, important to confirm that isolates are indeed anaerobic (rather than facultative). Motility, ability to produce indole, lipase, nitrate reductase, and urease, resistance to bile, and fermentation of carbohydrates are important assays (Table 35-5; see p. 291). Definitive identification may require the use of microbiochemical test systems.

TABLE 35-3 Colonial and Cellular Morphology of *Bacteroides* Species

Bacteroides Species	Colonial Morphology
B. asaccharolyticus	Cells short, spherical to rodlike; colonies 0.5-1 mm diameter, round, convex, opaque, light gray, becoming black with age
B. fragilis	Cells singly or in pairs, rounded ends; colonies 1-3 mm diameter, circular, entire, low, convex, translucent to semiopaque; rare β-hemolysis
B. levii	Cells in pairs, short chains; colonies minute, circular, entire, low, convex, buff to light brown, becoming dark brown with age
B. ovatus	Cells generally oval, singly or occasional pairs; colonies 0.5-1 mm diameter, circular, entire, convex, pale buff, semiopaque, mottled
B. uniformis	Cells single, pairs, occasional filaments and vacuoles; colonies 0.5-2 mm diameter, circular, entire, low convex, gray to white, translucent to slightly opaque
B. thetaiotaomicron	Cells pleomorphic, single, pairs; colonies punctiform, circular, entire, convex, semiopaque, whitish, soft, shiny
B. vulgatus	Cells single, short chains, pleomorphic with swellings or vacuoles

TABLE 35-4 Response of Gram-Negative Anaerobes to Antimicrobial Potency Disks

	Kanamycin 1000 μg	Vancomycin 5 μg	Colistin 10 μg
B. fragilis group	R	R	R
B. ureolyticus group	S	R	S
Fusobacterium spp.	S	R	S
Porphyromonas spp.	R	S	R
Prevotella spp.	R	R	V

R, Resistant; *S*, susceptible; *V*, variable.

PREVENTION AND CONTROL

Most *Bacteroides* spp. are susceptible to clindamycin and metronidazole, but susceptibility to ciprofloxacin is variable and bimodal. Minimal inhibitory concentrations (MICs) suggest tetracycline resistance.

SUGGESTED READINGS

Berg JN, Fales WH, Scanlan CM: Occurrence of anaerobic bacteria in diseases of the dog and cat, *Am J Vet Res* 40:876-881, 1979.

Collins JE, Bergeland ME, Myers LL, Shoop DS: Exfoliating colitis associated with enterotoxigenic *Bacteroides fragilis* in a piglet, *J Vet Diagn Invest* 1:349-351, 1989.

Jang SS, Hirsh DC: Identity of *Bacteroides* isolates and previously named *Bacteroides* spp. in clinical specimens of animal origin, *Am J Vet Res* 52:738-741, 1991.

Kraipowich NR, Morris DL, Thompson GL, Mason GL: Bovine abortions associated with *Bacteroides fragilis* fetal infections, *J Vet Diagn Invest* 12:369-371, 2000.

TABLE 35-5 Biochemical Characteristics of Some Members of the Genus *Bacteroides*

Bacteroides Species	Bile Sensitivity	Esculin Hydrolysis	Indole Production	Black Pigment	Fermentation of: Arabinose	Glucose	Lactose	Maltose	Rhamnose	Salicin	Sucrose	Trehalose
B. fragilis	Pos	Pos	Neg	Neg	Neg	Pos	Pos	Pos	Neg	Neg	Pos	Neg
B. asaccharolyticus	Neg	Neg	Pos	Pos	Neg	Neg	Neg	Neg	Neg	Neg	Neg	Neg
B. levii	Neg	Neg	Neg	Pos	Neg	Pos	Pos	Neg	Neg	Neg	Neg	Neg
B. distasonis	Pos	Pos	Neg	Neg	Neg	Pos	Pos	Pos	(Pos)	Pos	Pos	Pos
B. ovatus	Pos	Pos	Pos	Neg	Pos	Pos	Pos	Weak pos	Pos	Pos	Pos	Neg
B. uniformis	Weak pos	Pos	Pos	Neg	Weak pos	Pos	Pos	Weak pos	(Neg)	Pos	Weak pos	Neg
B. vulgatus	Pos	Pos	Neg	Neg	Pos	Pos	Pos	Pos	Pos	Neg	Pos	Neg
B. thetaiotaomicron	Pos	Pos	Pos	Neg	Pos	Pos	Pos	Pos	Pos	(Neg)	Pos	Neg

Neg, Negative; *(Neg),* most negative; *Pos,* positive; *(Pos),* most positive.

Chapter 36

The Genus *Dichelobacter*

The genus *Dichelobacter* was created to accommodate the former *Bacteroides nodosus,* the cause of ovine footrot. The genus name derives from the two-clawed hooves of its primary hosts. *Dichelobacter nodosus* is the single species of veterinary importance. The organism is also of intrinsic importance in microbial physiology and evolution as a slowly growing anaerobic, gram-negative bacterium. It has been placed in the family Cardiobacteriaceae, with the genera *Cardiobacterium* and *Suttonella* (which contain opportunistic human pathogens), and has no close phylogenetic relatives among the anaerobes.

DISEASE AND EPIDEMIOLOGY

Dichelobacter nodosus causes footrot in sheep and is occasionally recovered from interdigital infections in cattle, pigs, and goats. The disease in sheep is a mixed infection, but the essential causative agent is *D. nodosus.* It is probably noteworthy that footrot, especially in cattle, is rarely an etiologic diagnosis, so dogma is not necessarily congruent with current fact.

Footrot is characterized by rapid onset of severe lameness, manifesting initially as interdigital dermatitis. Affected animals often become recumbent (Figure 36-1), are unable to feed efficiently, and will lose weight and productivity; decreased milking by ewes, reduced fertility, and discontinuity in wool fibers also occur. Affected rams often fail to serve their intended purpose.

Disease is most common in sheep with poorly maintained hooves. Cracking of overgrown and underrun hooves allows invasion by *D. nodosus.* Warm, wet conditions encourage bacterial growth, contributing to both severity of individual cases and spread within the flock. High stocking densities increase incidence. Infected animals are important sources of continued infection in a flock.

Footrot is likely the most economically significant bacterial disease of sheep in most wool- and lamb-producing countries. Surveys suggest that the prevalence of footrot is nearly 30%, ranking it among the top five ovine infectious diseases. Costs are difficult to estimate, but effects on meat and wool quality, as well as the labor-intensive

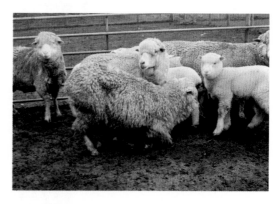

FIGURE 36-1 Sheep affected with footrot, unable to stand. (Courtesy Julian I. Rood.)

nature of treatment regimes, suggest that economic losses are substantial.

PATHOGENESIS

A well-defined experimental model is in place for ovine footrot. Sheep inoculated with *D. nodosus* grown on solid medium develop severe footrot within 28 days. Assessment of the extent of disease is based on severity of inflammation and degree of invasiveness.

Unraveling of the mechanisms of pathogenesis has been hampered by lack of genetic methods for manipulation of *D. nodosus,* but type IV fimbriae, extracellular proteases, and a 27 kb pathogenicity island (the *vrl* locus) are putative contributors. Polar type IV fimbriae confer twitching motility and are composed of monomeric pilin subunits encoded by *fimA,* which is essential for virulence in sheep (Figure 36-2). *fimA* mutants do not exhibit twitching motility, no longer secrete proteases, and are completely avirulent.

Virulent strains produce two acidic extracellular serine proteases, encoded by *aprV2* and *aprV5,* and a basic protease, encoded by *bprV.* Closely related protease genes are found in benign isolates. Differences in biochemical properties, thermostability, and elastase activity of these proteases provide a basis for differentiating virulent and benign strains of *D. nodosus.* These differences also suggest a role for proteases in the disease process, but this role has not been elucidated.

Chromosomal loci designated *vap* and *vrl,* which were among the first pathogenicity island-like loci to be identified in pathogenic bacteria, have been associated with virulence. The *vap* region is found in most virulent strains, but *vrl* is perhaps a more likely indicator of virulence. Results of genetic analysis suggest that the *vap* region arrived via an integrase-mediated plasmid insertion. The *vap* locus appears to be involved in regulation of protease production.

Similarly, the *vrl* locus may have become a part of the *D. nodosus* genome by horizontal transfer, with site-specific integrase-mediated insertion into a small rRNA gene. The region contains at least 19 genes that appear to comprise an operon. Banked, virulence-associated sequences from other bacteria are not related to those in *vrl,* and thus the functional role of this locus remains unknown.

DIAGNOSIS

Diagnosis is often based on clinical signs and gross lesions. Initially the area between the toes becomes moist and reddened, with ensuing invasion of the hoof sole and undermining and separation of horny tissues. The organism may infect one or more feet at the same time. Lesions have a characteristic foul-smelling exudate.

Not all lame sheep have footrot. Footscald (ovine interdigital dermatitis) affects the skin between the claws or toes and is caused by *Fusobacterium necrophorum,* sometimes in company with *Arcanobacterium pyogenes.* Skin is reddened without accompanying odor, and although the hoof is not involved, this condition can progress to footrot. Infection of deep structures of the hoof by *A. pyogenes* results in foot abscesses that are accompanied by a white to black purulent discharge with the odor of footrot. Laminitis, traumatic injuries, and foreign bodies lodged between the toes may also be misdiagnosed as footrot.

Infection can be readily confirmed by bacteriologic culture and identification and typing of isolates. *Dichelobacter nodosus* cells are fairly large, pleomorphic, slightly curved, and occur singly or in pairs. They may be distended at one or both ends. Colonies are grayish white and 0.5 to 3 mm in diameter. Colonial morphology ranges from papillate or beaded (B type, from typical ovine footrot) to mucoid (M type, less virulent, from noninvasive disease) to circular (avirulent, often due to repeated in vitro passage). The organism is near inert in traditional biochemical tests, failing to hydrolyze esculin, produce indole, or

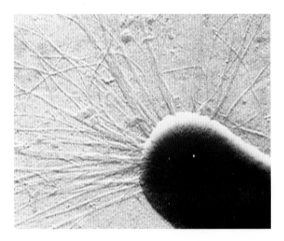

FIGURE 36-2   Fimbriae of *Dichelobacter nodosus.* (Courtesy J. Glenn Songer.)

ferment carbohydrates. It can be separated from other agar-pitting gram-negative anaerobic bacilli (*Bacteroides ureolyticus* and *Bacteroides gracilis*) by its failure to produce urease and its hydrolysis of gelatin. Agglutination reactions based on pilus antigen provide the basis for classification of *D. nodosus* into serogroups A through I.

PREVENTION AND CONTROL

Prevention is preferable to treatment or control. This begins by refraining from buying sheep with footrot or from a footrot-affected flock or from livestock markets where clean and infected sheep commingle. Sheep should not be allowed access for at least 2 weeks to trails, corrals, and dipping areas used by infected sheep. Animals should always be transported in vehicles that have been properly cleaned and disinfected. The feet of all new arrivals should be trimmed and treated, and then reexamined periodically during quarantine.

Routine trimming of feet (at least twice annually) reduces bacterial accumulation in cracks and crevices, removes infected hoof, and facilitates killing of the organism by air and various medications. Trimming without further treatment may *increase* disease severity during an outbreak. Trimming instruments should be disinfected between animals.

Zinc sulfate and copper sulfate should be used in footbaths or foot soaks. Detergent can be added to increase penetration into hoof cracks. Drying agents may be used around feed or water troughs to reduce moisture and decrease disease spread. Zinc sulfate (0.5 g per animal per day for 21 days) may be useful in treatment and prevention, especially in zinc-deficient animals.

Penicillin and streptomycin in combination are effective in treating footrot, as are procaine penicillin G or long-acting penicillin products. Long-acting tetracyclines also have been used. Oxytetracycline or penicillin in alcohol has been used topically.

Vaccination with whole cells or purified fimbriae provide serogroup-specific protection against footrot. Vaccination is preventive but also effects cures, and should be applied before the start of the wet season. Antigenic competition and pilus antigenic variation limit the effectiveness of vaccines; efficacy ranges from zero to 100%, with an average of 60% to 80%.

Resistance to footrot may be genetic, and it is often recommended not to keep ewe lambs from ewes that have had multiple cases of disease.

SUGGESTED READINGS

Billington SJ, Johnston JL, Rood JI: Virulence regions and virulence factors of the ovine footrot pathogen, *Dichelobacter nodosus, FEMS Microbiol Lett* 145: 147-156, 1996.

Egerton JR, Ghimire SC, Dhungyel OP, et al: Eradication of virulent footrot from sheep and goats in an endemic area of Nepal and an evaluation of specific vaccination, *Vet Rec* 151:290-295, 2002.

Jelinek PD, Depiazzi LJ, Galvin DA, et al: Eradication of ovine footrot by repeated daily footbathing in a solution of zinc sulphate with surfactant, *Aust Vet J* 79:431-434, 2001.

Kennan RM, Dhungyel OP, Whittington RJ, et al: Transformation-mediated serogroup conversion of *Dichelobacter nodosus, Vet Microbiol* 92:169-178, 2003.

Lewis CJ: Contagious ovine digital dermatitis, *Vet Rec* 152:667, 2003.

Rood JI: Genomic islands of Dichelobacter nodosus, Curr Top Microbiol Immunol 264:47-60, 2002.

Chapter 37

The Genus *Fusobacterium*

The genus *Fusobacterium* is in the class Fusobacteria, order Fusobacteriales, and family Fusobacteriaceae. The 13 current species are non–spore-forming, anaerobic, gram-negative fusiform or pointed rods, and the genus name derives from this morphotype (Figure 37-1). The major metabolic end product is butyric acid and most species have a characteristic rancid butter odor in culture.

DISEASE AND EPIDEMIOLOGY

Members of the genus *Fusobacterium* are normal inhabitants of the oral cavity and gastrointestinal

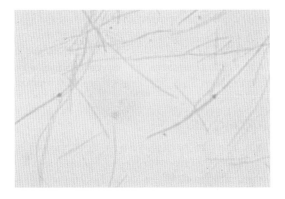

FIGURE 37-1 Gram-stained smear of *Fusobacterium nucleatum* ssp. *fusiforme,* showing the typical fusiform morphology from which the genus derives its name. (Courtesy Public Health Image Library, PHIL #3044, Centers for Disease Control and Prevention, Atlanta, date unknown, V.R. Dowell.)

tract of animals and humans, and the source of infection is usually endogenous. Virulent species include *Fusobacterium necrophorum* (ssp. *necrophorum* and ssp. *fundiliforme*), *Fusobacterium equinum,* and *Fusobacterium nucleatum* (ssp. *nucleatum,* ssp. *polymorphum,* ssp. *vincentii,* ssp. *fusiforme,* and ssp. *animalis,* and newly proposed subspecies *canifelium*).

Subspecies of *F. necrophorum* are the fusiform organisms most frequently isolated from veterinary specimens, where they cause a variety of necrotic infections (Table 37-1). These organisms are normal inhabitants of the intestinal tract, and are frequently encountered on other mucous membranes. The source of infection is usually endogenous. Enteric infections are not uncommon in swine, especially in conjunction with infection by *Brachyspira hyodysenteriae.* Hoof infection in horses is frequently called "thrush." Necrotic stomatitis occurs in cattle, as do metritis and mastitis. Calf diphtheria (Figures 37-2 and 37-3) is a common presentation of *F. necrophorum* infection of the bovine mouth, larynx, and trachea, and necrotic laryngitis also occurs in feedlot cattle. It is a secondary invader in various primary ulcerative conditions in sheep, and is commonly associated with *Arcanobacterium pyogenes* in interdigital dermatitis and reproductive tract problems. The organism also complicates infections by fowl poxvirus.

Other organisms of clinical significance are *F. equinum,* which has been isolated from tracheal

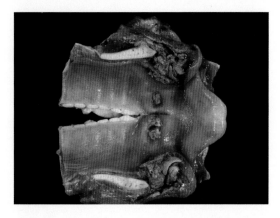

FIGURE 37-2 Gross lesions of *Fusobacterium necrophorum* infection (diphtheria) in a calf. (Courtesy Edward G. Clarke.)

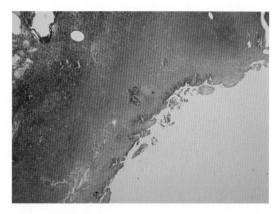

FIGURE 37-3 Diphtheritic tonsillitis, a hallmark lesion of *Fusobacterium necrophorum* infection (calf diphtheria). (Courtesy Stephen Rushton.)

TABLE 37-1 Fusobacteria of Veterinary Significance

Fusobacterium Species	Associated Diseases
F. necrophorum	Bovine footrot, mastitis, metritis, liver abscesses; calf diphtheria; ovine interdigital dermatitis; "bullnose" in swine; equine thrush; avian diphtheria; necrobacillosis in rabbits; lamb septicemia; ovine, bovine abortion
F. equinum	Tracheal washes and pleural effusions of horses with lower respiratory tract disease, including necrotizing pneumonia and pleurisy
F. nucleatum	Sporadic ovine and bovine abortion; soft tissue infections of companion animals
F. russii and *varium*	Soft tissue infections in companion animals

washes and pleural effusions of horses with lower respiratory tract disease, including necrotizing pneumonia and pleurisy. Horses that have been recently transported are at increased risk. The name *F. nucleatum* ssp. *canifelinum* has been proposed for organisms recovered from pleuritis in dogs and cats and from cat- and dog-bite wounds in animals and humans.

The single most important disease associated with *F. necrophorum* infection may be bovine liver abscesses (Figure 37-4). Organisms of biotype A (*F. necrophorum* ssp. *necrophorum*) are of greatest virulence, and are most often found in bovine liver abscesses, in pure culture. Biotype B (ssp. *funduliforme*) is isolated from the rumen (including rumenal wall lesions). When *F. necrophorum* ssp. *funduliforme* is found in liver abscesses, it is usually in mixed culture. The uncommonly isolated biotype AB is of intermediate virulence, and biotype C strains are avirulent.

Aggressive grain-feeding programs produce abscesses in livers of as many as one third of animals slaughtered from some feedlots. Reduced feed intake, reduced weight gain, decreased feed efficiency, and decreased carcass yield, as well as liver condemnation at slaughter, are sources of economic loss to producers. *Fusobacterium necrophorum* is the primary cause, but is frequently in combination with *A. pyogenes*. Animals rarely show signs in association with liver abscessation.

Fusobacterium necrophorum is a not uncommon cause of hepatic abscessation in humans, as well. Other members of the genus, including *F. nucleatum*, may also cause disease in animals (see Table 37-1).

PATHOGENESIS

Fusobacterium necrophorum is an opportunist, multiplying and producing lesions from a point of initiation in damaged tissue. Infections are frequently mixed and invariably necrotic. A potent leukotoxin is involved directly (through local tissue damage) and indirectly (through effects on immune cells) in lesion production, and immunization against this molecule provides a measure of protection against *F. necrophorum*–induced

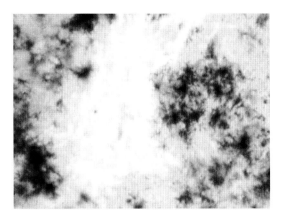

FIGURE 37-4 Large numbers of fusiform organisms in a direct smear from a bovine liver abscess. (Courtesy Raymond E. Reed.)

liver abscesses. Encapsulation is also apparently involved in virulence, in that strains with capsules are more virulent for mice than nonencapsulated strains. Other extracellular products include hemagglutinin, adhesins, proteases, and DNase, but these have no more than a speculative role in pathogenesis.

Mechanisms have not been completely elucidated in all cases, but products of *F. necrophorum* likely play important roles in establishment of liver abscesses. Proteases, dermonecrotic factor(s), and leukotoxin are all likely to be involved. The steps by which liver abscesses are generated are reasonably clear. High-energy feedlot rations push evolutionarily established rumen function to its very boundaries, and a common result is ruminal acidosis. Sudden changes to high-energy diets, dietary indiscretions, changes in feeding schedules that allow cattle to become excessively hungry, and feeding very little roughage contribute to this condition. Ruminal damage as a result of acidosis is a predisposing factor for hepatic abscessation; this damage is intensified by foreign objects, sharp particles, or hair in feed.

One consequence of rumen wall damage is establishment of infectious foci in rumen wall, and *F. necrophorum* is the principal contributor. From these primary lesions, *F. necrophorum* gains access to portal circulation and the liver is showered with septic thrombi, leading to infection and abscess formation (see Figure 37-4). The extensive vascularization of the liver (and therefore its high Eh) and its nonspecific immune defenses (in the form of Kupffer and other phagocytic cells) make

this an inhospitable environment for *F. necrophorum* and other organisms. Leukotoxin may offer protection from phagocytosis, as may soluble antiphagocytic substances from other organisms in the often-mixed populations in abscesses. Lysosomal enzymes and oxygen metabolites from disrupted phagocytes may damage liver parenchyma, resulting in circulation deficits in microenvironments in which *F. necrophorum* can multiply. Facultative organisms growing in company with *F. necrophorum* may, in using oxygen, provide the same sort of reduced Eh microenvironment. Intravascular coagulation induced by lipopolysaccharide (LPS) and platelet aggregation factors may also contribute to local ischemia.

DIAGNOSIS

Specimen collection, handling, transport, and processing are crucial (see Chapter 35). Direct examination of specimens by Gram staining reveals long gram-negative fusiform rods with a characteristic beading (Figure 37-5). Isolation methods are much the same as those suggested for *Bacteroides* spp. Colonies are usually quite small, smooth, and yellowish white, and may be α- or β-hemolytic (Table 37-2). Fusobacteria may be rapidly differentiated from other anaerobic gram-negative rods by a few simple tests. They are resistant to vancomycin (5 μg potency disk), susceptible to kanamycin (1000 μg potency disk), and colistin (10 μg potency disk), produce chartreuse fluorescence under long-wave ultraviolet illumination, and fail to produce catalase or

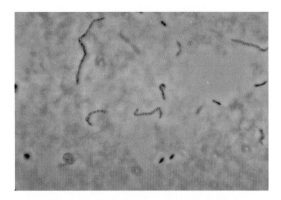

FIGURE 37-5 Phase-contrast photomicrograph of *Fusobacterium necrophorum,* showing the typical beaded-rod appearance. (Courtesy Public Health Image Library, PHIL #3109, Centers for Disease Control and Prevention, Atlanta, 1965, L.V. Holdeman.)

TABLE 37-2 Colonial Morphology of *Fusobacterium* Species

Species	Colonial and Cellular Morphology
F. necrophorum	Colonies 1-2 mm diameter, circular, convex to umbonate, often with bumpy, ridged to uneven surfaces ("breadcrumb-like"), translucent to opaque, opalescent, with scalloped to erose edges; some with α- or β-hemolysis Cells long, filamentous, tapered to rounded ends
F. nucleatum	Colonies 1-2 mm diameter, circular to slightly irregular, convex to pulvinate, translucent, flecked Cells tapered to pointed ends, sometimes with tapered swellings
F. equinum	Colonies 1-2 mm diameter, circular, convex to umbonate, cream colored with entire or undulate margins Cells pleomorphic to coccobacillary with rounded ends, some curved, stain irregularly
F. russii	Colonies 0.5-1 mm diameter, circular, smooth, shiny, entire, convex, translucent Cells thin filaments in palisades
F. varium	Colonies punctiform to 1 mm diameter, flat-to-low convex, translucent, gray or white centers, colorless edges Cells pleomorphic, coccoid, rod shaped, unevenly staining

TABLE 37-3 Biochemical Characteristics of Animal Pathogenic Fusobacteria

Fusobacterium Species	Indole Production	Bile Susceptibility	Esculin Hydrolysis	Lipase Production	Glucose Fermentation
F. necrophorum	Pos	(Pos)	Neg	(Pos)	(Neg)
F. nucleatum	Pos	Pos	Neg	Neg	(Neg)
F. equinum	Pos	Neg	Neg	Pos	Neg
F. russii	Neg	(Pos)	Neg	Neg	Neg
F. varium	(Pos)	Neg	Neg	Neg	Pos

Neg, Negative; *(Neg),* most negative; *Pos,* positive; *(Pos),* most positive.

reduce nitrate. Differentiation of species within the genus can be based on biochemical characteristics (Table 37-3).

Liver abscesses are detected only at the time of slaughter, because cattle, even those that carry hundreds of small abscesses or several large abscesses, seldom exhibit clinical signs. Occasionally, cattle may exhibit abdominal pain, or the rupture of a superficial abscess or erosion and perforation of the caudal vena cava could lead to extensive spread and massive infection of other organs and death.

PREVENTION AND CONTROL

Fusobacterium spp. are usually susceptible to erythromycin, tetracyclines, penicillins, and sulfonamides. Tylosin is commonly used in bovine feedlot rations to prevent liver abscesses. Surgical intervention may be required in certain circumstances.

A bacterin-toxoid is available for prevention of bovine footrot, and experimental evidence suggests that antileukotoxin immunity is critical in preventing *F. necrophorum* infection of bovine livers.

SUGGESTED READINGS

Citron D: Update on the taxonomy and clinical aspects of the genus *Fusobacterium, Clin Infect Dis* 35(Suppl 1):s22-s27, 2002.

Dorsch M, Love DN, Bailey GD: *Fusobacterium equinum* sp. nov., from the oral cavity of horses, *Int J Syst Evol Microbiol* 51:1959-1963, 2001.

Nagaraja TG, Sun Y, Wallace N, et al: Effects of tylosin on concentrations of *Fusobacterium necrophorum* and fermentation products in the rumen of cattle fed a high-concentrate diet, *Am J Vet Res* 60:1061-1065, 1999.

Nagaraja TG, Beharka AB, Chengappa MM, et al: Bacterial flora of liver abscesses in feedlot cattle fed tylosin or no tylosin, *J Anim Sci* 77:973-978, 1999.

Nagaraja TG, Chengappa MM: Liver abscesses in feedlot cattle: a review, *J Anim Sci* 76:287-298, 1998.

Saginala S, Nagaraja TG, Lechtenberg KF, et al: Effect of *Fusobacterium necrophorum* leukotoxoid vaccine on susceptibility to experimentally induced liver abscesses in cattle, *J Anim Sci* 75:1160-1166, 1997.

Chapter 38

The Genera *Prevotella* and *Porphyromonas*

*P*revotella spp. and *Porphyromonas* spp. are obligately anaerobic, non–spore-forming, nonmotile, pleomorphic rods. Both genera have taxonomic placement in the class Bacteroides, order Bacteroidales; however, *Prevotella* spp. are members of the family Prevotellaceae, whereas *Porphyromonas* spp. are classified in Porphyromonadaceae. The species in these genera were formerly included in the genus *Bacteroides*.

Prevotella spp. are pigmented or nonpigmented asaccharolytic bacteria. Their growth is inhibited by 20% bile, nitrate is not reduced to nitrite, and most are indole negative. More than 20 species inhabit the oral and gastrointestinal cavities of man and other animals. *Prevotella* spp. comprise one of the largest groups recovered from the rumen and hindgut. They may play an important role in the utilization of plant-origin polysaccharides and in metabolism of proteins and peptides.

Porphyromonads may be pigmented or non-pigmented and are asaccharolytic to weakly saccharolytic. Indole is produced and nitrate is not reduced to nitrite. Generic taxonomy is evolving rapidly, with 13 currently recognized species. *Porphyromonas* spp. are found primarily in the oral cavity of man and animals.

DISEASE AND EPIDEMIOLOGY

Prevotella melaninogenica (Bacteroides melaninogenicus), so named because of its colonial pigment, is isolated (in pure or mixed culture) from suppurative lesions in a variety of animals. It is frequently associated with *Fusobacterium necrophorum* and *Arcanobacterium pyogenes* in bovine footrot. *Prevotella melaninogenica* is a common isolate from various lesions in dogs and cats, and is often involved in life-threatening infections. *Prevotella intermedia* and *Prevotella nigrescens* cause abscesses, naturally and experimentally, often (in the former case) in company with facultative anaerobes or aerobes.

The normal oral residence of many *Prevotella* spp. is reflected in their common isolation from dog- and cat-bite wounds, perhaps explaining in part their frequent recovery from various soft tissue infections in cats and dogs. *Prevotella heparinolytica* is common and *Prevotella zoogleoformans* and *Prevotella oralis* are occasional in such lesions.

Prevotella melaninogenica is not uncommon as a cause of acute tonsillitis in children, and subcutaneous inoculation of mice with strains recovered from these lesions produces abscesses, whereas this is seldom the case with isolates from the normal respiratory mucosa. Sputum IgA titers against *Prevotella intermedia* are significantly elevated in humans with acute exacerbation of chronic bronchitis.

Prevotella spp. are also found in lower respiratory tract disease in horses, again frequently in company with facultative anaerobes. Significant numbers of anaerobic bacteria are isolated only after the fifth day of illness. Pleural fluid from these animals is usually culture negative, but transtracheal aspirates and lung tissues collected at necropsy frequently yield *Prevotella heparinolytica* and pigmented *Prevotella* spp. as well as *Porphyromonas* spp. Isolation of pulmonary anaerobes from horses augurs against recovery.

Porphyromonas gingivalis causes marked lung inflammation in humans, and this condition can progress to severe bronchopneumonia with lung abscesses. This organism originates in the oral cavity, and is a significant cause of human aspiration pneumonia and lung abscess. The mortality rate is 25% in mice inoculated intratracheally with *P. gingivalis*. Surviving animals evidence a marked recruitment of neutrophils, with substantial reduction in bacterial populations within 48 hours. Despite this, mice develop acute necrotizing bronchopneumonia, often with abscessation. Increased lactate dehydrogenase (LDH) in pulmonary lavage fluids suggests severe parenchymal damage, and extensive influx of serum albumin is compatible with injury to alveolar capillary membranes.

On the whole, *Prevotella* spp. are less invasive than *Fusobacterium* spp., and are seldom found other than transiently in the bloodstream. *Prevotella* spp. and *Porphyromonas* spp. are among the most common microorganisms isolated from human tubo-ovarian abscesses, and pigmented members of these genera are predominant among anaerobes causing infection and inflammation of the parotid salivary gland.

Porphyromonas levii is a common cause of summer mastitis in cattle, ranking third behind *F. necrophorum* and *Peptostreptococcus indolicus* among the anaerobes. Isolates of *P. levii* are common on conjunctivae and teat tips among clinically healthy animals, suggesting that contributing factors are required for development of clinical disease. Incidence is significantly higher during the pasture period, and the distinctly seasonal distribution coincides with seasonal activity of symbovine insects, such as headflies (*Hydrotaea irritans*). *Porphyromonas levii* is also isolated in conjunction with *Actinomyces* spp. from pleural effusions in dogs and in conjunction with fusobacteria from bovine and ovine footrot.

Porphyromonas gingivalis, as well as *P. intermedia*, are involved in the onset of periodontal disease in humans and domestic animals. *Porphyromonas gingivalis* is common in active periodontitis sites, and patients with periodontitis have higher antibody titers against it. *Prevotella intermedia* is frequently isolated from subgingival sites in periodontitis and various forms of gingivitis. It also is found in dental crevices of periodontally healthy subjects. Many new species have been described recently. *Porphyromonas cangingivalis, Porphyromonas cansulci, Porphyromonas gingivicanis, Porphyromonas creviorcanis, Porphyromonas canoris,* and *Porphyromonas gulae* have been associated with periodontitis in animals.

Prevotella nigrescens, a close relative of *P. intermedia,* seems to be associated with endodontic infection and adult gingivitis, whereas *P. intermedia* is more common in periodontal lesions.

Odontogenic mandibular and maxillary abscesses in domestic rabbits are consistent, in bacteriologic characteristics, with periodontal disease in humans, although they are typically caused by *Prevotella heparinolytica* and other *Prevotella* spp. not ordinarily involved in human disease.

Animal strains (from the oral cavities of cats, dogs, and other carnivores) resolve into a biotype of *P. gingivalis* that is different from the biotype containing human strains. Feline *P. gingivalis* is 75% DNA homologous with human *P. gingivalis,* and is one of multiple species of porphyromonads isolated from the feline oral cavity and oral-associated disease. *Porphyromonas macacae* biotype *salivosa* and *Porphyromonas circumdentaria* also are found occasionally.

Domestic sheep develop a form of periodontitis called "broken-mouth," characterized by premature spontaneous exfoliation of teeth and accompanied by malnutrition, weight loss, and systemic health problems. Oral microbes in periodontally diseased sheep are consistent with findings from humans with periodontitis. Affected animals yield cultures of *P. gingivalis* and *P. intermedia,* and elevated serum IgG titers to these organisms vary directly with the number of teeth lost and decreases in body weight.

There may be an association between periodontal disease and cardiovascular disease in humans. Hematogenous dissemination from chronic subgingival periodontal infections may infect vascular endothelium, contributing to atherosclerosis and increasing the risk of myocardial ischemia and infarction. *Porphyromonas gingivalis* causes platelet aggregation in vitro, suggesting a contribution to thrombotic effects in vivo. Results of experimental studies in animals suggest that atheromagenesis is amplified in the presence of periodontal pathogens. Polymerase chain reaction (PCR) examination of atherosclerotic plaque has revealed *P. gingivalis.*

PATHOGENESIS

Attempts to understand the pathogenesis of *Prevotella* spp. and *Porphyromonas* spp. infections in animals are based in large part on inference from studies relating to human disease. Most of this information relates to periodontal infections. Necrosis and osteoclastic resorption of alveolar bone underlie the process of tooth loss.

Invasion of gingival and junctional epithelial cells is a likely virulence mechanism. *Prevotella nigrescens* invades human epithelial cells in a process that requires microfilament integrity but is not affected by impaired microtubule organization. Invasiveness may be a means of immune evasion by *P. nigrescens.*

Inflammation in periodontitis may be caused in part by lipopolysaccharide (LPS), and host responses to LPS are mediated by CD14 and LPS-binding protein. *Prevotella intermedia* proteases cleave these molecules, modulating the effects of LPS in periodontal infections.

Hemagglutinin, fimbriae, proteases, and LPS may play roles in pathogenesis of *P. gingivalis* infections. These black-pigmented anaerobes are no different from other bacteria in their requirements for iron, and hemoglobin or hemin from red blood cells could be a major source of exogenous iron. Hemolytic and hemagglutinating activities of *P. intermedia* and *P. nigrescens* differ with the erythrocyte species, and are in general greater in the former than the latter. Hemolytic activity of *P. intermedia* is also greater than that of *P. gingivalis.* The hemagglutinin gene *(phg)* of *P. intermedia* is also present in some strains of *P. nigrescens.*

Porphyromonas gingivalis requires both iron and protoporphyrin IX, which it obtains preferentially from hemoglobin. Gingipains are cell surface arginine (Arg)– and lysine (Lys)-specific proteases produced by *P. gingivalis*, and these molecules have adhesin domains that may play a role in colonization. Targeting of proteolytic activity to host-cell surface matrix proteins and receptors leads to death of epithelial, fibroblast, and endothelial cells, with ensuing inflammation and vascular disruption. The Arg-specific proteolytic activity is essential for rapid hydrolysis of hemoglobin, so the major role of the gingipain complexes may be vascular disruption and subsequent binding and degradation of hemoglobin for heme assimilation.

Gingipains also may also play a part in immune avoidance by *P. gingivalis.* Proinflammatory cytokines and cellular receptors may be rapidly and efficiently degraded adjacent to the infection site, whereas lower protease concentrations distal to the area may promote inflammation, with resulting tissue destruction and bone resorption. In fact, immunization against the gingipains protects against experimental challenge with *P. gingivalis.*

Gingipains apparently play a role in abscess formation, as well, at least during experimental infection of mice, possibly by suppressing the function of neutrophils. Mutants have reduced neutrophil-suppressive activities, and immunization against gingipains diminishes abscess formation.

Proteases of *Prevotella* spp. cleave IgA in the hinge region, leaving intact monomeric Fab and Fc fragments. In vivo activity of *Prevotella* spp. IgA proteases is elevated in sera from adults with periodontal disease.

DIAGNOSIS

Diagnosis of infections by these species is based on anaerobic culture and identification of isolates. Species in both genera require hemin and/or vitamin K_1 and their optimal growth temperature is 37° C. Specimens should be plated onto prereduced media. Supplemented brucella agar (which contains hemin and vitamin K_1), supplemented phenylethyl alcohol agar (PEA), *Bacteroides* bile esculin agar, and kanamycin-vancomycin laked sheep blood agar are routinely used for isolation. Colonies of most species form slowly. *Prevotella* spp. surface colonies on blood agar vary from minute to 2 mm in diameter. They are generally circular, entire, convex, shiny, and smooth, and may be translucent or opaque, and gray, light brown, or black. Hemolysis is variable from strain to strain. *Prevotella melaninogenica* cells are rod-like and may be somewhat pleomorphic. Colonies are 0.5 to 2 mm in diameter, circular, entire, convex, and shiny, with dark centers and gray to light brown edges. Colonies become much darker on continued incubation, and this pigmentation is best observed after cultivation on PEA agar. A few strains are hemolytic and all fluoresce under ultraviolet illumination.

On blood agar, colonies of *Porphyromonas* spp. are usually smooth, shiny, convex and 1 to 3 mm in diameter. Colonies of most species are pigmented because of protoheme production. *Porphyromonas gingivalis* cells are coccobacillary, with some rod-shaped forms. Colonies are 1 to 2 mm in diameter, convex, and produce a black pigment after 7 to 10 days' incubation. Identification is according to biochemical properties (Table 38-1). As with *Prevotella* spp., pigmentation is best observed after cultivation on PEA agar.

Rapid, presumptive identification to genus level is based on growth response to special-potency antibiotic disks (vancomycin 5 µg, kanamycin 1000 µg, and colistin 10 µg), bile susceptibility, indole production, nitrate reduction,

and phenotypic properties, such as brick red fluorescence under long-wave ultraviolet illumination, and pigment production (see Table 38-1). Identification to species is according to biochemical properties (Table 38-2).

PREVENTION AND CONTROL

Vaccines are not available for prevention of infections by *Prevotella* spp. or *Porphyromonas* spp. *Prevotella* spp. strains from rabbits are generally susceptible (based on in vitro testing) to clindamycin, penicillin, and ceftriaxone, and about half are susceptible to ciprofloxacin, but most are unlikely to be susceptible in vivo to trimethoprim-sulfamethoxazole. Given that these organisms are often encountered in mixed culture, single-agent therapy may not be efficacious unless directed against both facultative and strict anaerobes (as with cefoxitin). Therapy that eliminates aerobes or facultative anaerobes (e.g., *Streptococcus pyogenes* and *Escherichia coli*) may allow emergence of encapsulated *Prevotella* spp. in abscesses and progression to chronic infection. *Prevotella* spp. and *Porphyromonas* spp. from cats and dogs are likely to be sensitive in vivo to the lincomycin family, the penicillin family, chloramphenicol, and cephaloridine.

Molar dental disease in horses is often at an advanced stage when diagnosed, and permanent restoration of diseased teeth is not workable. Bacteremia and septicemia may result from dentogenous sinusitis or occur as a sequel to normal dentosurgical procedures.

Parotid salivary gland and other abscesses in humans, as well as similar conditions in animals, are treated by surgical drainage and administration of parenteral antimicrobials. Application of dental hygienic measures is indicated in dogs or cats with periodontal disease.

TABLE 38-1 Rapid Differentiation of the Genera *Prevotella* and *Porphyromonas*

	Prevotella	*Porphyromonas*
Susceptibility to vancomycin	R	S
Susceptibility to kanamycin	R	R
Susceptibility to colistin	V	R
Growth in 20% bile	N	N
Spot indole production	V	(Pos)
Pigmentation	(Pos)	(Pos)
Brick red fluorescence	(Pos)	P
Nitrate reduction	N	N

Neg, Negative; *Pos,* positive; *(Pos),* most positive; *R,* resistant; *S,* susceptible; *V,* variable.

TABLE 38-2 Differentiation Among *Prevotella* Species and *Porphyromonas gingivalis*

	Acid from:			Glycine	Acid from:
	Glucose	*Cellobiose*	*Lactose*	Aminopeptidase	*Arabinose*
Porphyromonas gingivalis	Neg	ND	ND	ND	ND
Prevotella heparinolytica	Pos	Pos	ND	Pos	Pos
P. oralis	Pos	Pos	ND	Pos	Neg
P. zoogleoformans	Pos	Pos	ND	Neg	ND
P. melaninogenica	Pos	Neg	Pos	ND	ND
P. intermedius	Pos	Neg	Neg	ND	ND

Neg, Negative; *Pos,* positive; *ND,* not determined.

SUGGESTED READINGS

Berg JN, Fales WH, Scanlan CM: Occurrence of anaerobic bacteria in diseases of the dog and cat, *Am J Vet Res* 40:876-881, 1979.

Choi J, Takahashi N, Kato T, Kuramitsu HK: The isolation, expression and nucleotide sequence of the *sod* gene from *Porphyromonas gingivalis, Infect Immun* 59:1564-1566, 1991.

Love DN, Johnson JL, RF Jones RF, Calverley A: *Bacteroides salivosus* sp. nov., an asaccharolytic, black-pigmented species from cats, *Int J Syst Bacteriol* 37:307-309, 1987.

Love DN, Redwin J, Norris JM: Cloning and expression of the superoxide dismutase gene of the feline strain of *Porphyromonas gingivalis*: immunological recognition of the protein by cats with periodontal disease, *Vet Microbiol* 86:245-256, 2002.

Norris JM, Love DN: The association of two recombinant proteinases of a feline strain of *Porphyromonas gingivalis* with periodontal disease in cats, *Vet Microbiol* 71:69-80, 2000.

Norris JM, Love DN: Serum antibody responses of cats to soluble whole cell antigens of feline *Porphyromonas gingivalis, Vet Microbiol* 73:37-49, 2000.

O'Brien-Simpson NM, Veith PD, Dashper SG, Reynolds EC: *Porphyromonas gingivalis* gingipains: the molecular teeth of a microbial vampire, *Curr Protein Pept Sci* 4:409-426, 2003.

Privalle CT, Gregory EM: Superoxide dismutase and O_2 lethality in *Bacteroides fragilis, J Bacteriol* 138: 139-145, 1979.

Chapter 39

The Genera *Mycoplasma* and *Ureaplasma*

Mycoplasmas and ureaplasmas, members of the family Mycoplasmataceae, are the smallest prokaryotes and are related phylogenetically to members of the genera *Clostridium, Streptococcus,* and *Lactobacillus.* Members are distinct from other bacteria in their small genome size (0.58-1.35 Mb, which accounts for their limited metabolic options for replication and survival), and lack of cell wall synthesis (which places them in the class Mollicutes [soft skin] and renders them resistant to antimicrobials that interfere with cell wall synthesis). Mollicutes are of gram-positive lineage, but absence of a cell wall makes them unable to retain crystal violet/Gram's iodine, so Gram staining is not part of the identification process.

Mycoplasmas and ureaplasmas have complex nutritional requirements because of their limited biosynthetic capabilities, and depend in vivo on the host microenvironment. Most genes for amino acid and cofactor biosynthesis were lost during evolution. Exogenous fatty acids and sterols are required; the latter separates the family Mycoplasmataceae from similar organisms and is useful in their identification because it renders them sensitive to digitonin.

This group of organisms is widely distributed in humans, mammals, birds, reptiles, fish, and plants, and requires intimate association with host cell surfaces for growth. Until recently, these agents were considered to be strict pathogens of the mucous membranes, associated mainly with respiratory, arthritic, or genitourinary tract diseases. That dogma has changed with recognition of a new group, the hemotrophic mycoplasmas or hemoplasmas, which parasitize erythrocytes and are refractory to cultivation on solid media.

THE GENUS *MYCOPLASMA*

The genus *Mycoplasma* comprises more than 100 species, some of which cause chronic diseases in animals and humans. The majority of mycoplasmas have species-specific host-organism associations or tropisms for particular anatomic sites. The lack of a cell wall accounts for their plasticity and allows them to pass through filters with pore sizes as small as 450 nm, despite cell diameters ranging from 0.3 to 0.8 μm. Mycoplasmas are structurally simple, in that they consist of ribosomes and DNA bound by a trilaminar cytoplasmic membrane composed of sterols, phospholipids, and proteins. Most are facultatively anaerobic, except for the human pathogen *Mycoplasma pneumoniae,* which is a strict aerobe. They grow slowly, with a generation time of 1 to 6 hours.

Diseases and Epidemiology

Mycoplasma spp. infect a variety of animals, and some of diseases attributed to them have major economic impacts (Table 39-1). As a general rule, infections are spread among susceptible individuals through direct or droplet contact with oral, nasal, ocular, or genital secretions. Mycoplasmas are typically introduced into a group by the addition of clinically healthy carrier animals.

In poultry, the predominant mycoplasmal pathogens are *Mycoplasma gallisepticum, Mycoplasma synoviae, Mycoplasma meleagridis,* and *Mycoplasma iowae. Mycoplasma gallisepticum* infection commonly results in chronic respiratory disease in chickens. Clinical signs include nasal discharge, coughing, sneezing, tracheal rales, and conjunctivitis. Turkeys are more susceptible than chickens and often develop severe sinusitis (Figure 39-1). Other less common disease syndromes are keratoconjunctivitis, arthritis,

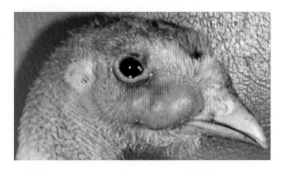

FIGURE 39-1 Turkey with sinusitis caused by *Mycoplasma gallisepticum.* (Courtesy Raymond E. Reed.)

salpingitis, and encephalopathy. *Mycoplasma synoviae* usually causes a subclinical upper respiratory infection but may result in airsacculitis and synovitis in chickens and turkeys. Some strains of *M. synoviae* produce subclinical infection, a characteristic that creates difficulty in the management

TABLE 39-1 *Mycoplasma* Species That Infect Domestic Animals

Species	Host(s)
M. agalactiae	Goats, sheep: contagious agalactia
M. alkalescens	Cattle: arthritis, mastitis
M. bovigenitalium	Cattle: infertility, mastitis
M. bovis	Cattle: arthritis, mastitis, pneumonia, abortions, abscesses, otitis media, genital infections
M. bovoculi	Cattle: conjunctivitis
M. californicum	Cattle: mastitis
M. canadense	Cattle: abortions, mastitis
M. capricolum ssp. *capricolum*	Goats, sheep: mastitis, septicemia, polyarthritis, pneumonia
M. capricolum ssp. *capripneumoniae*	Goats: contagious caprine pleuropneumonia
M. conjunctivae	Sheep, goats: infectious keratoconjunctivitis
M. cynos	Dogs: pneumonia
M. dispar	Cattle: bronchiolitis
M. equigenitalium	Horses: abortion?
M. felis	Cats: conjunctivitis, pneumonia Horses: pneumonia
M. gallisepticum	Chickens, turkeys: airsacculitis, sinusitis
M. gatae	Cats: chronic arthritis, tenosynovitis
M. hyopneumoniae	Pigs: enzootic pneumonia
M. hyorhinis	Pigs: polyarthritis, polyserositis
M. hyosynoviae	Pigs: polyarthritis
M. iowae	Turkeys: embryo mortality
M. meleagridis	Turkeys: airsacculitis, skeletal abnormalities, decreased growth
M. mycoides ssp. *capri*	Goats: arthritis, mastitis, pleuropneumonia, septicemia
M. mycoides ssp. *mycoides* (small-colony type)	Cattle, domestic water buffalo: contagious bovine pleuropneumonia
M. mycoides ssp. *mycoides* (large-colony type)	Goats, sheep: mastitis, septicemia, polyarthritis, pneumonia
M. ovipneumoniae	Goats, sheep: pleuropneumonia
M. pulmonis	Laboratory rats and mice: murine respiratory mycoplasmosis
M. synoviae	Chickens, turkeys: infectious synovitis

and control of disease outbreaks. Infections may result in financial loss to the industry through processing condemnations, as well as reduced growth efficiency and egg production. *Mycoplasma meleagridis* causes respiratory disease in young turkeys and is involved in stunting, poor feathering, and leg problems. *Mycoplasma iowae* infection is economically important in turkeys, and the organism has occasionally been isolated from chickens. In turkeys it has been associated with reduced hatchability and embryo mortality, whereas experimentally infected chickens and turkeys develop airsacculitis and leg abnormalities. Avian mycoplasmas are egg transmitted and may spread laterally by direct or indirect contact. The mode of transmission of *M. meleagridis* to the egg is venereal. Infection of the male thallus results in semen contamination, which leads to oviduct infection after mating. With all of the avian pathogenic mycoplasmas, disease severity is dependent on the virulence of the strain involved, the age and breed of the bird, the degree of stress, methods of management, and presence of concurrent bacterial or viral infections.

Three species of mycoplasmas commonly causing disease in swine are *Mycoplasma hyopneumoniae*, *Mycoplasma hyosynoviae*, and *Mycoplasma hyorhinis*. *Mycoplasma hyopneumoniae* is recognized as the etiologic agent of porcine enzootic pneumonia, which is characterized by high morbidity and low mortality that is commonly complicated by other opportunistic bacterial or viral infections. Enzootic pneumonia is an important economic problem affecting swine production worldwide. Clinical pneumonia is common in young animals but generally not seen in adults. *Mycoplasma hyopneumoniae* is transmitted from older to younger pigs by contact. Mechanical transmission by man and other animals is possible, and the organism may spread on the wind for several miles. Surveys conducted in different countries have revealed lesions of enzootic pneumonia in 30% to 80% of slaughter pigs. Feed conversion may be reduced by 14% to 20% and rate of gain by 16% to 30% in affected swine. The primary clinical sign is a sporadic dry nonproductive cough. Other signs may include fever, dyspnea, or impaired growth. Typical lesions are located in the apical and cardiac lobes of the lung, and consist of well-demarcated, dark red to purple areas in acute disease, or tan to gray areas in chronic disease. Microscopic examination reveals

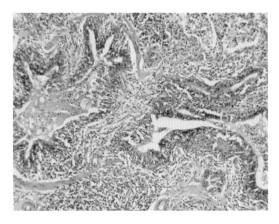

FIGURE 39-2 Porcine lung histopathology of chronic enzootic pneumonia caused by *Mycoplasma hyopneumoniae:* bronchioalveolar lymphoid hyperplasia. (Courtesy Peter Moisan.)

characteristic lesions that include suppurative bronchopneumonia, histiocytic alveolitis with peribronchiolar and perivascular lymphohistiocytic cuffing, and nodule formation typical of bronchoalveolar lymphoid hyperplasia (Figure 39-2).

Mycoplasma hyosynoviae is a common inhabitant of the upper respiratory tract that may occasionally be recovered from 3- to 6-month-old pigs with polyarthritis. Disease is sporadic and of low morbidity. *Mycoplasma hyorhinis* is a sporadic cause of polyserositis and polyarthritis, which is indistinguishable from Glasser's disease in pigs less than 3 months old. Infections are also sporadic in nature.

More than 20 species of *Mycoplasma* have been recovered from cattle. Many are purely commensal in nature, whereas others are responsible for a wide variety of clinical manifestations. *Mycoplasma mycoides* ssp. *mycoides,* isolated in 1898, was the first *Mycoplasma* species associated with animal disease. The small colony variant is the causative agent of contagious bovine pleuropneumonia (CBPP), one of the most important cattle diseases in history. The first veterinary college was founded to train practitioners to deal with CBPP. The disease has been eradicated from North America, Europe, and Australia, but remains endemic in parts of Africa and Asia. The disease is characterized by marked edema of the interlobular septa, with diffuse pneumonia and serofibrinous pleuritis (Figure 39-3). Infection spreads slowly within a herd, and may reach a peak morbidity rate of 50% only after several months. The disease may have acute or chronic manifestations.

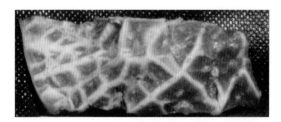

FIGURE 39-3 Contagious bovine pleuropneumonia, with marked interlobular edema and diffuse pneumonia (*Mycoplasma mycoides* ssp. *mycoides*). (Courtesy Raymond E. Reed.)

Mycoplasma bovis is among the most virulent mycoplasmas of cattle worldwide. It is most often associated with bronchopneumonia, and infection is believed to be a predisposing factor in the development of bovine respiratory disease complex, or shipping fever. *Mycoplasma bovis* is capable of systemic invasion, and arthritis and meningitis may be sequelae to mycoplasmemia. In addition, *M. bovis* has been associated with otitis media, mastitis, keratoconjunctivitis, endometritis, oophoritis, abortion, and seminal vesiculitis. In the United States alone, costs in the form of decreased weight gains and loss of production have been estimated at $32 million per year.

It is not clear whether mycoplasmas are primary pathogens or opportunistic invaders in cats and dogs. Results of one survey indicated that mycoplasmas are part of the oropharyngeal flora in 33% of cats; however, they are not normal inhabitants of the lower respiratory tract. Sporadic reports of mycoplasmal pneumonia, bronchial disease, bite wound abscesses, and pyothorax have been described. *Mycoplasma felis* is a significant etiologic agent of conjunctivitis in young cats, as well as a secondary invader in pneumonia. Mycoplasmas have been isolated from the upper respiratory tract of 25% of healthy dogs and from 21% of animals with pulmonary disease. *Mycoplasma cynos* is frequently recovered from chronic pulmonary mycoplasmosis in dogs. Mycoplasmas have been implicated as agents of canine infertility, but several studies have found no difference in mycoplasma recovery rates from the vagina or semen of fertile versus infertile dogs. There are several reports of endometritis associated with *Mycoplasma canis*.

Many mycoplasmas have been isolated from sheep and goats, but few are considered to be pathogens, and these are associated with pneumonia, mastitis, arthritis, genital infections, and conjunctivitis. The two most important diseases of small ruminants are contagious caprine pleuropneumonia and contagious agalactia. These are responsible for major losses in goat herds in Africa and Asia and are designated list B diseases by the Office International des Epizooties. *Mycoplasma capricolum* ssp. *caripneumoniae* is the primary etiologic agent of caprine pleuropneumonia, a severe disease that may result in 100% morbidity and 80% mortality upon initial exposure of animals in naive herds. Contagious agalactia caused by *Mycoplasma agalactiae* has been estimated to cause annual losses in excess of $30 million in European countries, mainly as a result of decreased milk production. Severe mastitis and a decline in milk production are the first clinical signs of this primarily lactational disease. It may progress to septicemia and death in 20% of affected animals, and keratoconjunctivitis and arthritis are common sequelae in survivors. The udder may undergo complete fibrosis, resulting in permanent agalactia. Young ruminants become infected as a result of suckling, which may result in arthritis.

Of the 10 *Mycoplasma* species recovered from horses, only *M. felis* is considered pathogenic. It is a demonstrated cause of pleuritis. Mycoplasmas have been isolated from equine fetuses, but their etiologic role has not been established. Other species are apparent commensals of the upper respiratory and lower genitourinary tracts.

Pathogenesis

Mycoplasmas have evolved unique strategies that allow them to survive and replicate in hosts. Some of their inherent properties may cause damage to host cells; their inability to synthesize many essential nutrients forces them into competition with host cells, altering cellular integrity and function. For example, nonfermenting mycoplasmas use the arginine dihydrolase pathway to generate ATP, and host cell protein synthesis grinds to a halt when arginine reserves are depleted.

Cytadhesins are among the major virulence determinants of mycoplasmas. One such is the P97 protein of *M. hyopneumoniae*. The organism attaches to cilia of respiratory epithelial cells, resulting in damage to and subsequent loss of cilia (Figure 39-4). Lung damage results, as the lungs become predisposed to infection by secondary bacteria and the effects of other irritants.

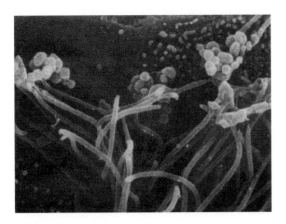

FIGURE 39-4 *Mycoplasma hyopneumoniae* associated with cilia in the porcine respiratory tract. (Courtesy Eileen Thacker.)

Cytadhesins have also been identified in *M. gallisepticum, M. synoviae,* and the human pathogen, *M. pneumoniae.*

Intimate association of mycoplasmas with the host cellular surface may lead to a buildup in the local concentration of cytotoxic metabolites and cytolytic enzymes. Hydrogen peroxide production is thought to play a role in the pathogenicity of some mycoplasmas, including *M. pneumoniae* and *Mycoplasma dispar.* Its production may induce oxidative stress in host cells, resulting in damage to the cellular membrane. Many *Mycoplasma* species have membrane-bound phospholipases that may release cytolytic lysophospholipids capable of disrupting host cell membranes.

Mycoplasmas produce at least three different types of modulins (molecular moieties that induce cytokine synthesis with pathologic consequences). Mycoplasmal lipoproteins play a key role in pathogenesis, stimulating monocytes and inducing secretion of proinflammatory cytokines and interleukins. The resulting pulmonary inflammation is characteristic of mycoplasma pneumonia. Infections are further characterized by initial infiltration of neutrophils, followed by an influx of macrophages and lymphocytes. The extent of neutrophil infiltration is directly correlated with disease severity because neutrophil attraction is controlled by chemotactic cytokines. Several mycoplasmas (*M. pneumoniae* and *Mycoplasma arthritidis*) function as superantigens, stimulating migration of inflammatory cells to infection sites, with subsequent release of cytokines. Certain mycoplasmas also can modulate immune functions,

including induction of bovine lymphocyte apoptosis by *M. bovis.*

An important characteristic of mycoplasma infections is chronicity, and this may be based in immune evasion. Antigenic variation may be utilized by mycoplasmas, including *M. bovis, Mycoplasma pulmonis,* and *M. gallisepticum,* to evade the immune response and cause chronic infection. Mycoplasmas have the genetic capability to alter, at high frequency, the structure and expression of membrane lipoproteins that are exposed to the host immune system. The exact mechanism underlying lipoprotein variation is not precisely understood.

Another virulence factor, which may be important in infections by *M. mycoides* ssp. *mycoides* and *M. dispar,* is a polysaccharide capsule, which may afford protection from phagocytosis.

Mycoplasma infection predisposes to infection with other pathogens, and mycoplasmas can act synergistically with these pathogens to increase disease severity. Studies indicate that *M. hyopneumoniae* potentiates pneumonia induced by porcine respiratory and reproductive syndrome virus. Mycoplasmas appear to play a role in accelerating the progression of human immunodeficiency virus infection to acquired immunodeficiency syndrome (AIDS).

Diagnosis

Culture is a specific method used to determine the infection status of an individual, but it is laborious, time consuming, and frequently inconclusive because of low sensitivity. Furthermore, isolation of mycoplasmas from clinical specimens does not confirm their etiologic status because they are widely distributed in normal animals. For optimum recovery, specimens should be collected early in the course of disease and processed within 48 hours of collection. Isolation media are complex and should ideally contain sterols, vitamins, amino acids, and a source of DNA or adenine dinucleotide. Penicillin or ampicillin and thallium acetate are added to inhibit the growth of contaminants. For optimal growth of mycoplasmas, the medium must be buffered at pH 7.3 to 7.8. No single medium formulation has been universally accepted; solid and liquid media are generally inoculated in parallel because some species grow better initially in a liquid medium. Incubation is at 37° C in a humidified environment, and most animal pathogenic species produce colonies after

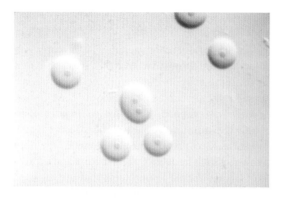

FIGURE 39-5   Colonies of *Mycoplasma bovirhinis,* showing characteristic "fried-egg" appearance. (Courtesy J. Glenn Songer.)

4 to 5 days' incubation. Agar plates are examined for colonies with a dissecting microscope, or under low power on an ordinary light microscope with decreased light intensity. Unstained colonies are 0.1 to 1 mm in diameter and usually have dense, elevated centers giving a "fried-egg" appearance (Figure 39-5). The use of Diene's stain may facilitate differentiation of mycoplasmal colonies from cell wall–deficient bacteria (L-forms), which have no sterols in their cellular membrane but can form cell walls under appropriate growth conditions. Mycoplasma colonies retain the blue of the Diene's stain, whereas bacterial colonies decolorize in 15 minutes.

Isolates are not easily identified to the species level. Presumptive identification to genus is through a requirement for sterols using the digitonin sensitivity test; digitonin has a deleterious effect on sterols in the medium. Digitonin-impregnated filter paper disks are placed on solid medium streaked for confluent growth with a pure culture of the test organism. Growth inhibition around the disk indicates digitonin sensitivity.

Acholeplasmas are mycoplasma-like organisms in the class Mollicutes that generally lack a cholesterol requirement, and are therefore insensitive to digitonin. Mycoplasmas may be further differentiated by their colonial morphology and size, host specificity, and assessment of phosphatase and proteolytic activity and ability to ferment glucose and hydrolyze arginine or urea (Figure 39-6).

Isolates are more commonly identified through immunologic methods, using rabbit hyperimmune antisera against each pathogenic species. Common procedures include immunofluorescence, immunodiffusion, and immunoperoxidase tests. The most common application is examination of intact colonies on solid media by fluorescent antibody staining, followed by microscopic evaluation (Figure 39-7). Immunohistochemistry also can be used to detect mycoplasmal antigen in

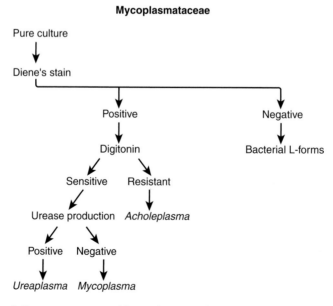

FIGURE 39-6   Differentiation among genera with veterinary significance in family Mycoplasmataceae. (Courtesy Ashley E. Harmon.)

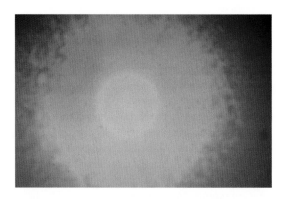

FIGURE 39-7 Fluorescent antibody staining of *Mycoplasma hyosynoviae* on agar. (Courtesy J. Glenn Songer.)

tissues, and a diagnosis of *M. hyopneumoniae* infection can be made through detection of the organism in pig lungs by a monoclonal antibody–based immunofluorescent assay.

Serology is a sensitive indicator of clinical infection and is the mainstay of most mycoplasma monitoring programs in poultry and swine production systems. Several simple serologic tests have been used successfully to detect mycoplasmal infections in domestic animals. Monitoring programs for *M. gallisepticum* and *M. synoviae* have been heavily dependent on serum plate agglutination, hemagglutination inhibition, and enzyme-linked immunosorbent assays (ELISAs). The latter method is used widely to examine sera from pigs suspected of infection with *M. hyopneumoniae*.

Development of polymerase chain reaction (PCR) techniques and availability of commercial test kits for diagnosis of *M. gallisepticum, M. synoviae,* and *M. hyopneumoniae* has made PCR a valuable adjunctive test in many diagnostic laboratories.

Prevention, Treatment, and Control

Prevention and control of mycoplasmosis are difficult because of mycoplasmal concealment from host defenses. Because many of these diseases may be stress related, management changes to minimize stress factors such as crowding, rapid feed changes, chilling, excessive heat, poor sanitation, transportation, and commingling. Segregation of new animals and assessment of their serologic status before addition to a herd or flock are also recommended.

For commercial poultry, methods include surveillance and eradication, vaccination, and use of

antimicrobials. Because of their economic impact, *M. gallisepticum* and *M. synoviae* are controlled in the U.S. commercial poultry industry by the National Poultry Improvement Plan voluntary testing program. The program consists of periodic serologic monitoring with depopulation of positive flocks. Control of avian mycoplasmosis through vaccination is limited because only a few vaccines are available. Control by chemotherapy is sometimes a necessary complement to biosecurity measures designed to minimize lateral or vertical transmission. Many antimicrobial agents, such as macrolides, tetracyclines, and fluoroquinolones, have in vitro activity against avian mycoplasmas, but resistance to enrofloxacin, oxytetracycline, tylosin, and erythromycin has emerged recently.

Selection of replacement stock from herds free of porcine enzootic pneumonia is the best way to prevent introduction of the disease into a herd. Once herd infection is established, control can be achieved by continual or pulse-dosing antimicrobial therapy with tylosin, tiamulin, chlortetracycline, or lincomycin. Effective control measures also depend on optimizing environmental conditions (air quality, ventilation, temperature). Management methods for control include periodic examination of lungs from slaughter animals, clinical inspections, serologic monitoring for infection, segregated early weaning programs, and all-in/all-out pig flow. Total eradication of *M. hyopneumoniae* from swine herds requires separate breeding of adult sows in isolation, based on the premise that *M. hyopneumoniae* is eliminated from the lower respiratory tract in adults. No animals younger than 1 year are present in a herd for more than 1 month. This method is often impractical and ineffective, and the most practical approach appears to be depopulation of infected herds and repopulation with enzootic pneumonia–free animals. Vaccination may be an alternative for disease control, but vaccines vary in their efficacy and apparently do not prevent infection.

Control measures for contagious bovine pleuropneumonia have traditionally involved eradication by way of test and slaughter protocols. Vaccination of susceptible cattle living in enzootic regions is now recommended. Antibiotic therapy is generally ineffective for control of this severe disease; it reduces clinical signs but promotes development of the carrier state. Once established in a herd, *M. bovis* infection often takes a protracted course and is difficult to control as a result of its resistance to antimicrobial therapy and lack of efficacious vaccines. Prevention and control measures in a feedlot setting are related to stress reduction and good management. Tilmicosin, tylosin, tetracyclines, lincomycin, spectinomycin, and florfenicol have the most potential for treatment. Newly purchased dairy cows or replacement heifers should be quarantined and tested for mycoplasmal mastitis before admission to the herd. There is no treatment for mycoplasmal mastitis, and positive animals should be culled. Waste milk from mastitic cows should not be fed to calves without pasteurization.

No vaccines are available for prevention of mycoplasmosis in dogs and cats. Extended antimicrobial therapy with macrolides, tetracyclines, chloramphenicol, or fluoroquinolones is advocated to eradicate infection. Immunity against mycoplasmas does not appear to develop, so affected animals should be segregated from healthy penmates.

Prevention and control of small ruminant contagious pleuropneumonia and contagious agalactia are best achieved by culling affected and in-contact animals. Antimicrobials may yield clinical cures but rarely eliminate these agents. In addition, *M. capricolum* ssp. *capripneumoniae* and *M. agalactiae* are becoming increasingly resistant to tetracyclines. Good husbandry practices should be implemented to include proper hygiene and decreasing periods of lactation. New vaccines are on the horizon and offer the possibility of more effective prophylactic measures.

HEMOTROPHIC MYCOPLASMAS

Eperythrozoon and *Haemobartonella,* wall-less bacteria that attach to and grow on the surface of red blood cells, were previously classified in the order Rickettsiales, family Anaplasmataceae, based on staining characteristics, obligate intracellular status, susceptibility to tetracyclines, and transmission by arthropods. Recent phylogenetic analysis of 16S rRNA gene sequences and electron microscopy findings have demonstrated that these hemotrophic organisms are closely aligned with species in the *M. pneumoniae* group and represent an entirely new clade of pathogens within the genus *Mycoplasma.* As a result, *Eperythrozoon ovis, Eperythrozoon suis,* and *Eperythrozoon*

wenyonii have been transferred as *Mycoplasma ovis, Mycoplasma suis,* and *Mycoplasma wenyonii,* respectively. The former *Haemobartonella felis, Haemobartonella canis,* and *Haemobartonella muris* have been reclassified as *Mycoplasma haemofelis, Mycoplasma haemocanis,* and *Mycoplasma haemomuris,* respectively. Based on genetic and clinical data, reclassification has also been proposed for the small form or California strain of *H. felis,* and the newly characterized haemotrophic bacteria from opossums, camelids and squirrel monkeys, as *Candidatus* M. haemominutum, *Candidatus* M. haemodidelphidis, *Candidatus* M. haemolamae, and *Candidatus* M. kahaneii, respectively. The *Candidatus* designation is a provisional nomenclatural status applied by the international bacterial nomenclature system. These results call into question the taxonomic affiliation of the remaining species of *Eperythrozoon,* namely *Eperythrozoon coccoides, Eperythrozoon ovis,* and *Eperythrozoon parvum* (Table 39-2).

Hemoplasmas are erythrocytic parasites that adhere to the surface of the red blood cell, often in a depression or infolding. Electron microscopic examination reveals that they lack a cell wall, and most are coccoidal shaped and less than 0.9 μm in diameter. They reproduce by binary fission, are resistant to penicillin and its analogs, and remain noncultivable in vitro.

Hemotrophic mycoplasmal interactions with host erythrocyte cell membranes are important features in pathogenesis. Several genes encoding adhesins have been identified, and electron microscopic examination reveals bacterial fibrils in depressions on the red cell surface. Depressions formed by the attachment of *Mycoplasma haemosuis* cause disruption of the erythrocyte cytoskeleton, leading to increased cellular fragility. The pathogenesis of anemia may also have an autoimmune component, in that hemoplasmas are removed from the surface of erythrocytes by splenic and lymph node capillary endothelial cells and by macrophages, before the red cells are returned to the circulation. Nonparasitized erythrocytes are phagocytosed in the spleen and lymph nodes, and autoantibodies on the erythrocyte membranes are IgM cold agglutinins that appear to be misdirected against the red blood cell membrane or the parasite–red blood cell membrane antigen complex. This immune-mediated osmotic fragility further contributes to the anemia.

TABLE 39-2 Features of Hemotrophic Mycoplasmas

Organism	Disease	Vector (if known)
Eperythrozoon coccoides	Murine eperythrozoonosis	Lice
Eperythrozoon ovis	Ovine, caprine eperythrozoonosis	Mosquitoes, sand flies, sheep ked (*Melophagus ovinus*)
Eperythrozoon parvum	Nonpathogenic (porcine origin)	
Mycoplasma (Eperythrozoon) suis	Porcine eperythrozoonosis or icteroanemia	Hog louse, mosquitoes (*Aedes aegypti*), biting flies (*Stomoxys calcitrans*)
Mycoplasma (Eperythrozoon) wenyonii	Bovine eperythrozoonosis	Ticks (*Dermacentor andersonii*)
Mycoplasma haemocanis (*Haemobartonella canis*)	Canine haemobartonellosis	Ticks (*Rhipicephalus sanguineus*)
Mycoplasma haemofelis (*Haemobartonella felis*, large form or Ohio strain)	Feline haemobartonellosis or infectious anemia	
Mycoplasma haemomuris (*Haemobartonella muris*)	Murine haemobartonellosis	Rat louse (*Polypax spinulosa*)
"*Mycoplasma haemodidelphidis*"	Severe anemia (opossum)	
"*Mycoplasma haemolamae*"	Anemia (camelids)	
"*Mycoplasma haemominutum*" (*Haemobartonella felis* small form, California strain)	Feline haemobartonellosis or infectious anemia	
"*Mycoplasma kahaneii*"	Mild anemia (squirrel monkey)	

Microscopic examination of blood smears stained with Romanovsky-type stains reveals small blue to purple coccoid-, rod-, or ring-shaped structures, 0.3 to 0.7 μm in diameter, occurring either singly or in chains on the surface of erythrocytes. Occasionally they may be free in the plasma. Microscopic examination has limitations because parasitemia is transient, often developing concurrently with clinical signs. Acridine orange staining is more sensitive than the Romanovsky stain. Blood smears should be carefully evaluated to distinguish mycoplasmas from other erythrocytic structures, such as Howell-Jolly and Heinz bodies, or basophilic stippling and stain artifacts.

Many infections are clinically inapparent and persist for years in latently infected animals. Even if treated, infected animals likely remain chronic carriers. Organisms are cleared from circulation by sequestration in the spleen, but stress, immunosuppressive disease, or splenectomy may be followed by appearance of infected erythrocytes in the bloodstream or clinical disease. Transmission frequently involves arthropod vectors such as, fleas, lice, ticks, mosquitoes, and biting flies.

Hemotrophic mycoplasmas infect a wide range of animal hosts, including primates. Wall-less, hemotrophic bacteria were also demonstrated in Brazilian AIDS patients.

Mycoplasma (Eperythrozoon) ovis

Mycoplasma ovis causes ovine eperythrozoonosis, a disease of worldwide distribution that affects sheep of all ages and, rarely, goats. The seasonal incidence suggests that infection may be related to changes in the arthropod population. Summer epizootics have high morbidity and low mortality, and affected animals are febrile, anemic, and develop cranial edema. Disease in lambs is especially severe, with a high mortality rate. Postmortem findings include anemia, hydropericardium, and an enlarged, soft spleen. Infected ewes appear to serve as a reservoir of infection for lambs. Experimental transmission has been accomplished through inoculation of susceptible animals with blood from infected animals. The incubation period was inversely proportional to the infecting dose, with the median being 7 days. Complement fixation and indirect fluorescent antibody tests may be used for diagnosis, and organic arsenicals and tetracyclines have been used to control and treat disease.

Mycoplasma (Eperythrozoon) suis

Mycoplasma suis is the etiologic agent of porcine eperythrozoonosis or icteroanemia. The disease was first described in 1934, and infections occur today in the Midwestern and southern United States,

Germany, and South Africa. Economic losses may be significant. Addition of tetracyclines to swine feeds as growth promoters has reduced morbidity and mortality from *M. suis* infection, and the true incidence and prevalence of disease are largely unknown. Organisms are transmitted by biting arthropods, transfer of contaminated blood, and in utero. The highest incidence of infection occurs during summer, which correlates with peak arthropod activity.

Four disease syndromes include acute hemolytic anemia in grower/finisher swine, decreased conception rates in sows, anemia and weakness in neonates, and poor weight gains in feeder pigs. The usual manifestation of the hemolytic syndrome is sudden death. Illness is characterized by anemia and fever. Necrosis of extremities may occur in colder climates and is attributed to the activity of cold agglutinins. Necropsy findings include icterus, serous effusion, splenomegaly, and watery blood. Affected sows exhibit fever and anorexia immediately before farrowing, and fever may persist into the postpartum period. First-breeding conception rates show a decline. Pigs less than 5 days of age may be pale, icteric, or generally unthrifty. Infected neonates are at an increased risk for developing respiratory or enteric disease. In feeder pigs, the classic icterus is usually not observed, perhaps in part because of the widespread use of medicated feeds. Affected animals may be mildly anorectic.

Diagnosis is based on clinical signs and history, direct microscopic observation of organisms attached to red blood cells in stained films, serologic test results, and molecular diagnostic test results. Serologic tests include the indirect hemagglutination inhibition (IHA) assay and the ELISA. The ELISA is more sensitive than IHA, but both tests have diagnostic limitations because of a marked variability in antibody response (piglets more than 3 months old and boars tend to have lower titers) and failure of these assays to accurately detect acutely and chronically infected pigs. Serologic tests continue to be routinely used to monitor infection, but they should be considered as indicators of herd rather than individual infection. Molecular approaches to diagnosis include a recombinant DNA probe and PCR tests, which may be useful in assessing the infection status of individual animals.

Identification and removal of carrier pigs that may serve as reservoirs are recommended.

No pharmaceuticals are currently approved for treatment of eperythrozoonosis, but administration of tetracyclines or arsenicals will eliminate acute signs and prevent mortality. These drugs will not totally eliminate the organism from infected pigs, which remain as carriers. No vaccines are available to prevent eperythrozoonosis.

Mycoplasma (Eperythrozoon) wenyonii

Mycoplasma wenyonii infection is common worldwide in cattle, but most cases are subclinical. The tick vector is *Dermacentor andersonii*. In adult cattle, mild anemia, fever, and myositis may occasionally be observed, although bulls may experience scrotal edema and decreased fertility and postpartum dairy heifers may have edema of the teats and hindlimbs. No serologic tests are available, so diagnosis is based on identification of organisms in blood smears. Prevention and control involve the use of acaricides and tetracyclines.

Mycoplasma haemocanis (Haemobartonella canis)

Mycoplasma haemocanis is the etiologic agent of canine haemobartonellosis, also referred to as infectious anemia of dogs, which occurs worldwide. Infection is of little consequence in healthy dogs, but latent infections can be activated by splenectomy or immune suppression. A severe illness, characterized by the finding of numerous parasitized erythrocytes, rapidly progressive anemia, and possibly death, may result in these individuals. Romanovsky-stained peripheral blood films reveal coccus-shaped organisms, either singly or in chains. Some chains may split, producing Y-shaped forms.

Experimental transmission of *M. haemocanis* by *Rhipicephalus sanguineus* has been demonstrated. These ticks may be vectors and reservoirs, as there is both transovarial and transstadial transmission of the bacterium. Iatrogenic transmission by blood transfusion from clinically normal carrier dogs has been documented, and indirect evidence exists for in utero and oral transmission.

Clinical signs are usually inapparent in otherwise healthy nonsplenectomized animals. These dogs develop mild disease and recover, but latent or chronic infection may result. Recrudescence into acute disease may result if they become concurrently infected with parvovirus, ehrlichiae, or

Babesia. Experimental infection of splenectomized dogs results in low-grade fever, anemia, anorexia, and malaise.

A diagnosis of canine haemobartonellosis depends on recognition of the organisms in stained smears of peripheral blood. Prevention of disease may be accomplished by the use of negative transfusion donor animals and elimination of blood-feeding arthropods. Oral administration of oxytetracycline, or intravenous injection of either chloramphenicol or thiacetarsamide sodium, has proven efficacious for the treatment of acute disease.

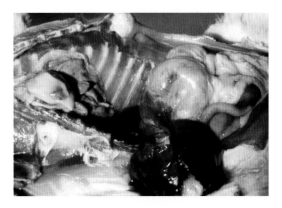

FIGURE 39-8 Gross lesions in a cat with feline infectious anemia (haemobartonellosis). (Courtesy Raymond E. Reed.)

Mycoplasma haemofelis (*Haemobartonella felis*)

First described in 1953, feline infectious anemia or haemobartonellosis, caused by *Mycoplasma haemofelis,* is a contagious disease of domestic and wild cats, and is associated with severe weakness, anemia, weight loss, depression, and sometimes death. The disease occurs worldwide. Not enough information is available on the epidemiology of this disease, but the infection rate may be as high as 30%. Epidemiologic studies have identified several risk factors for haemobartonellosis. The disease is more common in free-roaming cats less than 3 years of age. Concurrent illnesses, such as feline leukemia, increase the chance for developing illness. Flea infestation is another risk factor; however, vector transmission by arthropods has not been definitively established. Routes of transmission are oral, intraperitoneal, and through bite wounds. Vertical transmission may also occur.

Haemobartonellosis varies in clinical presentation from peracute to chronic. Peracute disease is associated with parasitemia and a severe, sometimes fatal, hemolytic anemia. At necropsy, infected cats appear pale and emaciated with splenomegaly and icterus (Figure 39-8). When disease is acute, fever, hemolytic anemia, depression, anorexia, and weakness are exhibited. Parasitemic episodes correlate with a decline in packed-cell volume. The chronic form of disease usually follows, with animals remaining anemic, lethargic, and anorexic. Recovered animals remain asymptomatic carriers, possibly for life.

Mycoplasma haemofelis produces a patent parasitemia. Attachment of a single organism to two or more red blood cells leads to erythrocyte sequestration in capillaries. The cause of hemolysis in feline haemobartonellosis is not completely understood, but a positive direct Coombs' test results and autoagglutination has been observed, suggesting immunopathogenesis. Parasite antigen adsorbed to erythrocytes sensitizes them to phagocytic cell engulfment, and selective removal by the spleen and bone marrow macrophages contributes to the anemia. Antibody in experimentally infected cats is a cold agglutinin, which is a factor in the development of clinical disease. As a result, the red blood cell life span is decreased by half.

Mycoplasma haemofelis is refractory to culture, so diagnosis depends on morphologic identification of the organisms on infected erythrocytes. Light microscopic examination is most common, but fluorescence microscopy (with acridine orange or fluorescent antibody staining) and electron microscopy are also used. Organisms are recognized as small blue cocci, rods, or ring forms on the edges or across the faces of Romanovsky-stained erythrocytes. As with any direct examination technique, false negatives occur and molecular applications (PCR and hybridization probes) have largely replaced microscopic methods for diagnosis of feline infectious anemia. Serologic testing is not currently available on a commercial basis.

Chemotherapeutic agents such as tetracyclines, chloramphenicol, macrolides, and fluoroquinolones appear to be effective in suppressing infection. Supportive care such as blood transfusions may be necessary to control the extreme anemia in some severely affected cats. Flea control should be practiced.

THE GENUS *UREAPLASMA*

Ureaplasmas, initially described as "T" (tiny) strain mycoplasmas, were discovered in the 1950s in human urogenital tract specimens. All members of the genus are membrane bound, do not utilize glucose or arginine, pass through 450 nm membrane filters, require cholesterol for growth, and form minute colonies (0.02-0.06 mm) on agar media. The property that differentiates them from mycoplasmas is the ability of ureaplasmas to hydrolyze urea. The seven named species are *Ureaplasma diversum, Ureaplasma cati, Ureaplasma felinum, Ureaplasma canigenitalium, Ureaplasma gallorale, Ureaplasma parvum,* and *Ureaplasma urealyticum.*

Ureaplasma diversum is a common inhabitant of the bovine vagina and, less frequently, of the uterus and oviducts. It is the etiologic agent of granular vulvitis in cows and heifers. The acute form is characterized by the formation of pale to red granular nodules in the vulvar mucosa and intermittent mucopurulent vaginal discharge. The agent has been implicated as a cause of abortions and stillbirths. Several studies have estimated the prevalence of *U. diversum* to be 36% to 64% at prebreeding and 54% to 76% at pregnancy examination. The exact route of transmission is unknown, but is thought to be venereal because bulls carry ureaplasmas as part of their normal preputial and urethral flora. Indirect transmission may occur via fomites, such as artificial insemination pipettes. Intrauterine infusion of tetracycline in affected cows has been beneficial in the restoration of fertility. *Ureaplasma diversum* has been implicated in bovine urinary and respiratory tract disease. Pneumonia and cystitis have been reproduced in cattle by experimental inoculation.

Ureaplasmas have been associated with disease in other species. Several reports tell of *Ureaplasma* isolation from sheep in association with spontaneous granular vulvitis and infertility. These organisms may be responsible for the formation of urinary calculi in goats. Ureaplasmas, most commonly *U. canigenitalium,* have been recovered from dogs with genitourinary tract infections and infertility problems. The role of ureaplasmas in feline pulmonary disease is poorly defined because *U. cati* and *U. felinum* have been isolated from the oropharynx of clinically normal cats. However, these agents are implicated as causative agents of feline urinary tract infections. *Ureaplasma gallorale* has been isolated from the upper respiratory tract of healthy chickens. Experimental challenge of chickens and turkeys with ureaplasmas has produced variable results. *Ureaplasma* sp. has been isolated from turkeys with infertility problems. In humans, *U. parvum* and *U. urealyticum* are etiologic agents of genitourinary infections. Several lines of evidence have suggested that they play a role in the etiology of nongonococcal urethritis. *Ureaplasma urealyticum* is the agent of a serious infection of neonates that can cause either a severe respiratory disease in utero or mild to severe meningitis.

Ureaplasmas are mucosal parasites. Although generally considered opportunistic pathogens, the extent of their pathogenicity is poorly understood. They can produce ammonia from the hydrolysis of urea, and urease activity is essential to generation of ATP. Urea production may be an important virulence mechanism in host tissue damage. *Ureaplasma diversum* cultivated in bovine oviduct tissue cultures stops the action of cilia and produces deciliation and desquamation of the epithelium. High levels of ammonia may contribute to lesion development.

Ureaplasmas require urea for growth but are inhibited by the higher alkalinity resulting from urea metabolism. Thus isolation media must be highly buffered. In any case, ureaplasmas are difficult to isolate. Colonies usually develop after 24 to 72 hours of incubation. Unlike those of *Mycoplasma,* typical "fried-egg"–type colonies are uncommon. On agar medium containing manganese sulfate, ureaplasmas produce brown colonies as a result of the deposition of manganese on the colonial surface. Lack of growth on media without urea differentiates them from mycoplasmas. Serotyping of isolates can be accomplished by an immunofluorescence assay, and PCR is available as a sensitive detection assay.

Granular vulvitis may resolve spontaneously, but many treatments have been attempted. Intrauterine infusion of tetracycline solutions has been advocated. Artificial insemination instead of live cover may decrease transmission to cows.

SUGGESTED READINGS

Messick JB, Walker PG, Raphael W, et al: 'Candidatus Mycoplasma haemodidelphidis' sp. nov., 'Candidatus Mycoplasma haemolamae' sp. nov. and *Mycoplasma haemocanis* comb. nov., haemotrophic parasites from a naturally infected opossum (*Didelphis virginiana*), alpaca (*Lama pacos*) and dog (*Canis familiaris*): phylogenetic and secondary structural relatedness of their 16S rRNA genes to other mycoplasmas, *Int J Syst Evol Microbiol* 52:693-698, 2002.

Neimark H, Johansson KE, Rikihisa Y, Tully JG: Proposal to transfer some members of the genera *Haemobartonella* and *Eperythrozoon* to the genus *Mycoplasma* with descriptions of 'Candidatus Mycoplasma haemofelis,' 'Candidatus Mycoplasma haemomuris,' 'Candidatus Mycoplasma haemosuis' and 'Candidatus Mycoplasma wenyonii,' *Int J Syst Evol Microbiol* 51:891-899, 2001.

Nicholas RAJ, Ayling RD: *Mycoplasma bovis*: disease, diagnosis, and control, *Res Vet Sci* 74:105-112, 2003.

Robertson JA, Stemke GW, Davis JW, et al: Proposal of *Ureaplasma parvum* sp. nov. and emended description of *Ureaplasma urealyticum* (Shepard et al. 1974; Robertson et al. 2001), *Int J Syst Evol Microbiol* 52:587-597, 2002.

Tasker S, Lappin MR: *Haemobartonella felis*: recent developments in diagnosis and treatment, *J Feline Med Surg* 4:3-11, 2002.

Whitford HW, Rosenbusch RF, Lauerman LH, eds: Mycoplasmosis in animals: laboratory diagnosis, Ames, Iowa, 1994, Iowa State University Press.

Chapter 40

The Family Anaplasmataceae

The family Anaplasmataceae has been reorganized based on 16S rRNA gene sequences to include all species of α-*Proteobacteria* in the genera *Neorickettsia, Anaplasma, Ehrlichia,* and *Wolbachia; Aegyptianella* has been retained as a genus incertae sedis (Table 40-1). *Wolbachia* spp. are associated exclusively with invertebrates, and the genera *Eperythrozoon* and *Haemobartonella* have been transferred to the order Mycoplasmatales. The obligately intracellular Anaplasmataceae replicate within cytoplasmic vacuoles of host cells, such as erythrocytes, reticuloendothelial cells, bone marrow–derived phagocytic cells, endothelial cells, and reproductive tissues of insects, arthropods, or helminths. Most members have a trematode, tick, or other invertebrate vector host.

THE GENUS *NEORICKETTSIA*

Neorickettsia spp. are small, nonmotile, coccoid to crescentric, intracytoplasmic, gram-negative bacteria that are found within vacuoles of monocytes, macrophages in lymphoid tissues, and occasionally in enterocytes. They stain readily with Giemsa or Macchiavello stains and cannot be cultivated in cell-free media or in chicken embryos. Flukes serve as vectors, and all stages within the life cycle of flukes are infectious. The infectious cycle includes transovarial and transstadial transmission.

Neorickettsiae maintain their individual vacuolar membranes when they undergo binary fission, so intracellular inclusions may not be observed microscopically. Cell lysis leads to release of cell-free bacteria that can infect other host cells.

Species of note are *N. helminthoeca, N. (Ehrlichia) risticii,* and *N. (Ehrlichia) sennetsu.* Molecular and antigenic analyses have recently established a close relationship among these organisms and further similarities may exist in their modes of transmission.

Neorickettsia helminthoeca

Salmon poisoning disease was first recognized in the early nineteenth century by settlers in the Pacific Northwest when their dogs fell ill after consuming raw salmon. The causative agent, *N. helminthoeca,* was characterized in 1953, but could not be placed in a previously described genus based on the disease and morphologic characteristics. It is unique, in that it is the only obligately helminth-borne pathogenic bacterium. Canine mononuclear cells are infected after dogs ingest salmonid fish encysted with a fluke, *Nanophyetus salmincola* (Figure 40-1), infected with the organism. The disease is indigenous to

TABLE 40-1 Anaplasmataceae of Veterinary Importance

Organism	Host	Disease	Vector Reservoir	Infected Cells	Geographic Distribution
Aegyptianella spp.	Birds, reptiles, amphibians	Anemia, sudden death	*Argus, Amblyomma, Ixodes* spp. Unknown	RBC	Africa, Asia, South America, Southern Europe, South Texas
Anaplasma (Ehrlichia) bovis	Cattle	Bovine ehrlichiosis	*Rhipicephalus appendiculatus, Amblyomma variegatum, A. cajennense, Hyalomma excavatum* Rabbits, ruminants?	Mononuclear leukocytes	Africa, Asia, South America
Anaplasma caudatum, centrale, marginale, ovis	Ruminants	Anaplasmosis	*Boophilus, Dermacentor, Ixodes,* or *Rhipicephalus* species Ruminants, wild cervids	RBC	Worldwide
Anaplasma phagocytophilum (*Ehrlichia equi;* HGE agent, *E. phagocytophila*)	Humans, horses, small ruminants	Human and equine granulocytic ehrlichiosis, tick-borne fever	*Ixodes* spp. Deer, sheep, white-footed mice	Granulocytes	Worldwide
Anaplasma (Ehrlichia) platys	Dogs	Infectious cyclic thrombocytopenia	*Rhipicephalus sanguineus?* Ruminant?	Platelets	United States, Southern Europe, Middle East, Venezuela, Taiwan
Ehrlichia canis	Canidae	Canine monocytic ehrlichiosis	*Rhipicephalus sanguineus, Amblyomma americanum?* Canids	Mononuclear leukocytes	Worldwide
Ehrlichia chaffeensis	Humans, dogs, deer	Human monocytic ehrlichiosis	*Amblyomma americanum, Dermacentor variablis* Domestic dogs, white-tailed deer	Mononuclear leukocytes	United States
Ehrlichia ewingii	Dogs, humans	Canine granulocytic ehrlichiosis	*Amblyomma americanum* Canids	Granulocytes	United States
Ehrlichia muris	Mice	Not named	*Haemaphysalis flava* Not known	Mononuclear leukocytes	Not known
Ehrlichia (Cowdria) ruminantium	Ruminants	Heartwater	*Amblyomma* ticks Ruminants	Granulocytes, endothelium, macrophages	Sub-Saharan Africa, Caribbean
Neorickettsia helminthoeca	Canidae	Salmon poisoning disease	Ingestion of fluke-infested salmonid fish Fluke-infested fish	Mononuclear leukocytes	U.S. Pacific Northwest
Neorickettsia (Ehrlichia) risticii	Horses	Potomac horse fever equine monocytic ehrlichiosis	Ingestion of fluke infested insects Flukes	Mononuclear leukocytes, enterocytes	North and South America
Neorickettsia (Ehrlichia) sennetsu	Humans	Sennetsu fever	Ingestion of fluke infested fish Fluke-infested fish	Mononuclear leukocytes	Japan, Southeast Asia

HGF, Human granulocytic ehrlichiosis; *RBC,* red blood cell.

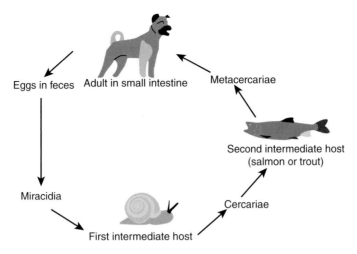

FIGURE 40-1 Life cycle of *Nanophyetus salmincola*. (Courtesy Ashley E. Harmon.)

river areas of the U.S. Pacific Northwest coast, from northern California to southwestern Washington State. Occasional cases associated with fish migration have been reported in British Columbia.

The raccoon and spotted skunk are the principal definitive hosts for the fluke. Adult flukes develop in the intestinal lumen within 6 days after ingestion in dogs, cats, foxes, bears, coyotes, opossums, otter, mink, lynx, and birds. Infected eggs shed in feces hatch and release a miracidium. The miracidium penetrates the first intermediate host, the snail *Oxytrema silicula*, where the cecariae (free-living trematode larvae) develop. Cercariae are liberated and penetrate the skin of the secondary intermediate host, which are fish, usually of the family Salmonidae, or Pacific giant salamanders. Metacercariae are found in the muscle, kidney, eye, and other organs of fish and salamanders. *Neorickettsia helminthoeca* is maintained by transovarial passage in the helminth and is found throughout the life cycle of the fluke, including free-swimming cercariae.

Salmon poisoning (Figure 40-2) generally affects only members of the family Canidae, but death of captive polar bears has been reported in association with salmon poisoning disease. After ingestion of infested fish, the trematodes attach to and penetrate deeply into the mucosa, particularly in the duodenum but also throughout the small and large intestines. The precise mechanism of infection remains to be elucidated, but superficial enteritis develops rapidly, and progresses to hemorrhagic enteritis. Bacteria spread by the hematogenous route to lymph nodes, spleen, liver, lungs, brain, and thymus. Acute disease is characterized by fever, depression, dehydration, anorexia, diarrhea, and lymphadenopathy. The case fatality rate in untreated dogs is 50% to 90% and the exact cause of death remains unknown. Recovered animals are immune to reinfection.

Difficulties related to bacteriologic culture of *N. helminthoeca* have been a detriment to studying disease pathogenesis. Recently propagation in a continuous cell line has facilitated antigenic and genetic analyses. Canine monocytes, canine leukocytes, mouse lymphoblasts, and a macrophage line support in vitro growth.

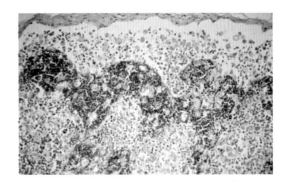

FIGURE 40-2 Lymph node with lesions of salmon poisoning, showing accumulation of bacteria-laden macrophages in the subcapsular sinus and among the medullary cords. Edema is evident. (Courtesy Raymond E. Reed.)

Antemortem diagnosis is based on detection of fluke eggs in feces, presence of compatible clinical signs, history of travel to the Pacific Northwest, demonstration of rickettsiae in lymph node aspirates, and serology. Trematode eggs are operculated and are passed in the feces 5 to 8 days after fish ingestion. They can be detected by direct smears or sugar flotation techniques. Macchiavello or Giemsa stains of lymph node aspirates reveal intracytoplasmic rickettsial bodies, but organisms are not detected by microscopic examination of circulating lymphocytes. Affected animals typically seroconvert 13 to 15 days postinfection, so several veterinary diagnostic laboratories offer serologic diagnosis by way of indirect fluorescent antibody or complement fixation tests.

Postmortem diagnosis is based on compatible gross and microscopic lesions. Changes are primarily associated with lymphoid tissues, and include lymphadenopathy, splenomegaly, and petechiation of the gallbladder, pancreas, and mucosae of the esophagus, urinary bladder, and intestinal tract. General lymph node enlargement is attributed to marked infiltration of macrophages. Microscopic lesions include depletion of mature lymphocytes from lymph node cortex and medulla, nonsuppurative meningoencephalitis, splenic follicular central hemorrhage and necrosis, and obliteration of thymic architecture. Coccoid bodies may be found within the macrophages.

Prevention of the disease involves not allowing raw or improperly cooked fish to be fed to dogs. Thorough cooking, or freezing at −20° C for 24 hours, kills *N. helminthoeca* and metacercariae. If infected raw fish is eaten, apomorphine should be administered as an emetic. Sick animals are given supportive care to control vomiting and diarrhea, and to maintain acid-base balance. Parenteral administration of tetracyclines is usually helpful, but there are no commercial vaccines.

Elokomin Fluke Fever

Elokomin fluke fever (EFF), which is similar to salmon poisoning disease, was first described in the Elokomin River valley of Washington State. The etiologic agent is suspected to be a less virulent strain of *N. helminthoeca*. The organism has been referred to as "*Neorickettsia elokominica,*" and EFF is also associated with ingestion of raw fish. Clinical features distinguishing this disease from salmon poisoning are incubation period, character of the febrile response, persistence of lymphadenopathy, low mortality, and lack of conferred immunity between the two diseases. The incubation period for EFF, at 5 to 12 days, is slightly longer than that for salmon poisoning. The period of elevated temperature is extended, lasting 4 to 7 days. Other clinical signs are identical to, but less severe than, those observed in salmon poisoning. Bears, in addition to dogs, appear to be susceptible to EFF. Serologic differentiation between EFF and salmon poisoning disease has been accomplished by way of the complement fixation test.

Neorickettsia (Ehrlichia) risticii

Neorickettsia risticii is the agent of Potomac horse fever (PHF), an acute diarrheic illness of equids, also known as equine monocytic ehrlichiosis or equine scours, because of the affinity of the organism for blood monocytes, tissue macrophages, and intestinal epithelial cells. The disease was first recognized in 1979 in areas bordering the Potomac River in Virginia and Maryland. Since then it has been diagnosed in most states within the continental United States, several Canadian provinces, and South America (Brazil, Venezuela, and Uruguay). Serologic evidence of PHF has been found in France, India, and Australia.

The epidemiology of PHF has remained obscure since its discovery more than 20 years ago. The disease appears to be restricted to low-lying regions in proximity to bodies of water, and there is a seasonal pattern with peak incidence occurring during summer. Arthropod vectors do not appear to be involved in transmission, but *N. risticii* is found in the feces of infected horses. Oral transmission has been demonstrated experimentally, but this route is not natural.

Neorickettsia risticii appears to be maintained in nature in a complex aquatic ecosystem. The infection cycle apparently involves an intermediate snail reservoir and a trematode cercarial vector. In the laboratory, researchers have infected mice and horses by intraperitoneal subcutaneous inoculation, respectively, with trematodes from snails. DNA of *N. risticii* has been found in virgulate cercariae from the freshwater snails *Juga yrekaensis* in northern California and *Elimia livescens* in Ohio. Such DNA has also been detected in metacercariae from aquatic insects, such as caddis flies, stoneflies, damselflies, mayflies, and dragonflies. Oral transmission of PHF has been demonstrated in horses fed caddis flies, and it is natural to speculate that transmission to horses involves accidental ingestion of insects harboring infected metacercariae. Potential helminth vectors include *Lecithodendrium* and *Acanthatrium* spp. These *N. risticii*–infected helminths have been found in the intestinal tracts of bats and birds, but no definitive reservoir host has been identified. Besides horses, other susceptible mammals include cattle, mice, dogs, and cats. In endemic locations, antibody titers to *N. risticii* have been found in goats, pigs, cats, dogs, and coyotes.

The primary clinical sign is acute, watery diarrhea. Mild colic, anorexia, fever, depression, edema, dehydration, laminitis, and leukopenia are additional findings. Rarely, abortion may result from infection in the unborn fetus. The case fatality rate is 5% to 30%. Fatalities result if severely affected horses are not treated promptly with electrolytes, fluids, and appropriate antimicrobial agents.

The watery diarrhea is a direct result of enterocyte infection. Degeneration of infected epithelial cells, with loss of microvilli, results in accumulation of cAMP and physical inability to conduct electrolyte transport in the colonic mucosa. Malabsorption of sodium and chloride ions and lack of water resorption lead to diarrhea.

A diagnosis of PHF is suggested in horses exhibiting nonspecific signs and diarrhea during the summer months in areas endemic for *N. risticii*. Several options are available for the diagnosis of PHF, including an indirect fluorescent antibody test. Rising titers with accompanying clinical signs suggests active infection. Detection of the organism in infected tissues has been accomplished using a modified Steiner silver stain, an immunoperoxidase method, or transmission electron microscopy. Definitive diagnosis of PHF formerly required isolation of *N. risticii* in cell culture, but polymerase chain reaction (PCR) amplification of DNA from peripheral blood or feces has proven to be a highly specific and sensitive means of diagnosis.

Commercial, inactivated vaccines for PHF are available but the antibody response to vaccination has been poor and there are consistent reports of vaccine failure in the field, particularly in endemic areas. Heterogeneous strains of *N. risticii* have been recovered from field-vaccinated horses suffering from clinical PHF. Thus it appears that both a deficiency in antibody response and heterogeneity among isolates are responsible for the present vaccine failures. Infections can be treated by intravenous administration of oxytetracycline early in the course of the disease.

Neorickettsia (Ehrlichia) sennetsu

The first neorickettsial pathogen of humans was identified in Japan in 1953. Sennetsu fever, caused by *N. (Ehrlichia) sennetsu*, is characterized by fever and swollen lymph nodes. The disease is very rare outside the Far East and Southeast Asia, with the majority of cases having been reported from western Japan. Epidemiologic studies suggest that infection is acquired through ingestion of raw gray mullet fish infested with the metacercarial stage of trematodes infected with *N. sennetsu*. This organism is infectious but nonpathogenic for horses, and inoculation with *N. sennetsu* has protected horses from PHF upon challenge with *N. risticii*. Laboratory mice are highly susceptible to infection.

THE GENUS *ANAPLASMA*

With the inclusion of the former *Ehrlichia bovis*, *Ehrlichia phagocytophila*, *Ehrlichia equi*, and *Ehrlichia platys*, the description of the genus *Anaplasma* was amended to include gram-negative, small coccoid to ellipsoid bacteria that live within cytoplasmic vacuoles of myeloid cells, neutrophils, and erythrocytes in peripheral blood, or in tissues of the mononuclear phagocyte organs. Organisms occur singly, or more commonly in inclusions called morulae, and stain bluish purple by Romanovsky methods. Biologic vectors are usually ticks. The genus now consists of species *Anaplasma bovis*, *Anaplasma caudatum*, *Anaplasma centrale*, *Anaplasma marginale*, *Anaplasma ovis*, *Anaplasma phagocytophilum*, and *Anaplasma platys*.

Anaplasma (Ehrlichia) bovis

A. bovis infects mononuclear cells of cattle and possibly sheep in tropical and subtropical regions of the world. Disease is characterized by anemia and weight loss, and, rarely, by abortion and death. Survivors are lifelong carriers. Organisms are infrequently observed within the cytoplasm of monocytes in peripheral blood smears. Tick vectors include *Amblyomma cajennense*, *Amblyomma variegatum*, *Rhipicephalus appendiculatus*, and *Hyalomma excavatum*. Serologic cross-reactions with *Ehrlichia ruminantium* have been documented.

Anaplasma caudatum

Bovine anaplasmosis in the United States may be caused by the intraerythrocytic bacteria *A. caudatum* and *A. marginale*. Organisms are transmitted biologically by ixodid ticks and mechanically by biting flies or veterinary procedures. Clinical and pathologic signs include anemia, icterus, splenomegaly, gallbladder obstruction, erythrophagocytosis, and hemosiderosis. Pregnant cows may abort. The natural history of infection is characterized by four sequential stages; an incubation period of 3 to 5 weeks is followed by patency, with clinical signs lasting 2 or more weeks, convalescence of 4 to 8 weeks, marked by increased hematopoiesis and recrudescence, and an indefinitely long carrier state during which hematologic values return to normal. Tetracyclines are used for elimination of the carrier state.

Anaplasma centrale

Anaplasma centrale produces a natural, persistent infection of bovine erythrocytes. As implied by the name, the bacteria are usually found in the center of red blood cells. Subclinical disease is common, but in some instances fever and anemia without icterus may result. The agent has been employed as an immunizing agent against *A. marginale* in endemic areas.

Anaplasma marginale

Initially described by Theiler in 1908 as a developmental stage of the protozoan *Babesia bigemina*, *A. marginale* is the primary cause of bovine anaplasmosis, an economically significant disease on six continents. Biologic transmission occurs when infected hard ticks in the genera *Boophilus*, *Dermacentor*, *Ixodes*, or *Rhipicephalus* feed on immunologically naive cattle. Mechanical transmission occurs through biting flies or blood-contaminated fomites such as used hypodermic needles or dehorning instruments. Cattle that recover from acute infection remain persistently infected for years, with microscopically undetectable levels of the organism. Carriers develop clinical disease when stressed. Persistence in primary hosts is fundamental to continued transmission because transovarial transmission of *A. marginale* in the tick vector does not occur. Anaplasmosis is enzootic in the southern Atlantic and Gulf Coast states, on the lower plains, and in western states, but occurs sporadically in northern states. Natural and biologic vectors are seasonal, so there is a correlation between disease outbreaks and vector seasons.

Anaplasma marginale causes fever, anorexia, weight loss, decreased fertility in bulls, and icterus. Acute disease is characterized by severe anemia, pale mucous membranes, and lethargy. Animals may be belligerent if hypoxia affects the brain. Cows in late pregnancy may abort. Animals less than 1 year old are susceptible to infection but relatively resistant to disease, whereas cattle older than 36 months of age usually experience severe disease with a 30% to 50% case fatality rate.

Anaplasmosis induced by *A. marginale* occurs in four stages. The *incubation period* comprises the time from introduction of the agent into a susceptible animal until 1% of the red blood cells are parasitized. This varies from 3 to 8 weeks and depends on the initial number of infecting organisms. During this time the animal remains asymptomatic. The first clinical signs become apparent during the *developmental stage*, when more than 15% of the erythrocytes are infected. Fever is the initial finding, followed by anorexia, depression, and lethargy. The length of this period ranges from 4 to 9 days. The *convalescent stage* varies greatly in length, from weeks to months, and extends from the appearance of reticulocytes in peripheral circulation until the blood values return to normal. Mortality may occur during the early convalescent stage. Necropsy findings are attributable to hemolytic anemia. Grossly, the blood appears thin and watery. Other findings include tissue pallor, icterus, hepatosplenomegaly, and enlarged gallbladder. The *carrier stage* may last for the remainder of the life of the animal.

Within the tick, the bacterium undergoes a complex developmental cycle that involves the gut initially and ultimately the salivary gland, from which transmission occurs during feeding. When the organism invades mature erythrocytes, replication occurs by binary fission within membrane-bound cytoplasmic inclusions and two to eight infective initial bodies are formed. These leave the red blood cells by exocytosis to infect other susceptible erythrocytes.

The severity of the disease is related directly to the proportion of the erythrocyte mass destroyed. Hemoglobinuria does not occur in anaplasmosis because the destruction of erythrocytes occurs intracellularly rather than intravascularly. Serum factors sensitize erythrocytes to phagocytosis by the monocyte-macrophage system and these opsonins increase in the circulation before the hemolytic crisis. Fetal hypoxia is responsible for abortion.

Persistence of *A. marginale* in fully immunocompetent hosts is mediated by antigenic variation in the organism's major surface proteins. Recently, *A. marginale* has been propagated in continuous culture in a tick embryo cell line. This system has been used as an infection model and for adhesion studies. Adhesion, infection, and transmission are mediated by major surface protein 1a.

A presumptive diagnosis of anaplasmosis is based on clinical signs and hematologic findings in animals in an endemic area. Serologic testing, direct examination of blood smears, and molecular methods are also useful. Rapid card agglutination, complement fixation, and enzyme immunoassays are available for serologic diagnosis. Phenotypic criteria for identification of ruminant erythrocytic *Anaplasma* spp. (*A. centrale, A. marginale,* and *A. ovis*) have for many years relied on subjective methods, such as the location of inclusion bodies in host red blood cells (Figure 40-3) and host pathogenicity (cattle vs. sheep). Recent studies have confirmed the suitability of 16S rDNA sequence analysis to define the species from blood samples.

Prevention and control measures include testing the herd and removing carriers, administering tetracyclines, vaccination, vector control, and good hygiene. Killed, whole-cell vaccines have reduced the severity of disease, and their use is advocated when mature susceptible cattle are to be shipped to an epizootically stable location. Reducing vector transmission through application of insecticidal sprays or dusts substantially reduces the biting insect population. Disease transmission can occur via blood-contaminated instruments, so disinfectants should be used to clean equipment between animals.

Anaplasma ovis

Anaplasma ovis induces anemia, depression, fever, and anorexia, with low mortality, in sheep and goats, following invasion and replication within erythrocytes. Cattle are not clinically affected. Infections have been documented throughout the world, but loss of livestock productivity and extent of infection remain poorly understood. Reports of acute infections in tropical and subtropical regions, where small ruminants are an important source of food, suggest that the disease may be widespread and of economic significance. Diagnosis has been based primarily on finding organisms in Giemsa-stained blood smears. A DNA probe has been used to identify infected animals, but this method is useful only in the acute stages of illness because limited sensitivity of the probe prohibits detection of persistently infected carrier animals. A competitive inhibition enzyme immunoassay has been developed for detection of infected animals.

Anaplasma phagocytophilum

This new species was created to accommodate the former *Ehrlichia equi, E. phagocytophila,* and the unnamed agent of human granulocytic ehrlichiosis (HGE). These gram-negative, pleomorphic, coccoid to ellipsoidal organisms infect bone marrow–derived cells. The preferred habitat is the cytoplasm of host granulocytes, where it forms microcolonies or morulae containing up to 20 individual organisms that may be detectable in peripheral blood. Tick vectors include *Ixodes* spp. White-tailed deer and white-footed mice may act as reservoirs in nature. Besides horses, ruminants, and humans, dogs appear to be susceptible to the agent.

Equine granulocytic ehrlichiosis (EGE) is an infectious, noncontagious disease of horses first described in the 1960s in northern California. It is characterized by fever, anorexia, depression, limb edema, jaundice, petechiation, and ataxia. Most horses are affected during the late fall, winter, and spring. In the United States, the disease has been reported with increasing frequency in the Pacific Northwest, Colorado, Florida, New Jersey, Minnesota, Wisconsin, Connecticut, and Illinois.

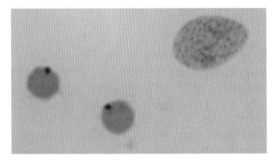

FIGURE 40-3 Blood smear from cow with anaplasmosis, showing two typically parasitized erythrocytes and an immature form. (Courtesy Raymond E. Reed.)

Brazil, Canada, and several European countries have confirmed cases of EGE. After tick exposure and an incubation period of 2 to 3 weeks, the horse develops a fever followed in a few days by limb edema. EGE is generally self-limiting, but rare complications such as myocardial vasculitis or secondary infections may develop. Hematologic abnormalities include thrombocytopenia, leukopenia, and anemia. Immunity involves cellular and humoral responses. Diagnosis is based on clinical signs, demonstration of cytoplasmic inclusion bodies in neutrophils, serology, and molecular methods. Organisms may be seen in stained blood films obtained on days 3 to 5 of fever during peak bacteremia. The inclusion bodies have a unique pleomorphic appearance with a spoked-wheel pattern. Indirect fluorescent antibody titers persist for more than a month after experimental infection, and a fourfold or greater increase in titer between paired serum samples is considered diagnostically significant. Recently, a specific and sensitive PCR assay has been made available in reference labs. No vaccine is available for EGE, so tick control measures are necessary to prevent disease. Therapy involves intravenous administration of oxytetracycline.

Tick-borne fever, caused by the former *E. phagocytophila,* is a disease of wild and domestic ruminants that is limited to parts of Europe. *Ixodes ricinus* is the primary vector where transmission is transstadial. Infected ticks transmit the bacteria to susceptible ruminant hosts. Persistently infected ruminants are probably efficient reservoirs of *A. phagocytophilum* during the acute and postacute phases of infection. Variations in tick density strongly affect the infection rate in ruminants. Tick-borne fever has an incubation period of up to 2 weeks. Clinical signs include fever, anorexia, failure to thrive, decreased milk production, and rarely, stillbirth and abortion. Infection tends to predispose to secondary infections because tick-borne fever causes immunosuppression. Diagnosis is based on residence in an endemic region, clinical signs, demonstration of the organism within neutrophils during the febrile stage of illness, and positive indirect immunofluorescence test to detect antibody titers. Therapy and prevention are similar to EGE.

HGE is an emerging disease that occurs primarily in the northeastern and upper Midwestern United States, as well as in Scandinavia and Switzerland. Disease is usually characterized by an acute, sometimes fatal febrile syndrome, commonly accompanied by myalgia, arthralgia, headache, and malaise. Laboratory findings include leukopenia, thrombocytopenia, and anemia.

Anaplasma phagocytophilum has developed strategies to survive intracellularly. The organism produces proteins that extend the longevity of host cells, thus ensuring that this pathogen has adequate time to multiply. The newly recognized proteins delay apoptosis in neutrophils. Because cytoplasmic vacuoles do not fuse with lysosomes inside the cell, the agent is insulated against several destructive features of host lysosomes. The respiratory burst, one of the primary methods of antimicrobial activity of neutrophils, is also inhibited by *A. phagocytophilum.*

Diagnosis is virtually impossible based on clinical and epidemiologic findings. Disease should be considered when patients present with acute febrile illness in an appropriate geographic area and during the seasons when the required vector ticks are active.

In vitro studies have suggested that quinolone antibiotics and rifampin may be alternative agents for patients intolerant to tetracyclines.

Anaplasma (Ehrlichia) platys

Canine infectious cyclic thrombocytopenia, caused by *A. (Ehrlichia) platys,* is so named because parasitemia and thrombocytopenia are of a cyclical nature, occurring at 10- to 14-day intervals. A tick vector is suspected *(Rhipicephalus sanguineus),* but to date none has been confirmed. First reported in the United States, the geographic distribution now includes southern Europe, the Middle East, Venezuela, and Taiwan. Although *A. platys* infects platelets, it is generally of low pathogenicity. Affected animals are febrile, depressed, and anorexic. Rarely, more severe symptoms such as uveitis, epistaxis, lymphadenopathy, and petechial or ecchymotic hemorrhages of the oral mucosa and skin may occur. In some instances, coinfection with other infectious agents (e.g., *E. canis*) may potentiate the clinical effects of both. Thrombocytopenia is the principal hematologic change associated with acute ehrlichial infection and it has been suggested to be immune mediated. Mild regenerative anemia also may occur. The anemia has been associated with inflammation and is attributed to low-grade hemolysis, sequestration of iron by macrophages, and decreased erythropoiesis.

Diagnosis may be accomplished by finding the organisms within platelets during examination of stained blood smears. However, this method is unreliable because *A. platys*, if present, is in low numbers. Other tests include an indirect fluorescent antibody test to detect serum antibodies and a PCR assay to detect the agent in platelets. Because of the probable involvement of a tick vector, vector control measures are recommended for disease prevention. Tetracyclines are effective for therapy.

THE GENUS *EHRLICHIA*

Ehrlichia are pleomorphic coccoid to ellipsoid gram-negative bacteria. They reside and multiply by binary fission within membrane-bound cytoplasmic vacuoles derived from an early endosome of host mononuclear and polymorphonuclear leukocytes and endothelial cells (Figure 40-4). These organisms enter and maintain distinct cytoplasmic compartments forming inclusions (morulae) that do not fuse with each other or with lysosomes. A larger reticulate cell and a smaller dense core form are observed by electron microscopy. *Ehrlichia* spp. stain bluish purple with Romanovsky-type methods, including Giemsa, Wright, and Diff-Quik. Ticks are the usual vectors.

Infection of the vertebrate host occurs when the infected tick ingests a blood meal and salivary secretions contaminate the feeding site. The emended genus now includes the five species *E. canis, Ehrlichia chaffeensis, Ehrlichia ewingii, Ehrlichia muris,* and *Ehrlichia ruminantium;* the last was previously known as *Cowdria ruminantium.* Other organisms formerly classified in the genus, including *E. equi, E. phagocytophila, E. platys, E. risticii,* and *E. sennetsu,* have been transferred to new genera.

Definitive diagnosis of infections by these agents may be difficult. Clinical and hematologic abnormalities are often nonspecific. A variety of serodiagnostic tests are available, but the diagnostic value of most remains unevaluated. Isolation and growth of ehrlichiae is difficult, time consuming, and of limited availability. Specific and sensitive assays, such as PCR and sequencing, are now used for detection of ehrlichiae.

Ehrlichia canis

First reported in Algeria in 1935, canine monocytic ehrlichiosis caused by *E. canis* is a common and widespread disease of tropical to temperate parts of Asia, Africa, North America, and Europe. Other names for this disease are tropical canine

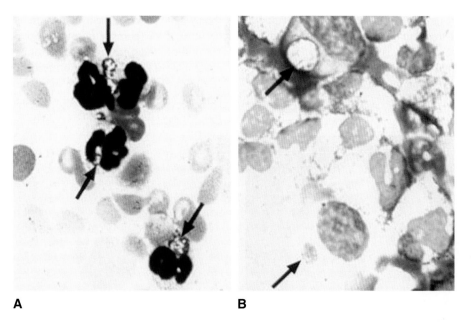

A   **B**

FIGURE 40-4   Granulocytic **(A)** and monocytic **(B)** infection by *Ehrlichia chaffeensis.* Arrows point to organisms within granulocytes and monocytes, respectively. (Courtesy Public Health Image Library, PHIL #87, Centers for Disease Control and Prevention/National Center for Infectious Diseases, Atlanta, 1997.)

pancytopenia, canine hemorrhagic fever, tracker-dog disease, and Nairobi bleeding disorder. In the Vietnam War era, the illness received considerable attention as a cause of mortality in U.S. military dogs stationed in Southeast Asia.

Members of the family Canidae are the vertebrate hosts and the brown dog tick, *R. sanguineus,* is the primary arthropod vector. Experimental transmission has been accomplished with *Amblyomma americanum.* Ticks become infected when they feed on bacteremic dogs. Transstadial, but not transovarial transmission occurs in the tick. *Ehrlichia canis* disseminates from the gut of the tick to the salivary gland, where bacteria are injected into a susceptible host as the tick feeds. Larvae, nymphs, and adults can transmit the bacterium.

The clinical course of disease has been divided into three phases. The *acute phase,* which begins after an 8- to 20-day incubation period, is characterized by fever, anorexia, depression, lymphadenopathy, oculonasal discharge, and dyspnea. Hematologic changes at this time include thrombocytopenia, leukopenia, and anemia. The acute phase generally resolves spontaneously, and is followed by the *subclinical phase.* During this 2- to 4-month period, the animal appears clinically normal, and immunocompetent dogs eliminate *E. canis.* The *chronic phase* develops in dogs that are unable to eliminate the organism. Hemorrhage, epistaxis (Figure 40-5), emaciation, and peripheral edema are frequent observations with chronic disease. Disease severity is related to the breed of the dog infected. German shepherds are at a higher risk for developing severe disease manifestations.

Recently, natural *E. canis* infection was described in cats. Clinical manifestations were polyarthritis and pancytopenia. Serologic and molecular evidence supported the diagnosis.

Canine mononuclear cells are attracted to the site of tick bites, as part of the normal inflammatory response, and this facilitates the infection process. Ehrlichiae are carried to lymph nodes by the monocytes, from whence they escape into systemic circulation. They localize in endoreticular cells of lymph nodes, spleen, and liver, where replication occurs in mononuclear macrophages and lymphocytes. Organisms are released by both exocytosis and cell lysis. Hematologic changes are associated with immune and coagulation dysfunction that are directly related to the infection. Thrombocytopenia has been attributed to vasculitis and associated increased platelet consumption or sequestration. Antiplatelet antibodies are apparently directed against platelet glycoproteins, thus playing a role in platelet aggregation inhibition. Epistaxis is a result of hemorrhages in the lungs or nasal mucosa because *E. canis*–infected cells are found in the microvasculature of the lung.

Diagnosis is based on clinical signs, hematologic abnormalities, demonstration of morulae in peripheral monocytes (Figure 40-6), detection of serum antibodies, and demonstration of the agent in blood, by culture or molecular assays. Clinical signs may be variable through the course of the disease, and morulae are usually difficult to detect because of low parasite numbers. Approximately 4% of the blood smears evaluated from dogs in the acute stage of illness have demonstrable inclusions. In the absence of other clinical signs, anorexia and generalized depression, coupled with characteristic but nonspecific hematologic changes, are suggestive of ehrlichiosis. Various serologic tests are

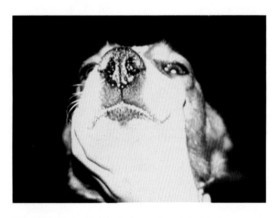

FIGURE 40-5 Epistaxis in canine ehrlichiosis. (Courtesy Raymond E. Reed.)

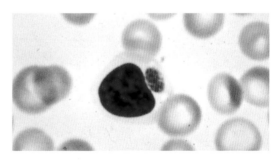

FIGURE 40-6 *Ehrlichia canis*–infected lymphocyte. (Courtesy Raymond E. Reed.)

available for diagnosis, the gold standard being the indirect immunofluorescence assay; however, cross-reactions with other species often preclude definitive diagnosis. Cell culture isolation of the agent is both sensitive and specific, but requires 1 to 4 weeks and is performed in only a limited number of reference laboratories. PCR amplification of ehrlichial DNA is gaining acceptance as an adjunct to serologic testing. A recently developed, highly specific and sensitive PCR assay for *E. canis* has been used to confirm the presence of disease in dogs with clinical signs but without morulae on blood smears.

Prevention involves tick control because vaccines are currently unavailable. Tetracycline chemoprophylaxis has been used to control disease in endemic regions. *Ehrlichia canis* may not be eliminated by doxycycline therapy.

Ehrlichia chaffeensis

The first isolation of *E. chaffeensis* was from Army officers at Fort Chaffee, Arkansas. This agent proliferates exclusively in monocytes and macrophages and is the cause of human monocytic ehrlichiosis. Severe disease manifestations may also occur in dogs, and natural infection has also been reported in coyotes, domestic goats, and lemurs. The white-tailed deer is recognized as a complete and sufficient host for maintaining the transmission cycle of *E. chaffeensis*, although dogs are potential reservoirs. The primary tick vector is *A. americanum,* but *E. chaffeensis* has also been found in the American dog tick, *Dermacentor variabilis.* There is no evidence of transovarial transmission in ticks.

Diagnosis can be accomplished by cultivation in a canine cell line. Serologic testing by indirect immunofluorescence assay (IFA) cannot consistently distinguish infection with *E. chaffeensis* from that by *E. canis*. Molecular detection and characterization of ehrlichial DNA by PCR and sequencing is necessary to definitively diagnose this disease. Like *E. canis,* this organism may not be eliminated by doxycycline therapy. Animals may remain PCR positive after treatment with doxycycline at a dose and duration generally considered to be efficacious for the treatment of ehrlichial infections.

Ehrlichia ewingii

Canine granulocytic ehrlichiosis was first reported in 1971. The etiology was initially ascribed to a less virulent strain of *E. canis,* but in the 1990s was found to be a new species, *E. ewingii*. Once thought exclusively to be a canine pathogen, the bacterium has recently been shown to infect humans. Subclinically affected dogs may provide a reservoir for human infection. Natural infection has been confirmed in deer, who may serve as an important reservoir for *E. ewingii*.

Amblyomma americanum, the Lone Star tick, is the only confirmed vector. However, *E. ewingii* DNA has recently been detected by PCR assay in *R. sanguineus* and *D. variabilis*.

Granulocytic ehrlichiosis has been reported in dogs from the southern United States (North Carolina, Virginia, Mississippi, Tennessee, Arkansas, Kentucky, Georgia, and South Carolina), as well as Missouri, Oklahoma, New York, Wisconsin, Minnesota, and California. Most *E. ewingii*–infected dogs have polyarthritis, fever, and thrombocytopenia; however, ataxia and paresis may also be present.

Morulae may be identified in neutrophils (Figure 40-7). The agent has been refractory to in vitro culture, and this has limited development of specific serologic testing. Cross-reactivity with *E. canis* antigens has been demonstrated. *Ehrlichia ewingii* can be confirmed in a clinical setting by use of a species-specific PCR assay, which is available in several reference laboratories.

Ehrlichia muris

Ehrlichia muris was originally isolated in Japan from the spleen of a wild mouse. The organism causes fever, lymphadenopathy, and splenomegaly when injected intraperitoneally into laboratory mice. There is serologic cross-reaction with *E. chaffeensis* and *E. canis*.

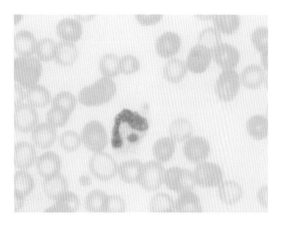

FIGURE 40-7 Neutrophil inclusion in blood smear from a dog with ehrlichiosis. (Courtesy Karen W. Post.)

Ehrlichia (Cowdria) ruminantium

Ehrlichia ruminantium comprises a clade of closely related bacteria, the majority of which cause heartwater disease in ruminants. Several of these strains have recently been associated with a disease in dogs reminiscent of canine ehrlichiosis.

Ehrlichia ruminantium is a small, pleomorphic, coccoid to ellipsoid, gram-negative rod that resides in membrane-bound vacuoles in the cytoplasm of vascular endothelial cells. During intracellular residence, the organisms are 0.2 to 0.5 μm in diameter and stain dark blue with Giemsa. Occasionally, they are found in densely packed clusters containing up to 50 organisms. Reproduction is by binary fission.

Heartwater is an infectious, noncontagious tick-borne disease of domestic and wild ruminants. Its name derives from the extensive pericardial effusion that may be a finding at necropsy. The disease was first recognized in the early 1800s in South African cattle and sheep, but it was not until 1925 that the causative agent was described by E.V. Cowdry. This often fatal disease is widespread in sub-Saharan Africa, Madagascar, and the eastern Caribbean. It is a serious constraint to animal production within endemic regions.

The epidemiology of heartwater is not completely understood, but the agent is known to be transmitted by ticks of the genus *Ambylomma*. These three-host ticks have a variety of hosts, ranging from birds to tortoises to mammals. Major vectors in Africa are *Amblyomma hebraeum* (the bont tick) and *A. variegatum*, while *A. cajennense* and *Amblyomma maculatum* serve as important vectors in the Western Hemisphere. Transstadial transmission occurs in vector ticks; transovarial transmission is infrequent.

Some animals such as the black wildebeest, springbok, and blesbok may serve as reservoirs. The various domestic hosts differ in their disease susceptibility. Goats and sheep are generally considered to be more susceptible to heartwater than cattle. Imported breeds of cattle, goats, and sheep tend to be more susceptible than indigenous breeds. In particular, Angora goats and Jersey or Brahman cattle are highly susceptible. Calves and lambs less than 3 weeks of age are highly resistant to disease, but become most susceptible in the early stages of sexual maturation.

Heartwater has peracute, acute, subacute, and chronic manifestations that depend on host susceptibility and virulence of the infecting strain. Peracute disease is characterized by fever, convulsions, prostration, and sudden death. The acute form is most common, with fever and nervous signs predominating. The animal initially appears listless and anorectic, and circling and walking with a stiff or unsteady gait follow, with progression to paddling movements, opisthotonos, nystagmus, and convulsions. Death ensues unless treatment is administered early in the course of the disease. Subacute and chronic forms of disease have been reported in animals with some natural resistance. Clinical signs are similar to those in acute disease, but are milder. At gross necropsy, hydropericardium, hydrothorax, pulmonary edema, splenomegaly, and occasionally hemorrhagic gastroenteritis may be found. *Ehrlichia ruminantium* may be observed in preparations taken from the cerebral cortex, hippocampus, and intimal surfaces of the large veins.

Ehrlichia ruminantium introduced by the tick bite is cleared from circulation by phagocytic cells, and subsequent replication takes place in lymph nodes and spleen. Infected cells rupture, resulting in bacteremia and subsequent infection of the vascular endothelial cells. The organism has a distinct predilection for endothelial cells of vessels in the brain. Damage to these cells results in increased intracerebral pressure, which accounts for the wide variety of central nervous system signs. Lesions of myocardial degeneration and pulmonary edema are reflections of vascular injury. Complement or the products of arachidonic acid metabolism may generate vasoactive compounds, with subsequent increases in capillary permeability.

Diagnosis of heartwater is difficult because clinical signs are not pathognomonic and may be confused with other diseases. Presumptive diagnosis is based in part on a history that includes residence in an endemic region and infestation with *Amblyomma* ticks. Consistent clinical signs and gross lesions and microscopic demonstration of organisms in brain endothelial cells, either in smears or sections, aid in confirming a diagnosis. Reproduction of heartwater by inoculating susceptible animals with blood or brain biopsy material from infected animals also has been used to establish a diagnosis. A range of serologic tests is affected by false-positive and false-negative results. *Ehrlichia ruminantium* apparently has antigens that cross-react with several other ehrlichiae. The recent discovery of two new *E. ruminantium* genotypes (Omatjenne and Ball 3) may also contribute to serologic discrepancies. A highly specific and sensitive PCR assay detects *E. ruminantium* in blood, but is not yet widely available.

Control of tick infestation is the most useful preventive measure and depends on intensive use of acaricides. Prophylactic administration of a live blood vaccine is practiced in some regions. Blood from infected animals is given intravenously to animals younger than 4 months of age, the rationale being that these animals have innate resistance to disease. Infection at an early age results in immunity that is boosted by continuing tick challenge as the animal matures. Removal of carrier animals is essential to break the infection cycle. Successful establishment of the agent in bovine endothelial cell cultures and in an *Ixodes scapularis* cell line has led to development of inactivated vaccines, but phenotypic variation among field isolates is apparently responsible for limited efficacy. Tetracyclines will effect a cure if administered early in the course of illness.

The potential for introducing heartwater and its vectors into the United States through international trade and travel is high. Many areas are climatically suitable for the survival of *A. variegatum,* and indigenous *Amblyomma* spp. can transmit disease. Recently, *E. ruminantium*–infected ticks were collected from African tortoises imported into the United States. A bont tick, which is exotic to the United States, was portered into the country by a tourist returning from Africa.

THE GENUS *AEGYPTIANELLA*

This genus incertae sedis contains intraerythrocytic bacteria that cause disease in fowl and amphibians. For many years these organisms were thought to be *Babesia*, but electron microscopic evaluation eventually demonstrated their true rickettsia-like nature. The five proposed species are *Aegyptianella pullorum, Aegyptianella botuliformis, Aegyptianella minutis, Aegyptianella bacterifera,* and *Aegyptianella ranarum.*

Aegyptianella pullorum is the etiologic agent of aegyptianellosis in chickens, turkeys, ducks, and geese. Aegyptianellosis has primarily been confined to parts of Africa, Asia, and southern Europe; sporadic cases have been documented in South America and southern Texas. The vectors are soft ticks of the species *Argus* and infection is transstadial. Severe disease manifests as anemia, diarrhea, anorexia, fever, and high mortality. Diagnosis is through the examination of Giemsa-stained blood smears. *Aegyptianella* spp. appear in erythrocytes as purple to reddish, spherical to ring shaped, intracytoplasmic inclusions that are approximately 4 μm in diameter. Each inclusion may contain up to 25 initial bodies that reproduce by binary fission. Disease prevention requires tick control, and tetracyclines are apparently effective therapeutic agents.

Aegyptianella botuliformis is another avian pathogen, having been recovered from guineafowl in Africa. This agent does not infect domestic fowl, suggesting host-specificity. *Amblyomma* spp. and *Ixodes* spp., as well as *Argus* spp., may serve as vectors.

In 1999, the new species *A. minutis* was discovered in blood smears from a mountain fluvetta, a bird indigenous to Malaysia. It was named for its small size (1 μm diameter).

Aegyptianella bacterifera and *A. ranarum* are blood parasites of amphibians. Tick vectors are not involved in transmission.

SUGGESTED READINGS

Castle MD, Christensen BM: Isolation and identification of *Aegyptianella pullorum* (Rickettsiales, Anaplasmataceae) in wild turkeys from North America, *Avian Dis* 29:437-445, 1985.

Dumler JS, Barbet AF, Bekker CPJ, et al: Reorganization of genera in the families Rickettsiaceae and Anaplasmataceae in the order *Rickettsiales:* unification of some species of *Ehrlichia* with *Anaplasma, Cowdria* with *Ehrlichia* and *Ehrlichia* with *Neorickettsia,* descriptions of six new species combinations and designation of *Ehrlichia equi* and "HGE agent" as subjective synonyms of *Ehrlichia phagocytophila, Int J Syst Evol Microbiol* 51:2145-2165, 2001.

Harrus S, Bark H, Waner T: Canine monocytic ehrlichiosis: an update, *Compend Cont Educ Pract Vet* 19:431-444, 1997.

Madigan JE, Pusterla N: Ehrlichial diseases, *Vet Clin North Am Equine Pract* 16:487-499, 2000.

Mebus CA, Logan LL: Heartwater disease of domestic and wild ruminants, *J Am Vet Med Assoc* 192:950-952, 1988.

Peter TF, Burridge MJ, Mahan SM: *Ehrlichia ruminantium* infection (heartwater) in wild ruminants, *Trends Parasitol* 18:214-218, 2002.

Rikihisa Y: The tribe *Ehrlichiae* and ehrlichial diseases, *Clin Microbiol Rev* 4:286-308, 1991.

Chapter 41

The Genera *Chlamydia* and *Chlamydophila*

Members of the order Chlamydiales are gram-negative obligate intracellular bacterial pathogens that parasitize hosts from humans to amebae. The family Chlamydiaceae has recently undergone extensive taxonomic revision, and the two proposed genera are *Chlamydia* and *Chlamydophila*. The genus *Chlamydia* would include *Chlamydia trachomatis, Chlamydia suis,* and *Chlamydia muridarum.* Six species assigned to the genus *Chlamydophila* are *Chlamydophila abortus, Chlamydophila caviae, Chlamydophila felis, Chlamydophila pecorum, Chlamydophila pneumoniae,* and *Chlamydophila psittaci.* This newly proposed nomenclature is not yet widely accepted.

Chlamydiae were once thought to be protozoa, and later were thought to be viruses because of their ability to pass through 450 nm filters. Ultimately, it has become clear that chlamydiae are bacteria. Molecular analysis of rDNA has confirmed them to be gram negative. Chlamydial cell walls contain cytoplasmic and outer membranes, but unlike other bacteria have no peptidoglycan layer. The cell wall also contains a genus-specific lipopolysaccharide. All chlamydiae encode an abundant major outer-membrane protein (MOMP), which is the principal determinant for serologic classification of isolates.

Some strains of *C. psittaci* and *C. trachomatis* are considered to be "energy parasites," because host-derived ATP meets their energy needs.

This may, in fact, be a requirement for all members of the family Chlamydiaceae.

The order Chlamydiales has a developmental cycle (Figure 41-1) that is unique among prokaryotes, with two morphologically distinctive forms. The elementary body is the smaller (300-400 nm), infectious form, whereas the reticulate body is larger (800-1000 nm) and noninfectious. Elementary bodies are similar to spores, in that they are designed for survival in the environment. The reticulate body is metabolically active and capable of replication.

DISEASES AND EPIDEMIOLOGY

The Chlamydiaceae are pathogens of mammals, birds, and reptiles, and most have specific host or disease associations (Table 41-1). The host may serve as a natural reservoir of infection because many chlamydiae inhabit hosts in an asymptomatic state. Chlamydiae are spread by direct contact or through aerosols and do not require an alternate vector.

Chlamydia trachomatis is a human pathogen. Various strains are etiologic agents of prevalent sexually transmitted diseases and are the main causes of preventable blindness (trachoma) worldwide. Cervical infections, pelvic inflammatory disease, ectopic pregnancy, and infertility may affect women. Infants, infected in the birth canal, may develop pneumonia or conjunctivitis. In most cases, the conjunctivitis is self-limiting,

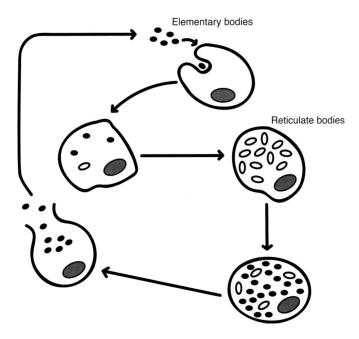

Elementary bodies

Reticulate bodies

FIGURE 41-1   Life cycle of chlamydiae. (Courtesy Ashley E. Harmon.)

TABLE 41-1   Chlamydial Diseases and Host Relationships

Current Name	Previous Name	Primary Hosts	Route(s) of Entry	Clinical Disease(s)
Chlamydia trachomatis	Same	Humans	Genital, rectal, ocular, pharyngeal	Arthritis, conjunctivitis, pneumonia, STD, trachoma, TMJ disease
Chlamydia suis	*Chlamydia trachomatis*	Pigs	Pharyngeal	Asymptomatic, conjunctivitis, enteritis, pericarditis, pneumonia, polyarthritis, rhinitis
Chlamydia muridarum	*Chlamydia trachomatis*	Mice, hamsters	Genital, pharyngeal	Asymptomatic, pneumonitis
Chlamydophila psittaci	*Chlamydia psittaci*	Birds	Ocular, pharyngeal	Conjunctivitis, encephalitis, enteritis, myocarditis, pneumonia, airsacculitis, hepatitis
Chlamydophila pneumoniae	*Chlamydia psittaci*	Humans, horses, koalas	Ocular, pharyngeal	Alzheimer's, atherosclerosis, conjunctivitis, cystitis, pneumonia
Chlamydophila abortus	*Chlamydia psittaci*	Ruminants, pigs	Genital, oral	Abortion, stillbirths
Chlamydophila caviae	*Chlamydia psittaci*	Guinea pigs	Genital, ocular, pharyngeal, urethral	Conjunctivitis
Chlamydophila felis	*Chlamydia psittaci*	Cats	Genital, ocular, pharyngeal	Conjunctivitis, pneumonitis, rhinitis
Chlamydophila pecorum	*Chlamydia psittaci*	Ruminants, pigs, koalas	Oral	Abortion/infertility, arthritis, conjunctivitis, cystitis, encephalitis, enteritis, pneumonia

STD, Sexually transmitted disease; *TMJ*, temporomandibular joint.

but in some instances it results in blindness. In males, urethritis and lymphogranuloma venereum predominate. The latter condition is characterized by swollen lymph nodes in the groin. A secondary consequence of infection, more common in men than in women, is arthritis or Reiter's syndrome. This organism has also been found in the temporomandibular joint (TMJ) of patients with TMJ disorder.

Diagnosis of swine chlamydial infections is relatively rare, especially in the United States, partly because most veterinary diagnostic laboratories do not routinely examine tissues for the presence of chlamydiae. The swine chlamydia *C. suis* were initially referred to as *C. trachomatis*, based on shared biologic characteristics; these organisms are susceptible to sulfadiazine and form glycogen-containing intracellular inclusions. Most infected animals remain asymptomatic. However, pneumonia, rhinitis, polyarthritis, conjunctivitis, pericarditis, and enteritis have been reported. Pre- and postweaning intestinal disease in pigs has been described, and affected animals have mild coughs, weight loss, and diarrhea. It is noteworthy that chlamydial infections have been detected in the intestines of clinically normal pigs and chlamydial antibodies have been identified in a high percentage of apparently healthy animals.

Chlamydia muridarum contains two strains, isolated from hamsters and mice, that previously belonged to *C. trachomatis*. The hamster strain may be avirulent, and murine infection may be inapparent or manifest as pneumonia.

Chlamydophila psittaci is primarily a pathogen of birds, with infections documented in more than 150 species worldwide. The disease has been given several names. Psittacosis is a disease of psittacine (parrot-type) birds. Ornithosis is the same disease affecting nonpsittacine birds. Other names used are avian chlamydiosis or parrot fever. Six serovars have been isolated from birds (A-F) and two from mammals (M56 and WC); virulence among serovars is variable. Serovar identification is useful for epidemiologic purposes. Most (50%-80%) of a flock will exhibit clinical signs when infection is caused by a highly virulent strain. Signs include anorexia, fever, conjunctivitis, production of yellowish green gelatinous droppings, and decreased egg production. Morbidity from less virulent strains is only 5% to 20%. Mortality attributed to highly virulent strains ranges from 10% to 30%, but is only 1% to 4% with less virulent strains. Lesions are similar, regardless of virulence, although they are less extensive with strains of lower virulence; airsacculitis, lung congestion, fibrinous pleuritis and/or pericarditis, hepatitis, splenomegaly, and enteritis are common. Recovered birds may shed chlamydiae in feces and nasal discharges for extended periods and pose a health threat to people.

Bacterial infection of humans with *C. psittaci* is also referred to as psittacosis. Infection usually occurs following inhalation of aerosolized bacteria from droppings, feathers, or tissues of infected birds. Transmission also may be mouth to beak, although cases acquired in this fashion are no doubt underreported, for obvious reasons. Most human disease results from exposure to infected cockatiels, parakeets, parrots, and macaws, and contact with birds through work or hobbies is a significant risk factor. The incubation period is 4 to 15 days, and the disease is a flulike illness with sudden onset of fever, chills, headache, weakness, and muscle aches. Some people also may have a dry cough, chest pain, breathlessness, and, in severe cases, pneumonia. Psittacosis in humans can be treated with antibiotics, and diagnosis is usually confirmed by blood tests and chest radiographs. Person-to-person transmission does not occur.

Three biovars of *C. pneumoniae* have been designated TWAR, Koala, and Equine. Biovar TWAR, derived from the laboratory designation of the first conjunctival and respiratory isolates (TW-183 and AR-39, respectively), is strictly a human pathogen. The organism causes bronchitis and pneumonia. Seroepidemiologic studies, direct detection of the organism within lesions, and isolation of the organism from atherosclerotic plaques have associated this strain with cardiovascular disease. Recently, researchers have suggested a connection to Alzheimer's disease, which is based on the ability of *C. pneumoniae* to infect blood vessel endothelial cells and cause inflammation.

Biovar Koala strains have been isolated exclusively from ocular and urogenital sites of koalas, and do not appear to be highly virulent. The single strain of biovar Equine was isolated from the upper respiratory tract of a horse with a serous nasal discharge. Experimental inoculation of horses with this strain leads to asymptomatic infection.

Chlamydophila psittaci isolates associated with abortion in sheep, goats, cattle, and swine are now called *C. abortus*. These strains are endemic among ruminants and are colonizers of the placenta.

Enzootic ovine abortion is the most common disease attributed to this organism, and is reported in the United States, South Africa, and Europe. The disease is characterized almost exclusively by a loss of lambs in late pregnancy, although weak or dead lambs may be born at term. Retained placenta and vaginal discharge are common clinical signs. Chlamydiae are present in high numbers in fetal membranes and in vaginal discharge; under these conditions, disease is spread to other ewes by the oral route. Bacteria can persist in ewe lambs for up to 2 years before causing abortion. The organism may have a broader than believed host range in that it has apparently been recovered from abortions in horses, rabbits, guinea pigs, and mice. Pregnant women working with infected sheep are at increased risk of abortion.

Chlamydophila caviae, which contains guinea pig strains formerly designated *C. psittaci,* is an agent of conjunctivitis. The infection is noninvasive, and attempts to infect other species of laboratory rodents have been relatively unsuccessful.

Feline strains of *C. psittaci* have been reclassified as *C. felis.* The organism is endemic among domestic cats worldwide and is a well-recognized cause of conjunctivitis, rhinitis, and, to a lesser degree, pneumonia. Of these syndromes, acute, chronic, or recurrent conjunctivitis is the most common clinical presentation. Experimental ocular inoculation of cats consistently results in acute conjunctivitis. Some experimentally infected animals develop persistent gastrointestinal or genital infections as a result of colonization of those mucosal surfaces. Whether chlamydiae are responsible for naturally occurring feline gastrointestinal or reproductive disease remains to be determined; however, infections at these sites may be a means by which disease is transmitted. Zoonotic infection has been linked to endocarditis, glomerulonephritis, chronic cough, and flulike illness in humans.

Chlamydiae isolated from mammals, but not associated with a specific host, have been assigned to the species *C. pecorum.* This organism causes infertility and genitourinary disease in koalas. Sporadic bovine encephalomyelitis, also known as Buss disease, affects young cattle and buffaloes, and is characterized by encephalitis, peritonitis, and fibrinous pleuritis and occurs worldwide. The incubation period is 1 to 4 weeks, and affected animals are anorectic and febrile. Hypersalivation,

dyspnea, and ataxia are frequently observed, and mortality is 50%. Organisms are located in the brain, spinal cord, and lymph nodes, indicating systemic infection. Enteritis and arthritis in swine and sheep have occasionally been attributed to infection with *C. pecorum.*

Chlamydiosis has been described in chameleons, turtles, tortoises, crocodiles, and snakes. Manifestations include pericarditis, hepatitis, enteritis, pneumonia, and splenitis. Most of these strains remain uncharacterized.

PATHOGENESIS

The major determinants of chlamydial pathogenesis are complex and remain largely unknown. They are apparently not acutely toxigenic, in that infection is, in many cases, inapparent and persistent. Serious disease is a function of several processes, including attachment, intracellular growth, persistence and dissemination, directed remodeling of the intracellular environment, and modulation of the host immune response.

Elementary bodies initiate infection by binding to receptors on microvilli of host cells. The identity of the receptor remains elusive and may vary with the chlamydial species and strain. Heparan sulfate glycosaminoglycans appear to be involved in the attachment process. Putative chlamydial adhesins include MOMP, a heat-labile cytadhesin, heat shock proteins, and outer-membrane protein OmcB.

The exact mechanism by which chlamydiae enter cells is not well characterized, and again may be dependent on the infecting species. In any case, entry is by receptor-mediated endocytosis, pinocytosis, or phagocytosis. Once inside a host cell, chlamydiae do not leave the cytoplasmic vacuole in which they enter. Within 8 hours of cellular invasion, disulfide crosslinks among the elementary bodies are reduced, and they begin to reorganize into reticulate bodies that can synthesize their own RNA and proteins. Chlamydial protein synthesis appears to be crucial in avoiding phagolysosomal fusion. Replication, by binary fission, continues for 18 to 24 hours, and the vacuole with the accumulated reticulate bodies is called an inclusion. Twenty-four hours postinfection, the reticulate bodies begin reorganizing into elementary bodies. The infected cell ultimately ruptures and releases elementary bodies that infect other cells. Infection is facilitated by chlamydial glycolipid exoantigen (GLXA), an outer-membrane component that is secreted into the microenvironment of chlamydia-infected cells and appears to make neighboring cells more susceptible to infection.

Because chlamydiae are not totally eliminated by the host immune response, reinfection and host damage continue. Possible determinants of chlamydial growth and survival in host cells include sustained iron channeling from host to phagosome, steady availability of tryptophan (an essential amino acid), avoidance of lysosomal degradation, and modulation of calcium ions, nitric oxide, and superoxides within the macrophage.

Repeated chlamydial infection increases the severity of the inflammatory response and promotes chronic inflammation at focal sites of infection. Pathogenesis is due in part to the cellular response of chlamydia-infected nonimmune cells, in particular the mucosal epithelial and vascular endothelial cells. Host responses involve production of cytokines, proinflammatory chemokines, and growth factors that result in local tissue damage.

DIAGNOSIS

Chlamydial infections can be diagnosed by cytology, serology, culture, and direct detection of organisms by molecular methods or immunohistochemistry.

Giemsa, Gimenez, or Macchiavello stains are used for cytologic examination of lesion impression smears. Chlamydial inclusions appear dark purple with Giemsa, and red with Gimenez and Macchiavello stains, against contrasting backgrounds. Cytologic testing is relatively insensitive for diagnosis of chronic or persistent infections.

The many serologic tests developed for diagnosis of chlamydiosis reflect the strain-to-strain differences in pathogenicity and the immune response of hosts. These methods include various iterations of enzyme immunoassays, complement fixation, and latex agglutination. Limitations of serologic results, including lack of titers in the acute phase of disease and diagnostically positive titers in clinically normal individuals with persistent infections, necessitate additional confirmatory testing. A fourfold increase in titer between paired acute and convalescent phase sera suggests active disease. In birds, elementary body agglutination is the most useful serologic method

because it detects only IgM activity and is indicative of early infection.

Chlamydiae are obligate intracellular pathogens and cannot be cultivated on artificial media. Cell culture remains the most specific method for diagnosis. Embryonated chicken eggs were historically used for this purpose, but have been replaced by cell culture methods. McCoy and HeLa-229 cells are among the most frequently used cell lines. The basic procedure involves centrifugation of the inoculum onto the cell monolayer, incubation for 48 to 72 hours, and demonstration of intracytoplasmic inclusions by Giemsa, Macchiavello, or Gimenez stains (Figure 41-2). Species within *Chlamydia* and *Chlamydophila* are distinguished by use of group-specific fluorescent antibody staining or polymerase chain reaction (PCR) assays. Sensitivity of culture ranges from 70% to 85% with adequate specimens. Chlamydiae are relatively labile, so refrigeration and prompt transport are important.

The direct fluorescent antibody test (Figure 41-3) and enzyme immunoassays are the procedures most commonly used to detect antigens in clinical specimens. Both assays use antibodies prepared against either the chlamydial lipopolysaccharide (LPS) or MOMP. Antigenic determinants on LPS are shared with other bacteria, so antibody tests using this target are less specific. Anti-MOMP monoclonal antibodies are species specific.

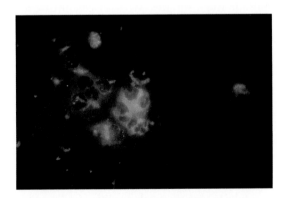

FIGURE 41-2 Photomicrograph of inclusion bodies of *Chlamydia trachomatis* in a monolayer of McCoy cells. (Courtesy Public Health Image Library, PHIL #3802, Centers for Disease Control and Prevention, Atlanta, 1975, E. Arum and N. Jacobs.)

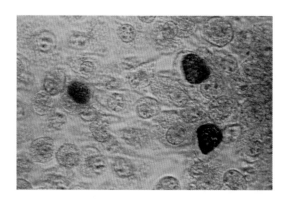

FIGURE 41-3 *Chlamydia psittaci* in a direct fluorescent antibody–stained impression smear of infected mouse brain. (Courtesy Public Health Image Library, PHIL #3021, Centers for Disease Control and Prevention, Atlanta, 1971, Vester Lewis.)

Molecular diagnostic methods include PCR assays and commercially available nucleic acid probes. These tests are less sensitive than culture, but have specificity in the range of 90%. Genus- and species-specific assays are necessary for reliable diagnosis, and these are only available in a limited number of reference or research laboratories. Immunohistochemical methods can be applied to fixed tissues obtained at necropsy or to biopsy specimens.

PREVENTION AND CONTROL

Prevention of avian chlamydiosis calls for segregation of new birds on addition to aviaries or poultry production facilities and serologic testing to identify infected birds for culling. Ideally, birds should be reared in confinement to eliminate contact with potential reservoirs or vectors, such as wild birds.

State and federal regulations may impose quarantines on the movement of infected birds. The U.S. Department of Agriculture–Animal and Plant Health Inspection Service (USDA-APHIS) regulates importation of pet birds to ensure that exotic poultry diseases are not introduced into the United States. During the 30-day quarantine period, psittacine birds must receive a medicated feed containing chlortetracycline as a precautionary measure against chlamydiosis.

General sanitation should be practiced to prevent the transfer of fecal matter, feathers, food, and other materials from one cage or house to another. Disinfection of rooms and cages should follow removal of all organic matter. *Chlamydophila psittaci* is susceptible to most disinfectants and detergents, as well as heat. Quaternary ammonium compounds, 70% isopropyl alcohol, chlorophenols, and bleach (diluted 1:100) are all effective disinfectants.

No commercial vaccines induce long-lasting protection against disease. Antimicrobial treatment of infected poultry is required before slaughter. Control of outbreaks of avian chlamydiosis involves isolation of affected birds and treatment with tetracyclines.

Psittacosis is reportable as a human disease, and a plethora of public health guidelines include avoidance of contact with wild birds; not breathing dust from dried bird droppings, feathers, or cages; pre-use dampening of garden materials, including mulch, that could be contaminated with bird droppings; wearing gloves and dust mask before using any garden materials that could be contaminated with bird droppings; using dust masks when mowing lawns; not handling sick birds; and using dust masks, protective eyewear and gloves when disposing of dead birds.

Commercial vaccines are available for prevention of ovine enzootic abortion. Disease control measures include culling of infected animals, administrating long-acting tetracyclines to pregnant ewes, isolating aborting ewes, immediately removing placental membranes after lambing, and disinfecting pens where abortions have occurred.

Maternal antibodies to *C. felis* usually protect kittens from infection until 7 to 9 weeks of age. Killed and modified live vaccines do not entirely prevent colonization of the mucosa but do minimize the replication of the bacteria and lessen the severity of respiratory disease. Segregating affected individuals and treating affected and in-contact cats with tetracyclines may be necessary to control disease in a cattery.

There is no specific means for preventing and controlling sporadic bovine encephalomyelitis. The agent is susceptible to tetracyclines and tylosin, but effective dosage regimens have not been established. Disease is irreversible when central nervous system signs become apparent.

SUGGESTED READINGS

Eidson M: Psittacosis/avian chlamydiosis, *J Am Vet Med Assoc* 221:1710-1712, 2002.

Everett KD: *Chlamydia* and *Chlamydiales:* more than meets the eye, *Vet Microbiol* 75:109-126, 2000.

Everett KD, Bush RM, Andersen AA: Emended description of the order *Chlamydiales,* proposal of *Parachlamydiaceae* fam. nov. and *Simkaniaceae* fam. nov., each containing one monotypic genus, revised taxonomy of the family *Chlamydiaceae,* including a new genus and five new species, and standards for the identification of organisms, *Int J Syst Bacteriol* 49:415-440, 1999.

Stephens RS: The cellular paradigm of chlamydial pathogenesis, *Trends Microbiol* 11:44-51, 2003.

Wyrick PB: Intracellular survival by *Chlamydia, Cell Microbiol* 2:275-282, 2000.

Chapter 42

Coxiella burnetii

*C*oxiella burnetii was originally named *Rickettsia burnetii,* and it shares rickettsial characteristics, including obligate intracellular growth, failure to stain by Gram's method, and transmission, in some cases, by ticks. Recent 16S rRNA gene sequencing has demonstrated that these bacteria are more closely related to the genera *Francisella* and *Legionella* than to the family Rickettsiaceae, with which they are taxonomically placed.

The organism is the cause of "Q fever" (query fever) that was first described as a cause of febrile illness in abattoir workers in Queensland, Australia, in 1937. Burnett and Freeman, working in Nine Mile, Montana, described a febrile illness in guinea pigs following tick exposure, and in 1938, the "Ninemile agent" was found to be identical to the agent of Q fever. *Rickettsia burnetii* was subsequently reclassified into the new genus *Coxiella,* in honor of Herald R. Cox, who initially isolated the organism in the United States.

Coxiella burnetii is a small pleomorphic rod-shaped bacterium (0.2-0.4 µm wide and 0.4-1 µm long) with a cell membrane similar to that of gram-negative bacteria. The organism multiplies in phagolysosomes of infected cells and can undergo phase variation, with antigenic changes in the lipopolysaccharide (LPS). Phase I is the highly infectious, natural phase; a complex carbohydrate on its surface blocks antibody interaction with surface proteins. LPS is modified upon in vitro cultivation, and the organism enters phase II, exposing surface proteins to antibodies and producing a less virulent form.

DISEASES AND EPIDEMIOLOGY

Q fever is a zoonotic disease that is endemic throughout the world, except for New Zealand. *Coxiella burnetii* is widely distributed in nature and has been identified in arthropods, birds, reptiles, fish, and mammals, including humans. All reservoirs of *C. burnetii* have not been identified, although livestock, such as ruminants, are primary reservoirs and pet cats and dogs have been linked to urban outbreaks of Q fever. Intermittent shedding may occur in vaginal discharges, feces, urine, milk, and birth products. Arthropods facilitate a sylvan life cycle in reservoir animals, and transmission by ticks and other arthropods to domestic animals and rarely to humans has been documented.

Disease may follow respiratory or digestive exposure. Domestic animals and humans are most commonly infected by inhalation of contaminated aerosols of dried placental materials, birth fluids, and excreta of infected animals. Humans are often very susceptible, and the infectious dose is perhaps as low as one organism. Within herds, infection may also be maintained by inhalation of contaminated dust or through contact with fomites. Consumption of raw cow's or goat's milk may result in asymptomatic infection in humans.

The extraordinary stability of *C. burnetii* outside the host is associated with the small sporelike forms observed by electron microscopy. The bacterium is resistant to elevated temperatures, ultraviolet light, desiccation, and disinfectants such as 0.5% sodium hypochlorite, quaternary ammonium compounds, and phenolics. Environmental survival favors wind-borne transmission, often over long distances. These factors also make *C. burnetii* a putatively attractive target for use in biological warfare and bioterrorism.

Q fever is an occupational disease of farmers, veterinarians, and abattoir workers. It became a notifiable disease in the United States in 1999, but reporting is not required in many other countries; accurate estimates of worldwide incidence are not available, and underestimation seems likely in light of the frequently insidious nature of the disease.

Acute Q fever is less common. The incubation period is 2 to 4 weeks, and the resulting disease is a self-limited flulike syndrome, with severe headache, malaise, fever, myalgia, and chills. Complications such as pneumonia, hepatitis, pericarditis, myocarditis, meningoencephalitis, gastroenteritis, pancreatitis, optic neuritis, lymphadenopathy, and skin rash are uncommon. Mortality is usually low in the absence of complications. The route of infection may determine the predominant manifestation of acute disease.

Endocarditis may develop years after acute infection. Chronic illness occurs in approximately 5% of patients, and most frequently involves not only the heart but also arteries, bones, and liver. Patients at risk for chronic disease include those with preexisting cardiac valve defects, transplant recipients, patients with cancer, and those with chronic kidney disease. The case fatality rate for chronic Q fever may be as high as 65%. Contracting Q fever during pregnancy may result in abortion or premature birth, and intrauterine transmission may occur.

Coxiella burnetii usually causes inapparent or mild disease in domestic animals. Sporadic abortions have been reported in sheep, goats, and cattle. Infertility or birth of weak offspring is a rare sequel to ruminant infection. Companion animals may be infected, but rarely exhibit clinical disease; however, abortion in cats and the birth of weak puppies have been described. Human illness has resulted from exposure to infected, pregnant, or parturient queens and bitches.

PATHOGENESIS AND VIRULENCE

Pathogenesis of Q fever is poorly understood because most infections are self-limited and no reliable animal models exist for chronic disease. Development of disease is directly correlated to overall condition and immune status of the host. Monocytes and macrophages are the only known target cells in humans and other animals, and are responsible for the dissemination of *C. burnetii*. Infection of alveolar macrophages follows respiratory exposure. Kupffer cells in the liver are also susceptible, and may become infected through hematogenous dissemination of the organism or, rarely, as a consequence of the digestive route of exposure. After hematogenous spread, the organism may localize and replicate in the female reproductive tract and mammary glands. Endocarditis may occur in patients with preexisting valvular defects caused by the recruitment of infected monocytes at the site of vascular injury.

Efficient invasion and replication within host cells is an important virulence attribute. The infectious, phase I form binds to human monocytes and macrophages via the complex of a leukocyte response integrin and an integrin-associated protein. Following phagocytosis, phagosomes fuse with lysosomes, and these early phagolysosomes continue to fuse, resulting in large vacuoles. *Coxiella burnetii* withstands the low pH of the phagolysosome, and bacterial metabolism and multiplication are enhanced in the acidic environment. Protein secretion is induced specifically within hours of exposure to acid pH, and this may reflect a means of communication between the bacterium and host cells.

Replication, through binary fission, occurs exclusively within the phagolysosome. A complex intracellular life cycle leads to formation of two different developmental stages, called small-cell and large-cell variants. Small-cell variants are metabolically inactive and correspond to the extracellular form of the bacterium, which is resistant to osmotic effects. The large-cell variants are metabolically active and correspond to the intracellular form. Small-cell variants are released from the infected cell either by lysis or exocytosis and infect adjacent host cells.

Induction of persistent infection is also a virulence factor. Slow intracellular multiplication (with a generation time up to 20 hours) of *C. burnetii* may in part explain why the organism does not damage the host cell despite the persistent infection.

The T-cell–dependent immune control of Q fever does not result in total elimination of the agent, and immunosuppression can cause a relapse of infection in apparently recovered patients or laboratory animals. Acute Q fever is associated with cytokine overproduction. Tumor necrosis factor-α (TNF-α) and interferon-γ (IFN-γ) may play important roles in the host defense processes leading to the elimination of the organism. *Coxiella burnetii* induces TNF-α–mediated apoptosis in macrophages during the late stages of the infection, and the response to IFN-γ may be similar. Apoptosis of infected macrophages may constitute a mechanism by which the host confines infection.

DIAGNOSIS

The signs and symptoms of Q fever are not specific, and accurate diagnosis without appropriate laboratory testing is difficult. Currently, diagnosis is based on a combination of direct cytologic examination of specimens, propagation of the organism, serology, demonstration of compatible microscopic lesions, and detection of the organism by molecular methods.

Examination of modified Ziehl-Nielsen–stained smears from placental tissue or vaginal discharges reveals small clumps of red coccobacilli. Gimenez or Giemsa staining is also useful, as is immunoperoxidase staining of paraffin-embedded tissues. Immunofluorescence-based techniques may be used to demonstrate *C. burnetii* in placental smears. Electron microscopy also may be used to detect organisms in affected placental tissues (Figure 42-1).

Many laboratory-acquired infections have been described, and the ready transmissibility of the agent requires that isolation of *C. burnetii* be attempted only under biosafety level 3 conditions. Historically, the organism was propagated in yolk sacs of embryonated chicken eggs. Extracts of infected spleen, inoculated into eggs, cause embryonic death after 7 to 9 days, and organisms can be detected by Giemsa, Gimenez, or direct fluorescent antibody staining. The bacterium is now more routinely cultivated in a variety of cell lines, including monkey kidney, mouse macrophage, and Vero.

Microscopic lesions of Q fever include inflammation, and granulomatous lesions are observed

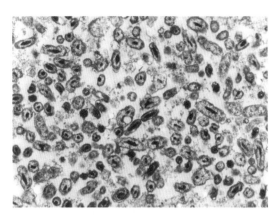

FIGURE 42-1 Electron photomicrograph of *Coxiella burnetii*–infected caprine placenta. (Courtesy Raymond E. Reed.)

in lungs, liver, and heart. Interstitial pneumonia, hepatitis, and myocarditis are common. Placentitis, fetal pneumonia, and hepatitis are common in cases of abortion.

Definitive diagnosis is often based on serology. Acute and convalescent sera, collected 2 to 4 weeks apart, are examined by complement fixation, microagglutination, indirect immunofluorescence, or enzyme-linked immunosorbent assay (ELISA). Antigenic variation of *C. burnetii* can be useful in distinguishing acute from chronic disease. In acute cases, the antibody titer to phase II antigens is usually higher than that to phase I antigens, often by several orders of magnitude, and is first detected during the second week of illness. In chronic Q fever, the reverse is true; high levels of antibody to phase I in later specimens, in combination with constant or falling phase II antibody titers and other signs of inflammatory disease, suggest chronic infection. Antibodies to phase I and II antigens may persist for months or years after initial infection.

Determination of titers of antibody isotypes other than IgG, namely IgA and IgM, can increase the accuracy of diagnosis. Elevated IgM titers indicate recent infection; in acute Q fever, patients will have IgG antibodies to phase II antigens and IgM antibodies to both phase I and phase II antigens. Increasing IgG and IgA titers to phase I antigens often indicate Q fever endocarditis.

DNA probes and polymerase chain reaction (PCR) assays are also available. The latter can detect *C. burnetii* DNA in both cell cultures and clinical materials, and is much more sensitive than standard culture techniques.

PREVENTION AND CONTROL

In the United States, Q fever outbreaks have resulted mainly from occupational exposure of veterinarians, meat-processing plant workers, sheep and dairy workers, livestock farmers, and researchers at facilities housing sheep. Prevention and control efforts should be directed primarily toward these individuals and environments, and should include public education on sources of infection; appropriate disposal of placentae, birth products, fetal membranes, and aborted fetuses; restriction of access to barns and laboratories used in housing potentially infected animals; and pasteurization of milk and milk products before consumption.

A vaccine for Q fever protects humans in occupational settings in Australia, but is not commercially available in the United States. A vaccine has been marketed in Europe for cattle and goats, but is not widely used because it protects only if administered to uninfected animals.

Doxycycline is the treatment of choice for acute Q fever in humans. Antibiotic therapy is most effective when initiated within the first 3 days of illness and continued for up to 3 weeks. Therapy should be continued in the case of relapse. Excellent in vitro activity of fluoroquinolone antibiotics suggests that they may be useful in vivo. Chronic Q fever endocarditis is much more difficult to treat effectively and often requires use of multiple drugs. Administration of doxycycline and hydroxychloroquine for 1.5 to 3 years is a superior regimen to administration of doxycycline in combination with quinolones for at least 4 years; the former allows fewer relapses, but requires routine eye exams to detect accumulation of chloroquine. Surgery to replace damaged valves may be required in some cases.

Antimicrobials such as tetracylines have been used to control herd outbreaks of Q fever.

SUGGESTED READINGS

Fournier PE, Marrie TJ, Raoult D: Diagnosis of Q fever, *J Clin Microbiol* 36:1823-1834, 1998.

Maurin M, Raoult D: Q fever, *Clin Microbiol Rev* 12:518-553, 1999.

Norlander N: Q fever epidemiology and pathogenesis, *Microbe Infect* 2:417-424, 2000.

Chapter 43

The Family Rickettsiaceae

Rickettsioses are some of the oldest diseases known to man. On one hand, epidemic typhus was responsible for large outbreaks of plaguelike illness in ancient Greece. On the other hand, rickettsioses comprise some of the most recently recognized emerging infectious diseases.

Bacteria classified in the family Rickettsiaceae have recently undergone extensive taxonomic revision. Initial phylogenetic and taxonomic studies were based on morphologic, antigenic, and metabolic characters. Analysis of data from 16S rRNA gene sequence studies has resulted in amendment of the description of the family Rickettsiaceae to include organisms that are obliged to reside in host-cell cytoplasm or nucleus and are not bound by vacuoles. As a result, the genera *Ehrlichia*, *Cowdria*, *Neorickettsia*, *Coxiella*, and *Wolbachia* have been removed from the family. Three genera now included are *Rickettsia*, *Orientia*, and *Piscirickettsia* (Table 43-1).

Members of the family are morphologically and biochemically similar to other gram-negative bacteria. These coccobacillary to short rods are usually 0.8 to 2 μm long and 0.3 to 0.5 μm wide, and cannot be stained by Gram's method. Presumptive identification is achieved by microscopic examination of clinical specimens stained with Giemsa or Gimenez stains.

THE GENUS *RICKETTSIA*

The genus *Rickettsia* includes some of the most highly virulent bacteria known. Historically, it has been divided into the typhus and the spotted fever groups. The former contains the human pathogens *Rickettsia typhi* and *Rickettsia prowazekii*, whereas the spotted fever group contains species *africae*, *akari*, *australis*, *conorii*, *felis*, *honei*, *japonica*, *montana*, *rickettsii*, and *rhipicephali*, most of which are human pathogens. Dogs may be naturally infected with rickettsiae (*R. akari*, *R. conorii*, *R. montana*, and *R. rhipicephali*), as well as cats (*R. typhi*, *R. felis*, and *R. conorii*), but no overt signs of disease are exhibited. Dogs and cats may serve as sentinel species for these rickettsiae.

The phylogeny of this genus has recently been delineated by sequence analysis of 16S rDNA, and of genes for citrate synthase, rickettsial outer-membrane proteins, and cytoplasmic antigenic protein genes. As a result, the genus *Rickettsia* currently contains 21 species with several agents described as species incertae sedis.

Rickettsia rickettsii

Rickettsia rickettsii is pathogenic for humans and other animals, and causes Rocky Mountain spotted fever (RMSF) in the former. RMSF was first recognized in 1896 in humans residing in the Snake River Valley of Idaho, where it was originally known as "black measles" because of its characteristic rash. It was a dreaded and frequently fatal disease that affected hundreds of people in the region. The geographic distribution of RMSF has grown to encompass most of the continental United States, as well as portions of

TABLE 43-1 Pathogenic Rickettsiaceae That Affect Animals

Agent	Disease	Incidental Host	Reservoir Host	Vector	Geographic Distribution
Rickettsia rickettsii	Rocky Mountain spotted fever	Humans, dogs	Rodents	*Dermacentor* spp. ticks, *Amblyomma cajennense Rhipicephalus sanguineus*	Western Hemisphere
Rickettsia felis	Cat flea typhus	Humans	Norway rat, domestic cat, opossum	*Ctenocephalides felis* (cat flea)	Western Hemisphere, Europe
Rickettsia conorii	Boutonneuse fever Mediterranean spotted fever, Israeli spotted fever, Astrakhan fever	Humans	Rodents, dogs	*Rhipicephalus* spp. ticks	Southern Europe, Africa, Asia
Rickettsia typhi	Murine typhus	Humans	Rats, opossums, cats	*Xenopsylla cheopis* (rat flea)	Worldwide
Rickettsia prowazekii	Epidemic typhus	Domestic animals	Flying squirrels, humans	Human body louse, flying squirrel louse, squirrel flea	Worldwide
Orientia tsutsugamushi	Scrub typhus	Humans, dogs	Birds, rats	Mites	Eastern Asia, northern Australia, western Pacific Islands
Piscirickettsia salmonis	Piscirickettsiosis	Salmonid fish	Unknown	Unknown	Chile, Norway, Ireland, Canada

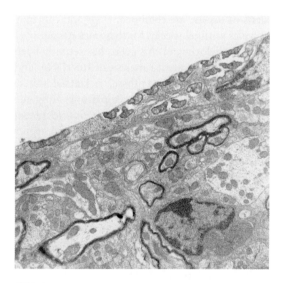

FIGURE 43-1 Transmission electron photomicrograph of multiple *Orientia tsutsugamushi* free in the cytoplasm of a murine capillary endothelial cell. (Courtesy Public Health Image Library, PHIL #928, Centers for Disease Control and Prevention, Atlanta, 1977, Edwin P. Ewing, Jr.)

southern Canada, Central America, Mexico, and South America. Thus RMSF has become a misnomer.

Rickettsia rickettsii is a very small gram-negative intracellular bacterium that ranges in size from 0.2×0.5 μm to 0.3×2 μm. These organisms are difficult to see in tissues stained by routine methods, and generally require the use of special staining methods (i.e., immunohistochemical or fluorescent antibody). The bacteria are present in the cytoplasm of infected cells (Figure 43-1).

DISEASE AND EPIDEMIOLOGY

Howard Ricketts established the identity of the etiologic agent of RMSF and described basic epidemiologic features of the disease, including the role of the tick. Humans and dogs are accidental hosts, and are the only species that display clinical illness. Natural transmission among dogs or humans, or between dogs and humans, does not occur in the absence of a vector.

RMSF, like all other rickettsial infections, is a zoonosis. Many of these diseases require a vector (e.g., a mosquito, tick, or mite) in order to be transmitted from the animal to human. Ticks are the natural hosts of RMSF, serving as both reservoirs and vectors of *R. rickettsii*. Transmission is primarily by bites, but may occur following exposure to crushed tick tissues, fluids, or feces. Only members of the tick family Ixodidae (hard ticks) are naturally infected with *R. rickettsii*. These ticks have four stages in their life cycle (egg, larva, nymph, and adult), across which transmission can occur. Transovarial transmission also occurs. Larval or nymphal ticks can become infected during feeding. Furthermore, male ticks may transfer *R. rickettsii* to female ticks through body fluids or spermatozoa during the mating process. The infected tick can maintain the pathogen for life.

The risk of exposure to a tick carrying *R. rickettsii* is relatively low because only 1% to 3% of the tick population carries *R. rickettsii*, even in areas where most human cases are reported. Transmission of rickettsiae by feeding ticks requires 6 to 20 hours of attachment and feeding.

The two major vectors of *R. rickettsii* in the United States are the American dog tick (*Dermacentor variabilis*) and the Rocky Mountain wood tick (*Dermacentor andersoni*) (Figure 43-2). The former is widely distributed east of the Rocky Mountains and also occurs in limited areas on the Pacific Coast. Dogs and medium-sized mammals are the preferred hosts of adult *D. variabilis*, although it feeds readily on other large mammals, including humans. It is the species most often responsible for transmitting *R. rickettsii* to humans and dogs. Dogs are sensitive indicators of the presence of disease, and they represent important transport hosts because they bring ticks into contact with humans.

Dermacentor andersoni is primarily found in the Rocky Mountain states and in southwestern Canada. The life cycle of this tick may require as long as 2 to 3 years for completion. Adult ticks feed primarily on large mammals, and larvae and nymphs feed on small rodents. Other tick species can be naturally infected with *R. rickettsii* or serve as experimental vectors in the laboratory (*Rhipicephalus sanguineus* and *Amblyomma americanum*), but these species are unlikely to play a major role in the ecology of *R. rickettsii* in the United States. In Mexico and South America,

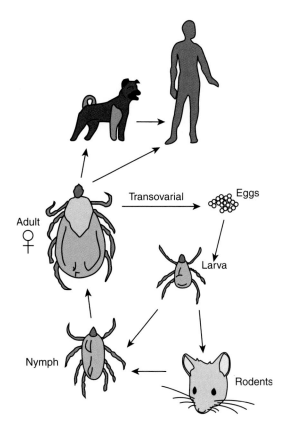

FIGURE 43-2 Natural history of *Rickettsia rickettsii* infection.

however, *Amblyomma cajennense* and *R. sanguineus* are commonly involved in transmission of RMSF to humans.

Human RMSF has been a reportable disease in the United States since the 1920s, and in the past 50 years there have been 250 to 1200 cases reported annually. It is likely that many more cases go unreported. More than 90% of patients with RMSF are infected from April through September, when the prevalence of adult and immature ticks is at its highest.

More than half of RMSF cases occur in the south Atlantic region of the United States (Delaware, Maryland, Washington, D.C., Virginia, West Virginia, North Carolina, South Carolina, Georgia, and Florida). Infection also occurs elsewhere in the country, including the Pacific Coast (Washington, Oregon, and California) and western south-central (Arkansas, Louisiana, Oklahoma, and Texas) regions. The highest incidence of RMSF is in North Carolina and Oklahoma, which, combined, accounted for 35% of all cases reported to the Centers for Disease Control and Prevention (CDC) from 1993 through 1996.

RMSF is the most severe and frequently reported rickettsial illness of humans in the United States. Initial symptoms include sudden onset of fever, headache, and muscle pain, followed by development of rash. The disease can be difficult to diagnose in the early stages, and without prompt and appropriate treatment it can be fatal; the case fatality rate is 3% to 5%.

Dogs are the only susceptible domestic species. Infection occurs more commonly in dogs younger than 2 years of age and in purebreds, especially German shepherds and English springer spaniels. The latter may have a genetic deficiency of phosphofructokinase production and are more likely to develop fulminant disease. Illness occurs most frequently between March and October.

Canine disease may be clinical or subclinical. Fever, occurring 4 to 5 days after contact with an infected tick, is the most consistent finding. The incubation period ranges from 2 days to 2 weeks. Cutaneous lesions include hyperemia and edema of the extremities, and pinna of the ears, lips, penile sheath, and scrotum. Petechial and ecchymotic hemorrhages may be found on the oral, genital, or ocular mucous membranes. Other clinical findings are vague and may include polyarthritis, myalgia, abdominal pain, vestibular deficits, anorexia, and altered mental status. In the latter stages of illness, necrosis of the extremities or nasal planum has been reported.

PATHOGENESIS

Rickettsial replication occurs only in host cells, despite their ability to independently synthesize proteins. Rickettsiae attach to a protein-dependent receptor on the host cell membrane, with rickettsial outer-membrane protein A functioning as an adhesin. The organisms stimulate their own uptake and, unlike some other similar organisms, they have not adapted to an intravacuolar environment. Rickettsiae must escape from the phagosome to survive intracellularly; soon after engulfment they lyse the phagosomal membrane and are released to the cytosol, where they acquire their nutrients and proliferate by binary fission.

Rickettsiae produce several enzymes that cause host-cell injury. Infected endothelial cells produce reactive oxygen species that damage membranes through lipid peroxidation. Phospholipase A_2, produced by *R. rickettsii* and several spotted fever group organisms, degrades phospholipids in cell membranes, causing hemolysis and other toxic/degenerative effects. *Rickettsiae rickettsii* can block host cell apoptosis, interfering with a host defense mechanism aimed at confining infection by intracellular bacterial pathogens.

Rickettsiae associate primarily with vascular endothelial and vascular smooth muscle cells, causing necrotizing vasculitis and perivasculitis as hallmark lesions. Hemorrhages, effusions, and, in severe cases, acute circulatory failure follow cellular degeneration. The swollen endothelium contains large numbers of bacteria that are released as the cells degenerate. Thrombosis occurs in affected vessels, with interstitial accumulation of neutrophils and mononuclear cells in lungs, liver, kidneys, heart, and perivascularly in the brain. Thrombocytopenia and disseminated intravascular coagulopathy may occur. Increased plasma loss results in edema. These processes also lead to development of the rash that is typical of RMSF and causes tissue damage.

DIAGNOSIS

Laboratory procedures to aid in the diagnosis of RMSF including microbiologic cultivation, serology, immunodetection, and molecular methods. Isolation of the organism from tissues or body fluids is preferred, but is time consuming and not widely available; biosafety level 3 containment and personnel with extensive experience are required. Serologic assays are the methods most frequently used for diagnosis of RMSF. They include indirect immunofluorescence assay (IFA), a latex agglutination test, and enzyme immunoassays. IFA, generally considered the reference standard, is the test currently used by the CDC and most state public health laboratories. It can be used to detect IgG or IgM antibodies in early (acute) and late (convalescent) samples. Most patients have increased IgM titers by the end of the first week of illness. Diagnostic levels of IgG generally do not appear until 7 to 10 days after the onset of illness, and the existence of low levels of specific antibody in nondiseased individuals emphasizes the importance of demonstrating a rising titer. A direct fluorescent antibody assay can be applied to rash biopsies. This test may not always detect the agent because of nonuniform distribution of rickettsiae in lesions. The sensitivity is only approximately 70%, even in laboratories with experience in performing this test, but can be useful in patients who have not seroconverted. This test is offered by the CDC, a few state health departments, some university-based hospitals, and commercial laboratories in the United States. Polymerase chain reaction (PCR) assays have been applied successfully to samples of peripheral blood, plasma, buffy coat, and fresh or paraffin-embedded tissue.

Treatment decisions should be based on epidemiologic and clinical clues because there is no widely available laboratory assay that provides rapid confirmation of early RMSF. Routine clinical laboratory findings suggestive of RMSF may include normal white blood cell count, thrombocytopenia, hyponatremia, or elevated liver enzyme levels.

CONTROL, PREVENTION, AND THERAPY

Dogs that reside near wooded areas or areas with high grass are at increased risk of infection. Reducing exposure to ticks, via topical or systemic tick control products, or prompt, careful tick removal is the most effective way to reduce incidence of RMSF. Regular applications of acaricides to kennels or other dog housing areas will control the tick population. Persons exposed to tick-infested habitats should search out and remove crawling or attached ticks. No licensed vaccine is available for RMSF.

Early diagnosis based on clinical and epidemiologic findings and early treatment with the appropriate antibiotic are essential to control infection. If the patient is treated within the first 4 to 5 days of onset, fever generally subsides 24 to 72 hours after initiation of treatment with an appropriate antibiotic. Failure of clinical disease to respond to tetracycline therapy argues against a diagnosis of RMSF. Resolution of fever may be delayed in severely ill patients, especially in cases of damage to multiple organ systems. Preventive therapy in non-ill patients who have had recent tick bites is *not* recommended and may, in fact, only delay the onset of disease.

Doxycycline is the drug of choice for patients with RMSF. Therapy is continued for at least 3 days after fever subsides and until there is unequivocal evidence of clinical improvement, generally for a minimum total course of 5 to 10 days. Severe or complicated disease may require longer treatment courses. Chloramphenicol is an alternative therapeutic drug for RMSF, but requires careful monitoring of blood levels because of its side effects.

Other Rickettsial Diseases

The term *typhus* comes from the Greek word "typhein," which means to smoke, and is a reference to the "smoky" or clouded mental status exhibited by patients affected by epidemic typhus, murine typhus, cat flea typhus, or scrub typhus.

EPIDEMIC TYPHUS

Rickettsia prowazekii is the etiologic agent of epidemic typhus, a louse-borne disease of humans worldwide. Disease usually occurs among people living in crowded, unsanitary environments. Symptoms are flulike, and include fever, headache, chills, myalgia, and arthralgia. A rash may appear 1 week after the onset of symptoms. Cases in the eastern and southeastern United States are attributed to contact with flying squirrels infested with fleas or lice.

MURINE TYPHUS

Murine typhus, caused by *Rickettsia typhi,* is distributed widely throughout the world, especially in the warm and humid coastal environments of the tropics and subtropics. In the developed world, the infection is found along the eastern coasts of the south Atlantic states of the United States, the Caribbean, and Pacific coasts, as well as Hawaii. It is also found around the Mediterranean and on the Atlantic coast of Africa. Although generally coastal in distribution, the disease may well spread away from the coast via major routes of transportation.

This zoonotic disease, in which rats function as an asymptomatic reservoir, is vectored by the Oriental rat flea *(Xenopsylla cheopis).* Domestic cats, opossums, and cat fleas have also been implicated in a transmission cycle. Transmission may be by flea bites, but also by contact with flea feces, by aerosolization, or by rubbing into a flea bite.

Murine typhus is a relatively mild disease, although about 10% of patients require intensive care and the case fatality rate is 1% to 4%. Tetracyclines remain the drug of choice for treatment.

CAT FLEA TYPHUS

Cat flea typhus is a recently described human disease associated with *Rickettsia felis* infection. The agent is stably maintained by transovarial transmission in the cat flea. The complete description of disease is not available because there have been so few clinical cases reported in humans. Cats may be naturally infected while remaining asymptomatic.

THE GENUS *ORIENTIA*

Orientia (Rickettsia) tsutsugamushi is the agent of scrub typhus, a febrile illness of humans that is endemic in eastern Asia, Japan, the western Pacific islands, and Australia. Disease is transmitted to humans by chigger bites, and bacteria are maintained in the mite population through transovarial transmission. Rodents and birds may serve as reservoirs of infection for mites, but are not believed to be important reservoirs for human disease. Rare subclinical infections have been reported in dogs. The agent resides free in the cytosol of infected cells.

THE GENUS *PISCIRICKETTSIA*

Since 1939, rickettsial agents have been associated with recurring epizootics of disease in a variety of fresh- and saltwater fish. In the early 1990s, *Piscirickettsia salmonis* became the first "rickettsia-like" bacterium to be recognized as a fish pathogen. It infects a wide range of salmonid fish, causing a systemic infection associated with high mortalities. Disease outbreaks have occurred in Chile, Norway, Ireland, and Canada. *Piscirickettsia salmonis* has not been found in nonsalmonid fish. This gram-negative, nonmotile, pleomorphic (but predominantly coccoid) bacterium is found within membrane-bound vacuoles in host cells. It has been placed alone in the class Piscirickettsiacae and, based on 16S rDNA gene sequence analysis, is closely related to organisms in the genera *Francisella* and *Legionella*.

There is little information regarding the source, reservoir, and mode of transmission of this agent. Several studies have suggested horizontal transmission. Gills and skin appear to be routes of entry.

Piscirickettsiosis is emerging as a disease with significant economic impact. Illness occurs within 6 to 12 weeks of smolt placement. Mortality rates may reach 100%. Clinical signs are nonspecific and include anorexia, lethargy, erratic swimming behavior, and exophthalmia. Raised skin lesions that become hemorrhagic may be present. Granulomatous lesions are present in the kidney,

spleen, and heart. "Crater-form" liver lesions, gill hyperplasia and necrosis, and gut necrosis are consistently observed with *P. salmonis* infection.

The diagnosis of piscirickettsiosis is made through cytologic examination of kidney impression smears, histologic examination of tissue lesions, immunohistochemistry, serology, and molecular detection methods. Histologic examination of affected tissues reveals small coccoid organisms within the cytoplasm of monocytes and macrophages.

Stress appears to be a predisposing factor to piscirickettsiosis, so reducing stocking density, immediate removal of moribund fish, and leaving a pond fallow for a period of time may control epizootics. Infected salmonids respond poorly to antibiotic treatment. This may be caused in part by the variability in dosage received by fish in a pond setting. No effective vaccine is commercially available; however, an experimental subunit vaccine has proven efficacious.

Piscirickettsia-like organisms have been associated with increased mortality rates in a wide variety of fish species, including white sea bass, black sea bass, tilapia, blue-eyed plecostomus, and dragonet. Three of these piscirickettsia-like organisms have already been reported in nonsalmonid fish species in North America. The bacteria are not known to infect human or other terrestrial animals. Clinical signs consist of red skin rashes that may reach up to 1 inch in diameter. Laboratory analysis reveals gram-negative curved intracellular bacteria with ringed or rod forms.

SUGGESTED READINGS

Campbell RS: Pathogenesis and pathology of the complex rickettsial infections, *Vet Bull* 64:1-24, 1994.

La Scola B, Raoult D: Laboratory diagnosis of rickettsioses: current approaches to diagnosis of old and new rickettsial diseases, *J Clin Microbiol* 35:2715-2727, 1997.

Madigan JE, Pusterla N: Ehrlichial diseases, *Vet Clin North Am Equine Pract* 16:487-499, 2000.

Mauel MJ, Miller DL: Piscirickettsiosis and piscirickettsiosis-like infections in fish: a review, *Vet Microbiol* 87:279-289, 2002.

Raoult D, Roux V: Rickettsioses as paradigms of new or emerging infectious diseases, *Clin Microbiol Rev* 10:694-719, 1997.

Walker DH, Vilbuena GA, Olano JP: Pathogenic mechanisms of diseases caused by *Rickettsia, Ann N Y Acad Sci* 990:1-11, 2003.

Warner RD, Marsh WW: Rocky Mountain spotted fever, *J Am Vet Med Assoc* 221:1413-1417, 2002.

Three

Veterinary Mycology

Chapter 44

Introduction to Veterinary Mycology

Fungal diseases of nonhumans were reported nearly two centuries ago, and among the first was infection by *Beauveria bassiana,* a fungal pathogen of silkworms that nearly destroyed the Chinese silk industry in the early nineteenth century. After many decades of relative neglect, modern veterinary mycology has become part of the mainstream of veterinary micro-biology. Frequency of diagnosis of mycoses in domestic animals has increased in concert with the pattern in human medicine. This is partly because of advances in veterinary oncology, in which immunosuppressive treatments predispose to fungal infection. In addition, the increased number of effective antifungal agents for use in animals has increased interest in detection, identification, and characterization of animal-associated fungi.

Fungi are unicellular or multicellular chemo-heterotrophic eukaryotes. Their cell walls contain cellulose, chitin, glucan, chitosan, and/or mannan. For practical purposes they may be grouped into yeasts, molds, and fungal-like agents. *Yeasts* are oval to spherical single cells; they reproduce by budding, a phenomenon in which a progenitor cell pinches off part of itself to produce another identical cell. *Molds* are multicellular filamentous fungi that consist of masses of threadlike fila-ments called hyphae that grow by elongation of their tips into an intertwining mat called the mycelium (Figure 44-1). *Fungal-like agents,* as

exemplified by *Prototheca* and *Pythium* species, have traditionally been discussed with mycotic agents because they produce elements that resem-ble fungi in tissue, and some may form yeastlike colonies on mycologic media.

The individual reproductive bodies of fungi are called spores. During the evolutionary process, most fungi relied on a combination of asexual and sexual reproduction for survival. Asexual spores are produced by mitosis. The two main types of asexual spores are sporangiospores and conidia (Figure 44-2). Many of the lower fungi of the class Zygomycetes produce sporangiospores that are contained in a closed structure called the spo-rangium. Conidia are naked spores borne on hyphae and produced by fungi such as *Aspergillus* and *Penicillium* spp. Sexual spores are produced through fusion of the protoplasm and nuclei of two cells by meiosis, and include ascospores, basidiospores, and zygospores (Figure 44-3). Sexual spores and the protective structures that surround them serve as the basis for fungal classification.

Pathogenic fungi are categorized into four groups based on sexual reproduction, even if sexual reproduction has not been observed. These groups correspond to phyla within the kingdom Fungi and comprise the ascomycetes, basidio-mycetes, zygomycetes, and deuteromycetes (fungi imperfecti). The first three groups produce sexual spores, but the deuteromycetes are "imperfect,"

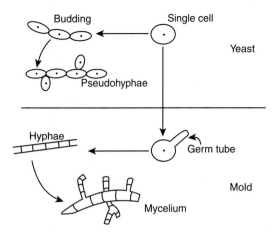

FIGURE 44-1 Yeast and mold forms of fungi. (Courtesy Ashley E. Harmon.)

in that they have no known sexual state. The genera comprising the deuteromycetes are called "form" genera, because they are characterized without the use of sexual structures. Taxonomy of the veterinary pathogenic fungi is presented in Table 44-1.

Mycology is often descriptive, and the importance of morphology in the identification process mitigates in favor of a clear understanding of mycologic terminology (Table 44-2). The *mycelial mat* is known as the thallus, but this term is specifically reserved for colonial growth that arises from a single spore. Some of the medically significant fungi, such as *Histoplasma capsulatum* and *Blastomyces dermatitidis,* are *dimorphic,* in that they can exist in either the yeast or mold form; yeast forms are present at 37° C and the mold

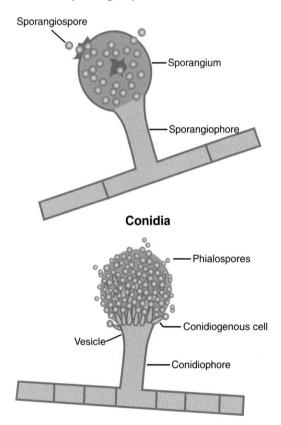

FIGURE 44-2 Sporangiospores and conidia, the two main types of asexual spores. (Courtesy Ashley E. Harmon.)

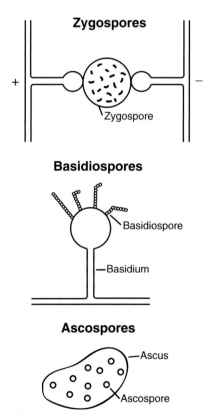

FIGURE 44-3 Sexual spores (ascospores, basidiospores, and zygospores) are produced through fusion of the protoplasm and nuclei of two cells by meiosis. (Courtesy Ashley E. Harmon.)

TABLE 44-1 Taxonomy of the Veterinary Pathogenic Fungi

Taxonomic Designation	Representative Genera	Veterinary Disease
	Phylum Zygomycota, Class Zygomycetes	
Order Mucorales	*Absidia, Mucor, Rhizopus*	Abortion, zygomycosis
Order Entomophthorales	*Basidiobolus, Conidiobolus*	Nasal infection, zygomycosis
	Phylum Ascomycota, Class Ascomycetes	
Order Saccharomycetales	*Pichia* (teleomorphs of some *Candida* spp.)	Numerous mycoses
Order Onygenales	*Arthroderma* (teleomorphs of dermatophytes)	Ringworm
Order Eurotiales	Teleomorphs of some *Aspergillus* spp.	Aspergillosis
Order Microascales	*Pseudoallescheria boydii* (teleomorph of *Scedosporium apiospermum*)	Mycetoma
Order Pyrenomycetes	*Gibberella* (teleomorph of some *Fusarium* spp.)	Mycotic keratitis
	Phylum Basidiomycota, Class Basidiomycetes	
Order Tremellales	*Filobasidiella* (teleomorph of *Cryptococcus neoformans*)	Cryptococcosis
	Phylum Deuteromycota, Class Deuteromycetes	
Order Cryptococcales	*Candida, Cryptococcus, Malassezia, Trichosporon*	Numerous mycoses
ORDER MONILIALES		
Family Moniciliaceae	*Aspergillus, Coccidioides, Sporothrix*	Numerous mycoses
Family Dematiaceae	*Alternaria, Bipolaris, Cladosporium, Curvularia, Exophiala*	Chromoblastomycosis, mycetoma, nasal granuloma, phaeohyphomycosis

TABLE 44-2 Glossary of Mycologic Terminology

Term	Definition
Aerial hyphae	Hyphae that develop above the agar surface
Anamorph	Asexual form of a conidial fungus
Annelide	Cell that produces conidia; as the conidium is released, a ring of cell wall material is formed
Anthropophilic	Fungi that almost exclusively infect humans; examples are *Epidermophyton floccosum* and *Trichophyton rubrum*
Arthrospore	Asexual spore produced by fragmentation of existing hypha into separate cells; examples are *Coccidioides immitis* and *Geotrichum candidum*
Ascospore	Sexual spore produced in a saclike structure (ascus), characteristic of true yeasts
Ascus	Round saclike structure that contains ascospores
Asexual	Reproduction by division or redistribution of nuclei but without nuclear fusion
Basidiospore	Sexual spore formed on the basidium
Blastoconidium	Blastospore; conidium formed by budding along hypha, pseudohypha, or single cell; examples are *Candida albicans* and *Cryptococcus neoformans*
Budding	Process of asexual reproduction in which new cells develop as outgrowths of the parent cell; examples are yeasts
Capsule	Colorless, mucopolysaccharide sheath on the cell wall; example is *Cryptococcus neoformans*
Chlamydospore	Thick-walled resistant cell formed as a result of enlargement of an existing hyphal cell; examples are *Histoplasma capsulatum* and *Candida albicans*
Chromoblastomycosis	Chronic fungal infection characterized by nodular, cutaneous lesions; contain dark brown sclerotic bodies when examined microscopically
Clavate	Club shaped; examples are macroconidia of *Microsporum nanum*
Cleistothecium	Closed, round structure in which asci and ascospores are held until their release; example is *Pseudallescheria boydii*
Columella	Swollen tip of sporangiospore projecting into sporangium in some Mucorales; examples are *Rhizopus* and *Mucor* spp.

Continued

TABLE 44-2 Glossary of Mycologic Terminology—cont'd

Term	Definition
Conidiophore	Specialized hypha or cell on which conidia are produced; examples are *Aspergillus* and *Penicillium* spp.
Conidium	Asexual spore; examples are *Aspergillus* and *Penicillium* spp.
Dematiaceous	Fungi that possess dark hyphae; examples are *Sporothrix schenckii* and *Ochroconis (Dactylaria) gallopava*
Dermatophtye	Member of genus *Microsporum, Trichophyton,* or *Epidermophtyon;* infects hair, skin, or nails
Dichotomous	Division of hyphae into two equal branches of same diameter as original hypha; examples are *Aspergillus* spp.
Dimorphic	Fungi that exist in yeast and mycelial forms; examples are *Blastomyces dermatitidis* and *Histoplasma capsulatum*
Echinulate	Spiny; examples are macroconidia of *Microsporum* spp.
Ectothrix	Arthrospores located on outermost portion of hair shaft; examples are *Microsporum* spp.
Endothrix	Arthrospores located within hair shaft; examples are *Trichophyton* spp.
Fungus	Filamentous or unicellular, achlorophyllic organism with true nucleus enclosed in membrane and containing chitin in cell wall
Fusiform	Spindle shaped; examples are macroconidia of *Fusarium* spp.
Geophilic	Fungi that reside in soil; examples are *Microsporum gypseum* and *Coccidioides immitis*
Germ tube	Tubelike outgrowth produced by germinating cells; develops into hypha; example is *Candida albicans*
Hyaline	Transparent, clear, or colorless, usually in reference to hyphae; examples are *Fusarium* and *Penicillium* spp.
Hypha	Individual, threadlike filament comprising vegetative fungal growth
Macroconidium	Larger of two sizes of conidia, usually multicellular; examples are *Microsporum gypseum* and *Microsporum nanum*
Microconidium	Smaller of two sizes of conidia, usually unicellular; examples are *Trichosporon verrucosum* and *Trichosporon mentagrophytes*
Mold	Multicellular filamentous form of fungus; consists of masses of hyphae that grow together into a mycelium; examples are *Aspergillus* spp. and zygomycetes
Muriform	Conidium with longitudinal and transverse walls; examples are *Alternaria alternata* and *Curvularia* spp.
Mycelium	Mass of branching filaments (hyphae) that makes up vegetative growth of fungus
Mycetoma	Fungal tumor of cutaneous and subcutaneous tissues with triad of clinical signs (swelling, draining sinuses, grains, or granules in exudates)
Mycosis	Disease caused by a fungus
Phaeohyphomycosis	Fungal infections whose tissue form is dark-walled hyphae; usually associated with dematiaceous fungi
Phialide	Flasklike structure that produces conidia; examples are *Aspergillus* and *Phialophora* spp.
Propagule	Unit that is able to give rise to another organism
Pseudohypha	Chain of yeast cells; result of budding and elongation without detachment, forming hyphalike filament; examples are *Candida albicans* and *Trichosporon* spp.
Rhizoid	Short, branching hypha that resembles a root; examples are *Rhizopus* spp.
Ringworm	Superficial skin infection caused by dermatophytes; derived from ringlike lesions once thought to be caused by wormlike organisms
Sclerotic bodies	Large, round, brownish, thick-walled cells with vertical and horizontal septa; found in tissue sections from animals affected with chromoblastomycosis
Septate	Having cross-walls; examples are *Aspergillus* spp.
Sessile	Direct hyphal attachment; no stalk involved.
Sexual state	Part of life cycle during which organism reproduces by fusion of two nuclei; in mycology, also known as the "perfect state"
Spherule	Large round structure containing spores; examples are *Coccidioides immitis* and *Rhinosporidium seeberi*

TABLE 44-2 Glossary of Mycologic Terminology—cont'd

Term	Definition
Sporangiophore	Spore-bearing structure, usually closed, on which sporangium develops; examples are *Rhizopus* and *Mucor* spp.
Sporangiospore	Asexual spore produced within a sporangiophore
Sporangium	Closed, often spherical, structure that contains sporangiospores; examples are zygomycetes
Spore	Propagule that develops asexually within a sporangium or by sexual reproduction (ascospore, basidiospore, or zygospore)
Sterigmata	Specialized hypha that bears a conidium; examples are *Aspergillus* spp.
Teleomorph	Sexual form of conidial fungus
Thallus	Vegetative body of a fungus
Tuberculate	Knoblike projections from a cell; examples are macroconidia of *Histoplasma capsulatum*
Vesicle	Swollen or bladderlike cell produced at terminal end of condiophore; examples are *Aspergillus* spp.
Yeasts	Unicellular, budding fungi; examples are *Malassezia pachydermatis* and *Candida albicans*
Zoophilic	Fungi associated with animals
Zoospore	Motile asexual spore
Zygospore	Thick-walled sexual spore produced by zygomycetes

form is present at 25° C. *Dematiaceous fungi* are dark colored, containing melanin in hyphal or conidial cell walls. *Dermatophytes* invade hair, nails, and claws.

Fungal diseases may be grouped in several ways. *Opportunistic fungi* seldom cause disease without some underlying predisposing factor, such as trauma or immunosuppression. *Pathogenic fungi* cause disease without a predisposing factor, and may be grouped into the superficial or cutaneous, subcutaneous, and systemic mycoses. *Superficial* and *cutaneous mycoses* are associated with hair, nails, and keratinized layers of the skin. *Subcutaneous mycoses* affect mainly dermis, bone, muscle, and fascia. *Systemic mycoses* represent a group of fungi that invade internal organs following hematogenous dissemination from the lungs. Each group will be covered in detail in subsequent chapters, as will fungal-like agents such as *Rhinosporidium seeberi, Pythium insidiosum, Prototheca,* and *Pneumocystis carinii.*

Mycoses should be included in the differential diagnosis of any chronic condition that has failed to respond to treatment or for which the etiology is unknown. Accurate diagnosis is facilitated by understanding and applying criteria by which one can distinguish among contamination, colonization, and infection. Animals are typically covered with hair or feathers that provide an ideal environment for fungal colonization that can take place in the absence of frank disease. In the initial assessment of a suspected case of fungal infection, the practitioner should determine if the symptoms are compatible, if fungal elements are observed in host tissue or sterile body fluids, if fungi are recovered from the specimens, and if fungi detected microscopically in tissue sections or other clinical specimens are compatible with those detected by culture.

PRACTICAL PROCEDURES FOR DIAGNOSIS OF FUNGAL DISEASES

Given a basic knowledge of mycology, many fungal infections can be presumptively diagnosed in the veterinarian's office. This requires recognition of basic fungal elements (hyphae, yeasts, or spherules) and minimal equipment and reagents; the practitioner will need a microscope with oil immersion lens, 10% potassium hydroxide (KOH) in glycerol, india ink, a hematologic stain, such as Diff-Quik, glass slides and cover slips, and a book containing an atlas of medical mycology.

Obtaining the proper specimen for diagnosis is of paramount importance. General guidelines are much the same as those for bacterial specimen collection and include aseptic collection techniques, collection from sites representative of the disease

TABLE 44-3 Collection of Clinical Specimens for Diagnosis of Fungal Disease

Specimen	Container	Comments
Hairs	Paper envelope (dry conditions inhibit overgrowth of bacterial or saprophytic fungal contaminants)	Wash and dry affected area with soap and water. With forceps, epilate hairs from the periphery of an active lesion. Pull hairs in the direction of growth to include the root. Look for broken, stubby hairs, which are often infected. Useful for diagnosis of dermatophytosis.
Skin	Paper envelope	Clean skin with alcohol gauze sponge (cotton leaves too many fibers). Scrape the periphery of an active lesion with a sterile scalpel blade. Also, obtain crusts and scabs. Useful for diagnosis of dermatophytosis.
Nails	Paper envelope	Proven nail infections in animals are rare. Cleanse affected nail with alcohol gauze. Scrape with a scalpel blade so that fine pieces are collected. Also, collect debris under the nail. Useful for diagnosis of onchyomycosis.
Biopsy	Sterile tube in sterile saline or water	Normal and affected tissue should be included. Important to prevent specimen desiccation.
Urine	Sterile tube	Centrifuge and use sediment for direct examination and culture. Useful for diagnosis of histoplasmosis.
Cerebrospinal fluid	Sterile tube	Useful for diagnosis of cryptococcosis. Make india ink preparation to observe encapsulated yeasts.
Pleural/ abdominal fluid	Sterile tube	If fluid contains flakes or granules, they should be included because these are actual colonies of organisms.
Transtracheal/ bronchial washings	Sterile tube	Centrifuge and use sediment for direct examination and culture. Useful for diagnosis of systemic mycoses.
Nasal flush	Sterile tube	Centrifuge and use sediment for direct examination and culture. Useful for diagnosis of nasal aspergillosis and guttural pouch mycosis.
Ocular fluid	Sterile tube or syringe	Examine directly. Inoculate onto plated fungal media immediately after collection. Useful for diagnosis of ocular blastomycosis.

process, collection before antifungal therapy, and collection of an adequate volume of material. Procedures are detailed in Table 44-3.

Microscopic examination of clinical materials and isolates obtained by fungal culture is used extensively in fungal identification. Most specimens suspected to contain fungi are initially examined in wet mounts to prevent morphologic distortion of fungal morphology. Wet mounts in KOH are incubated for 30 minutes at room temperature; KOH acts as a clearing agent, digesting the proteinaceous components of host cells and leaving the polysaccharide-containing fungal cell wall intact and more apparent. After digestion, mounts are examined at 100× and 400× magnification for fungal elements. The microscopic appearance of fungi and fungal-like agents in direct examination of clinical material is given in Table 44-4.

Fluorochrome stains, such as calcofluor white, bind to cellulose and chitin in the fungal cell wall and may facilitate detection of fungi. On wet preparations of specimens or on smeared and dried clinical materials, these nondifferential stains are examined with ultraviolet (UV) illumination. Fungi and *Pneumocystis* cysts appear bright blue or green, depending on the type of UV filter used. Hematologic stains can be applied to exudates, and allow examination of fungi without distortion. They are especially useful for demonstration of yeasts. Gram stains are generally not used because they distort fungal morphology.

Fungal specimens should be inoculated onto media that ensure adequate fungal growth and preclude the growth of bacterial contaminants. Traditional media for primary isolation include Sabouraud dextrose and potato dextrose agars. These have a high sugar content and acidic pH

TABLE 44-4 Microscopic Appearance of Fungi and Fungal-Like Agents in Clinical Specimens

Disease	Microscopic Examination Method	Appearance
Aspergillosis	Wet mount (lactophenol cotton blue or KOH)	Septate hyphae with dichotomous branching; may see fruiting heads
Blastomycosis	Wet mount	Thick, double-walled budding yeasts with broad bases of attachment to mother cells
Candidiasis and other yeast infections	Wet mount	Budding and nonbudding yeasts; pseudohyphae may be present
Coccidioidomycosis	Wet mount	Spherules with and without endospores
Cryptococcosis	India ink	Encapsulated yeasts
Dermatophytosis	Wet mount	Hairs with arthrospores (endothrix or ectothrix), hyphae or sheath of spores around skin and nails
Histoplasmosis	Hematologic stain	Small yeasts with narrow necks of attachment to mother cells, often within macrophages
Mycetoma	Wet mount	Dark brown chlamydospores and hyaline hyphae in crushed granules
Phaeohyphomycosis	Wet mount	Dark hyphae
Pneumocystosis	Hematologic stain	Cysts and trophozoites
Protothecosis	Wet mount	Spherical to oval nonbudding, small and large cells containing two or more autospores
Rhinosporidiosis	Wet mount	Spherules (some large) with and without endospores
Sporotrichosis	Hematologic stain	Small oval to round to cigar-shaped yeasts
Zygomycosis	Wet mount	Broad, relatively nonseptate hyphae

KOH, Potassium hydroxide.

that inhibit most bacteria but are supportive for fungi. Media may be made more selective by addition of antibiotics such as chloramphenicol, gentamicin, penicillin, or streptomycin to further inhibit bacterial growth. Cycloheximide, an antifungal agent, may be added to potato dextrose or Sabouraud dextrose agar to prevent overgrowth of saprophytic fungi. Mycosel (or Mycobiotic) are two commercial formulations containing cycloheximide. Because this agent can be inhibitory to some pathogenic fungi (e.g., most zygomycetes, *Cryptococcus neoformans,* and *Aspergillus fumigatus*), it is advisable to use media with and without cycloheximide for fungal specimen processing. Plates are routinely incubated at 25° to 30° C for up to 6 weeks. If dimorphic fungi are suspected, enriched media such as brain-heart infusion agar with 5% blood are incorporated. Blood enrichment and 37° C incubation temperatures promote the growth of the yeast phase. For isolation of the ringworm fungi, a partially differential and selective medium is used. Dermatophyte test medium contains antibiotics, cycloheximide, and an indicator to demonstrate a rise in pH, consistent with the growth of

dermatophytes. Processing schemes for clinical materials appear in Figures 44-4 and 44-5.

Historically, the identification of molds has involved the examination of macroscopic and microscopic characteristics. Macroscopic features, such as colonial morphology, surface color, and pigmentation, are often helpful in identification. Microscopic structures, such as spores and spore-bearing cells, are an essential part of the identification process. Slide cultures are especially useful in the identification of many fungi in that they provide a means to determine conidial ontogeny. Molds that fail to sporulate are often impossible to identify by this method.

Identification of yeasts is based on both morphology and physiologic reactions. Presumptive identification of yeasts is possible because of the incorporation of chromogenic substrates into agar-based media. Several yeast identification systems are commercially available, although identification of rare or atypical isolates may require the participation of a reference laboratory.

Other methods for laboratory diagnosis of mycoses include histologic examination of fixed biopsy material to which fungal stains have been

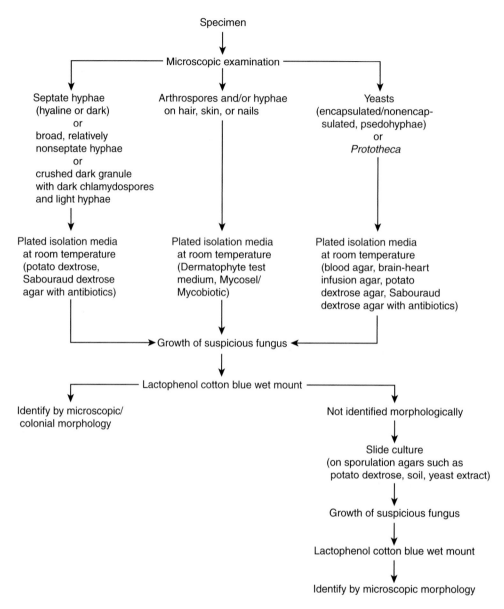

FIGURE 44-4 Processing scheme for clinical specimens: cutaneous and subcutaneous mycoses.

applied. Although most fungi can be visualized in tissue with hematoxylin and eosin stains, the use of special stains enhances their detection. The most widely used stains are Gomori methenamine silver, which stains fungi gray to black, and periodic acid–Schiff, in which fungal elements stain pinkish red.

Latex agglutination and enzyme immunoassay tests are widely used in the detection of fungal antigens in clinical specimens. Exoantigen identification of fungi involves the detection of cell-free antigens produced by the organism in cultures. Exoantigen tests exist for the systemic fungi and for *Pythium insidiosum*. Molecular methods (such as polymerase chain reaction and nucleic acid probes) have been applied to diagnosis and identification and will likely become more important in the future.

Diagnostic details are discussed in chapters on specific agents.

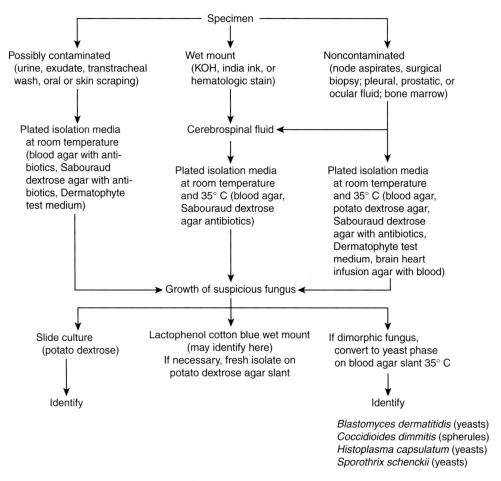

FIGURE 44-5 Processing scheme for clinical specimens: systemic mycoses. *KOH*, Potassium hydroxide.

SUGGESTED READINGS

Larone DH: *Medically important fungi: a guide to identification,* ed 4, Washington, DC, 2002, American Society for Microbiology.

McGinnis MR: *Laboratory handbook of medical mycology,* New York, 1980, Academic Press.

Murray PR, ed: *Manual of clinical microbiology,* ed 7, section 6, Mycology, Washington, DC, 1999, American Society for Microbiology.

Sutton DA, Fothergill AW, Rinaldi MG: *Guide to the clinically significant fungi,* Baltimore, 1998, Williams & Wilkins.

Chapter 45

The Cutaneous Mycoses

The cutaneous mycoses of animals include a wide variety of diseases of the integumentary system and its appendages. Although fungal infection is usually restricted to these areas, pathologic changes may occur elsewhere in the animal because of the presence of the agent and its metabolites. The great majority of these mycoses are caused by the dermatophytes ("skin plants"), or so-called ringworm fungi. In the strictest sense, *dermatophytosis* is an infection caused by a dermatophyte in the keratinized tissues, which include hair, feathers, stratum corneum layers of the skin, and, to a lesser degree, the nails, claws, and horns. Yeasts and normally saprophytic filamentous fungi cause cutaneous infections resembling dermatophytoses, and these are collectively referred to as the *dermatomycoses*.

Dermatophytes are generally grouped into three categories based on their host preference and natural habitat (Table 45-1). *Zoophilic organisms* are pathogens of animals or birds, but may infect humans through contact with infected animals. *Geophilic species* are soil-associated organisms, whereas *anthropophilic species* are near-exclusive pathogens of humans, rarely infecting animals.

The common etiologic agents of the animal dermatophytoses are classified into the anamorphic (asexual or imperfect state) genera *Microsporum* and *Trichophyton*. When members of these genera reproduce sexually, by producing ascomata with asci and ascospores, they are classified in the teleomorphic (sexual or perfect state) genus *Arthroderma*, in the family Arthrodermataceae, within the order Onygenales, and phylum Ascomycota. A third dermatophytic genus, *Epidermophyton*, is anthropophilic, although it has been isolated on occasion from dogs. Dermatophytes isolated from domestic animals are listed in Table 45-2.

Animal dermatomycoses include nondermatophytic superficial and cutaneous fungal infections

TABLE 45-1 Classification of Dermatophytes Isolated from Domestic Animals Based on Host Preference and Natural Habitat

Anthropophilic	Geophilic	Zoophilic
Epidermophyton floccosum	Microsporum gypseum	Microsporum canis
Trichophyton rubrum	M. nanum	M. equinum
T. schoenleinii	M. persicolor	M. gallinae
T. tonsurans	M. vanbreuseghemii	Trichophyton mentagrophytes
T. violaceum	M. cookei	T. simii
Microsporum audouinii		T. verrucosum
M. megninii		

TABLE 45-2   Dermatophytes Isolated from Domestic Animals

Agent	Cat	Dog	Cattle	Sheep	Horse	Chicken	Pig
Microsporum audouinii		R					
M. canis	F	F	R	O	O		R
M. gallinae	R	R	R			F	
M. gypseum	O	F			F		R
M. nanum							F
M. persicolor		R					
M. cookei		R					
M. vanbreuseghemii		R					
Trichophyton equinum		R			F		
T. megninii		R					
T. mentagrophytes	O	F	O	O	O		O
T. rubrum		R					R
T. schoenleinii	R				R		
T. simii		R				F (India)	
T. tonsurans		R					R
T. verrucosum	R	R	F	O	O		R
T. violaceum	R	R					
Epidermophyton floccosum		R					

Blank, Not reported; *F,* frequent; *R,* reported; *O,* occasional.

with organisms such as *Malassezia* spp. and *Trichosporon* spp. These are quite common and often result from an alteration of skin flora or immune status in the host.

DERMATOPHYTOSES: THE GENERA *MICROSPORUM* AND *TRICHOPHYTON*

The genus *Microsporum* includes 17 conventional species, the most significant of which are *Microsporum canis, Microsporum gallinae, Microsporum gypseum,* and *Microsporum nanum.* This genus is characterized by large, rough thick-walled multiseptate macroconidia that are borne from expanded ends of undifferentiated hyphae or short pedicles, and are released by rupture of the supporting cells. They vary in shape from fusiform to obovate, and the microconidia are sessile or stalked, clavate, and usually arranged singly along the hyphae. These species attack hair and skin, and *M. canis* is the most common dermatophyte of domestic animals.

Trichophyton mentagrophytes, Trichophyton equinum, and *Trichophyton verrucosum* are the most common veterinary pathogens among the 20 species in the genus *Trichophyton. Trichophyton* spp. differ from those of the genus *Microsporum* in their cylindrical, clavate to cigar–shaped, thin-walled or thick-walled smooth macroconidia that are produced rarely and in small numbers.

Some isolates may be sterile, and sporulation is induced only during growth on specific media. Microconidia are one celled and round or pyriform. They are numerous and are solitary or arranged in clusters. Microconidia are often the predominant type of conidia produced by *Trichophyton* spp. These species attack hair, skin, nails, horns, and claws.

DISEASES AND EPIDEMIOLOGY

Dermatophytoses are among the few communicable fungal diseases, and may be acquired from contact with other infected animals or from fomites. Geophilic dermatophytes reside primarily in the soil, resisting degradation by soil bacteria by means of antibacterial substances in their cell walls; their spores are heat resistant. Animal infections by geophiles result from contact with contaminated soil, where macroconidia on shed hairs play an important role in animal infection. Infections are sporadic and not transmitted readily between animals, occurring typically in autumn after the fungus has multiplied on the hair during the warmer summer months. Biting insects may also be involved in transmission. Geophilic species may be ancestral to the pathogenic zoophilic and anthropophilic dermatophytes, based on their ability to decompose keratin and their consequent close association with animals through living in hair and feathers.

Zoophilic dermatophytes are parasites of the skin of animals and not known to live in the soil; soil survival is possible, especially if embedded in hair, feathers, or skin scales. This is especially common in catteries, where recurrent ringworm infections may be common. Zoophilic dermatophyte infections are most often observed in young animals that are kept in proximity to one another. Predisposing factors include hot, humid conditions; trauma; and poor nutrition. Conidial survival in the environment depends directly on moisture. Although extremely resistant to freezing, spores tend to be susceptible to desiccation and high environmental temperatures. Spores may also remain viable on skin and hair after an animal recovers from clinical disease. Mice and rodents may further serve as a source of infection by leaving infected hairs around barns.

Clinical signs of dermatophytosis vary with the infecting strain and immune status of the host. Typical disease is characterized by alopecia, erythema, scaling, crusting, annular-ringed lesions, and vesicles or papules. As a rule, infections caused by *Trichophyton* spp. are usually more severe than those caused by *Microsporum* spp. because more inflammation is associated with the former.

Feline ringworm is usually caused by *M. canis* and cats serve as the primary reservoir for this dermatophyte. Animals are often asymptomatic and may thus pose a public health risk. In fact, feline ringworm is frequently subclinical, and attention may be drawn to the animal only after a diagnosis of ringworm is made in its owner. The main site of infection is the head. Clinical signs range from circular areas of stubbled hair, alopecia, and mild scaling to severe folliculitis and generalized hair loss. Disease is most common in kittens, which have immature immune systems, and in adults with debilitating disease or immune deficiency. In Persian cats, granulomatous dermatitis and panniculitis (pseudomycetoma) characterized by a relapsing skin disease with ulcerated nodules and yellow granular discharge caused by *M. canis* has been described. Rarely these pseudomycetomas may progress intraabdominally. Feline otitis caused by *M. canis* is often characterized by a persistent waxy, ceruminous otic discharge in both external auditory canals. Dermatophytosis should be included in the differential diagnosis of feline otic conditions, particularly when otitis becomes chronic or is refractory to treatment.

Canine ringworm is characterized by circular lesions up to 2.5 cm in diameter on any part of the body, but most commonly on the face, elbows, and paws. Agents frequently recovered are *M. canis, M. gypseum,* and *T. mentagrophytes.* Hairs become brittle, the skin appears dry and scaly, and crusts and scabs are present. In severe infections caused by *T. mentagrophytes,* kerions may develop. These are lesions of intense inflammation that exhibit swelling, ulceration, and purulent exudation. Canine dermatophytic pseudomycetoma, with subcutaneous nodule formation, has been reported.

Trichophyton equinum and *M. gypseum* are the two most common agents of equine dermatophytosis. The disease presents as multiple, dry, scaly raised lesions on any part of the animal. Areas that are groomed, or those upon which tack is placed, may be more frequently involved. Inflammation and production of exudates cause hair to mat together, and enlarged lesions create a "moth-eaten" appearance. Infections often become chronic and subclinical, but recrudesce in response to stress.

Ringworm is a common disease of cattle, with most infections being caused by *T. verrucosum.* Calves are more susceptible than adults, and incidence is higher in winter, possibly because of crowding and increased contact with carrier animals or contaminated debris in barns. Lesions are circular, scattered, and accompanied by skin scaling and alopecia. Large circumscribed plaques may develop, with the formation of thick scabs and crusts. Severe inflammation, pruritus, and secondary bacterial infection may occur. Spontaneous resolution of infection follows this stage.

Ringworm was only recently recognized as a common disease of sheep. Ovine dermatophytosis has been on the increase, especially in the show lamb arena in the United States, where it is referred to as "club-lamb fungus." A sheep-adapted strain of *T. verrucosum* has been identified as the etiologic agent. The infection is spread through direct contact with infected animals, contaminated grooming instruments, or infective materials lodged in wood fences and other materials in show barns or farm sites that have held infected lambs. Lesions generally appear a few weeks after contact and begin as clearly demarcated, scaly, scab-covered, or hairless areas on the face, ears, and wool-less areas of the neck, or as matted areas in the wool of unshorn or long-fleece sheep. Lesions vary in size from pinpoints to 3 inches in diameter. Disease is usually self-resolving within in 2 to 4 months after exposure, although wool may not grow back for an additional 2 to 5 months.

Ringworm infection of poultry is called "favus" and is attributed to *M. gallinae.* "White comb" is another name given to the small white patches on the comb of infected male birds. These areas may enlarge and coalesce so that the entire comb becomes covered with a thick white coating. The disease may occasionally extend into the feathers, leading to emaciation and death.

Dermatophyte infection of swine is common, whether animals are raised in confinement or outdoors. *Microsporum nanum* accounts for most cases of disease, followed by *M. gypseum, M. canis,* and *T. mentagrophytes,* although other agents have been reported. Large white breeds such as the Yorkshire are most frequently affected, and all age groups may be involved. Incidence appears to be greater where stocking density and humidity are high and sanitation is poor. Ringworm lesions may be located anywhere on the body, and are small, circular, roughened, and mildly inflamed. They begin as circumscribed spots that expand centrifugally and may involve large areas of the body. The skin becomes reddish or light brown, and crusts may form, but usually no loss of hair occurs. The disease is self-limiting and lesions resolve rapidly (usually within 2-3 months), leaving only areas of slight scaling and discoloration.

Because ringworm is a zoonotic disease, the veterinarian should be aware of human symptoms (which are similar to those in animals), and advise clients to seek the help of a physician if dermatophytosis is suspected. In addition, clients should further be advised of the increased susceptibility of children, and to discourage the handling of infected pets.

PATHOGENESIS

The dermatophyte structure most commonly associated with contagion is the spore, which is found within or attached to the exterior of infected hairs and within skin scales. Dermatophytes gain entry to the skin through minor trauma such as abrasions. They do not invade or survive on living cells or in areas of intense inflammation. Spores germinate and the fungus grows on the stratum corneum of the skin and nails, in the nonviable keratin above the zone of keratinization of actively growing hair (anagen phase), and in the keratinized stratum corneum around the hair follicle. Affected skin becomes scaly or crusty and infected hairs become brittle and dry. Fungal growth keeps pace with that of the hair, but once the hair enters the telogen phase, fungi stop growing and the infection of that hair resolves.

The ability to invade keratinized tissues and the possession of several enzymes, such as proteases, keratinases, and elastase, are major virulence factors of these fungi. Proteases are produced during the invasion process, weakening the hair shaft and resulting in breakage and stubble. There is evidence for in vivo secretion of a 315 kD keratinolytic subtilisin-like serine protease by *M. canis,* with resulting keratolysis. There may be a relationship between the clinical severity of *M. canis* infections and extent of keratinase production in vitro. Specimens from symptomatic dogs and cats contain significantly higher keratinase activity than those from asymptomatic animals. Strains with high in vitro keratinase activity induce infections in guinea pigs that were more acute than those caused by strains with low keratinase activity. The same relationship was not observed for elastase, lipase, or DNase.

Infection by geophilic or zoophilic dermatophytes evokes an intense inflammatory response. This is detrimental to fungal growth, which stops or moves to the next hair follicle and results in the circular spread of the lesion with healing in the center. Genesis of dermatophytic skin lesions may be associated with the host immune response, which is characterized by interferon-γ (IFN-γ) release. Inflammation is produced by activated lymphocytes and macrophages that are involved in the delayed type hypersensitivity reaction when these fungal agents reach the dermis.

The two major classes of dermatophyte antigens are glycopeptides and keratinases. The protein portion of the glycopeptides stimulates cell-mediated immunity, whereas the polysaccharide portion stimulates humoral immunity. Keratinases elicit delayed-type hypersensitivity responses. Inflammation has also been associated with the production of fungal elastases.

DIAGNOSIS

Diagnosis of dermatophytosis is based on demonstration of consistent clinical signs, examination of affected hair with a Wood's lamp, microscopic examination of hair or skin specimens, and fungal culture. Hairs infected with *M. canis* fluoresce green when illuminated with long-wave ultraviolet light. Microscopic examination is based on wet mounts of hair, skin, or nail scrapings in 10% potassium hydroxide (KOH), and the appearance of infected hairs depends on the causative agent. Hyphae invade the hairs, and arthrospores are produced by hyphal fragmentation. Ectothrix formation is associated with *M. canis, M. gallinae, M. gypseum, M. nanum, T. equinum, T. mentagrophytes,* and *T. verrucosum.* Arthrospores appear as a sheath surrounding the hair or as chains on the hair surface. Endothrix formation is not typically observed with the common animal dermatophytes. For culture, clinical material should be inoculated onto dermatophyte test medium (DTM), a selective/differential medium containing cycloheximide and chloramphenicol or gentamicin to inhibit saprobic fungal and bacterial contamination. Other media additives include nicotinic acid, which is necessary for the recovery of *T. equinum,* and inositol and thiamine, which are growth factors for *T. verrucosum.* This medium further contains a phenol red indicator. As dermatophytes grow, proteolysis results in the liberation of excess ammonium ion, raising the pH, and changing the medium from yellow to red (Figure 45-1). Some fungal contaminants, such as *Alternaria* spp., may grow on DTM, but they are morphologically dissimilar to the dermatophytes. Cultures are routinely incubated at 25° to 30° C, unless *T. verrucosum* is suspected because this dermatophyte grows optimally at 37° C. Plates are examined weekly for up to 4 weeks.

Routine procedures for dermatophyte species identification rely on examination of the colony (pigmentation on the surface or reverse sides, texture, topography, rate of growth) and microscopic morphology (size and shape of macroconidia and microconidia, presence of spirals, pectinate branches, and nodular organs) (Figures 45-2 and 45-3). These criteria, however, may be insufficient because of variable colonial appearance. Many agents, especially in the genus *Trichophyton,* fail to sporulate in vitro, and require special media to stimulate spore production. Physiologic tests such as, nutritional requirements (amino acids and vitamins), temperature tolerance, urease production, and in vitro hair perforation, may be used as adjuncts to identify these species correctly. Although molecular methods have been developed (such as polymerase chain reaction [PCR] assay),

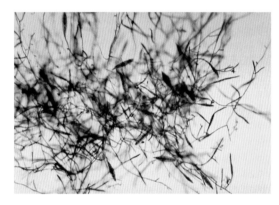

FIGURE 45-2 *Microsporum canis* macroconidia. (Courtesy Public Health Image Library, PHIL #3209, Centers for Disease Control and Prevention, Atlanta, 1969, Leanor Haley.)

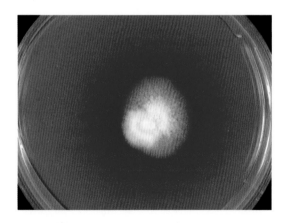

FIGURE 45-1 *Microsporum canis* on dermatophyte test medium. (Courtesy Karen W. Post.)

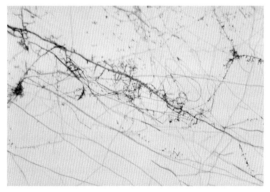

FIGURE 45-3 *Trichophyton mentagrophytes* macroconidia. (Courtesy Public Health Image Library, PHIL #3213, Centers for Disease Control and Prevention, Atlanta, 1969, Leanor Haley.)

and serologic tests (to quantitate dermatophyte antibodies), they are not routinely commercially available.

PREVENTION AND CONTROL

For prevention and control of dermatophytoses, the veterinarian must take into consideration the source of infection, the etiologic agent, and the infection site. It is important to locate the animal reservoir for infections attributed to the zoophilic dermatophytes. Dogs and cats infected with *M. canis* may be easily examined with a Wood's lamp, whereas it is more difficult to detect animals affected by *T. mentagrophytes* because infected hairs will not fluoresce. Good hygiene, sanitation, and fungicidal sprays and washes have been effective in controlling these infections. Carpeted areas should be vacuumed, environmental surfaces (cages, litterboxes), brushes/combs and transportation vehicles disinfected, and contaminated bedding removed.

Another means of preventing dermatophytosis involves the use of vaccines. This is an effective strategy to control disease in cattle; large-scale vaccination programs in Europe have greatly reduced the prevalence of dermatophytosis. Vaccination of cats, particularly in breeding catteries with *M. canis* problems, has been attempted, but efficacy of these vaccines has been poor.

Several factors should be considered in therapy of dermatophytosis. Fungi seen in direct smears are not active in the disease process but are being removed from the skin as keratin is shed. The important fungal activity is confined to the invasion of new keratin; thus the zone of active infection is restricted to and protected by the overlying keratin layer. Antifungal agents should be able to penetrate the keratin (if tropical treatment) or be transported systemically throughout the body to attack the fungus from within.

Localized dermatophytosis may be self-limiting, with spontaneous resolution, may generalize to other areas of the body, or may spread to other animals and humans. Because of this zoonotic potential, treatment is usually indicated. Hair on and around lesions is clipped and topical antifungal therapy initiated. Topical therapy should be reserved for glabrous areas where the keratin layer is thin. Topical agents that have been used successfully include lime sulfur solution, thiabendazole, miconazole, econazole, clotrimazole, enilconazole, ketoconazole, itraconazole, povidone-iodine solution, tolnaftate, 50% captan powder, chlorhexidine solution, and 5% sodium hypochlorite solution. Topical therapy is not always effective. Because viable ringworm fungi have been demonstrated in normal keratin up to 6 cm from the margin of a lesion, systemic therapy is preferred because all sites of infection may be treated at the same time.

For generalized lesions, therapy also includes clipping, applying topical antifungal agents, and systemically administrating antifungals. Griseofulvin has been used extensively for systemic therapy, but requires active fungal metabolism and consequently is not recommended to treat the asymptomatic carrier state. Once the drug of choice for treatment of dermatophytosis, griseofulvin is less commonly used because of the availability of more effective and less toxic drugs. Ketoconazole, clotrimazole, itraconazole, terbinafine, naftifine, and amorolfine are systemic agents that have demonstrated in vitro activity against dermatophytes. Of these, terbinafine appears to be the most effective. Systemic treatment is continued until lesions have resolved and fungal cultures are negative.

Lufenuron is an insect development inhibitor because of its effects on chitin synthesis, and is approved for use in veterinary medicine for flea control. However, it has now been shown to be effective in treatment of cutaneous fungal infections in cats and dogs, providing an effective, safe, and rapid method for treating dermatophytoses and dermatomycoses.

DERMATOMYCOSES: THE GENERA *MALASSEZIA*, *GEOTRICHUM CANDIDUM*, AND *TRICHOSPORON BEIGELII*

Malassezia spp., *G. candidum*, and *T. beigelii* have been associated with animal dermatomycoses. Infections by *Malassezia* spp. are more common and are discussed in greatest detail.

THE GENUS *MALASSEZIA*

The genus *Malassezia* belongs to the phylum Basidiomycota, class Basidiomycetes, order Tremellales, and family Filobasidium uniguttulatum, and was formerly the genus *Pityrosporum*. These lipophilic yeasts are members of the normal cutaneous flora of animals and man and they act as opportunistic pathogens. The nine species currently recognized are *Malassezia furfur*,

Malasezzia pachydermatis, Malassezia sympodialis, Malassezia globosa, Malassezia obtusa, Malassezia restricta, Malassezia dermatis, Malassezia nana, and *Malassezia slooffiae.* The primary species of veterinary significance are *M. pachydermatis* and *M. nana,* but *M. furfur, M. globosa, M. sloofiae, M. dermatis,* and *M. sympodialis* have also been recovered from animal infections.

All species exhibit common physiologic and morphologic features. Reproduction is through unilateral budding, which leaves prominent scars on the mother cells. Buds may be formed on a wide or narrow base. Yeasts vary in shape from ovoid to globose to cylindrical. The cell wall is thick and consists of multiple layers.

Disease and Epidemiology

Malassezia pachydermatis normally resides on the skin, lips and anus, and in the vagina, anal sacs, and external ear canal of dogs. Animals are rarely colonized by *M. pachydermatis* alone; in nearly all cases, cultures from these locations also contain *M. furfur* and/or *M. sympodialis.* Because these yeasts are normal flora, interpretation of clinical significance when recovered from clinical specimens is often difficult.

Host-related factors allow this commensal to produce disease. Certain microclimatic conditions in the ear canal, including high humidity and excessive wax accumulation, favor yeast overgrowth and disease development. Several conformational factors, such as hairy or pendulous ears, add to a favorable growth environment within the ear canal. Disease may be exacerbated by allergic dermatitis and inflammation, which further contribute to the moist otic environment. Dermatitis also occurs when there are environmental alterations on the skin. Changes in the quality or quantity of sebum, the presence of other dermatoses, recent antibiotic or glucocorticoid therapy, or increased moisture may cause disruption of the epidermal barrier, leading to yeast proliferation.

In dogs, *M. pachydermatis* has been accepted as a cause of otitis externa and seborrheic dermatitis. Clinical signs in dogs include head shaking, pruritus, and offensive odor. In cases of chronic otitis, the external ear canal may become filled with a thick, waxy brown discharge. Superficial dermatitis can occur either as a regionalized disease (ventral abdomen, face, feet, neck, perineum, leg folds), or generalized disorder. Face rubbing and foot licking are common complaints, and the skin appears erythematous and scaly. Secondary alopecia and excoriation are commonly observed. Hyperpigmentation and lichenification occur along with seborrhea as the infection becomes chronic. There appear to be breed predispositions, with a higher occurrence among poodles, cocker spaniels, terriers, Chihuahuas, German shepherds, boxers, basset hounds, shih tzus, and Shetland sheepdogs.

Cats appear to be less susceptible to infections with *M. pachydermatis.* Affected cats may present with otitis, accompanied by a dark ceruminous exudate, chin acne, or generalized exfoliative erythroderma. Clinical disease is frequently associated with immune suppression and internal malignancy.

Until recently, *M. pachydermatis* was thought to be the only organism within the genus to be associated with animal disease. However, there are now reports of chronic otitis externa in dogs caused by *M. furfur* and *M. obtusa,* and otitis externa in cats caused by *M. sympodialis* and *M. nana.* Bovine otitis externa may be associated with *M. globosa, M. nana, M. slooffiae, M. furfur,* and *M. sympodialis* because of the higher frequency of isolation of these species from cattle with otitis than from healthy animals. Tinea versicolor is primarily a human disease that is characterized by *M. furfur* infection of the stratum corneum. However, the infection also manifests as superficial lesions on the udders of milking goats. Lesions are circular, flat, slightly thickened, minimally inflamed, and have scaly edges. They appear as dark areas on light-colored udders or light areas on dark-colored udders.

Malassezia pachydermatis may be an emerging zoonotic pathogen. An outbreak of disease in a neonatal intensive care unit was theorized to have originated with attending nurses colonized by pet exposure; poor hygienic practices resulted in infection of the infants.

Pathogenesis

The opportunistic nature of *M. pachydermatis* has been demonstrated. This commensal yeast may become a pathogen whenever the microclimate of the skin or ear canal is altered. The details of this process are poorly understood. Adherence plays an important role in pathogenesis, because it allows the yeasts to resist physical forces that might otherwise result in their removal from the host. Attachment to cornified epithelial cells is mediated through lipids, and germination follows attachment. As conditions become favorable, *M. pachydermatis* proliferates. Sebum-altering lipases are produced by the yeasts as they grow, creating a favorable environment for the yeast. *Malassezia pachydermatis* strains isolated from dogs with otitis or dermatitis also produce proteinase, chondroitin-sulfatase, hyaluronidase, and phospholipase, which may contribute to disease. The assumption is that these enzymes are involved in the early steps of host invasion and in damage to host cells, although their exact mechanisms are currently unknown.

The host immune response to the yeast may contribute to pathogenesis, as IgE-mediated hypersensitivity augments the severity of disease. Pruritus and inflammation result from the presence of zymogens in the yeast cell wall, which activate the complement cascade in the host.

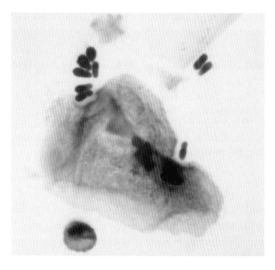

FIGURE 45-4 *Malassezia pachydermatis*, Gram stain. (Courtesy Karen W. Post.)

Diagnosis

Consistent clinical signs, history of poor response to antibiotics, glucocorticoids, or immunotherapy, and the demonstration of a high number of organisms from an affected area suggest a diagnosis of *Malassezia* otitis or dermatitis. However, definitive diagnosis relies on yeast identification and therapeutic response.

The most useful tool for diagnosis of *Malassezia* otitis or dermatitis is cytologic examination of affected areas. These yeasts have a characteristic, slightly elongated oval morphology with a thick wall and unipolar budding. *Malassezia pachydermatis* appears as footprint- or peanut-shaped yeasts (Figure 45-4). They are easily observed in impression smears stained hematologically and examined microscopically under high dry (40×) or oil immersion. Finding more than 10 yeasts per high-power field is considered to be diagnostic.

Culture alone is not a reliable means of diagnosis because a positive culture does not indicate infection. If cultures are attempted, *Malassezia* spp. may be recovered using fungal selective agars (such as Mycosel or Sabouraud dextrose) overlaid with sterile olive oil. *Malassezia pachydermatis* does not require lipid supplementation for growth, unlike other members of the genus. Media are incubated at 30° C for up to 1 week. Colonies are small, cream colored, raised to convex, and glossy. Phenotypic tests useful for differentiation of the species include Cremophor EL assimilation, growth on lipid-free medium, esculin degradation, catalase production, and growth on Dixon agar at 38° C.

Histopathology is of limited value in diagnosis; tissue processing may result in loss of the superficial layers of the stratum corneum, which is the primary location of the yeasts and active disease. The findings that remain (irregularly hyperplastic, spongiotic superficial, perivascular to interstitial dermatitis with parakeratotic hyperkeratosis) are not specific for *Malassezia*.

Prevention and Control

Therapy is aimed at the reduction of numbers of organisms as well as identification and amelioration of predisposing factors. For mild or localized disease, topical therapeutic options include shampoos and creams or dips containing miconazole or ketoconazole, selenium sulfide, and chlorhexidine. Systemic administration of an antifungal, such as ketoconazole, is often used for treating generalized disease. Newer therapy includes pulse administration and once daily administration of itraconazole for treating *M. pachydermatis* cutaneous infection in dogs. Adjunctive treatment may be needed in dogs with otitis. The main cause of long-term treatment failure is the inability to identify and control underlying dermatoses.

TRICHOSPORON BEIGELII

The genus *Trichosporon* belongs to the family Sporidiobolaceae, order Sporidiales, and phylum Basidiomycotina. These yeasts are isolated from

TABLE 45-3 Characteristics of Selected Veterinary Significant Yeasts

Genus	Pseudo-hyphae	True Hyphae	Blasto-conidia	Arthro-conidia	Urease	Growth at 25° C with Cycloheximide	Growth at 37° C on Potato Dextrose Agar
Candida	Pos	Pos	Pos	Neg	Neg	Var	Pos
Geotrichum	Neg	Pos	Neg	Pos	Neg	Neg	Neg
Malassezia	Neg	Neg	Neg	Neg	Pos	Pos	Pos
Trichosporon	Pos	Pos	Pos	Pos	Pos	Pos	Pos

Neg, Negative; *Pos,* positive; *Var,* variable.

soil, water, and vegetables, as well as mammals and birds. Seventeen species are recognized, but *Trichosporon beigelii* is the most significant pathogen.

Piedra, a fungal infection of the hair shaft, has on rare occasion been reported in horses and monkeys. Disease is characterized by the formation of small white to light brown nodules that appear on the hairs of the mane and tail. Infection begins under the cuticle of the hair, and nodules develop with yeast growth. The hair shaft may rupture or be weakened to the point of breakage, resulting in hair loss. Treatment consists of clipping hairs in the affected areas and topical application of fungicides.

Trichosporon beigelii may cause outbreaks of severe mastitis in dairy cows. Outbreaks were linked to the use of contaminated intramammary infusion products and outcomes ranged from substantial decreases in milk production to agalactia to death.

A nasal mass is the only feline infection with *Trichosporon pullalans.* The cat presented with a small mass occluding the left naris. The mass was surgically excised, and follow-up treatment consisted of parenteral administration of ketoconazole.

Diagnosis is based on microscopic examination and culture of infected hairs. Examination of clinical materials in 10% KOH reveals hyphae and arthrospores surrounding the hair shaft, and occasional budding blastospores may be observed. *Trichosporon* spp. are inhibited by cycloheximide, so Sabouraud dextrose or potato dextrose agar should be used as an alternative to selective media such as Mycosel agar. Plated media are incubated at 25° to 30° C and cream-colored yeastlike colonies appear within 5 to 7 days. Their surfaces become wrinkled and their centers heaped with extended incubation,

and they may have a tendency to adhere to the agar surface. *Trichosporon* spp. must be differentiated from *Candida* and *Geotrichum* spp., typically by examination of microscopic morphology of cultures on cornmeal-Tween 80 agar at 25° C and detection of urease production (Table 45-3).

GEOTRICHUM CANDIDUM

Geotrichum is a member of the phylum Ascomycota, order Saccharomycetales, and family Endomycetaceae. These yeasts are found worldwide as ubiquitous saprophytes of soil and decaying organic matter. They are also routinely isolated from dairy products and healthy human skin. The genus contains several species, the most common of which is *Geotrichum candidum.*

Geotrichosis (*G. candidum* infection) is frequently reported in reptiles and amphibians, but this fungus has only rarely been recovered from disease processes in domestic animals (dogs, cats, pigs, cattle, and horses). Cutaneous and disseminated disease has been described in dogs. Cutaneous lesions consist of discrete, nodular, well-circumscribed dermoepidermal masses that are located over the head and dorsal caudolumbar regions. Microscopic examination of dried, stained impression smears from the lesions reveals branched, septate filamentous hyphae admixed with inflammatory cells.

The pathogenesis of geotrichosis has not been fully elucidated in animals. Trauma or immunosuppression may play a role, and most human infections have been associated with underlying debilitating disease or immunocompromise.

This organism resembles the yeasts in its colonial morphology. Colonies are rapidly growing, dry, powdery to cottony, and white to cream colored. Aerial mycelia are occasionally produced. Colonies become slimy when disturbed on the

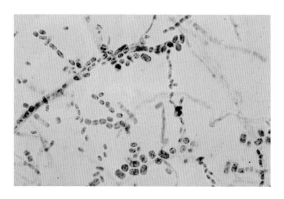

FIGURE 45-5 *Geotrichum* microscopic morphology. (Courtesy Public Health Image Library, PHIL #3056, Centers for Disease Control and Prevention, Atlanta, 1964, Lucille K. Georg.)

agar surface. Optimal growth is observed at 25° C. Most strains do not grow at 37° C.

Hyaline septate hyphae that fragment into arthroconidia are observed microscopically (Figure 45-5). Blastoconidia, conidiophores, and pseudohyphae are absent. Because the organism most closely resembles *Trichosporon* spp., it must be differentiated from them in the clinical laboratory. Phenotypic tests useful for separation appear in Table 45-3.

SUGGESTED READINGS

Guillot J, Bond R: *Malassezia pachydermatis:* a review, *Med Mycol* 37:295-306, 1999.

Weitzman I, Summerbell RC: The dermatophytes, *Clin Microbiol Rev* 8:240-259, 1995.

Chapter 46

The Subcutaneous Mycoses

Subcutaneous mycoses comprise a broad range of infections that involve the deeper layers of the skin, muscle, bone, or connective tissue. Common themes include typical association with injuries, etiologic agents usually found in soil or decaying vegetation, and infections of a chronic and insidious nature. The organisms establish themselves in the skin and produce localized infection of the surrounding tissues and lymph nodes; dissemination is rare. Organisms causing subcutaneous mycoses are dematiaceous or hyaline molds and dimorphic fungi, and the common diseases are sporotrichosis, epizootic lymphangitis, chromoblastomycosis, eucomycotic mycetoma, phaeohyphomycosis, and bovine nasal granuloma.

Some bacterial infections may be confused with the subcutaneous mycoses. These infections include actinomycotic mycetoma, botryomycosis, and mycobacteriosis, which are often readily managed by antimicrobial therapy, but subcutaneous mycoses are more difficult to treat. Thus it is important for the veterinarian to correctly establish the etiologic agent.

SPOROTRICHOSIS

Taxonomically, the genus *Sporothrix* is a member of the phylum Ascomycota, class Euascomycetes, order Ophiostomatales, and family Ophiostomataceae. There are three legitimate species but only one, *Sporothrix schenckii*, is an important pathogen of animals. *Sporothrix schenckii*

is a thermally dimorphic dematiaceous fungus, existing as a yeast form at 37° C in tissue and in a mycelial or mold form when cultivated at 25° C.

DISEASE AND EPIDEMIOLOGY

Sporotrichosis has been described worldwide but is most common in tropical and subtropical America. The organism is isolated from soil, living and decaying vegetation, peat moss, and wood, and disease follows inoculation of conidia into the skin by puncture wounds from thorns or bites. As a result, most cases present with localized skin and subcutaneous lesions with minimal systemic manifestations. The infection in humans is sometimes called "rose handler's disease."

Sporotrichosis is a relatively common disease of humans and animals. Naturally occurring disease has been documented in dogs, cats, horses, donkeys, mules, pigs, fowl, goats, and cattle, and is most common in the dog. Canine disease presents as one of three distinct clinical syndromes; cutaneous and disseminated disease is not rare, but lymphocutaneous is the predominant syndrome. Lesions begin at the point of entry and consist of subcutaneous nodules that ulcerate and heal. As the disease progresses, it follows the course of lymphatic vessels and may eventually involve the lymph nodes. The lesions usually are neither painful nor pruritic.

Feline sporotrichosis develops mainly in intact male cats that are allowed to live outdoors. Initially, lesions appear as small, draining puncture wounds and are commonly seen on the head or at the base of the tail. As the disease progresses, the lesions may become nodular, granulomatous, ulcerative, or necrotic, and systemic spread has been reported.

Hard, cutaneous nodules that develop along the lymphatics, usually on the medial surface of the legs, are commonly observed in horses. Nodules are 1 to 5 cm in diameter and may drain or ulcerate. Visceral or skeletal involvement may occur.

Sporotrichosis is zoonotic, and direct contact with lesions or contaminated bandages may result in human infection. Most human cases have come from contact with cats, often without a history of cat bites or scratches. Infected cats appear to continuously shed fungi in their lesion exudates and feces. In fact, *S. schenckii* has been isolated from domestic cats without clinical signs of sporotrichosis, reinforcing the zoonotic potential of feline disease. In contrast, canine sporotrichosis is considered to be of minimal zoonotic importance because few organisms are present in the tissues of most affected dogs.

PATHOGENESIS

Sporothrix schenckii conidia or mycelia generally gain access to the host through broken skin, either directly through some traumatic insult or indirectly through contamination of an existing wound. Upon entry, the mycelial or saprophytic form changes to the yeast or parasitic form as a result of the temperature increase and perhaps other in vivo signals. Lymphocutaneous manifestations of disease begin as single or multiple indurated, erythematous nodules that develop at the initial site of contact. The nodules contain microabscesses and granulomas. As the infection spreads along the lymphatics, papules appear, ulcerate, and drain. Regional lymph node involvement is not uncommon. Nodes may ulcerate and discharge pus. The limbs become swollen due to lymphangitis. A cutaneous form with no lymphatic spread also may be seen.

Virulence factors for *S. schenckii* include thermotolerance, production of extracellular enzymes, and adhesion. Ability to grow at 37° C is a virulence factor, in that it allows the fungus to invade deep tissues. Acid phosphatases are produced by the yeasts, mycelia, and conidia of *S. schenckii*. These enzymes may interact with macrophages to allow intracellular survival of the organism.

Two enzymes, proteinases I and II, hydrolyze human stratum corneum cells in vitro. Adhesion to extracellular matrix proteins may play a crucial role in the invasion process. Both the yeast cells and conidia of *S. schenckii* adhere to the extracellular protein fibronectin. Cell wall composition may play a role in fungal virulence because the more virulent forms show differences in cell-wall sugar composition with rhamnose-mannose molar ratios when compared with avirulent strains.

DIAGNOSIS

Diagnosis of sporotrichosis may be accomplished by several methods. Microscopic examination of direct mounts of feline specimens may reveal large numbers of small elliptical budding yeasts, referred to as "cigar bodies." These organisms are not plentiful in clinical materials obtained from infected dogs or horses. Histologic examination of punch biopsy specimens of cutaneous lesions provides a fairly rapid diagnosis, but care must be taken not to confuse *S. schenckii* with other yeasts. Definitive diagnosis is based on isolation of the organism from specimens.

Sporothrix schenckii forms colonies in 2 to 7 days on Sabouraud dextrose agar at room temperature. The mold colonies are cream colored, wrinkled, and leathery, and turn black or silvery gray with age (Figure 46-1). Microscopically, the mold appears as small, oval, hyaline, or dematiaceous conidia.

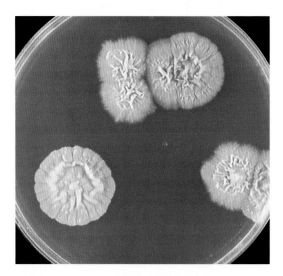

FIGURE 46-1 Agar plate culture of *Sporothrix schenckii,* incubated at 20° C. (Courtesy Public Health Image Library, PHIL #3196, Centers for Disease Control and Prevention, Atlanta, 1969, William Kaplan.)

These are arranged singly along the hyphae, or as "flower petals" at the end of short unbranched conidiophores (Figure 46-2). Conversion from the mold to the yeast phase is required for identification. The mold is plated on brain-heart infusion agar supplemented with 5% blood and incubated at 37° C in 5% to 7% CO_2 for 3 to 5 days. Yeast colonies are soft and white to cream colored (Figure 46-3).

Other diagnostic methods are available. Serologic tests are available for diagnosis of human disease and include latex particle agglutination, complement fixation, immunodiffusion, and indirect fluorescent antibody. However, these are not available for animal diagnostics. Recently, direct fluorescent immunohistochemical (IHC) techniques have been developed to specifically identify the organism in tissue sections and exudates. These IHC tests are offered by several veterinary diagnostic laboratories.

PREVENTION AND CONTROL

The organism is sensitive to direct sunlight and severe winter weather, but is fairly resistant to drying. Precautions should be taken when handling infected animals; gloves should be worn and handwashing, using cleansers with antifungal activity (e.g., chlorhexidine or povidone-iodine) should be practiced.

Historically, treatment of sporotrichosis in cats, dogs, and horses has involved oral administration of potassium or sodium iodide, and iodides remain the treatment of choice for equine infections. However, cats are very susceptible to iodide toxicosis, and individuals unable to tolerate iodide therapy have been treated with ketoconazole. Recently, itraconazole has become the drug of choice for treatment of canine and feline infections. Therapy should be continued for 3 to 4 weeks following clinical cure, or relapses may occur.

EPIZOOTIC LYMPHANGITIS

The thermally dimorphic fungus *Histoplasma capsulatum* var. *farciminosum* is the cause of epizootic lymphangitis of horses, donkeys, and mules. This fungus is assigned to the phylum Ascomycota, class Ascomycetes, order Onygenales, family Onygenaceae. The disease is limited to parts of North Africa, Europe, India, and Russia. The natural habitat of this fungus remains unknown, but infection is thought to be a result of skin trauma, perhaps by way of insect bites. Granulomatous, nodular lesions with a tendency to ulcerate are located in the skin and subcutaneous tissue, and along lymphatic vessels, primarily involving the neck and legs. Rarely, the disease may disseminate to internal organs.

Diagnosis is through the examination of wet mounts, cultures, or histopathologic examination of biopsy tissue obtained from closed nodules. Double-contoured, pear-shaped budding yeasts are observed in direct exams. These are usually found within macrophages or neutrophils. The mycelial form of the fungus requires up to 8 weeks for growth on plated media with and

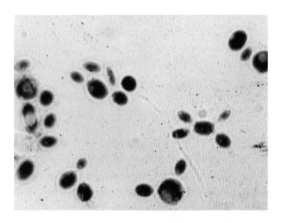

FIGURE 46-2 Micrograph of conidia of yeast phase of *Sporothrix schenckii*. (Courtesy Public Health Image Library, PHIL #3063, Centers for Disease Control and Prevention, Atlanta, 1964, Lucille K. Georg.)

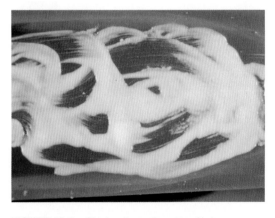

FIGURE 46-3 Slant culture of yeast colonies of *Sporothrix schenckii*. (Courtesy Public Health Image Library, PHIL #3062, Centers for Disease Control and Prevention, Atlanta, 1964, Lucille K. Georg.)

without cycloheximide, incubated at 25° C. Colonies are small, gray and flat, and have a tendency to peel off the agar surface in flakes. Microscopically, the fungus appears septate, with irregularly thickened hyphae. Chlamydospores and arthrospores may also be observed. The mycelial form must be converted to the yeast phase for definitive identification. The conversion process is slow, and yeast may require up to 4 weeks at 37° C in an environment of 10% to 20% CO_2 to grow, usually on Hartley digest agar. Ancillary diagnostic tests include an enzyme-linked immunosorbent assay (ELISA) and an indirect fluorescent antibody test.

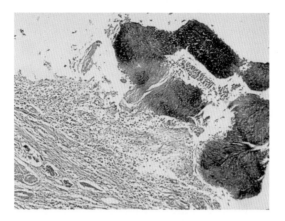

FIGURE 46-4 Histopathologic changes of the foot as a result of mycetoma. (Courtesy Public Health Image Library, PHIL #3103, Centers for Disease Control and Prevention, Atlanta, 1965, Martin Hicklin.)

DISEASES ASSOCIATED WITH DEMATIACEOUS FUNGI

Chromoblastomycosis

Chromoblastomycosis is a rare, chronic fungal infection of the subcutaneous and cutaneous tissues, caused by dematiaceous fungi that form thick-walled muriform cells known as sclerotic bodies. Etiologic agents recovered from animal infections are *Phialophora, Fonsecaea, Exophiala,* and *Cladophialophora* spp. These fungi gain entrance by traumatic implantation. Clinically, chromoblastomycosis appears as firm, protuberant, warty, ulcerative nodules that tend to remain localized on the feet and legs.

Eumycotic Mycetoma

Although the word *mycetoma* implies a fungal etiology, mycetomas can be of fungal or bacterial etiology. Mycetomas caused by fungi are eumycotic mycetomas, whereas those of a filamentous bacterial etiology are actinomycotic mycetomas. Agents associated with eumycotic mycetomas are dematiaceous fungi of the genera *Bipolaris, Curvularia,* and *Pseudallescheria* spp. Several canine and feline mycetomas associated with dermatophyte infection have been reported.

To be classified as a mycetoma, a triad of clinical signs (swelling, fistulas, and grains or granules) must be present. Clinically, mycetomas appear as subcutaneous swellings with draining tracts, and may resemble a chronic nonhealing abscess. Examination of the exudate reveals granules that are composed of aggregates of mycelium or bacterial colonies. The granules may vary in size, shape, texture, and color. Depending on the etiologic agent involved, granules may be white, black, or yellow.

Mycetomas are relatively rare. Infection progresses slowly and is limited to one area of the body (usually a foot or an area of the abdomen), and a large, fistulous tumor develops. As fistulas heal, tissue fibrosis occurs, leading to the formation of hard tumorlike masses that are characteristic of chronic mycetomas. Lesions on the extremities may lead to enlargement of the whole limb. The disease process may penetrate the periosteum and cause osteomyelitis (Figure 46-4).

Mycetomas have been reported in various animal species. Dermal disease and osteomyelitis have been reported in the dog and horse. Visceral and disseminated disease also has been documented.

Phaeohyphomycosis

Phaeohyphomycosis is a term applied to an infection caused by dematiaceous fungi, which grows in vivo as dark-walled hyphae, pseudohyphae, yeast cells, or any combination of these forms (Figure 46-5). Phaeohyphomycotic agents do not form grains or granules that characterize mycetomas, and lack the thick-walled, sclerotic bodies that characterize chromoblastomycosis. Phaeohyphomycoses are corneal, cutaneous, subcutaneous, or systemic, and the subcutaneous type is the most common. Organisms associated with animal infection are *Alternaria, Bipolaris, Cladophialophora, Cladosporium, Curvularia, Phialophora, Exophiala,* and *Phaeoacremonium* spp. Clinical signs include formation of pustules, abscesses, granulomas, or shallow ulcerated or

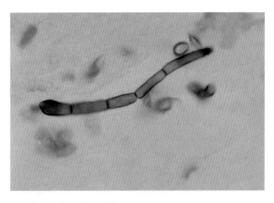

FIGURE 46-5 Dark-walled hyphae of a dematiaceous fungus. (Courtesy Public Health Image Library, PHIL #2949, Centers for Disease Control and Prevention, Atlanta, 1980, Libero Ajello.)

open lesions. Cases have been reported in dogs and cats.

Fungi that have been isolated from cats with subcutaneous phaeohyphomycosis include *Moniliella suaveolens, Bipolaris (Drechslera) spicifera, Stemplylium* sp., *Cladosporium* sp., *Alternaria alternata, Exophiala jeanselmei,* and *Phialophora verrucosa*. Ulcerative, subcutaneous, nodular, granulomatous lesions occur on the ventral abdomen, lips, feet, legs, and sternum.

Feline cutaneous phaeohyphomycosis may also be caused by *Cladophialophora bantiana*. Affected animals may present with breathing difficulty and swollen, ulcerated nodules, often on the dorsal nose and left nostril. Histologic examination of the nodule reveals cystic granulomatous dermatitis characterized by accumulation of neutrophils, macrophages, and giant cells. Pigmented, yeastlike fungal cells and hyphal elements are easily identified in hematoxylin-and-eosin–stained tissue sections, and *C. bantiana* is isolated. This infection can establish in immunocompetent cats, and, although antifungal therapy is useful, relapses are likely to occur.

Bovine Nasal Granuloma

Bovine nasal granuloma is characterized by the formation of granulomatous swellings in the nasal cavity and trachea of cattle. Clinical signs include dyspnea, inspiratory stridor, and bilateral, serous-to-mucopurulent nasal discharge. Pinkish white polyps may be visible on endoscopy of the nasal cavity, and direct examination of crushed polyps in KOH reveals dematiaceous and, in rare instances, hyaline hyphae and spherical bodies considered to be chlamydospores. For culture, pieces of polyp are placed in a 1:2500 dilution of Roccal D solution for 15 minutes to remove surface bacterial contaminants. The polyps are then rinsed several times in sterile saline and either crushed into small pieces using a sterile mortar and pestle or cut into small pieces with sterile scissors. The pieces are placed on Sabouraud or potato dextrose agar with and without antibiotics and incubated at 25° to 30° C for 3 to 5 days. Media containing cycloheximide should not be used because growth of the etiologic agents will be inhibited. *Curvularia* and *Bipolaris* spp. are most often recovered, and both grow rapidly and produce white colonies that become floccose, olive green, brown, or black, with dark reverse pigments. Large cylindric, brown, multiseptate smooth-walled macroconidia with rounded tips are produced on septate simple or branched conidiophores. The conidia of *Curvularia* usually contain up to four cells and are curved on their long axes as a result of swelling of a darker central cell. *Bipolaris* macroconidia are thick walled, contain four or more cells, and are not curved.

No successful transmission of disease by exposure of other animals to polyp-derived material has occurred. Natural infection usually begins following traumatic introduction of a saprophytic fungus into subcutaneous tissue, although biting insects may also be a source of infection. The fungus is localized in the subcutaneous tissue, and lesions usually begin as nodules that gradually enlarge and then ulcerate and drain. They can remain localized or spread in the subcutaneous tissues.

The dematiaceous fungi share in common the production of melanin, which may be a virulence factor. Melanin may play a role in fungal penetration of animal tissues because it appears to be important in hyphal tip protrusion. Other properties that may explain melanin's impact on virulence are its potential capability to shield fungal cell wall constituents from hydrolytic enzymes, its possible effect on redox buffering, and its ability to sequester host defensive proteins.

Diagnosis of disease involving a dematiaceous fungus requires direct examination, culture, and histologic examination of biopsy material. Fungal media containing cycloheximide (Mycosel, Mycobiotic, Dermatophyte test medium) will inhibit the growth of many dematiaceous fungi and should not be solely used for specimen culture. Potato dextrose or Sabouraud dextrose agar, with and without antibiotics, should be used instead. Hematoxylin-and-eosin or periodic acid–Schiff (PAS) stains are useful to visualize granules that are surrounded by an infiltrate of polymorphonuclear cells.

Infection may be controlled by surgical excision and antifungal therapy but is often unrewarding; it is common for lesions to reappear after surgical excision. Systemic antifungal agents, such as amphotericin B, itraconazole, and 5-fluorocytosine, are usually ineffective. Thus treatment is impractical, and affected animals are generally culled from the herd.

DEMATIACEOUS FUNGI

Pseudallescheria boydii/ Scedosporium apiospermum

Taxonomically the genus *Pseudallescheria* is placed in the phylum Ascomycota, class Euascomycetes, order Microascales, and family Microascaceae. The genus contains one species, *P. boydii*. This ubiquitous saprophyte is the teleomorph of *Scedosporium apiospermum* and *Graphium eumorphum*, but the *S. apiospermum* synamorph is most commonly isolated from clinical cultures. *Pseudallescheria boydii* has been isolated worldwide from water, soil, vegetation, animal manure, and sewage.

Pseudallescheria boydii is an animal pathogen. It has been reported to cause nasal granuloma, keratitis, and dermal eumycotic mycetoma in the horse, and keratitis, abdominal eumycotic mycetoma, and disseminated disease in the dog. Although cases of canine eumycotic mycetoma caused by *P. boydii* are infrequent, there appears to be a tendency for this fungus to infect the body cavity. Infection usually follows some form of trauma with subsequent soil contamination of the site.

Documented cases of *S. apiospermum* infection in animals are rare. Canine nasal granuloma often presents as chronic, bilateral nasal discharge that is unresponsive to antibiotics. Radiologic examination may reveal increased radiodensity and osteolysis in the nasal cavity. Biopsy specimens contained granules with numerous septate,

hyaline to pale brown hyphae, and *S. apiospermum* was recovered. The infection responded to oral ketoconazole.

Onychomycosis of horses has also been described in association with *S. apiospermum*, or the teleomorph *P. boydii*. The fungi have been isolated from lesions of white line disease, a condition that leads to deterioration of the hoof wall. Numerous fungi are found in the fissure cavities, the terminal horn of the white line, and the terminal horn–like laminae of the metaplastic white line–like tissue. The most susceptible region is the terminal horn of the hypertrophied white line and/or the terminal horn–like laminae of the metaplastic white line–like tissue.

Diagnosis is by culture and histopathology. Cottony, spreading colonies with aerial mycelia and a reverse white color grow moderately rapidly to maturity in 7 days. With age, the colonies change from white to grayish brown, with a reverse color of gray or black. *Pseudallescheria boydii* is inhibited by cycloheximide, whereas the asexual stage, *S. apiospermum*, is not inhibited. In the sexual phase, cleistothecia, ascospores, and asci may be observed, but prolonged incubation (up to 3 weeks) on potato dextrose or cornmeal agar is required for their development. Septate hyphae with conidiophores that bear unicellular, oval, truncate conidia, singly or in small groups, are observed.

Topical therapy with copper sulfate or naphthenate is often effective. Itraconazole, ketoconazole, and miconazole have the lowest minimal inhibitory concentrations (MICs) in vitro. There appears to be some resistance to amphotericin B, fluconazole, 5-fluorocytosine, griseofulvin, clotrimazole, and nystatin.

SUGGESTED READINGS

Dixon DM, Polak-Wyss A: The medically important dematiaceous fungi and their identification, *Mycoses* 34:1-18, 1991.

Dunstan RW, Reimann KA, Langham RF: Feline sporotrichosis, *J Am Vet Med Assoc* 189:880-883, 1986.

Tachibana T, Matsuyama T, Mitsuyama M: Characteristic infectivity of *Sporothrix schenckii* to mice depending on routes of infection and inherent fungal pathogenicity, *Med Mycol* 36:21-27, 1998.

Chapter 47

The Systemic Mycoses

BLASTOMYCOSIS, COCCIDIOIDOMYCOSIS, CRYPTOCOCCOSIS, HISTOPLASMOSIS

The systemic mycotic agents are inherently virulent and can cause disease in healthy individuals. The four veterinary pathogens in this group are *Blastomyces dermatitidis, Histoplasma capsulatum* var. *capsulatum, Coccidioides* spp., and *Cryptococcus neoformans,* which exhibit unique biochemical and morphologic features that enable them to evade host defenses and cause disease. Three of these pathogens, *B. dermatitidis, H. capsulatum,* and *Coccidioides*, are thermally dimorphic, growing as molds at 25° C and as yeasts at 37° C (Table 47-1). Blastomycosis, histoplasmosis, and coccidioidomycosis tend to be restricted to certain geographic regions (Figure 47-1).

The primary focus of infection for these fungi is the lung. In most cases, the respiratory infection is asymptomatic, resolves rapidly, and confers resistance to reinfection. In some cases, infection will disseminate to another organ. Each agent exhibits a unique pattern of secondary organ involvement. The etiologic agent and the host's immune status will determine the severity of infection.

TABLE 47-1 Characteristics of the Systemic Dimorphic Fungi

Agent	Ecology	Saprobic Form	Parasitic Form
Blastomyces dermatitidis	Slightly acidic soils and wood; possible association with animal excreta, water sources, beaver dams	Hyphae, oval to pyriform terminal and lateral conidia, 2-10 μm in diameter	Unencapsulated yeasts with thick refractile double walls; 5-20 μm in diameter
Coccidioides immitis	Alkaline desert soils with high levels of salt and carbonized organic materials	Hyphae with thick-walled or barrel-shaped arthroconidia alternating with thin-walled empty (disjunctor cells)	Spherules, 10-100 μm in diameter, with doubly refractile cell walls and containing endospores, 2-5 μm in diameter
Histoplasma capsulatum	Humid environments with highly nitrogenous soils, especially those contaminated with bird or bat droppings	Hyphae, globose microconidia, and tuberculate and nontuberculate macroconidia, 8-16 μm in diameter	Tiny, ovoid budding yeasts with narrow bases, 2-4 μm in diameter

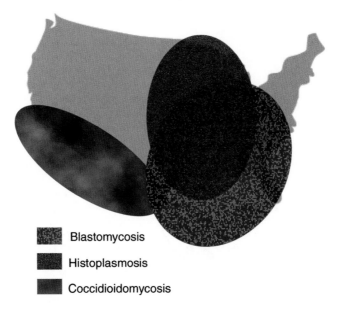

Blastomycosis

Histoplasmosis

Coccidioidomycosis

FIGURE 47-1 Geographic distribution of blastomycosis, coccidioidomycosis, and histoplasmosis. (Courtesy Ashley E. Harmon.)

BLASTOMYCOSIS

Blastomyces dermatitidis is taxonomically categorized in the phylum Ascomycota, class Euascomycetes, order Onygenales, and family Onygenaceae and causes blastomycosis. It is the sole species in the genus, but is closely related to *H. capsulatum*. The teleomorph has been discovered and designated as *Ajellomyces dermatitidis*, which is in the same genus as the sexual state of *H. capsulatum*. Ascospores are produced as sexual spores.

The first description of blastomycosis was by Gilchrist, at a meeting of the American Dermatologic Association in 1894. He reported pathologic findings from a biopsy that contained unusual budding yeasts from a patient with cutaneous lesions. In 1898, Gilchrist isolated the fungus from another patient with cutaneous disease and eventually named the organism *Blastomyces dermatitidis*. He then experimentally infected animals to successfully reproduce the disease, in fulfillment of Koch's postulates.

The distribution of *B. dermatitidis* is worldwide, with human disease having been diagnosed in Europe, South America, Asia, and Africa. The fungus is highly endemic in North America, where it is one of the principal systemic mycoses. Blastomycosis commonly affects individuals living in the Ohio, Missouri, Tennessee, and Mississippi river valleys, as well as in areas of the United States and Canada that border the St. Lawrence River and Great Lakes. Another distinct serotype of *B. dermatitidis* exists in Africa and parts of India.

Disease and Epidemiology

This thermally dimorphic fungus appears to be an inhabitant of soil and wood. Environments that are moist and shaded, have a high content of organic matter, and have slightly acidic pH seem to favor its growth. The ecologic niche of *B. dermatitidis* has been associated with water sources that change water levels. In highly endemic areas, shorelines may be an important reservoir for the fungus (Figure 47-2). Successful environmental isolations from rotting wood, decaying leaves, a beaver dam and lodge, a woodpile, twigs and roots, and tree bark have been reported. There may be an association of the organism with animal excreta; the fungus has been isolated from soil in chicken houses, from an abandoned mule stall, and from pigeon manure. Recovery of *B. dermatitidis* also has been documented from both the respiratory tract and feces of a dog with clinical disease, which suggests that yeast-phase cells may be recovered from the stool of dogs with pulmonary blastomycosis following transit through the gastrointestinal tract of swallowed infected sputum.

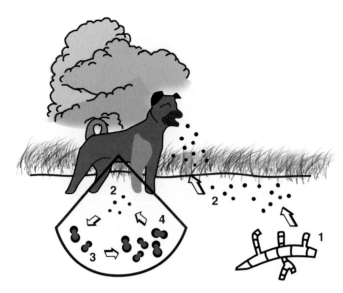

FIGURE 47-2 Natural history of the saprobic and parasitic life cycle of blastomycosis. Aerosolized mycelial fragments *(1)* or spores *(2)* from the environment are inhaled and deposited in alveoli of a susceptible host. The mature yeast form develops in the host *(3–4)* at 37° C. (Courtesy Ashley E. Harmon.)

Several epidemiologic studies of canine blastomycosis have been conducted. Risk groups include sexually intact males ages 2 to 4 years, large breeds, especially sporting or hound, and young, geriatric, or immunocompromised dogs. Other risk factors are residence in the southeastern, south-central, and upper Midwestern regions of the United States and proximity to river valleys or lakes. The highest risk for blastomycosis is in late summer, autumn, and early winter, which may reflect suitable temperatures for mycelial growth in the environment. The seasonal distribution may also reflect increased outdoor activity of animals during these times, and heat stress and an increase in dusty conditions may represent additional risk factors. In areas with endemic blastomycosis, infections in dogs can signal an increased risk for human infection. Whereas the prevalence of clinical versus subclinical disease in the dog is unknown, the incidence in dogs has been estimated to be approximately 10 times higher than in humans.

Zoonotic transmission of blastomycosis is uncommon. Percutaneous infection is most likely with the yeast phase. Cutaneous infection in humans has been reported as a result of bite wounds inflicted by dogs affected by *B. dermatitidis,* in which it is presumed that sputum was contaminated with yeasts. Veterinarians have developed disease after performing necropsies on infected dogs.

Man and dogs are the natural hosts of *B. dermatitidis,* but infection has been reported in a wide variety of species including domestic cats, horses, nonhuman primates, aquatic mammals, cattle, a ferret, wolves, a polar bear, a deer, a lion, a tiger, and a fruit bat. Two clinical forms of the disease exist: systemic or disseminated and cutaneous.

Prevalence of human blastomycosis in endemic areas may be as high as 0.5 to 4 cases per 100,000 individuals annually. Pneumonia and weight loss are the most common manifestations of disease. The acute pulmonary phase of blastomycosis may be subclinical or self-limiting, but if the disease progresses, pyogranulomatous inflammation develops in the lungs and at other sites. Blastomycosis has been reported in hunters and their dogs, suggesting that disease can develop in immunocompetent individuals.

Clinical signs associated with canine blastomycosis reflect the multisystemic nature of the disease and commonly include dyspnea, anorexia, depression, lameness, lymphadenopathy, or skin lesions. Ocular manifestations of blastomycosis (corneal opacity, uveitis, conjunctivitis, or blindness) occur in 30% to 40% of dogs with systemic disease. The prostate is often involved in males and there may be orchitis, but the intestinal tract is usually unaffected. Abnormalities in cell-mediated immunity develop in dogs, and nearly 25% of infections are fatal.

The prevalence of blastomycosis is lower in cats than in dogs. The disease is similar to that in dogs, being characterized by pyogranulomatous inflammation of an isolated organ system or as a multiorgan systemic disease. The lungs and eyes are the most commonly affected sites, and many infected cats have pulmonary lesions regardless of the other organs involved. Clinical signs consist of nasal discharge, cough, lethargy, and weight loss.

Blastomyces dermatitidis is not a common equine pathogen—there have been only two reported cases of disease. Clinical findings in affected animals include pyogranulomatous pneumonia, pleuritis, peritonitis, and cutaneous abscessation.

Pathogenesis

Infection develops when spores or mycelial fragments, aerosolized from soil, are inhaled and deposited in alveoli. The fungal elements develop into yeast forms within pulmonary alveoli at body temperature and subsequently multiply asexually by budding. At this time, some animals may exhibit acute respiratory distress. If the spore inoculum is too large or the animal is immunocompromised, hematogenous or lymphatic dissemination results, with subsequent infection of the skin, bones, lymph nodes, eyes, central nervous system, or reproductive tract.

Blastomyces dermatitidis evokes a strong inflammatory response in the host, characterized by an influx of neutrophils and mononuclear phagocytes. Yeast forms of *B. dermatitidis* may be located both inside and outside phagocytes at inflammatory foci, and replicate in normal macrophages. Macrophages are activated as part of the induced immune response, and delayed-type hypersensitivity develops within several weeks after the initial infection. Antifungal antibodies are also produced, but protective immunity resides within the cell-mediated arm of the response.

The organism possesses several key virulence attributes. Conversion from the mycelial to the yeast form confers an important survival advantage on the fungus. Whereas mycelia are readily phagocytosed and killed by neutrophils, yeasts appear resistant to neutrophils and mononuclear phagocytes during the early inflammatory process. The large size and thick cell wall of the yeast most likely contribute to this resistance.

Several constituents of the fungal cell wall are important virulence determinants. The major surface protein, termed WI-1, is a 120 kD adhesin that promotes attachment of spores to nonphagocytic cells and possibly to the extracellular matrix within the respiratory tract. It is somewhat of a conundrum that WI-1 appears also to promote recognition and killing of spores by phagocytes at the site of lung inflammation. Upon conversion of *B. dermatitidis* to the yeast phase, however, WI-1 expression is altered, minimizing recognition, ingestion, and killing of the yeasts by phagocytes. Because macrophages do not recognize the yeast cells, they freely invade tissues and disseminate via the bloodstream. Recent findings suggest that WI-1 modulates host immunity through blocking tumor necrosis factor-α (TNF-α) production by phagocytes, which further potentiates pulmonary infection. Shedding of WI-1 may also permit immune evasion by binding complement and opsonins, saturating macrophage receptors, impeding binding and phagocytosis of yeasts, and neutralizing phagocyte cytotoxic molecules. BAD-1, another adhesin, suppresses phagocyte proinflammatory responses of TNF-α. β-Glucan is a further cell wall constituent that initiates complement activation; canine complement enhances adherence of *B. dermatitidis* yeast to macrophages, and this adherence facilitates proliferation.

Diagnosis

In most animals, blastomycosis can be presumptively diagnosed by cytologic evaluation, which is based on finding the characteristic yeast form in preparations from fine-needle aspirates or touch preparations, and recovery of the fungus from clinical materials. Specimens suitable for disease diagnosis are exudates from draining tracts and lesions, transtracheal washes, fluid from the anterior chamber of the eye, prostatic fluid, and lymph node aspirates. The yeast ranges from 5 to 20 μm in diameter, is unencapsulated, and has a thick refractile, double cell wall (Figure 47-3).

Blastomyces dermatitidis does not remain viable for lengthy periods in clinical materials, so fungal cultures should be initiated immediately when blastomycosis is suspected. The yeast form, and in some strains the mycelial form, is sensitive to cycloheximide, so fungal media with and without cycloheximide should be used. Generally the fungus matures within 2 weeks, but it is recommended to hold cultures for 8 weeks before discarding them as negative. At 25° to 30° C, the mycelial form is quite variable. Colonies range

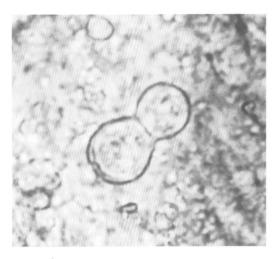

FIGURE 47-3 Smear from a foot lesion of blastomycosis demonstrating budding yeast. (Courtesy Public Health Image Library, PHIL #479, Centers for Disease Control and Prevention, Atlanta, date unknown.)

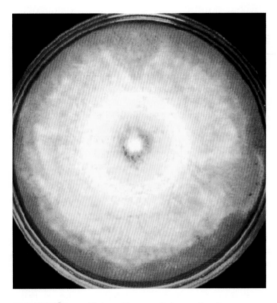

FIGURE 47-4 Plate with mycelial growth of *Blastomyces dermatitidis*. (Courtesy Public Health Image Library, PHIL #490, Centers for Disease Control and Prevention, Atlanta, date unknown, Libero Ajello.)

from flat and glabrous to cottony white or tan, and may have concentric rings (Figure 47-4). Visible spicules, consisting of aerial mycelia, may be evident within 1 week. Older cultures become brownish tan with a reverse tan pigment. The mycelial form is extremely infectious and great caution should be exercised when handling cultures.

Plates should be examined in a biological safety cabinet.

Because *B. dermatitidis* is a thermally dimorphic fungus, demonstration of conversion from the mycelial to the yeast form is required for definitive identification. After isolation of the mold, colonies should be plated onto an enriched medium such as brain-heart infusion agar with 5% sheep or bovine blood and incubated at 37° C for several weeks. Yeasts are waxy, wrinkled, and tan to cream. Some strains fail to convert in vitro, and it may be necessary to examine these strains with a specific oligonucleotide probe or by way of an exoantigen test to confirm the identity of the organism.

The yeast cells are the primary fungal structures found in tissue, although occasional mycelia may be observed. In hematoxylin-and-eosin–stained tissues, it may be difficult to see the forms. Use of fungal stains will aid in the visualization process.

Commercially available serologic testing may assist in diagnosis. Complement fixation and immunodiffusion tests generally lack sensitivity. An antibody test based on the immunodominant antigen WI-1 has good sensitivity and specificity but is not widely available. Titers become high, decline during treatment, and persist for months. A highly sensitive and specific DNA probe assay for confirmation of the identity of clinical isolates has been reported.

Prevention and Control

The risk for exposure to blastomycosis remains small even in areas where the disease is endemic, and few public health recommendations have been developed for disease prevention.

Amphotericin B lipid complex has been used to treat blastomycosis in dogs where it has proven to be both safe and effective. Treatment with itraconazole is also effective.

Because blastomycosis may pose an occupational hazard for veterinarians or veterinary technicians, precautions should be taken to decrease the likelihood of exposure when handling animals or tissues with suspected or confirmed blastomycosis.

COCCIDIOIDOMYCOSIS

Coccidioidomycosis affects numerous mammalian species and is caused by the dimorphic fungus *Coccidioides immitis*. It has the reputation as the most virulent fungal pathogen. Posadas and

Wernicke reported the first case of human disease in 1892, and at the time believed the causative agent to be a coccidian parasite. The true nature of *C. immitis* was not elucidated until 1900, and the original taxonomic reference has been carried through into today's name for the genus. Coccidioidomycosis has been referred to in the literature as San Joaquin Valley fever, Valley fever, desert disease or rheumatism, and Posadas disease. The U.S. government has classified this fungus among its select agents as a potential tool of bioterrorists.

Current taxonomic affiliation of the fungus is identical to that of *B. dermatitidis,* with the obvious exception of the genus. Two species of *Coccidioides* are currently recognized. Strains found mainly in Texas, Arizona, and endemic regions in South and Central America, formerly known as "non-California *C. immitis,*" have been classified as *Coccidoides posadasii,* whereas the specific epithet *C. immitis* has been reserved for the strains primarily recovered from the San Joaquin Valley in California. Teleomorphic states are unknown.

Disease and Epidemiology

Coccidioides spp. are residents of soil in certain arid and semiarid regions of North, Central, and South America. Endemic foci are located within the Lower Sonoran Life Zone in North America, which encompasses portions of Arizona, California, New Mexico, Texas, Utah, Nevada, and northern Mexico. Other endemic foci are in portions of Guatemala, Argentina, Paraguay, Colombia, and Venezuela. Climatic conditions in these regions are conducive to fungal propagation, with average rainfalls of 10 inches per year during a monsoon season, average summer temperatures of 100° F, and average winter temperatures of 35° F. The fungus can live indefinitely in alkaline soils where there is a high content of salt and carbonized organic material.

As a dimorphic fungus, *Coccidioides* spp. have an environmental or saprobic form and a parasitic tissue form. The mycelial form exists in the soil and is undetectable during the wet winter and spring, but actively grows in the upper layers of the soil during a hot, dry summer (Figure 47-5). Growth in the soil is directly affected by competition with

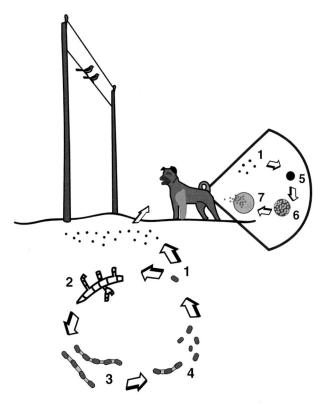

FIGURE 47-5 Natural history of the saprobic and parasitic life cycle of coccidioidomycosis. Mold to spherule transition occurs in a susceptible host at 37° C *(1–7)*. Arthroconidia in the environment *(1)* mature into mycelia, which fragment into arthrospores and are inhaled by the host. (Courtesy Ashley E. Harmon.)

other microorganisms. *Penicillium janthinellum* and *Bacillus subtilis,* which proliferate during the rainy season, appear to be important inhibitory organisms. Hyphae produce infective arthrospores that become aerosolized in the late summer and fall during dust storms or excavation. Winds may carry arthroconidia up to 400 miles from their point of origin. The fungus survives in rodent burrows, and rodents can apparently distribute it in the environment.

Naturally occurring coccidioidomycosis is seen most frequently in humans, dogs, horses, and llamas. Sporadic cases of disease have been reported in other species, including cattle, sheep, swine, cats, burros, desert rodents, a bottlenose dolphin, sea lions, sea otters, armadillos, a mountain lion, coyotes, chinchilla, Bengal tigers, non-human primates, and a snake.

In humans, more than half of the infections are asymptomatic. Clinical manifestations range from an influenza-like illness to severe pneumonia, and rarely, extrapulmonary disseminated disease. The last form is one of the most severe systemic mycoses, which may result in extensive tissue damage to the bones, joints, skin, and central nervous system. Coccidioidomycosis is uniformly fatal in the immunocompromised patient.

The high incidence of coccidioidomycosis in the dog may be a result of its propensity for sniffing or digging in the soil. Large and medium-sized male dogs are affected most commonly. Surveys of coccidioidomycosis in dogs indicate that 80% of dogs have primary pulmonary infection and 20% develop disseminated disease. Clinical signs noted at presentation vary widely and include dyspnea, anorexia, cough, weight loss, lameness, draining tracts, abscesses, lymphadenopathy, meningitis, and intermittent diarrhea. Extrapulmonary dissemination occurs most frequently to the bone and skin. A primary cutaneous form of the disease has been rarely reported and may have been preceded by trauma or wounds.

Pulmonary coccidioidal granuloma in cattle was first reported in 1937. Although frequently noted in slaughtered animals in the southwestern United States, the disease appears to be mild and self-limiting in ruminants, being confined to the bronchial and mediastinal lymph nodes. The lesions have been confused with those of tuberculosis. Infection is seen more often in feedlot animals than in those on pasture.

Unlike other herbivorous animals, horses and llamas may develop disseminated coccidioidomycosis. Equine coccidioidomycosis may have a gender-related predilection for females, and although a variety of breeds were affected, Arabians may be overrepresented. Abortion, mastitis, osteomyelitis, nasal granuloma, meningitis, pneumonia, and a visceral form (hepatic, splenic, and renal involvement) have been reported in the horse. Llamas appear to be highly susceptible to *Coccidioides* spp. Respiratory, dermatitis, osteomyelitis, meningitis, and polyperiarthritis syndromes have been recognized in this species.

Pathogenesis

Coccidioidomycosis is acquired through inhalation of infective arthroconidia. The arthroconidia are of a size (2-3 μm by 4-5 μm) that facilitates deposition in lung. The affinity for lung tissue is strong. After inhalation, the arthrospore, in the presence of phagocytic cells, increased CO_2, and 37° C temperature, differentiates by isotropic growth into a multinucleated spherule. Spherules reproduce through a process of endosporulation, with the wall of the spherule serving as the germinal center. The cytosol becomes compartmentalized into endospores, resulting from inward growth of the innermost stratum. Upon maturation, the spherule ruptures, releasing endospores that mature into new spherules. The exact mechanism by which the endospores are set free is still vague but chitinase and glucanases may be involved in spherule wall lysis. Disease initially begins in the lung but is usually self-limiting. In some individuals, hematogenous or lymphatic dissemination results in infection of the bone, skin, lymph nodes, and central nervous system. Because the organisms are removed primarily by mononuclear cells, this might explain why clinical disease and dissemination are more common in immunosuppressed individuals.

The fungus is extremely virulent. Its high fecundity promotes survival within the host, and in humans it may remain viable in lesions for up to 15 years' postinfection. Reactivation of these infections may be associated with chronic pulmonary disease, advancing age, and malnutrition.

Spherule size and composition may be virulence attributes of *C. immitis.* The size (up to 100 μm in diameter) of the spherule may allow it to escape engulfment by neutrophils and macrophages. The thick extracellular matrix is yet another deterrent to phagocytosis.

Coccidioides spp. cause extensive tissue damage in the lungs, and, if disseminated, to other affected organs and tissues. Components of the soluble conidial wall fraction contain humoral and cellular antigens, antiphagocytic properties, and proteolytic enzymes. These enzymes appear to be responsible for inciting tissue damage.

One enzyme, a 60 kD extracellular and cell surface serine protease, is associated with mycelia and conidia. Experimental evidence suggests that it is released from the fungus soon after inhalation and causes immediate damage to pulmonary tissue, perhaps primarily by way of its elastase activity. Several other proteolytic enzymes are found in the soluble conidial cell wall fraction. One in particular, AgCS, degrades immunoglobulins, elastin, glycoproteins, and collagen. End products of protein degradation may be neutrophil chemotaxins or chemotaxigens, and accumulation of these cells may contribute to tissue damage.

Hormone-binding proteins of *C. immitis* may also be important virulence factors. Men and pregnant women are apparently at increased risk for developing disseminated coccidioidomycosis, and in vitro studies have revealed that testosterone, progesterone, and estradiol stimulate the growth of *C. immitis* through their effect on spherule maturation. Investigators have found a direct correlation between rate of fungal growth and increasing β-estradiol levels in association with late pregnancy. In addition, cytosolic molecules of *C. immitis* can bind androgen, progestin, estrogen, and corticosteroids.

Coccidioides immitis produces urease, which may be a virulence factor. In nature, the enzyme aids in maintaining the alkalinity of the microenvironment necessary for fungal growth. Urease produced in the host may have deleterious effects on tissue.

Recent investigations have led to the discovery of a spherule outer-wall glycoprotein that functions as a major cell surface–expressed antigen. It elicits both cellular and humoral immune responses in individuals with coccidioidomycosis, and may function as an adhesin in colonizing pulmonary tissue.

Diagnosis

As with other fungal agents, the laboratory criteria for diagnosis are cultural, histopathologic, or molecular evidence of the presence of *Coccidioides* spp. Specimens for diagnosis include pus or exudates from lesions, transtracheal washes, and lymph node or bone biopsies. Wet mounts in 10% potassium hydroxide (KOH) will contain the tissue form of the fungus. Spherules are large (10-100 μm) and round, and have a thick, doubly refractile cell wall. Endospores inside the spherules have an average diameter of 2 to 5 μm (Figure 47-6).

The mycelial form of this organism is extremely dangerous to handle because of the production of numerous arthrospores, so cultures should be initiated on tubed rather than plated media. *Coccidioides* spp. grow on most routine fungal media and can grow in the presence of cycloheximide. Cultures may be incubated at 25° or 37° C with colonies of varying texture and color often appearing within 1 week. Colonies initially are white, moist, and membranous, and later turn cottony, with tan, brown, gray, pink, or yellow pigmentation. Microscopically, the mycelial phase consists of hyphae with thick-walled or barrel-shaped arthroconidia alternating with thin-walled, empty (disjunctor) cells (Figure 47-7). The fungus continues to grow as a mold in vitro and will not form spherules unless cultivated in defined media containing glucose and salts, such as Converse liquid medium. Spherules develop on incubation in liquid medium at 37° to 40° C and CO_2 concentrations up to 20%.

Microscopic examination of the mold reveals hyaline hyphae that are branched and septate. Thick-walled, barrel-shaped arthrospores appear

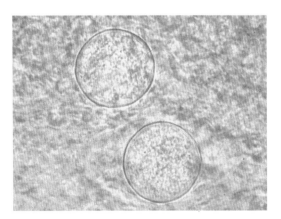

FIGURE 47-6 Smear of exudates showing spherules of *Coccidioides*. (Courtesy Public Health Image Library, PHIL #479, Centers for Disease Control and Prevention, Atlanta, date unknown.)

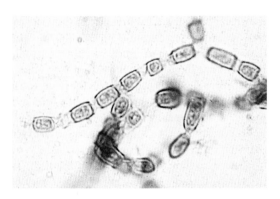

FIGURE 47-7 Arthroconidia of *Coccidioides*. (Courtesy Public Health Image Library, PHIL #476, Centers for Disease Control and Prevention, Atlanta, 1965, Hardin.)

alternatively in chains, separated by empty (disjunctor) cells. Arthroconidia of *C. immitis* may be confused with those of other fungi such as *Arthroderma, Malbranchea,* or *Geotrichum,* so confirmation of identity is necessary by use of DNA probes, immunodiffusion tests for exoantigen, or cultivation of spherules.

For decades, serologic tests have served as aids in the diagnosis and management of coccidioidomycosis. Although these have proved useful in human and veterinary medicine, they should not be the only diagnostic method chosen. Serology can be used for a presumptive diagnosis with compatible clinical signs when organisms are absent in cytologic preparations or biopsy materials.

The host generates cutaneous delayed-type hypersensitivity reaction to coccidioidin, so skin testing can also be used for diagnosis. Responses of dogs, horses, llamas, and nonhuman primates are similar to those in humans. Test results are positive after exposure to *Coccidioides,* including inapparent infection or resolution without intervention. A positive skin test may revert to negative in association with advanced disease, and is an indicator of poor prognosis. A negative skin test does not rule out coccidioidomycosis and should not preclude serologic and other tests to detect disease.

Other serologic tests detect circulating antibodies in serum or cerebrospinal fluid. Several techniques are available, including immunodiffusion, complement fixation, enzyme immunoassay, latex agglutination, or tube precipitin. These tests may be positive 2 to 4 weeks after infection. Rising titers in patients with active disease is indicative of a poor prognosis.

Prevention and Control

Contracting coccidioidal infection is an inherent risk associated with living in endemic regions. Although disease is not readily preventable, a better understanding of its epidemiology can assist in identifying and modifying risk factors. As the infective arthroconidia are inhaled, activities that increase exposure to dust should be avoided.

Because of the rise in population in endemic areas and the increasing number of senior citizens that may be at greater risk, there is renewed interest in developing effective vaccines. Experimental vaccines prepared from whole spherules or subunits are being developed and evaluated. Some protect mice and nonhuman primates.

Prevention of dissemination may be achieved by treatment with azole chemotherapeutics. Ketoconazole remains the drug of choice in veterinary medicine. Itraconazole has also been used with success.

CRYPTOCOCCOSIS

Cryptococcosis is a subacute to chronic mycosis of worldwide distribution caused by *Cryptococcus neoformans.* The fungus is unique among the systemic mycotic agents in that it does not share their geographic restriction. Unlike the dimorphic fungi, *C. neoformans* is monomorphic, growing as a yeast in infected tissue and in the environment. It is also the only encapsulated systemic mycotic agent.

The yeast was first recovered from peach juice in the late 1800s and given the name *Saccharomyces neoformans.* Current taxonomic placement of cryptococci is in the phylum Basidiomycota, order Sporidiales, and family Sporidiobolaceae. The teleomorphic phase is in the genus *Filobasidiella.* Although there are more than 30 species in the genus, only *neoformans* is pathogenic. Isolates of *C. neoformans* have been divided into four serotypes (A-D) based on capsular agglutination reactions. The authors of subsequent molecular typing studies have proposed that serotype A strains be designated as *C. neoformans* var. *grubii,* serotypes B and C strains be designated as *C. neoformans* var. *gattii,* and serotype D strains be designated as *C. neoformans* var. *neoformans.*

Diseases and Epidemiology

Cryptococcus neoformans var. *neoformans* and var. *grubii* are ubiquitous in the environment and have worldwide distribution. The yeasts are common inhabitants of soil and are found in large numbers in association with bird excreta, and in particular, pigeon droppings, that provide a major reservoir of the organism in urban areas. The high concentration of creatinine in bird droppings provides favorable growth conditions. Occasionally, organisms are isolated from substrates such as fermenting fruit and wood (Figure 47-8).

Cryptococcus neoformans var. *gattii* is found mainly in subtropical and tropical regions. Infections have been reported in Australia, New Guinea, Southeast Asia, southern California, Mexico, Cuba, Brazil, Argentina, Uruguay, Spain, Italy, Portugal, Kenya, and Zaire. Environmental isolations have indicated a specific association with *Eucalyptus* species. Decaying wood present in the hollows of these trees may provide a favorable substrate for growth.

Cryptococcus neoformans var. *neoformans* and var. *grubii* are responsible for most of the cases of cryptococcosis in immunocompromised patients, whereas *C. neoformans* var. *gattii* has been associated with infections in subjects with a normal immunologic status. Because the infection is acquired from environmental sources and not from infected animals, the agent is not considered

to be zoonotic. Animal-to-animal transmission has not been demonstrated.

Cryptococcus neoformans is an opportunistic pathogen of humans, causing especially severe illness in immunocompromised individuals. Disease prevalence is high in humans with cell-mediated immune deficiencies, and acquired immunodeficiency syndrome (AIDS), lymphoma, hematologic malignancy, and corticosteroid therapy are major risk factors, with a specific tropism for the brain and lungs. Cryptococcosis has increased in incidence with the increase in the number of patients with AIDS and those undergoing transplantation.

Cryptococcosis is the most common systemic fungal infection in cats. The nasal cavity is the primary site of infection. If the rostral portion of the nasal cavity is involved, mycotic rhinitis results, with clinical signs such as sneezing and nasal discharge. The fungus may invade the facial bones, causing distortion of the nasal cavity. If the caudal portion of the nasal cavity is affected, clinical signs of mycotic rhinitis may be absent and the fungus tends to spread to the olfactory bulbs, leading to meningitis. Hematogenous dissemination may result in cutaneous or ocular lesions. When nasal, respiratory, or cutaneous disease is diagnosed early, the prognosis is favorable with aggressive antifungal therapy. The prognosis remains grave for central nervous system or widely disseminated disease.

Genetic factors may predispose cats to cryptococcosis. Most studies have found no sex predilection, but Siamese cats have a higher incidence of disease than other breeds. Most infections occur in cats 3 to 7 years of age. Immunosuppressive viruses apparently do not predispose cats to cryptococcosis, but animals concurrently infected with a virus have a poor prognosis.

Cryptococcosis in dogs is less common than in cats. Purebred dogs 1 to 7 years old are most often affected. The common target organs include the respiratory tract, ocular tissues, skin, peripheral lymph nodes, and central nervous system. Systemic cryptococcosis affecting the kidney has been reported infrequently in dogs.

Many cryptococcal infections in horses have been meningitides or nasal granulomas. Lung infection was described in an aborted fetus, and granulomatous pneumonia in adult horses. The nasal passages are the most frequently reported site of infection, and cryptococcal rhinitis or nasal granuloma results. Animals may present with

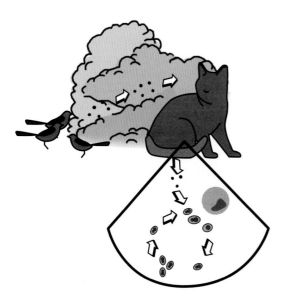

FIGURE 47-8 Natural history of the saprobic and parasitic life cycle of cryptococcosis. *Cryptococcus neoformans* remains in the yeast form in both environment (25° C) and host (37° C). (Courtesy Ashley E. Harmon.)

dyspnea, nasal discharge, and dysphagia. The disease remains relatively uncommon.

Avian cryptococcosis has been infrequently diagnosed, with only sporadic reports of disease in exotic and wild birds. Cryptococci have been isolated from pheasants with enterohepatitis; experimentally infected chickens develop granulomatous lesions in the liver, spleen, and lungs.

Cryptococcus neoformans var. *gattii* has a predilection for the respiratory and central nervous systems of apparently healthy domestic animals and humans. Disease has been reported in domestic and wild animal species including cats, dogs, goats, sheep, horses, koalas, Australian marsupial opossums, and a cheetah. In Spain, outbreaks of severe pulmonary and neurologic disease have been reported in goats.

Pathogenesis and Virulence Factors

Capsule formation by *C. neoformans* is limited during residence in an environment of high salt and sugar concentrations. This reduces the size of the yeast, allowing it to be readily aerosolized and facilitating alveolar deposition, which is the natural route of infection. Other modes of infection may be wound contamination or ingestion of contaminated dust. Once inside the lungs, capsular production is initiated. Dissemination to other organs is through hematogenous and lymphatic routes. Secondary spread to the central nervous system may also follow erosion of the cribriform plate.

Animals and humans suffering from debilitating diseases or receiving immunosuppressive therapy are more susceptible to infection. The marked predilection of individuals with T-cell dysfunction to disease indicates that antibody and neutrophil responses are inadequate to contain *C. neoformans*. Studies have confirmed that the organism has virulence factors that enable it to evade both phagocytic and humoral defenses.

The capsule of *C. neoformans* serves as its major virulence factor. The primary component is glucuronoxylomannan, a viscous polysaccharide. Once inside the host, the capsule thickens, and heavily encapsulated strains may simply be too large to be phagocytosed by macrophages. In the murine model, acapsular mutants are more susceptible to phagocytosis and killing than encapsulated yeasts. During an infection, the organism sheds capsule continuously into the

host's bloodstream and cerebrospinal fluid, and capsular antigen serves as the basis for many diagnostic tests.

Another putative virulence factor is phenoloxidase activity, which results in melanin production. The mechanism by which melanization plays a role in virulence has not been fully elucidated for *C. neoformans*, but in that it is a potent free radical scavenger, it may protect the yeast from neutrophil oxidants. In vitro, melanized yeast cells are less susceptible to amphotericin B–mediated oxidative damage.

Investigators have proposed additional virulence factors including production of phospholipases and mannitol. Phospholipases are involved in the membrane disruption processes that occur during host invasion, and experiments in mice have demonstrated an association between high phospholipase activity and virulence. Cryptococci produce mannitol both in vitro and in vivo, leading to speculation that it might contribute to brain edema and interfere with phagocyte killing, via scavenging of hydroxyl radicals.

Cryptococci are powerful activators of the alternative complement pathway. Incubation of encapsulated cryptococci in normal serum leads to binding of C3 to the capsule. Studies of both human and animal cryptococcosis showed that complement activation occurs in vivo. Experimental infections in animals with deficiencies of the complement system have provided insight into the importance of the complement system in resistance to cryptococcosis. Binding of C3 fragments to cryptococci in brain tissue is essentially absent, and this absence may explain the predilection of this organism for the central nervous system.

The macrophage plays a key role in cell-mediated immunity, and bronchoalveolar macrophages are the first line of defense. Although *C. neoformans* is not an obligate intracellular parasite, it may reside in the macrophage under some circumstances. The exact mechanism by which *C. neoformans* avoids killing by the macrophage is not completely understood. The fungus is relatively resistant to the oxidants generated as a result of the respiratory burst of these cells, and disease may be reactivated from latent foci in macrophages. In the absence of opsonins, macrophages do not bind the yeast because capsule masks ligands on the cell wall. The major opsonin promoting macrophage recognition is complement.

Diagnosis

The diagnosis of cryptococcosis can be established using fungal isolation, cytologic examination of body fluids, histologic examination of fixed tissues, and serologic tests.

Examination of impression smears of lesions, stained with india ink, reveals encapsulated yeast cells 2 to 20 μm in diameter that are oval or round with thin dark walls. Buds are on narrow bases. Characteristically thick capsules are produced.

When cultivated at 30° C on Sabouraud dextrose agar, colonies are small, convex, dull to mucoid, smooth, and cream to brownish (Figure 47-9). Identification is confirmed by characteristic growth on cornmeal agar, rapid urease production, inability to reduce nitrate, and brown pigmentation on Niger seed agar, which is due to the activity of phenoloxidase. Var. *neoformans* is differentiated from var. *gattii* through growth in L-canavanine-glycine-bromothymol blue agar and agar with D-proline and D-tryptophan.

Histologic examination of tissues using fungal stains reveals numerous small yeasts (Figure 47-10). These can be distinguished from *B. dermatitidis* in that cryptococci do not have a broad base of attachment between the bud and the parent cell. Mucicarmine or Alcian blue will stain the polysaccharide capsule of *C. neoformans* but will not stain *H. capsulatum*.

A commercial latex agglutination test for diagnosis of feline cryptococcosis is both sensitive and specific. Titers parallel the severity of infection, and the test may be useful in monitoring effects of therapy. Enzyme immunoassay reveals elevated levels of anticryptococcal antibodies in more than 80% of cats and dogs, at the time of diagnosis, or during or after successful therapy. Persistence of increased antibody titers in more than 50% of the cases following active infection suggest that this test could be a useful seroepidemiologic marker of previous infection.

Prevention and Control

The azole derivatives itraconazole and fluconazole have proven effective for managing cryptococcosis. Ketoconazole has been used alone or in combination with amphotericin B; 5-fluorocytosine also has been used. Amphotericin B is generally reserved for cases of life-threatening disseminated disease.

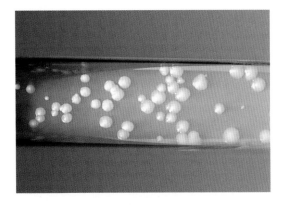

FIGURE 47-9 Slant culture of *Cryptococcus neoformans*. (Courtesy Public Health Image Library, PHIL #3208, Centers for Disease Control and Prevention, Atlanta, date unknown, William Kaplan.)

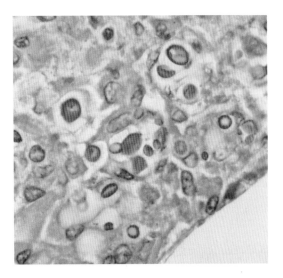

FIGURE 47-10 *Cryptococcus neoformans* in lung of AIDS patient. (Courtesy Public Health Image Library, PHIL #962, Centers for Disease Control and Prevention, Atlanta, 1984, Edwin P. Ewing, Jr.)

Treatment should be continued for 1 to 2 months past the resolution of clinical signs, or, if the titers are being monitored, until they have become undetectable or are decreased by at least two orders of magnitude.

Treatment of cryptococcal rhinitis has been largely unsuccessful. A favorable prognosis depends on early diagnosis, when the lesions are minimal and localized. Therapeutic measures have included surgical intervention, cryotherapy, and parenteral treatment with sodium iodide and amphotericin B.

Efforts are under way to develop vaccines against *C. neoformans,* with a focus on cell wall polysaccharides as candidate vaccines. The glucuronoxylomannan capsule of *C. neoformans,* in particular, stimulates antibodies against several epitopes.

HISTOPLASMOSIS

The three varieties of *H. capsulatum* are var. *capsulatum,* var. *duboisii,* and var. *farciminosum.* *Histoplasma capsulatum* var. *capsulatum* is the fungal pathogen responsible for histoplasmosis. This thermally dimorphic fungus exists as a mycelial form at 25° C and as a budding yeast at 37° C. The organism is a member of the phylum Ascomycota, class Ascomycetes, order Onygenales, and family Onygenaceae. The teleomorph is *Ajellomyces capsulatus.*

Histoplasmosis was first described in central America in 1905 by a pathologist named Darling. He performed an autopsy on a patient who had succumbed to an infection resembling tuberculosis and believed the agent he observed in lesions was a protozoan. The fungal etiology was discovered in 1929 when the organism was cultivated from human clinical specimens, and disease was reproduced in experimental animals.

The other varieties of *Histoplasma capsulatum* are also pathogenic. *Histoplasma capsulatum* var. *duboisii* is the agent of African histoplasmosis, which, as the name implies, is localized to the African continent. This clinically distinct form of histoplasmosis commonly involves the skin and bones rather than the lungs. Natural infection has been reported in nonhuman primates. *Histoplasma capsulatum* var. *farciminosum* is the cause of the subcutaneous mycosis epizootic lymphangitis in horses and mules.

Diseases and Epidemiology

Histoplasma capsulatum var. *capsulatum* flourishes in humid environments with highly nitrogenous soils, especially those heavily contaminated with bird or bat droppings. The first environmental isolation of the fungus was from soil near a chicken coop. This strong association with avian habitats has been further strengthened by the fact that *H. capsulatum* var. *capsulatum* grows well on shed feathers in vitro. The organism is routinely recovered in high numbers from soil samples where starlings roost (Figure 47-11). In fact, regions of the United States that have the highest starling population are the most highly endemic for histoplasmosis; these encompass the Tennessee, Mississippi, Ohio, Missouri, and St. Lawrence River basins. However, disease has been reported worldwide, and areas with high prevalence exist in Mexico, Panama, Guatemala, Honduras, Nicaragua, Colombia, Venezuela, Brazil, Peru, Indonesia, the

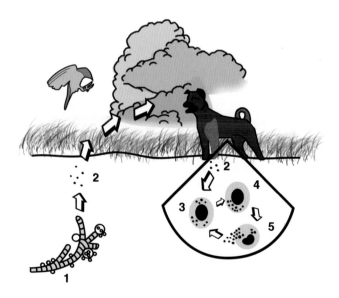

FIGURE 47-11 Natural history of the saprobic and parasitic life cycle of histoplasmosis. Environmental *Histoplasma capsulatum* grows in the mold form *(1)*. Microconidia or hyphal fragments *(2)* are inhaled or ingested by a susceptible host and convert to the yeast phase in host tissues *(2-5)* at 37° C. (Courtesy Ashley E. Harmon.)

Philippines, Burma, and Turkey. The disease is transmitted through the inhalation or ingestion of microconidia, and horizontal and interspecies transmission is unlikely.

Histoplasmosis is the most common human pulmonary mycosis in the United States. More than 95% of infections are either subclinical or mild self-limited respiratory infections. Rarely, acute primary disease may develop in healthy immunocompetent individuals who are exposed to a heavy inoculum of organisms. Disseminated histoplasmosis occurs in organs of the reticuloendothelial system and is caused by parasitism of the mononuclear phagocytes. This form of the disease tends to develop in elderly or immunocompromised patients, especially patients with AIDS or solid-organ transplant recipients. Long-term survival of the yeast within macrophages is responsible for later reactivation to cause life-threatening disease when host immunity is impaired.

Dogs seem to be the most susceptible of the domestic species, and young, outdoor sporting breeds are most commonly affected. The three forms of disease are pulmonary, in which involvement is limited to the lung; disseminated, in which multiple organs are involved; and clinically inapparent. Most canine infections are inapparent, but when clinical signs are evident, they usually reflect specific organ involvement and vary from mild respiratory signs to severe systemic disease. These signs may include coughing, dyspnea, anorexia, weight loss, depression, ascites, ulcerations of the oral or nasal mucosa, anemia, lymphadenopathy, thrombocytopenia, fever, and diarrhea. The organs most commonly affected are the gastrointestinal tract, skin, lymphatics, central nervous system, bone marrow, eyes, liver, and spleen. With disseminated disease, necropsy reveals numerous small, pale, necrotic granulomas scattered over serosal and cut surfaces of the lungs, liver, spleen, and lymph nodes.

Histoplasmosis is a rare, progressive, debilitating disease in the cat. Various studies have suggested that up to 44% of cats residing in endemic areas may harbor yeasts in their tissues. Most cases are characterized by weight loss, lethargy, and fluctuating fever. Less than half of the cats in one survey had clinical evidence of respiratory disease.

Histoplasmosis has been documented in other animal species. Pulmonary disease, anemia, and abortion have been described in the horse.

Avian histoplasmosis has been diagnosed in zoo birds, but is an infrequent occurrence in chickens and turkeys. Disease in cattle and pigs has been reported infrequently. Sporadic accounts of histoplasmosis in sea otters, dolphins, badgers, a Kodiak bear, and rodents have appeared in the literature.

Pathogenesis and Virulence Factors

In the environment, *H. capsulatum* var. *capsulatum* grows in an undifferentiated mold form. Upon inhalation or ingestion of the infectious forms (microconidia or hyphal fragments), the organism converts to the yeast phase in the host's tissues in response to elevated temperature. This mold-to-yeast shift is required for disease to develop. Yeasts engulfed by macrophages multiply intracellularly, and if the cell-mediated immune mechanism is overwhelmed, disease may disseminate via hematogenous or lymphatic routes.

Like the other systemic fungi, *H. capsulatum* var. *capsulatum* is well adapted to be infectious and pathogenic and has developed some unique virulence strategies. These features include dimorphism, entry into host macrophages and intracellular growth, melanin production, thermotolerance, and dormancy. The capacity to transform from the mycelial to the yeast form enables this fungus to withstand environmental challenges, including certain antifungal drugs and host defense mechanisms, and is critical for establishment of infection. Yeast forms in host tissues suggest that this form is more invasive and hardier.

The ability to survive and multiply inside macrophages is another virulence factor. To gain entry into phagocytes, yeasts use the CD11/CD18 family of surface adhesins to bind to the surface of the macrophage. Once inside the cell, the yeasts become engulfed in phagolysosomes. They withstand the acid proteases of the phagolysosome through alkalization of the pH-hostile environment. The increased pH may be caused by the action of fungal urease, or to release of ammonia or bicarbonate. Calcium-binding protein also may be involved in modulating phagolysosomal conditions, perhaps by chelation of calcium and restriction of the destructive power of lysosomal enzymes. Furthermore, yeasts appear to be able to impair the generation of the respiratory burst in macrophages, thereby avoiding damage from the toxic products that would be generated. Siderophores may be important for the acquisition of iron from transferrin, whereas the yeast resides in macrophages and derives its iron directly from cytoplasmic molecules. Iron is present as hemin in the intracellular environment of the macrophage and may also serve as a source of iron during infection.

Histoplasma capsulatum var. *capsulatum* conidia and yeasts can synthesize melanin-like pigments in vitro. It is theorized that melanin is an important antioxidant for this organism, as it is for other pathogenic fungi. Thermotolerance of *H. capsulatum* var. *capsulatum* may also be correlated with virulence.

Little is known about the impact of dormancy on pathogenesis, but following infection, the fungus likely persists somewhere in host tissues for life. In endemic regions, calcifications indicative of persistent organisms may be found on routine chest or abdominal radiographs. If the host's immune response is impaired, the fungus can reactivate to cause disease.

The immune system is usually highly effective in controlling the spread of the infection so the overwhelming majority of infected hosts effectively clear the fungus. Neutrophils do not appear to play a prominent role in host defenses, but macrophages exhibit a greater capacity to ingest yeast cells. Cell-mediated immunity is critical for clearance of the organism, and cytokine-activated macrophages inhibit fungal growth by limiting access to iron.

Diagnosis

Diagnosis is based on identification of the organism in clinical materials by culture or molecular detection methods or by cytology or histopathology, or through detection of anti-*Histoplasma* antibodies by serology.

Histoplasma yeasts are usually numerous in affected tissues. Fluids from exudative lesions, transtracheal washes, and aspirates of lymph nodes, bone marrow, or internal organs should be submitted for cytologic examination with hematologic stains and culture. Fungal organisms may occasionally be found in circulating leukocytes, histiocytes, or in urine sediment (Figure 47-12).

The detection of *H. capsulatum* var. *capsulatum* still depends largely on culture of the organism from clinical materials. Precise identification relies on visualization of the typical morphology and the demonstration of dimorphism. Specimens

should be refrigerated unless cultures can be initiated within a few hours of collection because the yeasts will become nonviable. The saprobic phase grows at temperatures below 35° C on a variety of fungal media, with and without cycloheximide. Colonies appear as white to brownish mycelial fungus after 14 days (Figure 47-13). Cultures should be held up to 6 weeks before discarding as negative. Microscopically, the organism produces characteristic tuberculate, hyaline oval to pyriform macroconidia up to 20 μm in diameter, and small, unicellular, hyaline globose microconidia

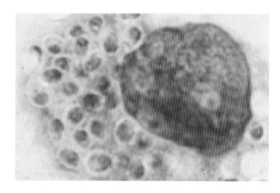

FIGURE 47-12 Histiocyte containing yeasts of *Histoplasma capsulatum*. (Courtesy Public Health Image Library, PHIL #453, Centers for Disease Control and Prevention, Atlanta, date unknown, D.T. McClenan.)

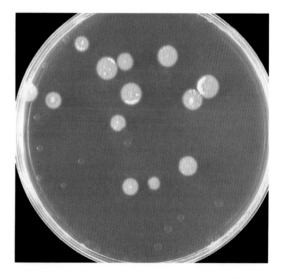

FIGURE 47-13 Plate depicting mycelial growth of *Histoplasma capsulatum*. (Courtesy Public Health Image Library, PHIL #3191, Centers for Disease Control and Prevention, Atlanta, 1969, William Kaplan.)

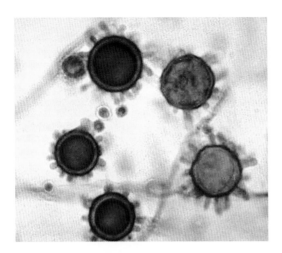

FIGURE 47-14 Asexual spores of *Histoplasma capsulatum* showing tuberculate macroconidia. (Courtesy Public Health Image Library, PHIL #299, Centers for Disease Control and Prevention, Atlanta, date unknown.)

(2-5 μm) (Figure 47-14). Isolates should be handled with caution in a biological safety cabinet because they are highly infectious. Several saprobic fungi, such as members of the genera *Chrysosporium* and *Sepedonium,* produce structures that resemble the tuberculate macroconidia of *H. capsulatum,* making visual identification somewhat difficult. The conversion to the yeast phase requires temperatures above 37° C, high humidity, increased CO_2 levels, and a blood-based enriched medium for growth (brain-heart infusion agar). Budding yeasts are tiny (2-4 μm in diameter), ovoid, and narrow based. Use of thermal dimorphism for identification may be problematic because conversion to the yeast phase is strain dependent and may take up to 1 month for completion. Molecular methods for identification of *H. capsulatum* should be used when thermal dimorphism cannot be demonstrated. PCR and DNA probe tests are available in some commercial reference laboratories.

The major diagnostic antigens of *H. capsulatum* var. *capsulatum* are the M and H antigens, glycoproteins that elicit both humoral and cell-mediated immune responses. A wide variety of tests are used in the laboratory for disease diagnosis but all have limitations. The complement fixation test detects antibodies against the M antigen and plays a significant role in the identification of infection. *Histoplasma* antigen detection in urine and/or serum has a variable range of sensitivity, depending on the clinical pattern, the chronicity of the infection, and the underlying condition of the patient. Generally the test is useful in cases of disseminated disease. Serologic testing by immunodiffusion also has utility. False-positive test results may be seen when patients are infected with other disseminated mycoses because of cross-reactions between shared epitopes. False-negative reactions may occur in immunocompromised individuals unable to mount an antibody response.

Prevention and Control

The drug of choice for control of clinical disease in dogs and cats is itraconazole because of its low toxicity. Other azole drugs, such as ketoconazole or fluconazole, may be beneficial. Amphotericin B can be given parenterally to dogs with severe intestinal lesions or life-threatening disease. The prognosis ranges from fair to good for animals with pulmonary disease and poor in cases of disseminated disease.

Environmental control measures have been used to eradicate the fungus. Disinfection of soil on contaminated premises has been accomplished through application of 3% formalin or 5% phenol. Elimination of starling roosts may control the source of infection.

Vaccination as a way of protecting hosts from histoplasmosis is a subject of ongoing research. Several components of *H. capsulatum* have protected mice against experimental infections.

SUGGESTED READINGS

Gionfriddo JR: Feline systemic fungal infections, *Vet Clin North Am Small Anim Pract* 30:1029-1050, 2000.

Hamilton AJ, Holdom MD: Antioxidant systems in the pathogenic fungi of man and their role in virulence, *Med Mycol* 37:375-389, 1999.

Hogan LH, Klein BS, Levitz SM: Virulence factors of medically important fungi, *Clin Microbiol Rev* 9:469-488, 1996.

Krohne SG: Canine systemic fungal infections, *Vet Clin North Am Small Anim Pract* 30:1063-1090, 2000.

Chapter 48

The Opportunistic Mycoses

Infection is a rare consequence of environmental exposure of animals to normally nonpathogenic fungi. Natural resistance to most of these agents is high, and most are of low virulence. However, agents of low virulence may act as pathogens when animals become stressed or otherwise debilitated, are treated with antibiotics, or following breakdown of the mucocutaneous barrier. Opportunistic fungi (a categorization without taxonomic standing) take advantage of these situations and cause infections. Most opportunistic mycoses are attributed to *Candida* and *Aspergillus* spp., and members of the class Zygomycetes.

THE GENUS *CANDIDA*

The genus *Candida* belongs to the family Cryptococcaceae (order Cryptococcales, class Deuteromycetes) and contains more than 200 species. Taxonomic relationships within the genus are poorly defined. They reproduce by budding and production of chlamydospores. Pseudohyphae may be absent, present in rudimentary form, or well developed. Hallmarks of the genus are failure to produce acetic acid, ballistoconidia, or arthrospores, and lack of red or orange pigmented colonies.

Diseases and Epidemiology

Candida spp. are normal inhabitants of the alimentary, upper respiratory, and genital mucosae of animals, and primarily associated with infections of the skin and mucous membranes; however, they can invade nearly every organ in the body.

Disruption of the epidermal barrier by trauma, antibiotic therapy, inflammation, immunosuppressive disease, or glucocorticoid therapy may allow the yeasts to overcome the normal cutaneous defense mechanisms.

Human infection often follows some sort of debilitation, such as hormone imbalance or application of immunosuppressive therapy. Infections are common in patients with acquired immunodeficiency syndrome (AIDS), and intravenous drug users are subject to endocarditis. Foreign bodies (such as catheters) can promote colonization, and hyperalimentation can predispose to infection.

Cutaneous candidiasis occurs infrequently in dogs and cats. In the dog, infection has been associated with *Candida albicans, Candida parapsilosis,* and *Candida guilliermondii*. Exfoliative dermatitis may be found on the muzzle, inguinal area, scrotum, and dorsal and lateral aspects of the feet. In addition, seborrhea, pruritus, and alopecia may be noted. *Candida albicans* has been associated with an outbreak of otitis externa in a pack of foxhounds, and localized and disseminated infections have been reported in cats. Many of the cats were concurrently infected with feline panleukopenia or feline immunodeficiency virus.

Gastroesophageal candidiasis, in association with gastric ulceration, has been described in foals and calves. Animals present clinically with signs of colic that are nonresponsive to medical treatment. *Candida albicans* or *Candida krusei* has been recovered from cultures of gastric fluid. Stress is an important predisposing factor.

Crop mycosis ("thrush") of poultry is caused by *C. albicans,* and serious outbreaks have been reported in many species of birds. The crop, mouth, esophagus, proventriculus, and gizzard are most frequently affected, and lesions consist of white plaques or pseudomembranes adherent to the mucosal surfaces (Figure 48-1, *A*). Superficial ulcers occur when plaques slough, and mortality may be high in young birds. Disease is frequently associated with other debilitating conditions such as intestinal coccidiosis or unsanitary, crowded housing.

The agent of candidiasis in swine is also *C. albicans,* and disease is associated with stress or immunosuppression and unsanitary housing conditions. Cutaneous and mucocutaneous disease has been described. Circular skin lesions are covered with thick, gray exudates, and alopecia may be apparent. In chronic infections the skin may become wrinkled and thickened. The lesions of mucocutaneous disease are similar to those observed in poultry, and are characterized by pseudomembrane formation. Similar gross lesions can be found in the javelina (Figure 48-1, *B*).

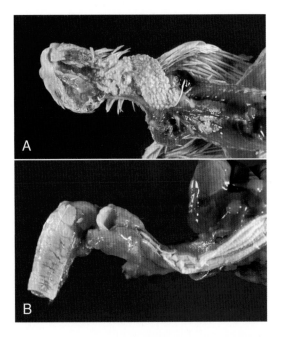

FIGURE 48-1 **A,** Crop mycosis caused by *Candida* sp. in a cockatiel. **B,** Esophageal candidiasis in a javelina. (Courtesy Gregory A. Bradley.)

Pathogenesis

Depression of cell-mediated immunity is likely an important factor in pathogenesis of candidiasis. Prolonged immunosuppression, neutropenia associated with chemotherapy, diabetes mellitus, and long-term glucocorticoid or antimicrobial treatments are predisposing factors. However, epithelial colonization can occur even in immuno-competent hosts, especially when an epithelial breach occurs. Virulence attributes include factors that mediate adherence to epithelial and endothelial cells, extracellular enzymes, and phenotypic switching.

Several types of adhesive interactions have been described. Candidal surface protein recognition of host-cell–surface carbohydrate results in a lectinlike interaction. Four structurally related adhesins, members of a class of glycosylphosphatidylinositol-dependent cell wall proteins, mediate attachment. Invasion of mucous membranes appears to follow adhesion of the yeasts to a debilitated surface, with subsequent development of pseudohyphae that invade the superficial epithelium.

Production of extracellular cytotoxic phospholipases and proteases correlates with virulence. Blastospores develop hyphae with phospholipase activity concentrated at their growing tips. This facilitates tissue invasion because host-cell membranes are injured as the yeasts germinate. Isolates that adhere most strongly to buccal epithelial cells and are most virulent for mice produce high levels of extracellular enzymes. Phospholipases, in particular, promote adherence of yeasts to host cells. Production of aspartyl proteinase facilitates penetration of keratinized epithelia.

Phenotypic or phase switching is a gene-regulated process whereby *Candida* spp. make the transition from budding to hyphal forms. Hyphae are commonly thought of as the invasive form, whereas the yeast form is responsible for colonizing epithelia. Tissue penetration and dispersal are mediated by a switch to the hyphal form. This process further enables the fungus to adapt to hostile environmental conditions. Phenotypic switching is accompanied by changes in antigen expression, perhaps allowing the organism to evade the host immune response.

Diagnosis

Isolation of *Candida* spp. from clinical specimens does not confirm candidiasis as the diagnosis.

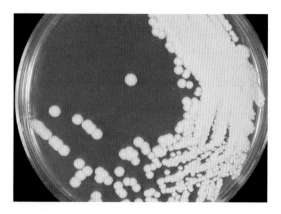

FIGURE 48-2   Colonial morphology of *Candida albicans*. (Courtesy Karen W. Post.)

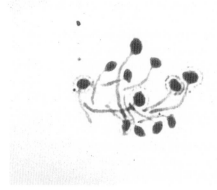

FIGURE 48-3   Germ tube production by *Candida albicans*. (Public Health Image Library, PHIL #1214, Centers for Disease Control and Prevention, Atlanta, 1967, Lucille K. Georg.)

The yeasts must be demonstrated either in a direct examination of lesion material or in tissues through histologic evaluation.

Candida spp. grow readily on a variety of nonselective fungal agars, such as Sabouraud dextrose or potato dextrose agars. Colonies are formed within 2 to 3 days at 25° to 30° C and are creamy, white, opaque, and circular (Figure 48-2). Yeast identification is based on microscopic morphology of organisms cultivated on cornmeal-Tween agar; on production of pigment, germ tubes, and urease; and assimilation and fermentation of carbohydrate.

Presumptive differentiation of *C. albicans* from other *Candida* spp. involves the germ tube test. The test is performed by placing several colonies from a nonselective fungal medium in animal serum and incubating at 37° C for 3 hours. Microscopic examination reveals short hyphal segments without constrictions, at the junction of the blastoconidium and the germ tube, in positive strains (Figure 48-3). Not all *C. albicans* strains produce germ tubes, so false negatives may occur.

Most *Candida* spp. can be differentiated through conventional or commercially available biochemical tests, or by molecular methods. Many commercial rapid tests are based on detection of preformed enzymes and provide presumptive identification in as little as 4 hours. Such tests are applicable only to the common yeasts. Molecular techniques are usually practiced only in mycology reference laboratories.

Prevention and Control

Prevention and control involve maintaining good sanitation and eliminating factors that predispose animals to infection. In cutaneous infections of large animals, crusts should be removed and topical solutions of povidone-iodine, copper sulfate, or copper naphthenate applied to the underlying areas. Treating yeast infections in small animals commonly involves azole drugs (ketoconazole, miconazole, itraconazole) given parenterally or applied topically in the form of a shampoo. Other agents useful for topical application include chlorhexidine and selenium sulfide. Crop mycoses can be treated by adding copper sulfate to the drinking water in poultry houses or administering nystatin in the feed. Therapy should be continued until 2 weeks after clinical signs are resolved.

THE GENUS *ASPERGILLUS*

Aspergilli were first described in 1729 by Micheli, a priest and botanist who thought that the chaining spores of these fungi resembled the brush used for sprinkling holy water, the "aspergillium." The genus contains more than 180 species and taxonomically is placed in the phylum Ascomycota, order Eurotiales, and family Trichomaceae.

Most cases of animal disease are attributed to *Aspergillus fumigatus, Aspergillus flavus, Aspergillus nidulans,* and *Aspergillus niger.* These fungi are ubiquitous in the environment and commonly isolated from plant debris and soil. Aerosol exposure to *Aspergillus* conidia is constant and inevitable.

Disease and Epidemiology

Human aspergillosis in the United States is the second most common fungal disease requiring hospitalization (after candidiasis). Single isolations of *Aspergillus* spp. from humans may be insignificant, but multiple positive cultures from immunocompromised individuals suggest invasive aspergillosis. Risk factors include leukemic granulocytopenia, corticosteroid or other drug therapy, smoking marijuana, and posttransplant neutropenia.

Manifestations of aspergillosis in animals include mycotic pneumonia, guttural pouch mycosis, chronic rhinitis, systemic disease, cutaneous disease, allergy, abortion, gastrointestinal aspergillosis, mastitis, and keratomycosis.

Fungi are introduced into poultry houses through spore-contaminated feed or litter. Fungi multiply rapidly under conditions of high humidity, and massive spore inhalation results in acute outbreaks of severe disease associated with high morbidity and mortality. Aspergillosis is sometimes referred to as "brooder pneumonia." Early lesions consist of small, caseous, white to gray nodules in the lungs or air sacs. Rapid fungal proliferation may line the air sacs with characteristic green hyphae. Acute aspergillosis occurs mainly in poults or chicks, and affected birds are dyspneic, anorexic, and febrile; death is rapid, usually within 48 hours. Chronic disease is seen in older birds, with clinical signs such as coughing, sneezing, ataxia, torticollis, corneal opacity, and emaciation. Trachea and bronchi may be filled with caseous exudate, and white to yellow circumscribed nodules may be visible in the brain. Although the respiratory system is the primary target, other manifestations include dermatitis, osteomycosis, ophthalmitis, enteritis, and encephalitis (Figure 48-4). *Aspergillus fumigatus* and *A. flavus* are the etiologic agents most often recovered from lesions.

Horses experiencing enteritis, typhlocolitis, and other diseases of the gastrointestinal tract can be predisposed to pulmonary aspergillosis. Inhalation of spores from moldy feed is probably the primary route of exposure, but cases have also been associated with carriage of spores to lung by migrating larval parasites.

Mycosis of the equine guttural pouch (auditory tube diverticulum) is a sporadic life-threatening infection characterized by necrotizing inflammation with formation of a diphtheritic membrane within the pouch. In most instances it is caused by *Aspergillus* spp. Infection begins on the roof of the pouch, and fungi proliferate and invade the

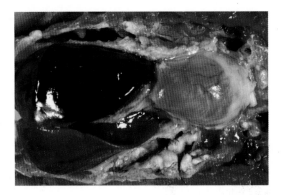

FIGURE 48-4 Aspergillosis in a hawk. (Courtesy M. Kevin Keel.)

internal carotid artery and vein and the glossopharyngeal nerve. Fatal hemorrhage follows erosion of the artery. Common clinical signs are epistaxis, dysphagia, parotid pain, abnormal head position, and unilateral mucopurulent nasal discharge. Endoscopic examination of the guttural pouch reveals a white diphtheritic membrane. Peak incidence is during the summer months, and stabled horses are at greater risk. Age, sex, and breed are not risk factors.

Canine rhinitis or nasal aspergillosis is a common disease that primarily affects previously healthy, young to middle-aged dolichocephalic and mesaticephalic breeds. *Aspergillus fumigatus* is the most frequently isolated species. Affected animals sneeze and have a persistent nasal discharge that is nonresponsive to antibiotics. The disease tends to be invasive and may involve the paranasal sinuses as well as the nasal cavity. Destruction of the turbinate bones with penetration into the brain may result. Immunosuppression is a consequence, rather than a predisposing condition, of infection in dogs. Golden retrievers and collies may be at greater risk than other breeds. Other risk factors are exposure to large numbers of spores and previous facial trauma.

Systemic aspergillosis has been reported in horses but rarely in dogs. Systemic or disseminated aspergillosis is seen almost exclusively in German shepherds and is not associated with prior upper respiratory disease.

Canine cutaneous disease with *A. niger* and *Aspergillus terreus* is uncommon and poorly characterized. Cutaneous lesions may result either from an extension of systemic disease or through inoculation during skin trauma. Immunodeficiency is an apparent predisposing factor in humans because disease seems to be most common in burn victims, neonates, transplant recipients, and individuals with cancer and AIDS.

Allergic disease results from an overexuberant immune response in a hypersensitive or atopic individual. Heaves in horses is a good example, and the recently described feline asthma is also associated with hypersensitivity to aspergilli. Clinical signs arise from responses in the upper respiratory tract, and include coughing and exercise intolerance.

Aspergillus spp. cause sporadic abortion in cattle and horses. Prevalence of bovine mycotic abortion has been estimated at 2% to 20%, which varies by geographic location and climate; rates are higher in colder regions and during winter, coincident with feeding of hay. Incidence may approach 10% in some herds. The primary lesions of mycotic abortion are in the placenta, which is generally thickened and leathery, with necrotic areas and fungal growth between the cotyledons. Fungi may invade the fetus and produce ringwormlike lesions (which are fungal colonies) on the skin surface. The fetus is usually expelled soon after death. *Aspergillus fumigatus* is recovered most frequently.

Mycotic gastritis is common in ruminants. *Aspergillus* spp., as well as zygomycetes, are usually recovered. Young calves are at greatest risk, and the clinical picture includes inappetance, rumen stasis, and pasty, scant, or loose feces. Acute necrohemorrhagic rumenitis and abomasitis are common.

Keratomycosis occurs more frequently in horses than in other domestic animals. Many different fungi are recovered from these infections, but *Aspergillus* spp. are the most common etiologic agents. Predisposing factors include trauma, corneal disease or surgery, and topical therapy with antibiotics or corticosteroids. In the affected animal, the cornea appears opaque and ulcerated. Endothelial plaques, which are characteristic of this infection, are located in the center of the cornea.

Pathogenesis

Healthy animals and birds can withstand substantial exposure to *Aspergillus* spores under natural conditions. Inhalation of massive numbers of spores, as may occur when feed or litter is heavily contaminated, may result in infection. Spores are an ideal size for alveolar disposition.

No single, true virulence factor has been identified, and the mechanisms responsible for protective immunity against *Aspergillus* spp. have yet to be elucidated. Proteases and other toxins may be involved in the pathogenicity of *Aspergillus* spp. The predominant protease is an elastase, which may cause lung damage by degrading structural barriers within the lung and facilitating invasion. Elastase-negative strains are relatively avirulent in a mouse model of invasive pulmonary disease. Extracellular proteinases of *Aspergillus ochraceus* are fibrinolytic and anticoagulative, and may explain the apparent affinity of aspergilli for blood vessels. Rapid release of toxic products may be a critical virulence factor in human infections, with most pertinent effects on macrophages. Gliotoxin, produced by some species, inhibits phagocytosis and T-cell activation and proliferation in vitro.

Equine systemic aspergillosis develops in concert with profound neutropenia associated with colitis. *Aspergillus* spp. invade the disrupted intestinal mucosa, and mycotic emboli disseminate to internal organs and brain. In horses with normal mucosal integrity, predisposing factors may be prolonged administration of steroids or antibiotics, immunosuppression from debilitating disease, and overwhelming exposure to spores.

Mycotic abortion follows infection by the respiratory or alimentary routes, with hematogenous dissemination of spores. Spores infect the placenta, and placental carbohydrates encourage germination, with subsequent hyphal invasion of fetal membranes and cotyledons. Fetal death and abortion result from impaired fetal circulation.

Aerosol exposure to *A. fumigatus* antigens induces marked inflammatory and immunologic alterations in the lungs of horses with chronic obstructive pulmonary disease (COPD), also known as heaves. Bronchoalveolar levels of IgE and IgG to somatic *Aspergillus* antigens are higher in COPD-affected than normal horses, suggesting the involvement of these antigens in the induction of airway immune responses. Increased degranulation of pulmonary mast cells probably contributes to the pathogenesis of heaves.

The pathogenesis of gastrointestinal infections is complex and multifactorial, and is affected by a variety of predisposing factors. Mycotic gastritis often follows injury to the gastric mucosal surface. In young calves, mucosal ulceration related to early ingestion of roughage and infection with bovine rhinotracheitis virus is an initiating factor. Prophylactic and therapeutic use of antibiotics in feed may be an additional risk factor. Mycotic rumenitis and omasitis are linked to the ingestion of moldy feed or hay, and have been described as sequelae to gastritis caused by grain overload. Normal flora of the forestomachs is altered and dietary carbohydrates serve as a source of nutrition for fungal proliferation. Decreased pH leads to erosion and ulceration of the mucosal epithelium, allowing fungal invasion. Penetration of the vasculature leads to thrombus formation and circulatory obstruction, with infarctions and necrosis.

Diagnosis

A diagnosis of aspergillosis should be approached with caution. These fungi are found widely in nature, and they are common contaminants of cultures. Aspergilli are also routinely isolated from the upper respiratory tract of healthy animals. Thus a diagnosis of invasive aspergillosis cannot rely solely on isolation of *Aspergillus* spp. from the site of infection. Repeated isolation of the same species from clinical materials and demonstration of tissue invasion with wet mount or histopathology are required.

Clinical materials are examined in potassium hydroxide (KOH). Key microscopic features useful for presumptive identification include production of septate hyaline hyphae (3-6 μm diameter) and dichotomous branching, which is characterized by formation of two equal hyphal branches of the same diameter as the original segment (Figure 48-5).

These fungi grow readily, usually within 3 days at 25° C, on a wide variety of laboratory media, but are inhibited by cycloheximide. Both macroscopic and microscopic features are used for identification of *Aspergillus* spp. Colonial morphology, including color, surface topography, reverse pigment, and growth rate, as well as thermotolerance, should be recorded. Most species initially produce white velvety or cottony colonies that change color with age. The colors vary by species through shades of green, brown, black, yellow, or orange (Figure 48-6). Key microscopic features include morphology of conidiophores, conidia, and phialides (Figure 48-7). Identification of these organisms to the species level may be extremely difficult because of the large number of species within the genus.

In tissues, aspergillosis causes acute inflammation with areas of ischemic necrosis. As in wet

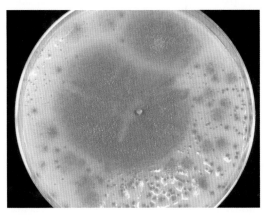

FIGURE 48-6 Colonies of *Aspergillus* sp. on potato dextrose agar. (Courtesy Karen W. Post.)

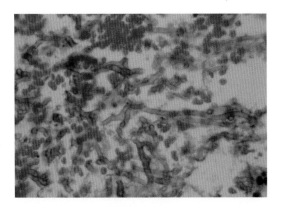

FIGURE 48-5 Dichotomous branching of *Aspergillus* in tissue. (Courtesy Peter Moisan.)

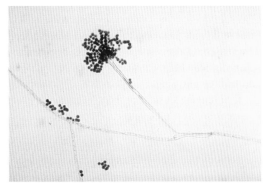

FIGURE 48-7 Phialoconidia of *Aspergillus fumigatus*. (Public Health Image Library, PHIL #300, Centers for Disease Control and Prevention, Atlanta, date unknown.)

mounts, the fungal hyphae appear hyaline, septate, and dichotomously branched. Invasion of blood vessels, infarction, and thrombosis may be seen. Occasionally, conidial heads may be observed. Special fungal stains may facilitate the visualization of *Aspergillus* in tissue. Application of immunohistochemistry techniques to aid in the diagnosis is a recent development.

Molecular methods of diagnosis have been developed for use in the human clinical setting, but are currently unavailable in veterinary medicine. Serologic diagnosis is offered through several veterinary teaching hospital laboratories, and test formats include enzyme-linked immunosorbent assay (ELISA), agar gel double diffusion, and counterimmunoelectrophoresis. False positives with each of these tests argues against their sole use for diagnosis. Detection of aspergillus galactomannan, the first antigen detected in body fluids of experimentally infected animals, correlates with compatible clinical findings and response to antifungal therapy; enzyme immunoassays and latex particle agglutination tests have been developed to detect this antigen in human serum. Detection of serum antibodies to *A. fumigatus* correlates with clinical findings in equine guttural pouch mycosis.

Prevention and Control

Prevention of poultry disease requires environmental sanitation and proper management. Daily cleaning and disinfection of feed and water containers prevents buildup of the mold in the environment. Reducing dust and improving ventilation in confinement situations will decrease the incidence of disease. Infection in young chicks or poults may be controlled through sanitation of incubators, hatchers, and incubator rooms. Control is best accomplished by removing moldy litter and feed. Spraying the ground around feed or water containers with bleach or copper sulfate solutions will help eliminate the infection. The addition of antifungal agents such as nystatin to the feed may be a useful preventive measure in an outbreak situation, but effective therapies are not available.

The prognosis is grave in the late stages of guttural pouch mycosis as a result of erosion of the carotid artery. Fatal complications include cranial nerve damage and cerebral penetration. Disease may resolve with early diagnosis and initiation of effective antimycotic therapy. Itraconazole appears to be an effective for treatment, although prolonged treatment (3-4 months' duration) is required.

Treatment of nasal aspergillosis in dogs has proved difficult. Therapeutic options include surgery, as well as systemic and topical antimycotic medications. Systemic administration of antifungal agents must be for a prolonged period, and the case-to-cure rate is only about 50%. Intranasal treatment may be more successful, and has improved management of this previously intractable condition. Different procedures, with varying degrees of invasiveness, have been developed to administer topical medications. Enilconazole, itraconazole, and fluconazole, delivered through tubes that are surgically placed into the nasal cavities and sinuses, have been the standard treatment. Recently, development of nonsurgically placed catheters allows infusion of the topical drug into the nasal cavities and frontal sinuses under general anesthesia. The long-term prognosis seems to be good for animals that are free of fungus at the end of antifungal drug therapy.

Management changes may prevent mycotic abortion. Decreasing time of confinement, improving ventilation, and limiting the feeding of moldy hay or poor silage decrease cows' exposure to the fungi. Keratomycosis may be managed through débridement and topical antifungals. Amphotericin B, nystatin, natamycin, ketoconazole, and miconazole have been used with success.

ZYGOMYCOSIS

Zygomycetes are in the phylum Zygomycota and are represented by organisms that have broad, relatively nonseptate, hyaline hyphae. Class Zygomycetes contains 6 orders, 29 families, 120 genera, and nearly 800 species. Zygomycosis is a granulomatous disease caused by members of two orders of zygomycetes, the Mucorales and the Entomophthorales. These organisms were first described as human and animal pathogens in the late 1800s, and their associated diseases are collectively referred to as mucormycoses and entomophthoromycoses. Zygomycotic agents cause cutaneous, pulmonary, gastrointestinal (Figures 48-8 and 48-9), or disseminated disease, as well as abortion. Disease is often severe because most of these agents have a pronounced angiotropism. Zygomycotic diseases occur in horses, dogs, cattle, sheep, goats, swine, several avian species, nonhuman primates, rabbit, mink, rodents, seals, gazelles, fish, reptiles, and amphibians.

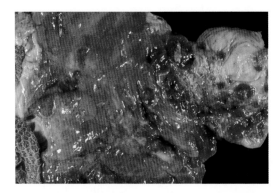

FIGURE 48-8 Zygomycotic necrotizing abomasitis. (Courtesy M. Kevin Keel.)

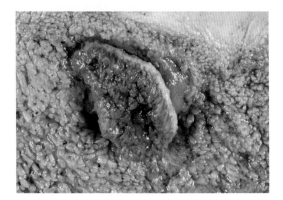

FIGURE 48-9 Zygomycotic ruminal infarct. (Courtesy M. Kevin Keel.)

Most species of zygomycetes are ubiquitous saprophytes that produce large numbers of airborne spores. They grow well in substrates high in sugars and nitrogen, reproducing by sexual and asexual means. The asexual phase occurs in a saclike structure called the sporangium and results in the production of sporangiospores. Zygospores are large and thick walled, and are formed by the sexual fusion of two compatible mycelia.

MUCORALES

The Mucorales contain 13 families, of which Mucoraceae, Mortierellaceae, Cunninghamellaceae, Saksenaceae, Syncephalastraceae, and Thamnidiaceae may be human or animal pathogens. The Mucoraceae are the agents most often associated with human and animal disease, so the term mucormycosis has been used extensively in the literature. Recently, the term mucormycosis has fallen into disfavor, and been replaced by zygomycosis. These fungi are distributed widely in the environment and are

isolated from soil, hay, grain, and animal manure. A columnella, or swollen extension of the sporangiophore, is morphologically characteristic of fungi in this order.

Disease and Epidemiology

Human mucormycosis is almost always associated with underlying conditions, such as diabetes mellitus. Disease can manifest as cutaneous, rhinocerebral, pulmonary, or gastrointestinal, or it may be disseminated. The case fatality rate is high.

The hallmark of disease caused by these organisms is angioinvasion. The major mode of transmission appears to be inhalation or ingestion of spores and traumatic percutaneous implantation, and infection can occur in virtually any body site. Zygomycosis is associated with infection of domestic poultry, ducks, cattle, pigs, horses, dogs, mink, ferrets, and rabbits. Disease manifestations include cutaneous lesions, abortion, gastrointestinal infection, mastitis, pneumonia, and disseminated disease.

Cutaneous infection presents clinically as chronic draining ulcerated tracts. Dissemination is common, especially to the gastrointestinal tract and respiratory system, as is regional lymphadenopathy.

Mycotic abortion and placentitis in ruminants are attributed to zygomycotic agents. The organisms most frequently isolated are *Mucor, Mortierella, Absidia, Rhizomucor,* and *Rhizopus* spp. *Mortierella wolfii* is apparently a cause of bovine abortion in New Zealand, where zygomycetes may account for about 20% of such abortions. The fetus is usually dead 12 to 24 hours before explusion. *Mucor* and *Absidia* spp. have been incriminated as agents of equine abortion.

Absidia, Mucor, and *Rhizopus* spp. are commonly associated with abomasal ulcers in ruminants and gastric ulcers in swine. The frequency of these infections has increased greatly as a result of the use of feed concentrates and antibiotic feed additives. Gross lesions consist of circumscribed areas of necrosis, surrounded by congestion, on gastric mucosa (see Figures 48-8 and 48-9). Fungal mycelial growth may be observed on the surface of the lesions.

Zygomycosis in dogs and cats is rare, with the gastrointestinal tract being most commonly affected. There appears to be no breed or sex predilection, but predisposing factors include concurrent debilitating disease (feline leukemia or panleukopenia, diabetes, malnutrition), intestinal trauma (bone perforation), and use of steroids or antibiotics. Clinical signs are vomiting, tenesmus, and diarrhea. Chronic granulomatous necrotic lesions involve the intestinal walls. Perforation with peritonitis or intestinal obstruction may result.

Fungal diseases caused by zygomycetes occur infrequently in a variety of avian species, including chickens, ducks, penguins, and parakeets. Younger birds appear at higher risk. Infections of the lung, heart, aorta, and vertebrae have been described. Postmortem lesions usually consist of multiple white circumscribed nodules scattered throughout the affected tissue.

Mycotoxins are produced by some species of Mucorales. *Rhizopus stolonifer* produces ergot alkaloids. Agroclavin, a metabolite of *R. arrhizus,* is toxic for ruminants. The mycotoxin rhizonin A, produced by *R. microsporus,* causes hepatitis in ducks and rats.

Pathogenesis

The Mucorales, as opportunists, require some breakdown in host defense to cause disease. Most disseminate rapidly because of their angioinvasive properties. Several virulence factors have been proposed. *Rhizopus, Rhizomucor,* and *Absidia* spp. are thermotolerant, a feature that allows these fungi to grow at the core body temperature of their hosts. Production of ketone reductase facilitates growth of *Rhizopus* spp. in acidic and glucose-rich environments, such as those seen with grain overload and diabetes. Proteases and lipases produced by other *Rhizopus* spp. may account for the rapid proliferation and invasiveness of these fungi in host tissues. *Absidia* spp. produce siderophores that facilitate iron scavenging and keratinase, which may allow penetration of unbroken skin.

Under favorable growth conditions of low pH, high glucose concentration, and increased iron content, spores germinate and form hyphae. The fungi invade, with extension along blood vessels, nerves, and fascial planes. Hyphae infiltrate the blood vessel walls, especially the arteries, which leads to infarction and necrosis.

The route of exposure may determine the clinical presentation. Cutaneous disease follows traumatic implantation of spores into the skin. Infection of the alimentary tract is most likely caused by ingestion of moldy feedstuffs. Inhalation of large numbers of spores may result in pulmonary disease. The pathogenesis of mycotic abortion may involve hematogenous dissemination of spores from the respiratory or gastrointestinal tract during a time of immunosuppression in the dam.

Diagnosis

As with other opportunistic fungal agents, diagnosis is based on demonstration of tissue invasion and repeated isolation of the same fungus from the site of infection. These fungi grow well on a variety of media but are inhibited by cycloheximide. Mucorales produce easily recognized, grayish, wooly colonies that fill a Petri dish within a few days' incubation (Figure 48-10). Differentiation of genera is based on presence (or absence) and location of rhizoids (rootlike structures along the vegetative hyphae), the nature of the sporangiophores in regard to branching, the shape of the columnella (the domelike region at the apex of the sporangiophore), the size and shape of the sporangia, and the appearance of the apophysis (the broad area near the apex of the sporangiophore below the columnella). Laboratory identification of the Mucorales to the species level is difficult. A variety of ancillary tests include carbon and nitrogen assimilation, fermentation, thiamine requirement, and maximum temperature of growth. Definitive identification of some zygomycetes requires mating studies and observation of the morphology of the zygospores. The hyphae of Mucorales may be observed in hematoxylin-and-eosin–stained tissues (Figure 48-11).

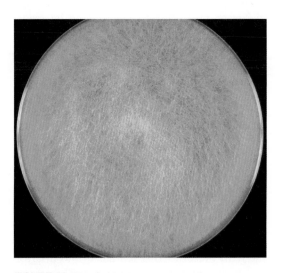

FIGURE 48-10 Colonial morphology of a zygomycete. (Courtesy Karen W. Post.)

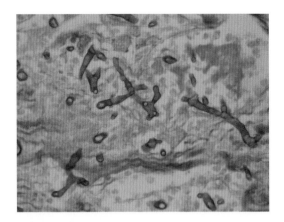

FIGURE 48-11 Zygomycete in rumen tissue. (Courtesy Peter Moisan.)

Prevention and Control

Prevention is difficult, and requires environmental modification to decrease exposure to airborne spores or decrease ingestion of spores; barns should provide adequate ventilation. Feeding of moldy hay, grain, or silage should be discouraged. Identification and control of the underlying risk factors are important.

Antifungal therapy and surgical intervention are required for control. Amphotericin B is the only antifungal agent with appreciable in vitro activity against the zygomycetes. Even with early diagnosis and aggressive therapy, the prognosis remains poor.

ENTOMOPHTHORALES: THE GENERA *CONIDIOBOLUS* AND *BASIDIOBOLUS*

Entomophthoromycoses are fungal diseases of the subcutaneous tissues or the nasal submucosa. In the older literature, the terms "mucormycosis" and "phycomycosis" were used to describe diseases caused by these agents. However, *Conidiobolus* and *Basidiobolus* are no longer grouped with the Mucorales, but are rather in the order Entomophthorales. In another previous taxonomic scheme, they were grouped in the class Phycomycetes, which is now replaced by the class Zygomycetes. Disease names based on the class, order, or genus now in current use for descriptive purposes are entomophthoromycosis, basidiobolomycosis, and conidiobolomycosis. Entomophthorales (from "entomon," the Greek word for insect) are primarily pathogens of arthropods, insects, reptiles, and amphibians.

Microscopic examination reveals broad, thin-walled, relatively nonseptate hyphae with irregular branches. The finding of these hyphae in haematoxylin-and-eosin–stained tissue sections suggests infection with Entomophthorales. A characteristic histologic change observed in entomophthoraceous infections is the eosinophilic cuff that surrounds individual hyphae. The cuff may be an antigen-antibody complex, and is known as the Splendore-Hoeppli phenomenon. It is usually difficult to visualize the fungal elements of these agents with routine fungal stains such as periodic acid–Schiff (PAS) or Gomori methenamine silver (GMS).

CONIDIOBOLUS SPECIES

Conidiobolus spp. are found in soil and decaying vegetation. They are isolated from the feces of cold-blooded animals and from insects. The fungus has worldwide distribution but tends to be concentrated in warmer climates, such as in India, Australia, equatorial Africa, Central America, Brazil, Colombia, and the southeastern United States, especially in those states bordering the Gulf Coast.

Disease and Epidemiology

Mammalian disease is rare. In humans, disease usually begins unilaterally in the nasal mucosa and manifests as polyp formation, with blockage of the passage. The infection spreads indefatigably, with characteristic facial swelling and lack of bone involvement

Conidiobolus coronata, Conidiobolus incongruus, and *Conidiobolus lamprauges* are associated with animal disease, and cases have been diagnosed in horses, mules, dogs, sheep, deer, non-human primates, and aquatic mammals. Infections are characterized by chronic sinusitis, and animals present clinically with subcutaneous masses on nasal mucosal surfaces.

Horses are the domestic species most frequently affected. Equine conidiobolomycosis, formerly referred to as rhinophycomycosis, is a pyogranulomatous infection of the nasal mucosa, resulting in nasal discharge, epistaxis, and dyspnea. Rarely, infection may involve the sinuses, larynx, or pharynx. Single or multiple granulomas are located on the external nares, nasal passages, or soft palate, and may interfere with eating and breathing.

The exact means by which warm-blooded animals become infected is unknown. Infection may be acquired through inhalation of either spores or insects, or through minor trauma such as insect bites. Animals are generally in good health at the time of infection.

Pathogenesis

Disease caused by this organism is relatively infrequent, suggesting that the fungus is of low virulence or that infection is difficult to acquire. Virulence factors of *Conidiobolus* include tissue-destructive enzymes and thermotolerance. A serine protease is involved in the discharge of conidia, and other proteases, secreted at the onset of infection, may lead to tissue degradation. This may favor invasion, and tissue breakdown products become available to the organism. Lipase and collagenase may also be important in invasion. *Conidiobolus* species grow at 37° C, and isolates from human disease grow more rapidly at this temperature than those from the environment. This differential may be an adaptation to growth in the mammalian host.

Diagnosis

Polyps or scrapings should be examined directly, by culture, and by sectioning and staining. Broad hyphae with lateral pegs (hyphae that form at right angles), and rare septations are seen in KOH mounts. Walls of the hyphae are refractile, and granular inclusions may be observed. The organism grows readily on potato dextrose or Sabouraud dextrose agar within 48 hours at 25° C. At first, colonies are white or gray, flat, and waxy or glabrous. With age, they become wrinkled, powdery, tan or brown, and produce aerial hyphae (Figure 48-12). The reverse side of the colonies is white. Large green, hemolytic colonies result from incubation on blood agar at 37° C. Ballistospores are formed, and the forcible ejection of spores from the sporangiospores on the agar surface results in those spores covering the sides and lid of the Petri dish. Distinguishing microscopic features include hyphae with few septa and unbranched sporangiophores that are slightly tapered toward their tips and resemble a beak and a corona, which results from spores giving rise to secondary spores.

Prevention and Control

Prevention of conidiobolomycosis is virtually impossible because the organism is widespread in the environment. Successful treatment of equine infections has involved intralesional injection of amphotericin B followed by systemic therapy with sodium and potassium iodide. Other agents used for treatment are trimethoprim-sulfamethoxazole and azole antimicrobial derivatives.

BASIDIOBOLUS SPECIES

Fungi in this genus are rare human pathogens, and *Basidiobolus ranarum* is the only species that has been associated with animal disease. This filamentous fungus has been cultured from decaying vegetation, fecal material of reptiles and amphibians, and insects. Most infections are reported from the tropics of Asia, South America, and Africa, with only a few cases from the United States.

Disease and Epidemiology

Basidiobolomycosis occurs mainly in healthy animals. Horses and dogs are the domestic species most frequently affected. Lesions in horses are more common on the lateral aspect of the trunk, ventral abdomen, neck, thorax, and head. Pruritic granulomatous lesions with a characteristic edematous surface usually develop at a site of trauma; these lesions may be confused with those in pythiosis. Subcutaneous ulcerative granulomatous lesions of the limbs and rare disseminated disease and gastrointestinal and respiratory infection have been described in dogs.

The mode of transmission for this organism remains to be confirmed. Infection may be acquired through inhalation, percutaneous inoculation, or ingestion of spores. As with *Condiobolus,* insects may play a role in transmission because they have been shown to carry spores on their body surfaces. Reptiles and amphibians pass spores in their excreta, which may be a source of infection

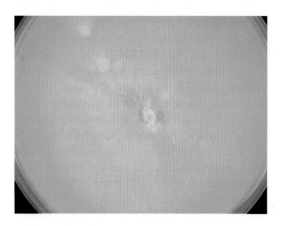

FIGURE 48-12 Colonial morphology of *Conidiobolus.* (Courtesy Karen W. Post.)

for animals. The stability of *Basidiobolus* spores in the soil is unknown, but entomophthoralean zygospores and conidia are usually quickly inactivated in the environment unless sheltered from sun and desiccation.

Pathogenesis

Virulence factors for this fungus are similar to those of *Conidiobolus* spp. *Basidiobolus* is relatively thermotolerant, and can grow, albeit poorly, at 37° C. Extracellular proteases and lipolytic enzymes are produced by *Basidiobolus*. One of these, a phospholipase C, attacks cell membranes and may be virulence factor. Cellular breakdown products may serve as a source of nutrition for the fungus.

Diagnosis

Diagnostic approach and methods are similar to those for conidiobolomycosis, and are based on direct examination, culture, and histopathology, which reveal wide thin-walled hyphae with few septations. The fungus grows rapidly on standard mycologic media such as potato dextrose or Sabouraud dextrose agars and reaches maturity in 5 days. Colonies are similar to those of *Conidiobolus* spp., in that they are flat, waxy and buff to gray. They become heaped or radially folded with age, and aerial hyphae are produced; some strains have a musty or earthy odor. Ballistospores are discharged onto the lid of the Petri dish. Microscopic examination of cultures reveals wide hyphae with occasional septa. Primary spores are formed singly on swollen ends of unbranched hyphae. Taxonomically characteristic smooth and undulant, thick-walled, intercalary zygospores with copulatory beaks are produced.

Prevention and Control

Appropriate treatment depends on the severity and location of the disease. Visceral basidiobolomycosis is appropriately treated by surgical resection of the lesion and administration of systemically active antifungal agents, but the prognosis is usually poor. Subcutaneous infections have been treated with azoles, amphotericin B, and potassium iodide. In vitro antifungal susceptibility testing has demonstrated the superior activity of itraconazole, miconazole, and ketoconazole to amphotericin B, fluconazole, 5-fluorocytosine, and potassium iodide.

DACTYLARIOSIS

Dactylariosis was first described in 1962 in association with an outbreak of encephalitis in turkey poults. A dematiaceous fungus, *Diplorhinotricum gallopavum,* was recovered from brain tissue of the affected birds. The organism was reclassified in 1968 as *Dactylaria gallopava,* and subsequent nomenclature revisions have placed the fungus in the genus *Ochroconis,* as *Ochroconis gallopavum.* The disease, however, is still commonly called dactylariosis. Because this mold lacks a known sexual state, it is a member of the class Deuteromycetes.

Disease and Epidemiology

Natural disease involving the central nervous system occurs in turkeys, chickens, snowy owl, quail, and grey-winged trumpeter. Affected birds exhibit torticollis, ataxia, opisthotonos, muscle tremor, and corneal opacity. Disease is infrequent and may result in high morbidity in commercial poultry flocks; mortality may approach 20%. On gross examination, necrotic granulomas are found in the cerebral cortex and may be characterized by a red-brown discoloration of the affected tissue.

Ochroconis gallopavum may be associated with disease in nonavian species, including feline encephalitis. It is a rare agent of human disease; it has been recovered from a brain abscess in a leukemic patient and from cases of cerebral phaeohyphomycosis in organ transplant recipients.

The fungus appears to be widely distributed in nature, and may be isolated from poultry litter and animal manure. Several reports document isolation of *O. gallopavum* from thermal effluent of nuclear power reactors, and from water and soil samples taken from in and around hot springs.

The epidemiology of dactylariosis is not fully understood. There appears to be a correlation between disease development and environmental conditions conducive to fungal growth. *Ochroconis gallopavum* favors moist, warm, and acidic conditions, similar to those found in a poultry house, and contaminated litter may serve as a source of infection. Outbreaks have been related to maintaining birds on bark, woodchip, or sawdust litter. Congenital infection in quail chicks has been attributed to incubator contamination. Young birds are at higher risk of developing disease.

Pathogenesis

The disease has been reproduced in poults by intratracheal inoculation of spore suspensions of *O. gallopavum*. Brain lesions in experimentally infected birds are similar to those in natural disease, suggesting fungal neurotropism.

Several virulence factors have been described. As a dematiaceous fungus, *O. gallopavum* produces melanin, which facilitates fungal penetration of animal tissues and shields fungal cell wall constituents from hydrolytic enzymes produced by host immune cells. Thermotolerance may also be a virulence factor, in that the ability of *O. gallopavum* to grow at or above 37° C, coupled with its ability to grow at physiologic pH, allows deep tissue invasion.

Diagnosis

Recovery of *O. gallopavum* from brain tissue of affected birds, and the presence of septate dematiaceous hyphae in sections of brain stained with hematoxylin and eosin, confirm a diagnosis of dactylariosis.

The fungus grows rapidly (usually within 48 hours) on Sabouraud dextrose agar at room temperature and up to 45° C. The organism is unable to grow on media containing cycloheximide. Colonies are dark brown, velvety, and flat or slightly wrinkled. An extensive, reddish purple to reddish brown diffusible pigment forms a halo around the colony, and the reverse side of the colony becomes a deep reddish purple. Other phenotypic characteristics include urease production, and hydrolysis of tyrosine and gelatin (although the latter may require up to 21 days). Microscopically, *O. gallopavum* is characterized by oval two-celled blastoconidia that are formed sympodially at the apices of the conidiophores, with the apical cells being markedly wider than the basal cell and usually constricted at the septum.

Prevention and Control

Prevention and control measures involve sanitation in both the poultry house and the hatchery environment. Litter should be changed frequently to prevent environmental buildup of the organism.

SUGGESTED READINGS

Ribes JA, Vanover-Sams CL, Baker DJ: Zygomycetes in human disease, *Clin Microbiol Rev* 13:236-301, 2000.
Sharp NJ, Harvey CE, Sullivan M: Canine nasal aspergillosis and penicilliosis, *Compend Contin Educ Pract Vet* 13:41-47, 1991.

Chapter 49

Fungal-Like Agents

RHINOSPORIDIUM SEEBERI

Rhinosporidium seeberi has for years been shrouded in taxonomic uncertainty. The organism, initially described as a coccidian parasite in 1900 by Seeber, was classified as both a protozoan and a fungus based on histochemical and morphologic characteristics. Most recently, molecular studies have demonstrated a taxonomic affinity with a novel group of amphibian and fish pathogens known as the "DRIP" clade (an acronym for *Dermocystidium*, rosette agent, *Ichthyophonus*, and *Psorospermium*). The DRIP clade is located at the point of divergence between fungi and animals. *Rhinosporidium seeberi* is currently classified as an aquatic protozoan of the class Mesmomycetozoea and order Dermocystida.

Rhinosporidiosis usually affects mucous membranes and leads to the development of polyploid masses located primarily on the nasal mucosa. There may be occasional involvement of the ocular conjunctivae or ear margins. This rare disease has been documented in humans, dogs, cats, cattle, horses, mules, pigs, and waterfowl. Although disease occurs worldwide, endemic foci are recognized in South America, Africa, India, Cuba, and Iran. Cases have also been reported in the southeastern United States, especially along the Gulf Coast.

Clinical signs of disease depend on the size and location of the polyps, which bleed easily. A blood-tinged mucopurulent, unilateral discharge may develop from the affected nostril. Dyspnea may occur from nasal obstruction as masses enlarge. Lesions do not appear to be painful. Polyps may appear pedunculated or sessile and are pink to purple. Cream-colored specks that are masses of sporangia may be observed within the polyps.

Little is known about the relationship between *R. seeberi* and its natural environment because the complete life cycle is unknown. Some members of the DRIP clade develop flagellated zoospores that are theorized to be infectious, and this is currently under investigation with *R. seeberi*. Epidemiologic studies have linked human infection to freshwater bathing or swimming. In animals, trauma may be a predisposing factor because oxen with rings in their noses have higher rates of infection than those without rings.

The organism has been extensively studied in its parasitic stages because it cannot be grown in artificial culture media. The in vivo life cycle is initiated with the release of mature endospores from spherules through a pore that develops in the spherule wall. These implant to infect host tissue, and gradually develop into spherules that mature, release endospores, and continue the life cycle. The exact mechanism of spherule formation and endospore release remains to be determined. However, watery substances stimulate the mature spherule to discharge endospores, supporting epidemiologic evidence that has linked *R. seeberi* to aquatic environments and further explaining the affinity of this organism for mucous membranes.

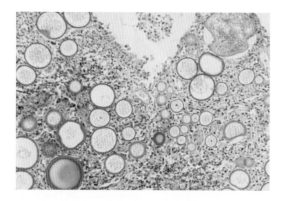

FIGURE 49-1 Micrograph of rhinosporidiosis. (Courtesy Public Health Image Library, PHIL #3107, Centers for Disease Control and Prevention, Atlanta, 1965, Martin Hicklin.)

Although polyps have been maintained in tissue culture medium for up to 15 days, actual propagation of the organism has not been successful. Diagnosis therefore is not based on culture of the organism but on the tissue appearance of the organism. In potassium hydroxide (KOH) mounts of crushed polyps, spherules with endospores (sporangium with sporangia) are observed. These spherules may be as large as 350 μm, much larger than those of *Coccidioides immitis* (Figure 49-1). *Rhinosporidium seeberi* is visualized in histologic sections with fungal stains such as periodic acid–Schiff and methenamine silver. The tissue response is inflammatory, with evidence of polymorphonuclear cellular infiltration and tissue necrosis. Scarring and granulation tissue are common findings.

Treatment consists of surgical excision followed by cautery. Injection of amphotericin B at the site of the polyp or topical treatment with dapsone may be efficacious. Relapses occur in up to 10% of the cases.

THE GENUS *PNEUMOCYSTIS*

Since its discovery in rats by Carlos Chagas in 1909, the taxonomic placement of *Pneumocystis* has been controversial. It was first described as a trypanosome and was later classified with the protozoa because of similarities in morphology and susceptibility to antiprotozoal drugs. Nucleotide sequence and gene structure data indicate numerous similarities to fungi, including the presence of β-1,3 D-glucan in its cell wall and homologous rRNA and mitochondrial sequences.

Despite the fact that *Pneumocystis* lacks the major fungal sterol, ergosterol, it has been placed in the kingdom Fungi, phylum Ascomycota, class Archiascomycetes, order Pneumocystidales, and family Pneumocystidaceae.

There are several *Pneumocystis* species, each residing in a specific mammalian host. Initially, the genus contained only one species, *P. carinii*, but molecular studies have revealed that this is in fact a group of heterogeneous organisms, genetically isolated from each other, that have undergone genetic and functional adaptation to each mammalian host. A nomenclature system that recognizes these differences uses the tripartite "special forms" (formae speciales) designations. The name of each is related to that of the host species from which it originated. Examples of this trinomial nomenclature are *P. carinii* f. sp. *equi*, *P. carinii* f. sp. *macacae*, and *P. carinii* f. sp. *suis*, for horse, macaque and swine strains, respectively. In 1999, *Pneumocystis jiroveci* was proposed for the human pathogenic strains, whereas *P. carinii* was reserved for organisms recovered from animals.

Pneumocystis is an opportunistic pathogen that causes severe pneumonia, usually in immunocompromised individuals. Naturally occurring pneumocystosis has been reported in rodents, rabbits, ferrets, mink, horses, dogs, cats, nonhuman primates, goats, and piglets. Disease is found in animals with acquired, inherited, or drug-induced immunodeficiency syndromes, but the exact host immunologic defects that permit proliferation of the organism are not known. In fact, the lack of resistance to *P. carinii* could be attributed to any defect in synthesis of or response to cytokines or in antigen processing by alveolar macrophages for T-cell presentation. Case fatality rate is high.

Because of the lack of an in vitro propagation system, the life cycle of this organism and the subsequent epidemiology of pneumocystosis have not been defined. It appears that the normal habitat is the lung and the only part of the life cycle that is known is that involving the mammalian lung. The proposed life cycle includes a sexual and an asexual growth phase. The two main developmental stages are the trophozoite and the cyst. Trophozoites are produced during the asexual growth phase and can probably replicate by binary fission. The haploid trophozoites also replicate sexually by conjugation, and produce diploid zygotes. Zygotes undergo meiosis and mitosis, resulting in precyst formation. Differentiation into a mature cyst results in the production of up to eight intracystic bodies that are released when the mature cyst ruptures and develop into trophozoites.

Transmission of infection does not occur between different mammalian species, and results of several studies suggest that humans do not contract pneumocystosis from animals. Animal investigations have documented airborne transmission, but the infectious form has not been identified. Recent findings suggest that immunocompetent hosts may play a significant role in the *Pneumocystis* life cycle. It has been hypothesized that the main source of *P. carinii* is individuals with the disease. Accumulating evidence shows that the mammalian host may acquire this organism early in life, in some cases immediately after birth. Transplacental transmission does not occur in the rat model.

Of the common domestic animal species, *P. carinii* infection has been reported most often in the horse. The majority of cases are in Arabian foals with combined immunodeficiency disease, or in foals that have been treated with immunosuppressive drugs. Infection with *Rhodococcus equi* may be an immunosuppressive factor. However, several cases have been documented in immunocompetent individuals. Foals are at risk because of the inherent immunodeficiency that occurs between 2 and 4 months of age, as maternal antibodies wane. Clinical signs are mainly limited to the respiratory tract and include cough, dyspnea, and exercise intolerance. There may be a history of poor response to antimicrobial therapy. Gross lesions include firm, meaty lungs with pink and yellow mottling. Lung parenchyma tends to resist being cut and bulges on cut section. Regional lymphadenopathy also may be observed.

Organisms proliferate extracellularly within the lung alveolus. Lung surfactant proteins adhere to the surface of *P. carinii* and tight adhesions are formed between adjacent organisms and type I alveolar epithelial cells. Diffuse alveolar injury ensues most likely from involvement of the host immune response through costimulation-dependent T-cell–mediated inflammation.

Antemortem diagnosis may be accomplished by careful cytologic examination of fine-needle aspirates of lung biopsy or bronchoalveolar

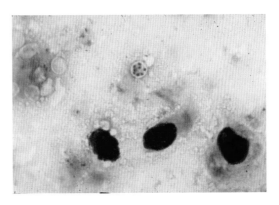

FIGURE 49-2 Giemsa stain of lung impression smear with *Pneumocystis carinii*. (Courtesy Public Health Image Library, PHIL #2998, Centers for Disease Control and Prevention, Atlanta, 1971, Mae Melvin.)

lavage materials. Organisms are small (3-5 μm in diameter) and may exist in low numbers. Wright-Giemsa–type stains best demonstrate trophozoites and intracystic bodies (Figure 49-2). Trophozoites appear as basophilic, dense, oval, or irregular structures having a lobed surface and a single nucleus. Intracystic bodies appear as aggregates of spherical to oval dense basophilic structures against a thick, foamy background. A direct immunofluorescence test can also be applied to bronchoalveolar lavage specimens. Diagnostic immunohistochemical kits are available for use on fixed tissues, and development of polymerase chain reaction (PCR) techniques has given a new alternative for identification of the organism. Serology is an antemortem method to determine exposure to *Pneumocystis*.

Subacute, interstitial pneumonia with diffuse, alveolar damage, marked macrophage infiltration, and intracellular cysts is observed histologically. Frothy "honeycombed" eosinophilic, intraalveolar material with lymphocytic/plasmacytic interstitial infiltrate suggests *P. carinii* pneumonia. Fungal stains, such as Gomori methenamine silver, stain the cyst form but not the trophozoite (Figure 49-3). The finding of clusters of nonbudding round to oval to crescent–shaped cysts that appear as "commas" or "parentheses" in alveolar exudates, is confirmatory.

Lack of ergosterol provides an explanation for the ineffectiveness of amphotericin B and several other triazoles in treating pneumocystosis. Treatment with trimethoprim-sulfamethoxazole

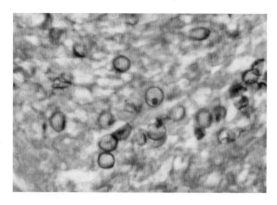

FIGURE 49-3 Cysts of *Pneumocystis carinii.* Methenamine silver stain. (Courtesy Public Health Image Library, PHIL #960, Centers for Disease Control and Prevention, Atlanta, 1984, Edwin P. Ewing, Jr.)

and pentamidine isethionate has resulted in clinical improvement of pneumonia.

THE GENUS *PROTOTHECA*

The genus *Prototheca* includes unicellular achlorophyllous algae, with a characteristic cellular morphology, that occasionally cause disease in animals and man. When *Prototheca* spp. were first isolated from tree slime in 1894 by Kruger, they were thought to be fungi because of their microscopic morphology. Based on cell-wall characteristics, the genus has been placed in the kingdom Plantae, phylum Chlorophyta, and family Chlorophyceae.

These ubiquitous saprophytes have been recovered from a wide variety of environmental sources, including water, mud, animal manure, sewage, and vegetation. Distribution is apparently worldwide, with disease having been reported in Africa, Asia, North America, Europe, and Australia. Two species, *Prototheca wickerhamii* and *Prototheca zopfii,* cause disease in lower animals, dogs, cats, cattle, deer, beaver, and fruit bats.

The life cycle of *Prototheca* spp. is similar to that of green algae, and it is speculated that *Prototheca* are *Chlorella* mutants. However, electron microscopic investigations have found structural differences between the two. Reproduction is asexual, by internal septation and release of sporangiospores from sporangia.

Prototheocosis in animals may be cutaneous, subcutaneous, or systemic, and may present in some cases as mastitis. Cutaneous infection with granuloma formation is the most common manifestation.

Infection may arise through traumatic implantation into cutaneous or subcutaneous tissue.

Canine protothecosis typically manifests as a disseminated disease, but may begin in the gastrointestinal tract. The gross pathology of systemic disease has led to the conclusion that ingestion, with subsequent hematogenous and lymphatic dissemination, is the route of infection. From electron microscopic observations, it has been found that algal cells in the form of sporangiospores and sporangia are contained within macrophages. Algae proliferate intracellularly and are spread to regional lymph nodes by macrophages. This explains the chronicity of the infection and the negative outcome of therapeutic efforts.

Natural infection in animals was first reported, in 1952, as bovine mastitis. *Prototheca* spp. are apparently common in the dairy environment and they can frequently be isolated from sites characterized by moisture and organic matter. *Prototheca* mastitis may involve individual animals or the entire herd, and infection is by the ascending route. Several outbreaks have been associated with the use of contaminated intramammary infusion products. Milk production is severely reduced, and chronicity and resistance to treatment often result in culling of affected animals from the herd.

Canine infections usually disseminate, so clinical signs depend on the anatomic sites affected. Lesions frequently develop in lymph nodes, intestine, liver, heart, kidneys, and eyes and rarely may involve the central nervous and musculoskeletal systems. Grossly white to gray foci are diffusely scattered throughout multiple organs and musculature. Treatment of disseminated protothecosis has been uniformly unsuccessful.

In order to obtain an accurate diagnosis, it is essential to recover the organism from clinical materials and to demonstrate tissue invasion or disease because these organisms have been isolated from specimens in the absence of disease. Cultivation is readily accomplished within 72 hours on routine fungal media without cycloheximide and also on blood agar (Figure 49-4). Isolates grow between 25° and 37° C as white to cream, dull, moist to mucoid yeastlike colonies. Following isolation, yeastlike colonies should be examined in lactophenol cotton blue wet mounts. The round to oval sporangiospores are characterized by hyaline cell walls and prominent nuclei.

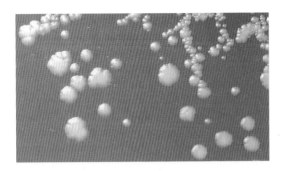

FIGURE 49-4 Blood agar plate with *Prototheca* colonies. (Courtesy Karen W. Post.)

Sporangia, varying from 7 to 25 μm in diameter, depending on their stage of development, and containing 2 to 20 sporangiospores are observed. Hyphal formation and budding do not occur. The cells of *P. zopfii* tend to be larger (14-25 μm in diameter) than those of *P. wickerhamii* (7-13 μm in diameter). *Prototheca* spp. can be identified through carbon assimilation tests in several commercial yeast identification systems. Antibodies in dairy cows can be detected by enzyme immunoassay. A strong serologic response may be present in infected cows.

On histopathology, varying degrees of nonspecific change are observed, including granulomas composed of areas of necrosis, lymphocytes, macrophages, plasma cells, few neutrophils, and high numbers of protothecal organisms. Fluorescent antibody and immunohistochemical techniques applied to paraffin-embedded tissues may aid in detection of the organism.

Cutaneous protothecosis has been treated successfully by surgical excision. Although isolates are susceptible to gentamicin, amphotericin B, nystatin, and polymyxin B in vitro, systemic administration of these agents does not produce a clinical response. In the dairy environment, disease may be controlled by improving management conditions, such as not using muddy loafing areas, culling infected animals that may shed organisms in their feces and serve as a source of infection, and using teat dips after milking.

THE GENUS *PYTHIUM*

Pythium spp. are members of the new kingdom Stramenopila, phylum Oomycota, and family Pythiaceae. These organisms are sometimes referred to as aquatic fungi because they produce chronic granulomatous disease and form hyphal-like structures in tissue. They are not considered true fungi because of the lack of chitin and ergosterol in the cellular structure and because biflagellate zoospores are produced. The genus contains more than 100 species, many of which are important plant pathogens, but only one, *Pythium insidiosum,* is a pathogen of warm-blooded animals.

Naturally occurring infection has been reported in horses, dogs, cats, cattle, and humans. Disease occurs in tropical, subtropical, and temperate climates throughout the world. In the United States, *P. insidiosum* is encountered most often along the Gulf Coast. However, sporadic isolations have occurred in North and South Carolina, Tennessee, Georgia, Missouri, Oklahoma, Kansas, Illinois, Wisconsin, New York, and New Jersey. There is no evidence to suggest animal-to-animal or zoonotic transmission.

Over the years, many unique names have been used to describe disease associated with this organism. Kerr reported a cutaneous disease of horses in 1829 that he named "bausette." In the 1890s, investigators described a similar equine disease in Florida known as "leeches." This disease was named for the granulomatous lesions with elongated, necrotic masses of tissue inside that resembled leeches. These necrotic masses were also called "kunkers." "Burusattee," from an Indian word meaning rain, is yet another cutaneous disease of horses reported from India during that same time. "Swamp cancer" became a popular term because of the association of disease with lakes and ponds in which horses would wade while grazing. In the older veterinary literature, the terms "hyphomycosis" or "phycomycosis" were widely used. The former originated with a report that the agent recovered from cutaneous lesions in horses was *Hyphomyces destruens,* and the latter was due to the fact that traditionally, granulomatous lesions containing hyphal elements were classified as "phycomycotic" infections. In the 1980s, the name *Pythium insidiosum* was proposed, and the disease became known by its current name, pythiosis.

The horse is most often affected by pythiosis. Subcutaneous and systemic disease has been described, but the cutaneous form predominates. Lesions are frequently located on the distal extremities and ventral abdomen, probably as a

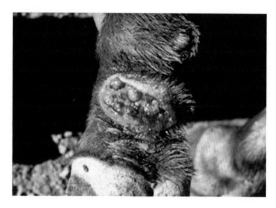

FIGURE 49-5   Equine leg lesion. (Courtesy Leonel Mendoza.)

result of the greater exposure of these areas to zoospores in the environment. Granulomatous fistulous lesions contain granular, yellowish, grayish, or coral-colored cores that are masses of viable hyphae. Lesions bleed easily, and an intense pruritus may result in self-mutilation. If left untreated, extremities may swell, with progress to gangrenous necrosis (Figure 49-5). Cutaneous lesions in dogs and cattle are nonpruritic and may lack the granular cores. Rarely, disease metastasizes to regional lymph nodes, bones, or lungs.

Intestinal pythiosis has been reported in dogs and horses. Infection is associated with the ingestion of contaminated grass or stagnant water. Clinical signs include bloody diarrhea, abdominal pain (colic), weight loss, and in the case of dogs, vomition. Organisms infiltrate the musculature of the stomach, small intestine, large bowel, and esophagus. Narrowing or obstruction of the intestinal lumen may result.

The life cycle of *P. insidiosum* has recently been elucidated. Wet environments are essential for reproduction of these organisms, whether in a lake or pond or in wet soil and grass. When a plant is colonized, sporangia mature and zoospores are released. These forms are motile by means of anterior and posterior flagella, and through a chemotactic mechanism find other plants. Zoospores secrete a sticky amorphous substance that acts as an adhesive and facilitates their encystment. Germ tube production is followed by development of hyphal filaments that invade plant tissue, produce sporangia, and continue the cycle.

The complete pathogenesis of pythiosis remains unknown. Zoospores are likely the infectious form for mammalian hosts; they have a strong tropism for equine and human hair and equine skin in vitro. It is believed that zoospores are attracted to small breaks in the epithelial or intestinal mucosal surface, where they encyst, form germ tubes, and produce hyphae that penetrate the host tissue and eventually cause disease. *Pythium insidiosum* does not exert sufficient pressure to penetrate undamaged skin by mechanics alone, but must effect a decisive reduction in tissue strength by proteinase secretion.

In vitro, production of motile zoospores is induced when the organisms are incubated at 37° C. Many investigators believe that zoospores are produced in nature during the warmer months, and this is consistent with the clinical findings that most cases of pythiosis are diagnosed in late summer to early fall.

Diagnosis of pythiosis involves several methodologies, including examination of wet mounts of clinical materials, culture, histopathology, and serology. Early diagnosis is of utmost importance if therapy is to be successful.

A recent study has dispelled an older recommendation requiring that specimens not be refrigerated. *Pythium insidiosum* can be recovered from specimens refrigerated for up to 5 days. Optimum isolation rates of *P. insidiosum* from equine tissues were obtained when fresh kunkers, rather than tissues, were plated onto a selective vegetable extract medium containing antibiotics. When samples cannot be cultured immediately, they can be kept at room temperature for up to 3 days, shipped on wet ice, and/or stored in solutions containing ampicillin and gentamicin.

Successful isolation depends on the inhibition of bacterial and fungal contaminants. *Pythium insidiosum* grows well on a variety of media, including potato dextrose and blood agar, with and without antibiotics. The organism may be inhibited by cycloheximide. Growth is more luxuriant at 37° C than at 25° C. In 24 to 48 hours, colonies appear as a thick flat mat of grayish white or yellowish white mycelia that have an undulated or radiating surface pattern (Figure 49-6). Hyphae are submerged into the agar, and microscopically are broad, 4 to 10 μm in diameter, hyaline, and initially have rare septations. Perpendicular branches, referred to as "lateral pegs," are observed (Figure 49-7). In older cultures, hyphal swellings, resembling sporangia and measuring 12 to 30 μm in diameter, are formed.

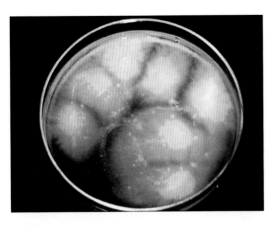

FIGURE 49-6 Plate culture of *Pythium*. (Courtesy Leonel Mendoza.)

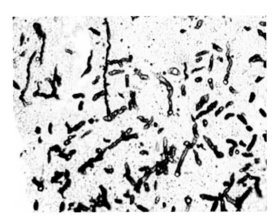

FIGURE 49-8 Pythiosis in tissue with fungal stain. (Courtesy Leonel Mendoza.)

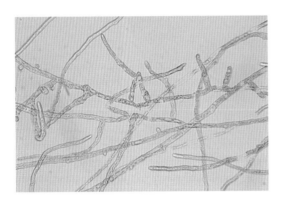

FIGURE 49-7 Microscopic morphology of *Pythium*. (Courtesy Leonel Mendoza.)

Definitive identification requires a positive exoantigen test (by immunodiffusion) and demonstration of zoospore production. The exoantigen test is performed on a limited basis at the Centers for Disease Control and Prevention (CDC). For zoospore production, agar blocks with vegetative mycelial growth are removed from plated media and placed into tubes with an aqueous yeast extract solution containing sterile grass blades. The tubes are incubated at 30° C in the dark for 5 hours. Grass blades are removed and examined microscopically for the presence of motile, biflagellate zoospores. Preliminary evaluation of a nested PCR assay suggests that it may become a useful identification tool.

The use of special fungal stains, such as periodic acid–Schiff, Gomori's methenamine silver, or Gridley's, has proven to be important in the visualization of *P. insidiosum* in tissue sections; these stains are superior to hematoxylin and eosin. Broad, relatively aseptate hyphae with perpendicular branches are apparent, as is an eosinophilic inflammatory response (Figure 49-8). Immunofluorescence and indirect immunoperoxidase techniques are also available for detection of *P. insidiosum* in fixed tissues.

Serologic tests have been developed for antemortem disease diagnosis. These are offered by several reference laboratories and include complement fixation, enzyme immunoassay, immunodiffusion, and Western blotting.

Pythiosis responds poorly to therapy. Wide surgical excision remains the treatment of choice. Early diagnosis is required because lesions tend to progress rapidly. *Pythium insidiosum* is susceptible in vitro to miconazole, fluconazole, and ketoconazole. These azole drugs should not be effective, because of the lack of their ergosterol target in *Pythium* cell membranes. However, successful antimicrobial therapy with a combination of terbinafine and itraconazole has been reported in the human medical literature. Use of these agents in veterinary medicine may not be feasible because of their cost. Recent reports from Australia and South America suggest that successful management of cutaneous equine disease can be achieved with commercial vaccines, but to be effective they must be initiated early. Immunotherapy in dogs has been unsuccessful to date.

MEGABACTERIOSIS

An organism of uncertain taxonomic position is associated with an avian disease widely known as megabacteriosis. This organism was originally characterized as a fungus, based on periodic acid–Schiff staining, but others described it as a large gram-positive bacterium. Recent molecular studies indicate that "Megabacterium" is indeed eukaryotic. It appears to be a novel yeast that is not closely related to any currently recognized species. The agent, previously referred to simply as avian gastric yeast, is now known to be an ascomycetous yeast and has been named *Macrorhabdus ornithogaster.*

Macrorhabdus ornithogaster is commonly associated with a wasting disease of budgerigars known as "going light syndrome." Affected birds progressively lose weight, despite having a good appetite. Other clinical signs are nonspecific and may include depression, regurgitation, diarrhea, and ruffled feathers. An acute form of disease may result in death within 12 to 24 hours. Necropsy reveals inflammation, ulceration, and distention of the proventriculus and, to a lesser extent, the ventriculus. Mucosal surfaces may be covered in a thick white mucous layer often containing frank blood.

Incidence of *M. ornithogaster* infection appears to be on the increase, and the disease is not limited to budgerigars. Infection has been reported in canaries, cockatiels, lovebirds, parrots, finches, ostriches, and chickens. The organism has been recovered from a canine bronchoalveolar lavage sample and a feline nasal flush. Mice have been experimentally infected by the oral route.

The method of natural transmission is likely fecal-oral, and close contact with an infected individual is apparently required. Genetic factors may be involved, and budgerigars seem particularly susceptible to disease. Prevalence of disease is higher in chicks from culture-positive parents than from negative parents, even when chicks with positive parents are raised by negative, surrogate parents.

Little is known about the pathogenesis of *M. ornithogaster* infections. Studies have been hampered by difficulties in propagating the organism in vitro. Yeasts can be isolated from clinically healthy birds, and stress may increase susceptibility to disease.

Macrorhabdus ornithogaster has infrequently been recovered from clinical materials inoculated onto plates of selective media containing blood or sodium azide and incubated in 10% CO_2 at 37° C. Flat, β-hemolytic colonies with irregular edges formed within 48 hours.

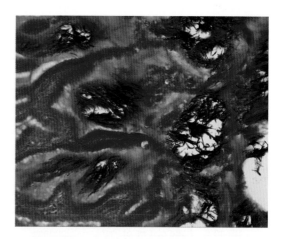

FIGURE 49-9 Proventriculitis resulting from *Macrorhabdus ornithogaster* infection. (Courtesy Karen W. Post.)

Definitive diagnosis is based on necropsy findings and histopathology because of the failure of culture to consistently recover the organism. Yeasts may be observed in stained smears (Gram's, Giemsa, Diff-Quik) of feces or proventricular scrapings, but shedding appears to be variable; false-negative results may be obtained if diagnosis is based solely on direct examinations. Histopathologic changes include layers of yeast lining the mucosal surface and sometimes within the glands of the proventriculus (Figure 49-9). There is usually minimal inflammation, and fibrosis of the submucosal layers is evident in chronic infections. Ulceration and mucosal necrosis also may be seen. The most common lesion of the ventriculus is degeneration of the koilin layer.

Control of *M. ornithogaster* infection has been through the oral administration of antifungal agents such as amphotericin B and nystatin. Other therapeutic options focus on lowering the pH of the gastric system in an effort to inhibit yeast growth. This can be accomplished by adding apple cider vinegar to drinking water or by orally administering probiotics.

SUGGESTED READINGS

Fredericks DN, Jolley JA, Lepp PW, et al: *Rhinosporidium seeberi:* a human pathogen from a novel group of aquatic protistan parasites, *Emerg Infect Dis* 6:273-282, 2000.

Hollingsworth SR: Canine prototothecosis, *Vet Clin North Am Small Anim Pract* 30:1091-1101, 2000.

Mendoza L, Taylor JW, Ajello J: The class mesmomyce-tozoea: a heterogenous group of microorganisms at the animal-fungal boundary, *Annu Rev Microbiol* 56:315-344, 2002.

Scanlan CM, Graham DL: Characterization of a gram-positive bacterium from the proventriculus of budgerigars *(Melopsittacus undulatus), Avian Dis* 34:779-786, 1990.

Stringer JR: *Pneumocystis carinii:* what is it exactly? *Clin Microbiol Rev* 9:489-498, 1996.

Thomas RC, Lewis DT: Pythiosis in dogs and cats, *Compend Contin Educ Pract Vet* 20:63-75, 1998.

Index

Page numbers followed by "f"
denote figures, "t" tables, and
"b" boxes.